Fluid Physiology and Pathology in Traditional Chinese Medicine

Fluid Physiology and Pathology in Traditional Chinese Medicine

STEVEN CLAVEY

BA(Colorado)
DipAdv Acupuncture (Nanjing)
Specialist in Traditional Gynecology
(Zhejiang College of TCM)

FOREWORD BY
DAN BENSKY D.O.

Churchill Livingstone

MELBOURNE EDINBURGH LONDON
MADRID NEW YORK AND TOKYO 1995

CHURCHILL LIVINGSTONE
Medical Division of Longman Group UK Limited
Distributed in Australia by Longman Australia Pty Limited, Longman House,
Kings Gardens, 95 Coventry Street, South Melbourne 3205, and by associated
companies, branches and representatives throughout the world.

First edition 1995

A catalogue record for this book is available from the British Library.
A Library of Congress Cataloging in Publication record is available for this title.

National Library of Australia Cataloguing-in-Publication Data

Clavey, Steven
  Fluid physiology and pathology in traditional Chinese medicine.

  Bibliography.
  Includes index.
  ISBN 0 443 04362 0

  1. Body fluids. 2. Medicine, Chinese. 3. Body fluid disorders. I. Title.

612.01522

Produced by Churchill Livingstone in Australia
Printed in Singapore

For Churchill Livingstone in Melbourne
Publisher: Judy Waters
Editorial: Pam Lewis
Copy Editing: Darryl Radcliffe
Desktop Preparation: Sandra Tolra
Typesetting: Friedo Ligthart, Designpoint
Indexing: Adrienne de Kretser
Production Control: Bob Stagg
Design: Churchill Livingstone

Preface

One reason for writing this book is to demonstrate how much valuable material may be found in ancient cultures of which we have yet to avail ourselves, and this material is often in areas where we believe that we are already highly advanced. Psychology is one example, where the writings of such people as Idries Shah and Robert Ornstein demonstrate a wealth and depth of psychological sophistication in Sufism far beyond our current cultural appreciation. Medicine is another where we in the West, dazzled by technology, are loath to credit clinical sophistication to a medicine whose diagnostic techniques employ nothing but the trained senses of the practitioner, and whose therapeutic armory is made up primarily of bare hands, simple needles and plants.

We—that is, those of us in 'modern developed nations'—also tend to assume that anything worth translating has already appeared in English. How far this is from the truth, and how much there is of value in cultures other than our own, many of our compatriots will never know due to ingrained culture-bound attitudes for which there is less and less room on a rapidly shrinking Earth.

But I can relate my own experience of amazement upon first surveying a library of traditional Chinese medical works and realizing that probably nine-tenths of this material was completely unheard of in the West. This amazement was matched by a feeling of urgency when the realization dawned that even more knowledge was not written, and could not be written, because it was in the form of practical skills: able to be passed on but not in words; able to be learnt but not from books.

Books however provide the essential bases of information, laying out a consistent set of principles through which practical learning can be developed. Few peoples hold to this more strongly than the Chinese, those indefatigable recorders, for whom the word 'classic'—*jing*—is the image of the lengthy warp threads on a loom, those lines which carry the essential experience of culture on and through weft after weft of succeeding generations.

In the practical area of Chinese medicine, the importance of this consistency cannot be over-emphasized. For more than twenty centuries, medical observations have been recorded in the same terms which are used today, carefully defined terms which for those actually engaged in the practice of traditional Chinese medicine retain their clinical significance to a remarkable degree. Thus a practitioner needing a new perspective on a difficult case has a tremendous breadth of resource material from which to draw: perhaps a modern journal, perhaps the essays of a physician first written fifteen hundred years ago. Compared to this, the acceptable clinical reference available for the modern Western doctor appears scant indeed, no matter how many double-blind trials and animal studies can be mustered. TCM, after all, depends upon the observation and recording of the effects of treatments upon *human* subjects, in all their variability, and it is the consistency in the terms of measurement used in this recording which ensures the value and usefulness of traditional Chinese medicine for the world of today.

It is for this reason that I believe that difficult-to-translate Chinese medical terms should as far as possible *not* be translated into English but rather left in pin-yin. Up until the present century, Chinese has been the medical language—the 'Latin' as it were—of Asia; doctors studying in Japan, Korea, Vietnam would look to Chinese texts for their learning material, would use Chinese terms and even Chinese characters to describe their cases. Only with the influx of Western medicine has this changed. But the Latin of Western medicine is not an appropriate vehicle for traditional Chinese medicine concepts, despite Manfred Porkert's heroic efforts; nor can English carry the rich connotations or the subtle relations between concepts in the original language. The appropriate vehicle already exists, the subtleties remain intact, the connections remain unbroken: I believe it is only fear of the strange formation of lines called 'characters' which push us scrambling for a familiar alternative. But at what price?

In this vein, where exception is taken to the admirable *Glossary* of Wiseman and Ellis, the disagreement is not with the concept of a glossary of TCM technical terms as such, but in the statement of principle that an unusual English term be chosen to signal a difficult-to-translate Chinese term. Since in both the case of an unusual English term and the case of an original pin-yin term the sphere of meaning must be learned by students of the subject, I believe we should stay as close to the original as possible, rather than adding an arbitrary step which alienates us from the rich tradition of our own profession. As more and more Western students of Chinese medicine take the next step of learning Chinese (which is far less difficult than generally imagined), such a policy should prove a boon. This is especially true as Chinese influence is almost certain to grow over the next century in a way very similar to that which has spread the use of Western medicine around the world during the last. We should be prepared.

Having said all this, it will be seen that throughout the present work common translations adopted in other English TCM books of quality have been retained in the interests of uniformity. This is particularly the case for formula names and the names of texts, where I have used Dan Bensky's translations, or—where a formula or text is not found in *Formulas and Strategies*—the style of translation is retained. Even technical terms whose meaning is unequivocal and the TCM connotations clearly understood I have given in English, such as damp, phlegm, blood-stagnation, wind, and cold. Zang and fu titles appear with an initial capital letter as has become the convention; less familiar terms appear in translation followed by pin-yin in brackets. The guiding principle throughout is to allow the reader's eye smooth passage over the text, while not sacrificing accuracy.

This is not a beginner's book. The reader is assumed to be familiar with material that is already well-represented in other English-language works on traditional Chinese medicine, and review of these areas is presented only as a basis for the introduction of a deeper level of discussion.

MELBOURNE, 1994   S.C.

Acknowledgments

There are several Chinese-language books that have proven indispensable throughout the preparation of the present work, and to the authors and editors of these I would like to express my especial gratitude. The books include the *Zhong Yi Tan Bing Xue* (TCM Phlegm Disease Studies) by Zhu Ceng-Bo (Hubei Science and Technology Press, 1984) and other articles by Dr. Zhu; the *Zhong Yi Zheng Zhuang Jian Bie Zhen Duan Xue* (Diagnostic Studies of Symptom Differentiation in Chinese Medicine) edited by Zhao Jin-Duo (People's Health Publishing, 1985); and the *Shi Re Lun* (Discussions of Damp-heat) by Jiang Sen (published by the Joint Publishing Company, Hong Kong, 1989).

I would also like to thank (the word is not strong enough) my internal medicine teacher at the Zhejiang College of TCM, Associate Professor Wu Song-Kang and his assistant Dr. Xi Ting-Hui, whose extraordinary kindness to a rather unpromising foreign student extended to transcribing every one of Professor Wu's methods for *each* breakdown in *every* category of internal medicine disease. In other words, they wrote a book for me, which coupled and compared with the volumes of case histories taken over the year at the College, provided the means of understanding not only Professor Wu's individual approach but its relationship to that of his famous teacher Ye Xi-Chun. My gratitude is unbounded—may I prove worthy of their effort.

Closer to home, I would like to thank Daryl Radcliffe for his untiring advice, and his repeated reading and editing of the text. Without his rarely equalled expertise in both the traditional Chinese medicine and the publishing fields the present work would be simply unreadable. Thanks to Judy Waters of Churchill Livingstone for her encouragement in the early stages of this book and the long discussions on the concept. Any errors or problems still remaining are the result of my own deficiencies.

Thanks are also due to Robby Todd for his incisive questioning and comments on details of pathology and treatment and the referral of the extremely interesting patient discussed in the case history in Chapter Seven; to Richard Coote for his perceptive comments leading to clarification of the text and for his unfailing humour, and to Lisa McPherson for keeping me honest.

But mostly, thanks to my wife Gabrielle and my children Lei Lei and Mark, for putting up without me for so many, many late nights.

To my parents, Elaine and Gordon,
in gratitude for their trust and
support always

Steven Clavey has studied Traditional Chinese Medicine in both Taiwan and the People's Republic of China, testing in the top 30 out of 1800 students on the Chinese written examinations when studying for certification in TCM gynecology. He is a consultant to the Australian government on matters relating to Chinese medicine, and he has been appointed by the federal Minister of Health to the Traditional Medicines Evaluation Committee, a committee which reviews the licensing of herbal products. He continues to be actively involved in teaching, the translation of Chinese medical texts and clinical practice, and he has published articles about Chinese medicine in both English and Chinese.

Contents

Foreword

Traditional Chinese medicine has always paid particular attention to the harmonious interaction of the various and sundry parts and materials that make up human beings. While previously slighted in the English language texts, the role of the fluids in the maintenance of health and development of diseases has always been considered a very important part of this matrix. In one way they can be considered the 'glue' that holds the entire edifice of traditional Chinese physiology together.

In this book, Steven Clavey approaches the fluids from all angles. He examines in detail the concepts and processes that make up fluid metabolism in traditional Chinese medicine. This not only includes the Organ functions related to fluids, but the difference between the various types of fluids and the relationship of the body fluids to the other major components of human life. His explanations of the differences between the pathological and physiologic states of different aspects in the body will clarify this important traditional concept. It covers the entire gamut of problems with fluids (such as sweat, urine, and edema). All types of fluid disturbances are discussed, including dampness and thin mucus. Still, it is the discussion of phlegm that will have a particularly big impact. The chapters and appendices that deal with this concept and its history in traditional Chinese medicine make up a landmark contribution.

This book contains much detailed clinical information that is extremely practical along with many useful tips from experienced practitioners. In addition, there is also much background information on the traditional Chinese natural philosophy. Knowing this type of information makes it much easier to comprehend traditional Chinese medicine and use it in the clinic.

One of the many facets of this book is its use of the comments and ideas of a host of medical authors from the time of the classics through the entire imperial era up to modern times. This makes the discussions fully fleshed out and three dimensional. It allows the reader to have a good idea how the great practitioners throughout Chinese history have grappled with the issues of fluid metabolism and pathology. Over and over again Steven Clavey demonstrates how much clinicians *need* to be conversant with premodern texts and applications of the nuances of basic theory to push their practices to the next level. Yet, in all discussions he takes a well-tempered, clear, and nondogmatic approach. As he says, "Each approach has its value: the modern viewpoint for its simplicity and familiarity to Western students of traditional Chinese medicine, the Classical for its precision and accumulated experience of some twenty centuries."

Not only is this a major contribution to the English literature on traditional Chinese medicine but a handy clinical reference. I am sure that it will have an immediate and salutary impact on the practices of all who read it carefully. It will be very useful to all who are interested in doing traditional Chinese medicine—students, novice practitioners, and those with more experience. I hope that it will serve as a model for future works.

DAN BENSKY, Seattle, 1994

Introduction

CHINESE MEDICINE AND THE MEDICINE OF THE WEST

Traditional Chinese medicine is the most vibrant and lively of the traditional medical systems still existing. Over a quarter of the world's population turns to Chinese medicine for a significant portion of their health care, and the numbers are increasing. Unlike the other traditional medicines it has proven so vibrant that it has spread far beyond its cultural borders and taken root right around the globe.

Part of the reason for this expansion is that Chinese medicine and Western medicine are not in competition. Areas covered in Western medicine are often those for which Chinese medicine has little to offer: the humble pap smear, for example, provides a far earlier indication of incipient cervical cancer than a standard Chinese diagnosis would offer. In other words, we cannot do without modern medicine. On the other hand, deficiencies and problems with modern Western medicine have become increasingly obvious over the last several decades, and are well described in its own literature and in the observations of social scientists. To a certain extent the problems arise from the very factors which underlie its strength: the ability to analyze molecular and cellular changes and to design therapeutic interventions which act at the same level. Because of this focus upon the microscopic level of disease however, it is virtually impossible (and in its own terms, meaningless) to consider the variety of factors which influence the daily functioning of the individual. Despite exhortations to family physicians to 'consider the whole person' Western medicine is simply not designed for this.

But Chinese medicine is. In effect, Chinese medical theory is a simplified physiology, the whole of which can be held in the mind of a practitioner while he or she considers the physical, social, meteorological and psychological factors affecting the individual patient and designs an approach which will bring them back into a normal range of health. Because of this, it is very well adapted indeed to deal with those aspects of health care which Western medicine is forced to ignore. Used in tandem or in combination, the two medicines cover the whole spectrum of health and disease, from molecular through to social and meteorological, in ways which allow the greatest strengths of each to contribute to a truly comprehensive system of health care. It is happening now, in China and in pockets in the West. Our descendants will be surprised that it was not always thus.

Chinese medicine in the West

At the present time, however, we in the West are not in full possession of the whole of Chinese medicine but rather a pastiche of segments. Some areas such as acupuncture, basic herbs and formulas, fundamental theory and so on, are relatively well-fleshed out, while others remain large blank spaces for those unable to read Chinese. For example, at the time of writing there has not yet appeared in English a complete textbook of Chinese 'Warm Disease' theory. In the face of such gaps, claims that we are able to 'adapt Chinese medicine for the West' may be an heroic expression of confidence, but are almost certainly premature. We have much work to do. So far, a large proportion of material about Chinese medicine comes from scholars who approach the subject from an historical or philological perspective. This is certainly important, but we need equally good scholarship from those who are writing from within the field, who view it as a living subject, who work with it and use it daily. Redressing this balance will bring us back into line with the main tradition in Chinese medical literature, whose major exponents have always been scholarly practitioners. Fortunately the range of good material is increasing and almost certainly will continue to do so.

Fluids in Chinese medicine

One of the large blank spaces in the non-Chinese TCM literature is in the area of fluid metabolism and pathology, despite the position of fluids as an integral part of the triad of 'qi, blood and body fluids' so well recognized by the Koho school of Kampo medicine. Not that fluids have been ignored in China itself, as I hope to show; indeed from the Sui Dynasty *Zhu Bing Yuan Hou Lun* (Generalized Treatise on the Etiology and Symptomatology of Disease) up to the present, fluid disorders have been exhaustively investigated and categorized, and treatments for these disorders devised by the exponents of every school of thought and within each department of TCM.

The detail and sophistication of these deliberations are staggering, and form the bulk of this present work. Disorders of sweating and urination, the formation of thin mucus, damp and phlegm, and the interaction of these with other pathological factors will all be discussed, and the Classical sources quoted. Differentiations and treatments, both Classical and modern, are provided in all categories, with case histories where appropriate and interesting.

Skills necessary in the use of TCM herbal therapy

Although the use of acupuncture for the treatment of specific fluid disorders is described variously throughout the present work, the emphasis is clearly on herbal therapeutics. Since this is the case, and because until recently herbs have been generally less well-represented in Western TCM educational institutions, it may be useful to review certain aspects of herbal therapy in traditional Chinese medicine, especially where these extend beyond standard acupuncture usage.[1]

Thorough knowledge of fundamental TCM theory

The extent to which basic theory comes into play with Chinese herbs is remarkable when compared to non-traditional medical systems such as naturopathy or modern

Western medicine. The essential pragmatism of the Chinese people is reflected in the focus on clinical reality: virtually everything in the basic theory is used at some point when diagnosing and prescribing herbs, from the yin and yang attributions of the seasons and cosmology and their reflections within the human body, to the energetic qualities of the Five Phases as expressed in the descriptions both of the organs and of the medicinal substances themselves.

Many of the aspects of fundamental TCM theory which are incidental to acupuncture suddenly leap into prominence in the study of herbal medicine. This is because in acupuncture the flow of qi in the channels is the medium through which a therapeutic effect is achieved. Thus an influence on the circulation of blood with this technique is almost always indirect, as the qi must be addressed first. If pathogenic fluids have accumulated, again it is through the medium of the qi that results are reached. Herbs, however, can act specifically on each of the circulating substances of the body (qi, blood or fluids), and also target specific zang-fu.

Tonification is a particular problem with acupuncture especially tonification of blood or yin-fluids, because it is necessary to indirectly encourage the production of these substances through improved zang-fu functioning, rather than directly supplementing the deficiency. Heat and cold also play a much more important part in herbal treatment than in acupuncture, because of the temperature qualities of the herbs.

Thus the accuracy of diagnosis is emphasized in herbal prescription, as the effect of a particular selection of herbs is very specific. Acupuncture can be effective, in many cases, even with a relatively hazy diagnosis, because of the general improvement to the harmony of qi flow throughout the body, and the influence this has on the functioning on the zang-fu. Attempting to apply herbs with a similar level of analysis of the pathology, however, can be disastrous.

Aspects of diagnosis essential to herbal therapy

At this point, an overview of diagnosis is useful in order to clarify concepts and procedures which are otherwise implicit in most Chinese medical works. There seems to be some confusion generally about the different types of diagnostic approach used in TCM, such as Illness Differentiation (Bian Bing), Syndrome Differentiation (Bian Zheng), the Four Methods of Diagnosis (Si Zhen), the Eight Principles (Ba Gang), the Etiological Differentiation (Bing Yin Bian Zheng), the Six Divisions (or the 'Six Channel System': Liu Jing Bian Zheng), the Wei Qi Ying Xue system, the San Jiao system, Zang Fu Differentiation, the Channel and Collateral diagnosis, and the Qi Xue Jin-Ye approach.

Diagnostic tools. These can be usefully envisioned as tools in a toolbox (which is TCM), tools which are brought out to perform specific jobs.

All patients will have two levels of diagnosis: an Illness Differentiation (sometimes called a diagnosis) and a Syndrome Differentiation. For example, (in the department of Internal Medicine) Gan Mao (the common cold) is the illness, while the syndromes involved in this type of illness could be wind-heat, wind-cold, either of the above combined with damp, or with summerheat, or with a constitutional qi deficiency or yin deficiency. These are the standard syndromes described in this illness, and each has a standard treatment principle and formula established.

Other departments have their own specialized illness differentiations. For example, in gynecology abnormal vaginal bleeding can be a) early period, b) heavy period, c) irregular menstruation, d) inter-menstrual bleeding, e) beng-luo (dysfunctional uterine bleeding), e) threatened miscarriage, f) postpartum hemorrhage, and so on. Each of these specific illnesses, again, has its own specialized approach. This example, in particular, should make clear how important a proper illness differentiation is to effective treatment.

Thus the study of different departments in TCM is primarily a study of the specific illnesses peculiar to each area, their differing pathologies, and their standard terminologies, differentiations and treatments. The Four Methods of Diagnosis are the tools used to obtain information, which is the basis for the Differentiation of Syndromes and the most general differentiation system is the Eight Principles (Ba Gang). These approaches will be used with all patients. Following this, and depending on the type of illness, the other more specialised tools of differentiation (detailed below) will be used:

The Etiological Differentiation identifies the pathogenic process involved (in particular exogenous factors, that is, factors that originate from the outside): for example the Six Pathogens, the Seven Emotions, dietary excess or external trauma.
The Six Channel System (Liu Jing Bian Zheng) is the tool used for exogenous wind-cold and its resulting conditions.
The Wei Qi Ying Xue and the San Jiao systems are used in combination for febrile disease differentiation.

For endogenous illnesses, that is, illnesses that originate from the inside, the following differentiation tools are employed:

The Channel and Collateral system identifies the channels or collaterals disturbed by obstruction (or in some cases, deficiency) and is most often used for local problems.
The Qi Xue Jin-Ye system identifies a problem at the level of one of the three media of communication between the zang fu. This is used for more general problems which have not, as yet, involved the zang fu themselves: eg qi deficiency, qi blockage, drooping qi, or rebelling qi; blood deficiency, blood stagnation, heat in the blood, or cold in the blood; lack of jin-ye fluids, accumulation of pathogenic fluids; and so on. This level of differentiation can also be used in combination with the level above or below it, for example with channels: qi blockage in the Liver channel, rebelling qi in the Stomach channel, or blood deficiency in the Chong and Ren channels; or for example with the zang fu: drooping Spleen qi, deficiency of Lung fluids (shang jin, which itself precedes shang yin), and so on.
The deepest level of endogenous differentiation is the zang fu differentiation, which again will often involve qi, blood and fluids, as these are the media with which the zang fu work.

There has, in the West, been an over-emphasis on zang fu diagnosis 'for historical reasons' as our Chinese comrades like to say, so that the zang fu are often brought into a differentiation when it is not necessary. The other side of the coin is the use of overly simplified differentiations, such as 'Five Elements', or as when a patient asks 'Am I Yin or Yang?'

Summary

An overview such as the above should hopefully provide an outline which puts these problems into context. The use of the proper tool for the job is essential for the accurate use of herbs, but it certainly does not hurt the effectiveness of an acupuncture or tui-na treatment either.

The area of fluid pathology straddles the entire range discussed above, from the surface through to the zang-fu, from acute exogenous disease through to chronic deficiencies. Without a good grasp of which diagnostic tool is most appropriate for the condition one is faced with in clinic, it is difficult to analyze the actual mechanisms at work producing the pathology. When one has a clear view of these mechanisms, the explanation for each and every symptom being experienced by the patient should also be clear.

Based upon this, a treatment strategy can be devised which is not only comprehensive but elegant and precise as well. The degree of success of the treatment demonstrates the degree of accuracy of the explanation, and the explanation itself is modified in accordance with the response of the patient. This may be worth remembering when, say, your edema patient fails to respond to simple diuretic herbs.

---

[1] It is an unfortunate symptom of the present political climate, particularly in the United States, that a discussion such as this, presenting basic information about herbs in the context of TCM, will likely be seen as a polemic 'against' acupuncture and 'for' herbs. There is no such intention. In fact, in many ways acupuncture is much more difficult to employ than herbs, for the following reasons.

In order to be consistently effective, acupuncture requires a proper diagnosis. If this is correct, a proper selection of points is required. If these are correct, each must be properly located. If these are correct, the technique of insertion must be comfortable for the patient at each point. At each point the proper depth and angle of the needle must be attained. If they are, the correct manipulation of the qi at each point must achieve the intended response. If it does, the needles must be retained for exactly the correct length of time. If they are, then the treatments must be repeated at just the right interval. If all of these goals are achieved, the acupuncture will be effective for that patient. To achieve these goals for each and every patient requires a level of consistent skill and application that truly deserves the name of 'art'.

Fluid physiology in traditional Chinese medicine

The concepts and processes involved in TCM fluid metabolism include the functions of the relevant organs, the difference between jin fluids and ye fluids, and the relationship of these body fluids to the qi, blood, jing-essence and shen. Each of these will be discussed in detail below.

BASIC CONCEPTS

Jin-ye

Jin-ye 津液, body fluids, is the general term for all the normal physiological fluids in the body, including internal fluids which may be secreted by the zang organs, such as tears, saliva, sweat, normal nasal mucus and Stomach or Intestinal fluids, and also the fluids which act to moisten the various tissues within the body, such as the skin, the flesh, the tendons, the bones and the marrow.

There are three points necessary to remember about jin and ye fluids:

1. They are substantial (i.e. they are material substances)
2. They are very sensitive to changes in the state of qi and blood, or changes in zang-fu functioning, or changes in the environment surrounding the body
3. The three factors qi, blood and body fluids form the only media of communication between the zang-fu and their related tissues and organs.[1]

Qi transformation

'Qi transformation' is a term which will be used extensively throughout this book. In TCM medical literature, it can refer broadly to all of the movements and changes of the qi in its circulation around the body, and includes all of the functioning of the zang and fu organs, and the rising and falling of qi and blood in the course of their travels. In *Zhong Yi Ji Chu Li Lun Xiang Jie* ('Detailed Explanation of TCM Basic Theory')—a modern text—qi transformation is defined as 'making one type of substance into many types of substance, or making many types of substance into one type of substance'. In a more narrow sense, it refers to the changes which occur during fluid metabolism in the various organs, through the action of the yuan qi, which Maciocia translates as 'Original Qi'. Yuan qi is distributed by the San Jiao from its source in the Kidney yang.

It is primarily in this latter sense that the term 'qi transformation' will be used in the chapters that follow.

NORMAL FLUID METABOLISM

The major functions in normal fluid metabolism, while functionally interwoven, can be artificially separated and listed for the purposes of discussion:

1. The Stomach accepts and holds food and fluids
2. The Spleen absorbs fluids[2]
3. The San Jiao provides a pathway for the passage of fluids, and also a pathway for the warming yuan (source 原) qi which allows the various qi transformations to occur around the body
4. The Lung qi provides regulation of fluid movement by its rhythmic descending action and also through the Lungs' motivating influence on the channel qi
5. The channel qi distributes nourishing fluids around the body
6. The Small Intestine initiates further separation of fluids from the solid waste carried down from the Stomach, while the Large Intestine accepts the remaining waste solids passed on by the Small Intestine, and performs a final extraction of fluids
7. The Urinary Bladder accepts impure fluids from all around the body, including the San Jiao, the Small Intestine and the descending action of Lung qi (which itself again includes the movement of channel qi)
8. The Kidney yang exerts a steaming action on these impure fluids in the Urinary Bladder, resulting in qi transformation
9. The Urinary Bladder qi transformation separates the still usable fluid qi from the impure fluids, and then recycles these usable fluids back into and through the body
10. The Urinary Bladder excretes the unreclaimable fluids as urine.

FLUID METABOLISM PROCESSES

After fluids are consumed, they are first taken in and held by the Stomach. It is the qi transformation functions of the Lungs, Spleen, San Jiao, Small Intestine, Kidneys and finally the Urinary Bladder, that transform these imbibed fluids into jin and ye fluids, to enable them to moisten and nourish the whole body; this will be looked at in detail below. The waste products of this metabolism are expelled from the body through the Urinary Bladder as urine, or through the pores as sweat; in this way the balance of fluids in the body is maintained.

The qi transformation mentioned above is a process of separating the murky (zhuo 浊) from the clear (qing 清) fluids. This does not happen just once, but is repeated again and again during the course of the fluids' movement through the body, in a double process of both increasing refinement on the one hand and conservation on the other. This is because even within the 'clear' fluids at any given point there remains a murky portion to be eliminated, and within the 'murky' fluids there is a clear portion which can be preserved. The clear fluids rise, the murky fluids descend, and this goes on in a constant rising and falling circulation within the body, along the San Jiao pathway for fluids.

In the *Su Wen*, Chapter 21, it says:

> When imbibed fluids enter the Stomach, its warming steaming action carries the essential qi to the Spleen. The Spleen then transports this qi, returning upward to the Lungs, where regulation of the fluid pathways is initiated [through the Lungs' clearing and rhythmic descent]: fluids are transported downward to the Urinary Bladder. The essential qi [of the fluids] is spread outward in the four directions, reaching the skin and pouring into the channels of the Five Zang organs. This is in accord with [the nature of] the four seasons and the yin yang of the five organs, and is part of the normal activity of the channels (jing mai).[3]

The interwoven process

After food and fluids enter the Stomach, the Spleen's qi transformation process absorbs fluid essence, separating clear and murky, and then Spleen transports the clear portion of the fluid qi up to the Lungs, while the murky solids and fluids pass downward with descending Stomach qi into the Small Intestine.

Once in the Lungs, the clear fluids lifted from the Spleen and the Kidneys again undergo qi transformation, and the even more refined clear fluids are circulated around the body by the combined action of the San Jiao, Lungs and the channel qi, to nourish and moisten the surface tissues, skin and hair, and similar tissues. Some of this fluid ends up being expelled from the body as perspiration, while the rest continues its flow in the channels. The murky portion from this Lung qi transformation is carried downward through the San Jiao by the Lungs' spreading and descending action, to the Urinary Bladder.

Those murky solids and fluids carried downward with the Stomach qi enter the Small Intestine, where they undergo a further qi transformation, and the fluid qi obtained from this extraction again passes into the San Jiao for distribution. The remaining almost completely solid dross passes down to the Large Intestine for a final extraction of fluids, while the murky fluids separated out by the Small Intestine are passed to the Urinary Bladder through the San Jiao, to undergo a last qi transformation. This occurs by virtue of the steaming action (zheng hua 蒸化) on these fluids by the Kidney yang, a portion of which must first pass through the Urinary Bladder[4] before continuing to circulate as yuan qi through the San Jiao.[5]

The steaming separates the reusable fluid qi from the murky fluids, and this clear fluid qi is then carried back up to the Lungs via the San Jiao and the Kidney channel itself, to begin the whole cycle once more. The remaining murky fluids are excreted as urine.

This process of qi transformation throughout the body, of fluids into qi and qi into fluids, has been analogously compared by the ancient Chinese medical authors to the rising of the qi of the earth as fog, and the falling of the qi of the heavens as rain.

ROLE OF ZANG AND FU ORGANS

Spleen and Stomach

Spleen, with its harmonious Earth-natured qi, plays an important part in the direction of fluid metabolism, exerting effects in three main areas: Spleen's zang organ function of transformation and transportation; Spleen acting as the harmonizing phase of Earth; and finally as the phase of Earth controlling the phase of Water.

Spleen transforms and transports. Spleen acts on the food and fluids warmed and ripened by the Stomach to absorb the essential qi of each. The *Yi Shu* ('Techniques of Medicine', 1817, by Cheng Wen-You) quotes an earlier work, the *Yi Can* ('Medical References', now lost) in this regard:

> The mechanism by which the Spleen is able to 'break up and mill' (xiao mo 消磨) water and grains is not that of a millstone which grinds, nor that of a pestle which pounds, but through the absorption of qi: foods never weigh it down! When foods enter the Stomach, they have qi and they have substance; the substance wants to descend, the qi wants to rise. The steaming action of the Stomach qi gleans half of the qi and the substance; once the Spleen qi begins to absorb, then the Stomach qi has assistance, and the jing-essence of the foods is completely obtained. The substance-without-qi is set free to be expelled, the pylorus (you men)[6] opens and the dross is eliminated.[7]

However, the warming transforming ability of the Spleen depends on the support of Kidney yang. As Zhao Xian-Ke says in his *Yi Guan* ('Key Link of Medicine', 1687): 'Fluids and food entering the Stomach are like water and grains in the midst of a stove: without fire they cannot cook. The Spleen's ability to transform depends completely on the insubstantial ministerial fire of Shao Yin, steaming from the lower Jiao; only with this can it begin to transform and transport'.[8]

This 'transport' function of the Spleen zang also includes the transport of fluids around the body. The statement in the *Su Wen* Chapter 45 that 'Spleen mainly helps Stomach move its jin and ye fluids'[9] refers to this aspect of Spleen functioning.

Zhang Xi-Chun, in his *Yi Xue Zhong Zhong Shen Xi Lu* ('Records of Heartfelt Experiences in Medicine with Reference to the West', published serially between 1918 and 1934) says: 'Spleen rules the ascent of the clear, and so transports jin and ye fluids upward. Stomach rules the descent of the murky, and so transports the dross downward'.[10]

The lifting of clear essence is one of the special characteristics of the Spleen, and is yet another part of its transport function; 'clear essence' includes both the essence of food, and the clear essence of fluid qi. Inability of the Spleen to transform, absorb and lift fluids has a direct effect on the fluid metabolism, slowing it and bringing about edema, heaviness of the limbs, scanty urine, and other similar symptoms. The *Ling Shu*, Chapter 8, confirms:

> If there is Spleen qi deficiency, then there will be lack of agility in the four limbs, and lack of harmony in the Five Zang; if the condition of the Spleen is one of excess (shi, e.g. impaired transportation through cold, qi obstruction, damp accumulation, and so on), then there will be abdominal distention and disruption to the flow of the menses, the bowels and the urine.

Another manifestation of the failure of Spleen qi to rise is dryness of the mouth, and occasionally even the eyes and the nose. This is characterized by dryness in the mouth without signs of deficiency in the rest of the fluids in the body. There may be, in fact, simultaneous signs of excess pathogenic fluid build-up due to damp development as a result of the weak Spleen qi, such as loose stool, excessive urination and leukorrhea.

Spleen as harmonizing Earth. The depth of the theories concerning the place of the Spleen as the harmonizing Earth is quite remarkable, as evidenced by the following quote from the *Si Sheng Xin Yuan* ('Secret Sources of the Four Masters') by Huang Yuan-Yu, in 1753:

> Spleen is the yin Earth, it is Tai Yin and controls rising; Stomach is yang Earth, it is Yang Ming and controls descent. The initiative to rise or descend derives from the meeting of yin and yang, and this [meeting] is in the qi of the center. The Stomach controls reception, the Spleen controls transformation. If the central qi is vigorous, [on the one hand] it can descend and is good at receiving, [while on the other] Spleen rises and promotes churning and ripening of the water and grain (Pi sheng er shan mo shui gu fu shou); essential qi nourishes life, and so there is no disease.
>
> If Spleen rises, then [the qi of the] Liver and Kidneys also rise, and therefore Water and Wood do not become obstructed; if Stomach descends, then [the qi of] Heart and Lungs can also descend, and therefore Metal and Fire have no blockage: Fire can descend so that Water does not chill the lower [body], Water rises so that Fire does not [over]-heat the upper [body].

The state of a healthy person, in being warm below and cool above, is a result of the proficient transportation of the central qi ... [which] harmonizes and benefits this mechanism of Fire and Water, and forms the axis for the rising and falling of Metal and Wood.[11]

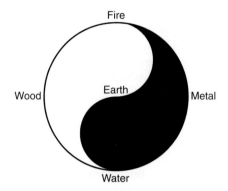

Fig 1.1 Relationship of the sequence of yin-yang growth and decline with the Five Phases

Figure 1.1 illustrates the relationship of the sequence of yin-yang growth and decline with the Five Phases. It should be looked at from the point of view of one standing on the earth facing South.[12] In this way the sun will rise on the left, proceed until directly overhead, then decline and set on the right, finally moving out of sight under the earth (which is the center of the universe in this traditional scheme).

Thus the rising yang energy of Wood corresponds with the rising sun in the East, birth and Springtime. This is why it is said that the 'Liver qi rises on the left'.

The sun directly overhead is yang energy at its peak, naturally corresponding to Fire, maturity and Summer.

Once the sun has passed its apex, yang begins to decline and the contracting yin influence begins, and the sun sinks to the right. This corresponds to the contracting yin energy of Metal, decline and Autumn. This is why it is said that the 'Lung qi descends on the right'.[13]

Having set, the sun moves out of sight below the earth, the activity of the world slows and quietens and yin energy predominates, naturally corresponding to Water, dormancy and Winter.

In the midst of all these changes of yin and yang, both daily and seasonal, Earth is constant, and thus the *Su Wen* Chapter 29 says: 'Spleen has no fixed time'. But Earth is not static: the nature of its energy is moderating and harmonious. While yang energy grows to its apex in the heavens, Earth balances it by remaining relatively yin: cool, nourishing, and still. As yin declines to its final dormant state, Earth retains a modicum of yang energy, warming the seeds of the future growth of yang.[14]

Earth, as the center, is the base upon which these permutations of yin and yang can occur. He Meng-Yao, in the *Yi Bian* ('Fundamentals of Medicine', 1751), explains:

> The Spleen zang-organ resides in the middle, and is the axis upon which ascent, descent, rising and falling occur. When food and drink enter the Stomach, Spleen transports its qi above and below, to the interior and the exterior, just like the earth extending its transformation throughout the Four Seasons. Therefore it belongs to Earth.[15]

The *Si Sheng Xin Yuan* ('Secret Sources of the Four Masters', 1753, by Huang Yuan-Yu) agrees: 'The Central qi is the axis of yin-yang's ascent and descent; this is why it is called Earth. [Through] the movement of this axis, clear qi spirals upward on the left and transforms into fire, and the murky qi twists downward on the right and transforms into water.'[16]

The functions of Earth itself also receive impetus from this ascent and descent of yin and yang. One example is the assistance Liver qi gives to Earth transport, described by He Meng-Yao:

> Everyone knows that Wood overcomes Earth: I alone promote the rising of Wood to cultivate Earth. Now the nature of Wood is that of growing Springtime qi, which is of the same origin as Stomach qi although different in name. This opening growing nature should be encouraged, because when Wood qi rises and opens, the Stomach qi rises and opens. When this opening has gone on for a long time, its producing effect becomes spent, and then it should be drawn back into the midst of Water and Earth, to provide the root for the emerging birth of the coming Spring. (A note appended to the above continues: If this is understood, then 'Metal overcoming Wood' actually becomes the source of Wood production, because

the opening dispersing nature of Wood is conserved [by Metal] and not allowed to dispel itself.) Where in all this is there any principle antagonistic [to the order of Heaven]?[17]

Zhou Xue-Hai, *Du Yi Sui Bi* ('Random Notes while Reading Medicine', 1898), relates this idea to overall treatment:

> Li Dong-Yuan says: 'When the Sages treated illness, they necessarily based this upon the seasonal principles of rising and falling, floating and sinking, and the appropriateness of these axial changes. The qi of the year must be primary to avoid impairing the harmony of Heaven.'
>
> The Classics say: [in treatment] accord with rising and falling, floating and sinking; but oppose cold, heat, cool and warmth.
>
> [Zhang] Zhong-Jing says if yang is vigorous and yin is deficient, purging will cure but sweating will kill; while if yin is predominant and yang deficient, sweating will cure but purging will kill.
>
> The general method of the Sages [can be shown by an] example: they would use a yang-lifting or dispersing-opening formula to assist Spring and Summer[-like] yang qi and make it rise and ascend, in this way reducing Autumn and Winter[-like] contracting-storing-killing-cold-cool qi. This is the great principle of ascent-descent, rising and falling. In the qi of Heaven and Earth, it is the ascent-descent, rise and fall [of yin and yang] which produce the seasons. In the treatment of disease, one cannot go against them, as those who follow the Heavens will prosper, and those who go against will die.
>
> In a person's body, there is also the qi of the four seasons, Heaven and Earth. They cannot be considered as exterior: people, in structure, are the same as Heaven and Earth.[18]

Spleen Earth controls Water. Under normal conditions, the meaning of the Five Phases concept of Spleen Earth controlling Kidney Water is the mutually influential relationship between these two organs. Only if Spleen Earth is vigorous will it be able to restrain Kidney Water, and prevent any abnormal activity on the part of Kidney Water. But when the function of Spleen Earth is weak, two things occur: on the one hand,

Spleen's own transformation will suffer and allow damp to form; on the other, Kidney Water loses Spleen's restraint and begins to move in a disordered fashion throughout the body.[19] Zhang Jing-Yue makes this comment: 'Water only fears Earth, so its control is in the Spleen ... a weak Spleen Earth not only cannot control Water, but is in turn restrained itself.'

Because the above relationship between the Spleen and the Kidneys has not been well represented in the English (or even the Chinese!) literature to date, it may bear further elucidation. The following short essay discusses this relationship in the context of treatment:

Mutual tonification of Spleen and Kidneys

The ancients had two phrases: 'Tonification of the Spleen is not as good as tonification of the Kidneys', and 'Tonification of the Kidneys is not as good as tonification of the Spleen'.

Now herbs that tonify the Spleen are all parching, and the Kidneys abhor dryness; while the herbs that tonify the Kidneys are moist, and the Spleen abhors moisture.

Average people have a way of both following and violating these principles, which is to use parching and moistening herbs together. But this completely misses the subtleties of Spleen and Kidney tonification!

Spleen is Earth; if Earth is deficient, it cannot guard against Water, and so water can flood without control, charging upward and causing symptoms such as the running piglet qi. It is important to note that this flooding water is originally Kidney water which is no longer in storage, and therefore it is pathogenic water which is disturbing the Spleen, and not True Essence (zhen jing) charging upward.

Thus the reason that herbs are used to nourish the Spleen is to settle the Central Prefecture and prevent further gushing upward. Not to mention that Earth produces Metal, which in turn produces Water, and so Kidney qi is naturally sufficient [as a result of this approach]. Hence the saying 'Tonification of the Kidneys is not as good as tonification of the Spleen'.

If Spleen Earth is already dry, then Kidney qi would naturally not dare to insult it [by allowing water to rush upward]; if both the Kidneys and the Spleen are peaceful, what need is there of [further] tonification?

As to the saying: 'Tonification of the Spleen is not as good as tonification of the Kidneys', there is even deeper meaning here!

[For example] in the case of Spleen and Kidney deficiency, if moistening Kidney tonics are used, will this not cause Spleen qi to become even more damp?

One must know that here [tonification of the Kidneys] is tonification of the fire within the Kidneys, and not tonification of water.

The books say: Wood produces sovereign fire, [but] sovereign fire is empowered by ministerial fire, [and only then] is Fire able to produce Earth. So we know that without this [ministerial] fire, Earth is unable to be produced.

The ancients compared this fire to the burning fuel under a stove, which is a particularly apt analogy: with a fire burning under the stove, the contents of the stove will naturally be cooked; and this is the same with Ming-men and the Stomach in the body.

Therefore Ba Wei Wan[20] is a miraculous formula for tonifying the Kidneys, because it uses the *Rou Gui* (Cinnamomi Cassiae, Cortex) and *Fu Zi* (Aconiti Carmichaeli Praeparata, Radix) among its ingredients to tonify Ming-men.

If one does not know this explanation, and wildly uses moistening herbs [to tonify the Kidneys], then the Spleen will become daily more defeated, and the appetite will decrease. How could the aim of a flourishing Kidney qi be attained in such a situation?'[21]

San Jiao

The functioning of the San Jiao, which Maciocia translates as Triple Burner or Three Burners, is described in the *Sheng Ji Zong Lu* ('Comprehensive Recording of the Sages' Benefits', 1117):

The San Jiao is the pathway of the fluids and food, and the location for all qi transformation. If the San Jiao is regulated in its course, then the vessels of the qi (qi mai) will be calm and even, and able to smoothly move the water and fluids into the channels so that they can be transformed into blood, and irrigate the whole body. If the San Jiao qi is obstructed, the pathways of the vessels will be blocked, and then the water and fluids will stop, gather, and be unable to move. [They will then] accumulate into phlegm and thin mucous.[22]

San Jiao has two exceedingly important activities in fluid metabolism. The first is to distribute the yuan (source) qi from the Kidneys, which is the basis for the process of qi-transformation in the organs of the upper, middle and lower Jiao. The second is to act as the pathway for the transformed fluids.

San Jiao is in a particularly good position to be able to fulfil these functions, because of its wide circle of relationships within the body: it derives warming yuan qi from the Kidneys, it links the Lungs, Spleen, Stomach, Small and Large Intestines, it drains into the Urinary Bladder, it has an interior-exterior relationship with the Pericardium and thus the Heart, and it is in same-name-channel relationship with the Gall Bladder (Shao Yang) and is thus influenced by the Liver. It is obviously in intimate connection with the state of qi and fluids, and, through the fluids, the blood.

Zhang Zhong-Jing, in the first chapter of the *Jin Gui Yao Lue* ('Essentials from the Golden Cabinet', *c.* 210 AD) also points out: 'The crevices (cou 腠) in the surface tissues on the exterior of the body and the organs are the place where the San Jiao moves and gathers the Original True [qi], the places which are suffused with qi and blood.' This again points to its connection with all parts of the body: the True qi from the Lungs, the Original qi from the Kidneys, the blood from the Heart; even the half-internal half-external position of Shao Yang is implied.[23]

The *Yi Yuan* ('Origin of Medicine', 1861) has a clear description of the nature of San Jiao energy:

San Jiao is full of the fire of True Yang (zhen yang). Its body (ti) is empty and moist, its qi dense and enshrouding. 'Jiao' means heat; with this heat completely filling and moving throughout the body cavity, it can move and regulate the fluid pathway. Because San Jiao comes out of the right Kidney, and Heart and Kidney

connect, thus San Jiao and Pericardium connect, and have an interior-exterior relationship.[24]

The *Nan Jing*, in the Sixty-sixth Difficulty, says: 'San Jiao is the 'director of separation'[25] for the yuan qi (San Jiao zhe, yuan qi zhi bie shi ye) ruling the free movement of the three qi (i.e. the zong qi of the chest from inspired air, the gu qi of the middle Jiao from foods, and the activated jing-essence qi of the lower Jiao) through the Five Zang and Six Fu'.

The *Ling Shu*, Chapter 36, says:

Of [the types of] qi emerging from the San Jiao: that which warms the muscles and the flesh, and fills out the skin, is the jin-fluid; while that which flows without moving is the ye-fluid (i.e. the thick and viscous fluids of the joints and bones, which 'flows' in the deep interior, but does not 'move' with the qi and blood around the body). When the weather is warm, or the clothing thick, the surface tissues open, and thus sweat emerges ... When the weather is cold the surface tissues close, the fluids [on the surface] (literally 'qi' and 'damp') do not move, and water flows downward to the Urinary Bladder, there to become urine or qi.

The *Nan Jing*, in the Thirty-first Difficulty, says: 'San Jiao is the avenue of water and foods, the beginning and the end of qi'.

From the above statements we can see that San Jiao is not only the pathway for yang qi transport but is also the route for the ascent and the descent of qi movement, controlling the qi transformation for the whole body, and indeed determining exactly where in the body the yuan qi will be distributed.

The San Jiao, furthermore, is crucial for the Urinary Bladder's function of excreting excess fluids from the body, both because the San Jiao drains murky fluids remaining from all of the qi transformations occurring elsewhere in the body into the Urinary Bladder, and also because the San Jiao is able to carry the recovered clear fluid qi back up through the body after Urinary Bladder's own qi transformation is complete.

The *Ling Shu*, Chapter 36, says, again:

If San Jiao does not drain, and the jin and ye fluids are not created by transformation, then food and fluids will together move in the midst of the Intestines and Stomach; the murky waste cannot return to the Colon [for expulsion], but remains in the San Jiao unable to seep into the Urinary Bladder. Then the lower Jiao becomes distended, and fluids flood and become edema.

The *Su Wen* is even more clear in Chapter 8: 'The San Jiao is the Official in charge of Irrigation: the place from which fluid pathways emerge.'

Finally, as the pathway for the ascent and descent of yin and yang, the San Jiao must be clear for Heart yang to descend and warm the Kidney yang, and for the Kidney yin to rise and nourish the Heart yin. The modern herbal formula textbook *Zhong Yi Fang Ji Yu Zhi Fa* ('TCM Formulas and Treatment Methods') comments:

The method of re-establishing Heart and Kidney communication is defined by the pathological mechanisms of this relationship. Heart resides in the upper Jiao, Kidneys in the lower Jiao. Under normal circumstances, the Heart yang should descend to connect with Kidney yin, and the Kidney yin should rise to benefit Heart yang, yin and yang coordinating each other.

This method mainly employs herbs which treat the two organs of the Heart and the Kidneys, combined with herbs that re-establish Heart and Kidney relationship such as *Yuan Zhi* (Polygalae Tenuifoliae, Radix), *Shi Chang Pu* (Acori Graminei, Rhizoma) and *Lian Zi* (Nelumbinis Nuciferae, Semen), as an auxiliary method. All of these type of herbs have the effects of harmonizing the Stomach, expelling phlegm and using fragrance to transform murky-damp. The rationale behind using middle [Jiao] harmonizers is [first] because middle Jiao is the axis of yin-yang ascent and descent—only if the middle Jiao is peaceful and harmonious can the yin and yang in the upper and lower [Jiao] be beneficially reconnected: this is the meaning of the saying that if the upper and lower connection is diseased, harmonize the middle. The second [reason] to use phlegm-expelling and damp-transforming herbs to reconnect Heart and Kidneys is that San Jiao is both the place where water and fluids travel, and also the avenue for the movement of qi to rise and fall, exit and enter. Phlegm-mucus and murky-damp obstructing the Shao Yang San Jiao will block the highway for yin and yang

ascent and descent. The use of fragrant-transforming and phlegm-expelling herbs will make the San Jiao open and free-flowing, so that this ascent and descent of yin-yang can return to normal.[26]

Lungs

The Lungs rule the qi throughout the body, above and below, inside and out. Thus the *Su Wen*, Chapter 10, says: 'All qi is controlled by the Lungs'. They are the source of the qi used by the body, because of the Lungs' ability to infuse the essential qi from food and drink with the clear qi of Heaven, while expelling the insubstantial murky qi through exhalation, which is why *Yi Zong Bi Du* ('Required Readings from the Masters of Medicine', Li Zhong-Zi, 1637) remarks: 'With inhalation, the [qi] is full, with exhalation, the [qi] is empty', and 'Lungs control ... the movement and transformation of clear and murky, acting as the bagpipes (tuo yue) of the body'.[27] This infusion of the clear qi of Heaven into the gu qi creates zong qi, which gathers in the chest, and provides part of the motive force both for breathing and for the movement of qi and blood through the channels (jing mai).

The activity of zong qi, as part of the channel qi (jing qi), is the mechanism by which the Lungs motivate the movement of fluid qi through the channels 'floating like a mist upon a river', being carried around the body like a bank of refreshingly moist fog to nourish all tissues and organs. In this way, too, the Lungs provide the motive force which enables murky fluids to be carried downward to the Urinary Bladder through the San Jiao.

Channel qi. One of the primary functions for the channels and vessels (jing mai) in the body is the movement of qi and blood, through which harmonization of yin and yang is accomplished. But where does the motive force for this movement come from? Let us look first at zong qi 宗气, which Maciocia translates as 'Gathering Qi'. In the *Ling Shu*, Chapter 71, it says: 'The zong qi gathers in the chest, can exit through the throat, or link (贯 guan) the vessels of the Heart with the movement of the breath.'[28] So zong qi is an essential part of the functional activity of the Heart and the Lungs.

Next we should look at the yuan qi, which Maciocia translates as 'Original Qi'. Yuan qi has its origin 'under the umbilicus, between the Kidneys'. The *Nan Jing* ('Classic of Difficulties'), in the

Eighth Difficulty, points out that 'The moving qi from below the umbilicus and between the Kidneys' is actually 'the foundation of the Five Zang and Six Fu, and the root of the Twelve Channels (jing mai).' Yuan qi is transformed from the jing-essence stored in the Kidneys, and is the fundamental driving force behind the body's vital activities.

Also, nutritive and protective qi depend upon the transformation of food and drink—the 'qi of food and fluids'—for their production. Nutritive qi travels in the vessels, as it is a nutritional substance which interacts closely with the blood; in fact, the one can transform into the other and back again depending upon local and systemic necessities (see the section on 'blood and jin and ye fluids' later in this chapter). Protective qi travels outside of the vessels, spreading out over the surface of both the body and the internal organs, and, besides its defensive functions, also regulates body temperature and the secretion of sweat, nourishes the tissues, and fills out the skin.

Both zong qi and yuan qi participate in motivating, sustaining and propelling the ceaseless circulation of nutritive and protective qi through the channels and vessels, permeating both the interior and exterior of the body, reaching every organ and tissue.

Thus the apparently simple function of 'moving qi and blood' is actually the result of the combined activities of zong qi, yuan qi, nutritive qi and protective qi, and, therefore, of the organs that produced them. The sum total of these activities is termed the 'channel qi': its substantial aspect made up of nutritive and protective qi (and the interaction with the blood), its directive aspect made up of zong qi and yuan qi. Through this continual movement around the body, yin and yang are maintained in concert, and the balanced harmony of qi, blood, and fluids is thus preserved.

Small Intestine and Large Intestine

The Small Intestine is connected to the lower opening of the Stomach, and receives both solid and fluid waste left over from the initial qi transformation process in the middle Jiao. The main job of the Small Intestine is to separate from this waste the still recoverable clear essence of food and fluids, which will then be recycled back into the body and used. The remaining solid waste is then passed downward into the Large Intestine, while the remaining murky fluids are carried to the Urinary Bladder through the San Jiao. Zhang Jing-Yue says:

> The Small Intestine resides beneath the Stomach, receiving the fullness of food and fluids from the midst of the Stomach, and separating the clear and the murky. Watery fluids go from here and pour into the front, solid wastes go from here and pass to the back [passage]. With Spleen qi transformation there is rising ascent, with Small Intestine transformation there is descent downward.[29]

If this function of the Small Intestine fails, excess fluids will pass into the Large Intestine, resulting in loose stool; while at the same time, due to a reduced amount of fluids passing to the Urinary Bladder, there will also be reduced urination. One method of treatment for diarrhea, therefore, is to promote this separation function of the Small Intestine, thus increasing the urination and reducing the fluid lost through the stool. On the other hand, loss of Small Intestine ability to absorb fluids can also result in murky fluids welling upward, leading to abdominal distention and pain, nausea and vomiting, scanty urination and constipation. In this case, promotion of the descent of Stomach qi can help re-establish Small Intestine functioning.[30]

Tang Rong-Chuan (1862-1918) expresses the individual view that once clear fluid essence is extracted from food in the Small Intestine, it rises to supplement Heart blood.[31]

Regarding the Large Intestine, Li Dong-Yuan, in his *Pi Wei Lun* ('Discussion of the Spleen and Stomach', 1249), says:

> The Large Intestine rules the jin-fluids, the Small Intestine rules the ye-fluids. It is only after receiving nourishing qi from the Stomach that the Large Intestine and the Small Intestine can move the jin and ye fluids to the upper Jiao, [thereafter] to irrigate the skin and suffuse the surface tissues (cou li) to make them firm. If eating and drinking is irregular, then the Stomach qi will be insufficient, and the Large and Small Intestine will have nothing to receive, thus the jin and ye fluids become as if desiccated.[32]

This quotation, besides mentioning the individual functions of the Stomach, Large and Small

Intestine, clearly demonstrates the concept of a functional yoke linking these three fu organs, a concept which is so pervasive in TCM that the three are often referred to simply as 'wei chang'—Stomach and bowels.

Otherwise, in terms of Classical text discussions of fluid metabolism physiology, the Large Intestine plays only a minor role: accepting solid waste from the Small Intestine, and passing it out of the body. The *Su Wen,* Chapter 8: 'Large Intestine, the Official of Passage; change and transformation exit here', upon which Zhang Jing-Yue comments: 'The Large Intestine resides below the Small Intestine and mainly expels waste, and thus acts as the passageway for the transformations of the [Small] Intestine and the Stomach'. There is the implication of a fluid reabsorption function in the *Zhong Zang Jing* ('Treasury Classic') when it says: '[If the Large Intestine is] exhausted, there will be unstoppable diarrhea—when the diarrhea does stop, then death ensues.'[33]

But it is in fluid pathology that the Large Intestine takes on a more important position, as fluids untransformed higher in the body pour into it and remain, causing borborygmus, abdominal distention and diarrhea. In later chapters this will be discussed in more detail.[34]

Kidneys

'Kidneys control Water' refers in broad terms to the Kidney storage of jing-essence, which Maciocia translates as 'Essence', and to the regulation of water metabolism.

The jing-essence stored in the Kidneys is of two types: constitutional and acquired. Constitutional Kidney jing-essence, which is the basic inherited energy at the root of a person's constitution, depends on supplementation from the acquired jing-essence for continued vitality. The acquired jing-essence is derived from the essential qi transformed from food and fluids and then distributed throughout the zang and fu organs. If the person is healthy, the Kidneys continually receive this essence from the Five Zang and Six Fu to be stored.

The Kidney yang produces yuan qi through its steaming action on the jing-essence of the Kidneys. The yuan qi then moves into the San Jiao, where one of its functions is to ensure the continuous and free movement of jin and ye fluids.

There thus exists a beneficial cycle whereby the Kidney jing-essence is transformed into yuan qi, which in turn powers the qi transformation process through which the acquired jing-essence can be obtained by the Kidneys and stored, to provide the fuel for future yuan qi. Part of the substance for the acquired jing-essence is made up of the jin and ye fluids.

Because the nature of the Kidneys corresponds to the particular energetic qualities of Water, fluids have a natural affinity for the Kidneys. So although Water is born of Earth, and Earth qi rises to Heaven, in the end the fluid qi always precipitates downward, and thus it is said: 'The source of fluids is in the Lungs, the root of qi is in the Kidneys'.

The warmth of Kidney yang supports Spleen yang, and thus the middle Jiao transformation of fluids, as described in detail above in the discussion of Spleen fluid metabolism.

The Kidneys, through the Urinary Bladder, also provide a draining function for the rest of the body, in the case of excess fluid build-up into pathogenic water. This is why the Sixty-first Chapter of the *Su Wen* says: 'The Kidneys are the floodgate of the Stomach, if the floodgate cannot move smoothly, the water will accumulate and gather with its kind'.[35]

Urinary Bladder

Urinary Bladder is the lowest organ in the body, and thus is the location to which fluids naturally sink. It is united with the Kidneys as the yang Water organ, and its function is to hold these fluids until they can be acted upon by the steaming action of the Kidney yang. This qi transformation process separates out reusable fluid qi from the rest of the fluids held in the Urinary Bladder, and this clear fluid qi is carried back up to the Lungs through the San Jiao and via the Kidney channel itself. The remaining murky fluids are excreted as urine.

There are three major sources of the fluids held by the Urinary Bladder. The first source is the middle Jiao, from which the murky fluids separated out in qi transformation are carried downward by the action of descending Lung qi through the San Jiao to the Urinary Bladder. The second source is the Lungs' qi transformation in the upper Jiao; and the third source is the Small Intestine, which separates reusable fluid qi from the dross carried downward from the Stomach, and then sends the murky fluid downward via the San Jiao to the Urinary Bladder.

The ability of the Urinary Bladder to excrete fluids as urine depends on the motive energy of Kidney yang supporting the qi transformation of the San Jiao. Thus it is said 'fluids are stored there (i.e. in the Urinary Bladder), only with qi transformation can they exit the body'. Zhang Jing-Yue comments on this in the *Lei Jing* ('Systematic Categorization of the *Nei Jing*', 1624):

> The source of this qi transformation is in the Dan Tian (Cinnabar Field), that which is named the lower Sea of Qi: the number one original Qi of Heaven is transformed and produced in this place. If the yuan (original) qi is sufficient, then transport and transformation is constant, the water passageways remain naturally open, and this is why qi is the mother of water. If the guidance of [the statement] 'with qi transformation they can exit' is appreciated, then the Dao of treating water diseases is more than half grasped.[36]

DEFINITION OF JIN-YE

'Jin-ye', while being a general name for all body fluids, is actually a composite term made up of 'jin' and 'ye', individual words which describe two types of normal fluids, differing in nature, function, and distribution. It is strictly differentiated in TCM theory from 'water', which is a pathological product of disrupted jin-ye physiology.[37]

Ye fluids

Ye fluids are distributed to the zang-fu, bones and joints, brain and marrow, but do not flow with the qi and blood. They are thick and viscous, move slowly, and function as a moistening lubricant and supplement to jing-essence, especially in the deep yin areas of the body, such as the joints and marrow.

As the *Ling Shu*, Chapter 36, remarks: 'The jin and ye fluids from the Five Grains can combine harmoniously and form a thick paste-like substance, which can seep into the spaces of the bones, and nourish and strengthen the brain and marrow.'

Jin fluids

Jin fluids follow the circulation of the qi and blood, and in fact assist their smooth flow, spreading throughout the surface of the body to warm and moisten the muscles, flesh and orifices, and flush the skin with nourishment. Jin-fluids are thin, clear and watery, and flow quickly and easily.

Again, the Thirty-sixth Chapter of the *Ling Shu* states: '[That which accompanies] the clear qi that issues through the San Jiao to warm the tissues and flesh, and suffuse the skin, is the jin.'

Earlier, in the Thirtieth Chapter of the *Ling Shu*, both jin and ye are defined in that classic question and answer style that characterizes the *Nei Jing*:

> The Emperor said 'We have heard it said that people have jing-essence, qi, jin-fluids, ye-fluids, blood, and mai (i.e. the activity of the vessels, hence 'pulse'). Previously we imagined that all were a single form of energy, but now there is this division into six separate terms, and we do not know why this is... What is jin?'
>
> Qi Bo said: 'That which issues from the subcutaneous tissues, that skin-moistening perspiration, is called jin.'
>
> 'What is ye?'
>
> Qi Bo said: '[When] food has entered [the middle Jiao] and qi is full to overflowing, that moistening nourishment that pours into the bones and allows the bones [and joints] to bend and straighten, that [fluid] which benefits and supplements the brain and marrow, and [even] moistens the skin, is known as ye'.

Zhang Jing–Yue, in the *Lei Jing* ('Systematic Categorization of the *Nei Jing*', 1624), comments upon the above quote, saying: 'Jin and ye are basically the same but also have a yin and yang differentiation: jin is the clear aspect of ye, while ye is the murky aspect of jin. Jin [can] become sweat, and moves in the surface tissues, and so it is yang; ye pours into the bones and tonifies the brain and marrow, and so it is yin.'[38]

Deficiency of jin and ye fluids, if mild, is called 'shang jin' (damage to jin fluids), and shows symptoms such as thirst and dry throat, dry stool, scanty urine, and dry lips, tongue and skin.

More severe deficiency of jin and ye fluids is called 'shang yin' (damage to yin), and will have the above symptoms plus scarlet tongue with cracks and little or no coat.

The next stage of deficiency will be yin failing to control yang, with resulting signs of fire flaring: nightsweats, flushing, insomnia, or even nosebleeds and coughing blood.

Abnormal accumulation of jin and ye fluids results from failure to circulate properly. Once these fluids cease moving, they are unable to carry out their normal physiological functions within the body, and thereafter form 'pathological fluids' such as water, damp, phlegm and yin.

It is discussion of these latter pathologies, and their treatment, that forms the bulk of this book.

RELATIONSHIP OF JIN AND YE FLUIDS TO QI, BLOOD, JING-ESSENCE AND SHEN

Qi and jin-ye fluids

Qi is yang, while jin and ye fluids are yin, and the relationship between them is virtually identical with (and certainly as crucial as) the relationship between qi and blood.

Qi depends on fluid as a 'carrier', much as it does on blood, and so can be weakened by excessive sweating, vomiting, diarrhea, or other fluid loss. At the same time, blockage of the flow of fluids will also impede the circulation of qi, and, if this fluid blockage leads to a pathological impairment of zang-fu functioning (such as the Spleen), the very production of qi can be at risk.

Qi can also directly transform into fluids, and fluids into qi, as happens when nutritive qi secretes sweat, or when the qi of the organs produce their respective fluids (as discussed in the next chapter), or when the final qi transformation occurs in the Urinary Bladder, when the last remaining clear portion of the fluids is transformed into qi by the vaporizing action of the warming yuan qi of the San Jiao, 'which then rises to warm and nourish the tissues of the zang-fu (zang fu zu zhi)'.

A good clinical example of fluid exhaustion damaging qi is dehydration from Summerheat, where not only is there dry mouth and thirst but also lassitude and exhaustion from a lack of jin and ye fluids to transform into qi. Treatment requires Bai Hu Jia Ren Shen Tang ('White Tiger plus Ginseng Decoction', Bensky, *Formulas and Strategies*, p. 71), the ginseng being added to the cooling White Tiger Decoction to replenish both the qi and the fluids.

The creation, development, transport, distribution, and finally excretion of jin and ye fluids, depend completely on two aspects of qi: movement and function.

The movement of qi, its rising and falling, its penetration to the interior and lifting to the surface, carries the jin and ye fluids to all parts of the body.

The various functions of qi, such as transforming, warming and consolidating, all play essential roles in the metabolism of fluids.

In order to be clear about this, it must be remembered that 'qi' has two, almost separate, meanings: a substance that moves around the body, and can be lost (e.g. with sweating or menstruation); and the level of functioning of a zang or fu organ, such as 'Spleen qi', 'Kidney qi' or 'Stomach qi'.

Qi and fluid production

The production of jin and ye fluids depends on the ability of the Spleen and Stomach to absorb the essence of food and fluids. If this activity is vigorous, the output of jin and ye fluids will be excellent; if the level of Spleen and Stomach functioning is inadequate, the production of jin and ye fluids will suffer and fluid deficiency may result. This is why in clinic a deficiency of both qi and fluids is not uncommon.

Qi and fluid movement and transformation

The distribution of jin and ye fluids and their transformation into sweat or urine for expulsion from the body is completely dependent upon the movement of qi in the body. This movement relies upon zang-fu qi (i.e. their functioning), of course: Spleen's dispersal of essence; Lungs' spreading, clearing and descent; the vaporizing function of the Kidneys; these are behind the rising and falling of jin and ye fluids through the San Jiao, and the movement of the qi and fluids from the interior to the surface, and back again.

In the *Lei Jing*, Chapter 3, section one, Zhang Jing-Yue says: 'If the yuan qi is sufficient, qi transformation is stable, and fluid metabolism is naturally free; this is why qi is the 'Mother of Fluids'.'

Therefore if the yuan qi, which is transported through the San Jiao, does not do its job, normal jin and ye fluids can stop flowing and become pathological water or damp.

Transformation into sweat and urine is the body's primary method of dealing with fluid excess, and any weakness or obstruction in this area of qi function, at any level, can lead to fluid accumulation. This, in Chinese, is called 'qi not moving (or transforming) water' (qi bu xing shui, qi bu hua shui). The reverse, though, is equally likely: fluids build up abnormally and occlude the flow of qi. This is called 'water stopping and causing qi blockage' (shui ting qi zhi). Either of these situations can eventuate in the creation of pathological fluids, such as water, yin, damp or phlegm. Treatment requires the simultaneous use of herbs to move qi, and herbs to promote fluid metabolism.

Blood and jin and ye fluids

The relationship between blood and jin and ye fluids is extremely close. Both blood and fluids are liquids, both can travel together within the vessels, and both function as moistening nourishers. Compared to qi, both are yin. Again, both have the same source: the essence of food and fluids.

The Eighty-first Chapter of the *Ling Shu* says:

Ying (nutritive) qi comes out of the middle Jiao and secretes jin and ye fluids like a life-giving fog. From above it pours into the confluences of the tissues, then seeps into the delicate collaterals (sun mai), where, if the jin and ye are harmonious, through the qi transformation of the Lungs and Heart they can become red blood. If this blood remains harmonious, it will first fill the delicate collaterals, then pour into the collaterals proper (luo mai). When these are full, the blood will pour into the major channels (jing mai) of the body, both yin and yang, ensuring abundance of protective nourishing qi and blood, flowing through the body with the rhythmic impetus of the Lung's breath.

The Seventy-first Chapter of the *Ling Shu* has a similar, though more succinct, description:

Bo Gao said: The Five Grains enter the Stomach and are digested. The waste, jin and ye fluids, and zong qi each go their own way: the waste is expelled from the lower Jiao, the jin and ye fluids issue from the middle Jiao, and the zong qi is expressed from the upper Jiao. This is why the zong qi gathers in the chest (the upper Sea of Qi), can exit through the throat, or link the vessels of the Heart with the movement of the breath. In the middle Jiao, the ying (nutritive) qi secretes jin and ye fluids, that pour into the vessels (mai) and transform into blood, which nourish the four limbs, and internally suffuse the Five Zang and Six Fu.

The *Tai Su* chapter called Shi Er Shui (12 Waters) carries on this account with a further description: 'The nutritive (ying) qi moves through the channels, like a mist. The blood in the channels [moves] like water in a canal. Therefore the twelve channels receive blood, and each is nourished.'

From these accounts we can see that after the jin-ye is produced in the middle Jiao, it is transported around the body through the San Jiao, and then acted upon by the Lungs and the Heart so that a portion of the fluids becomes blood.

In this context it is important to visualize the Lungs—anatomically surrounding the Heart—as being equivalent to the qi surrounding the vessels through which the blood is flowing. Part of the jin-ye goes to the Lungs, and part goes to the Heart; which is equivalent to saying that part of the jin-ye moves with the qi outside of the vessels, and part moves into the vessels, mixing with and becoming part of the blood.

That this does not happen only in the 'Lungs' and 'Heart' located in the upper Jiao, but can occur anywhere that there is the same structure of 'qi' surrounding 'blood', is shown by the quote above from the Seventy-first Chapter of the *Ling Shu*, describing the same transformation of fluids into blood taking place all over the body in the collaterals and the channels. The significance of this is demonstrated in the relationship between blood and sweat described below.

In pathological situations, blood and jin-ye fluids influence each other considerably. For example, when there has been excessive loss of blood, the jin and ye fluids outside of the vessels can permeate into the vessels to make up for the fluid loss. When this involves a large amount of fluids, however, the resulting depletion outside of the vessels can lead to a fluid deficiency, with typical symptoms of thirst, scanty urine, dry skin, and so on.

Blood stagnation in the channels and collaterals also leads to obstruction of the moistening effect of the jin and ye fluids on the surface, resulting in drying, thickening and roughening of the skin.

The opposite situation can also occur: when there has been severe damage to the jin and ye fluids, this can actually cause an exodus of fluids from the blood within the vessels to try to remedy the situation, leaving the vessels empty and deficient, a condition known in TCM as 'jin ku xue zao': jin withered and blood parched. This can lead to severe shen disturbance as the blood which normally should nourish the Heart becomes inadequate, as described in the *Shang Han Lun*: 'If someone with an established tendency to sweating is further encouraged to sweat, the result will certainly be [either] loss of concentration [or] panic.'[39]

In regard to the first case, since the earliest times the Classics have recorded the dangers of using diaphoresis as a method of treatment in cases of blood loss. The *Shang Han Lun* ('Discussion of Cold-Induced Disorders', *c.* 210AD), says: 'Diaphoresis should not be used for those who have lost a lot of blood; sweating will cause chills, shaking, and trembling.'[40]

The reason for the chills, shaking, and trembling is that:

1. Qi will also be lost with the sweat, and will be unable to warm the surface
2. The remaining blood has lost much of the moistening sustenance provided by the jin and ye fluids and the nutritive qi, and so the tendons and muscles malfunction due to lack of nourishment.

Again, in clause 86 of the *Shang Han Lun* appears the following: 'Diaphoresis should not be used for people with frequent nosebleeds; sweating will cause the arteries in the temples to spasm, the eyes to stare and lack free movement, and inability to sleep.'

The cause of these symptoms is, as above, the blood deficiency resulting from the withdrawal of fluids from the blood in the form of perspiration.

For those already sweating excessively, any treatment that may harm the blood, such as using 'blood-busting' herbs to disperse blood stagnation, is similarly contra-indicated; as the *Ling Shu*

Chapter 18 points out: 'Those with exhausted blood should not be encouraged to sweat; those with excessive perspiration should not [be treated with methods that may] harm blood.'

A rather less well-known example of the direct mutual influence of fluids and blood comes from the *Mai Jing* ('Pulse Classic'):

> The teacher said: A woman patient presents complaining that her last menses was scantier than before. What could be the reason for this?
>
> The answer is that if she has been sick with diarrhea, or sweating, or excessive urination, this is a quite normal reaction to these illnesses. And why should this be so? Because the jin and ye fluids have been damaged, the present period is scantier than the previous ones. On the other hand, a suddenly heavier period may be a sign of [some other] affliction [disturbing normal fluid balance], such as constipation or inability to perspire.[41]

The last two symptoms would suggest that the fluids were unable to move in their normal channels and have instead poured into the Chong and Ren, swollen the volume of blood, and resulted in a heavier menses.

Another pathological example in gynecology illustrating this close relationship between fluids and blood is the 'xue fen' and 'shui fen' syndromes, the first being amenorrhea followed by edema, the second being edema followed by amenorrhea.

The names of these syndromes first appeared in the *Jin Gui Yao Lue*, Chapter 14, but the better explanation occurs in the *Sheng Ji Zong Lu* ('Complete Record of the Sages' Benefits', 1117), Chapter 153:

> The meaning of 'xue fen' in the discourses is that as the menstruation is beginning to flow, cold-damp damages the Chong and Ren and causes the menses to cease. Qi accumulates and cannot move, and spreads into the skin [becoming pathological qi], the [pathological] qi and the [still normal] qi struggle, the menstrual blood separates and becomes water, which disperses causing cutaneous edema; hence the name 'xue fen' ('blood separating').

Treatment in the above case is primarily aimed at regulating menstruation, after which the edema will disperse by itself.

'Shui fen' results from Spleen weakness unable to control water, which accumulates internally and overwhelms the ability of the qi transformation function of the Urinary Bladder to deal with the problem by transforming the water into qi. The water spreads out through the lower Jiao, dispersing the blood and so stopping the menstrual flow, so that edema appears first, and then amenorrhea.[42]

Treatment in this case is exactly opposite that of xue fen: the Spleen must be strengthened and the qi-transformation of the Urinary Bladder encouraged, so that the water is dispersed, and then the menstruation will revert to its normal flow.

Jin and ye fluids and breast milk

That breast milk is merely transformed menstrual blood has long been a convention in TCM. Zhang Jing-Yue, in his Ming dynasty *Fu Ren Gui* ('Standards of Gynecology'), quotes an even earlier Song dynasty text when he says: 'A woman's breast milk is transformed from the qi and blood of the Chong and Ren channels, so that when it moves down it produces menstruation, and when it moves up it produces milk.'

Case history

A striking example of the relationship of breast milk to blood, and again of blood to fluids, can be found in the case of a woman with post-partum night-sweats who presented to me in 1986:

This 31 year old woman had given birth 16 days previously, since which time she had been suffering nightsweats so badly that she had to completely change her bedding every hour, soaking the beach towels that she had put down to such an extent that they had to be wrung out. Accompanying symptoms included thirst, frequent urination, exhaustion, poor appetite, a thready rapid pulse, and a slightly purplish tongue with a thin coat.

Her Western gynecologist, when consulted, suggested that this was normal, and that in any case there was little that he could do. TCM agrees that mild nightsweats for up to a week following parturition do not require treatment. This unfortunate lady, however, had more than doubled that time span, and to such an extreme degree that there was a very real danger that the situation could change for the worse.

I knew that even the earliest extant clinical handbook in TCM, the *Jin Gui Yao Lue* ('Essentials from the Golden Cabinet', *c.* 210 AD), had been very explicit about the dangers. In the first section of its chapter on post-partum diseases, it says that the results of severe post-partum sweating can be convulsions, vertigo, or (in less serious cases) acute constipation.

My differentiation was an exhaustion of qi and yin, and the treatment principle selected was to restore qi, nourish yin fluids and constrict perspiration. The prescription was based on Sheng Mai San ('Generate the Pulse Powder', *Formulas and Strategies*, p. 245).

The herbs were as follows:

Dang Shen	12 g	Codonopsis Pilosulae, Radix
Mai Men Dong	9 g	Ophiopogonis Japonici, Tuber
Wu Wei Zi	12 g	Schisandrae Chinensis, Fructus
Ma Huang Gen	9 g	Ephedrae, Radix
Duan Mu Li	15 g	Calcined Ostreae, Concha
Fu Xiao Mai	15 g	Tritici Aestivi Levis, Semen
Bai Shao	15 g	Paeoniae Lactiflora, Radix
Sheng Di	12 g	Rehmannia Glutinosae, Radix
Hong Zao	5 g	Zizyphi Jujubae, Fructus

After four packets of the above herbs, her energy was restored, and the perspiration greatly reduced. Another four packs of similar herbs and the sweating stopped completely.

Despite this success with the sweating and the prevention of a change to a more serious pathology, however, the damage to the fluids had already been done: her breast milk, which had been scanty at the start of the sweating, had completely dried up even before she started the herbs, and refused to flow again. But this was only to be expected. In that 'earlier text' mentioned above, the *Fu Ren Da Quan Liang Fang* ('The Complete Fine Formulas for Women') by the Song dynasty physician Chen Zi-Ming, it says: 'the reason that milk will be completely lacking is that the jin and ye fluids have been exhausted.'[43]

Jing-essence and jin and ye fluids

The *Su Wen*, Chapter 34, says: 'Kidneys are a Water Zang, and control jin and ye fluids'.

Kidney jing, which is yin, produces yuan qi through the vaporizing action of Kidney yang. The yuan qi then moves into the San Jiao, where one of its functions is to ensure the continuous and free movement of jin and ye fluids.

If the Kidney jing-essence should be deficient, it could result not only in meagre fluids but also in failure of jin and ye fluid distribution, leading to symptoms such as scanty dark urine, dry throat and parched skin (or in certain cases water accumulating into edema).

On the other hand, weak Kidney jing will be insufficient to allow Kidney yang to produce yuan qi, and this lack of qi to move the fluids upward will result in dry throat and mouth with thirst in the upper body, while below water builds up and causes frequent copious urination.

As we have seen above in the section on 'ye', ye fluids function as a moistening lubricant, moving into the deep yin areas of the body, and eventually the Kidneys, supplementing jing-essence and marrow and, indeed, forming their liquid material basis.

Herbal therapy illustrates this most clearly. Many of the herbs that tonify jing also have the ability to nourish and moisten jin and ye fluids, such as *Rou Cong Rong* (Cistanches, Herba), *Tu Si Zi* (Cuscutae, Semen), *Gou Qi Zi* (Lycii Chinensis, Fructus), *Shou Di* (Rehmanniae Glutinosae Conquitae, Radix), *Huang Jing* (Polygonati, Rhizoma) and *Shan Yao* (Dioscoreae Oppositae, Radix).

Furthermore, the idea behind using Spleen tonification to strengthen the Kidneys is to ensure healthy Spleen transformation so that jin and ye fluids (as well as jing-essence) are produced from foods, and this steady supply of ample jin and ye will be able to nourish the Kidney jing. This is the meaning of the saying 'The Later Heaven nourishes the Primal Heaven'.

Shen (spirit) and jin and ye fluids

Shen, which Maciocia translates as 'Mind', is produced from constitutional essence (xian tian zhi jing), but it also relies on the continual support of the acquired essence (hou tian zhi jing) derived from food and fluids, through the production of qi, blood, jing essence, and jin and ye fluids. All of these form the material basis of shen.

Speaking specifically of shen's relationship with jin and ye fluids, the Ninth Chapter of the *Su Wen* mentions that, besides depending on harmonious qi, 'the jin and ye fluids must complement each other, and then shen will manifest on its own.'

This implies that unhampered activity of the shen relies upon healthy fluids, and that loss of fluids can cause chaos within the shen. This is illustrated clinically when jin and ye fluids are damaged by excessive sweating, vomiting or diarrhea, and then symptoms such as palpitations, anxiety, delirium and even coma follow. Even excessive crying can damage first fluids and then the shen-ming of the eyes. The *Ling Shu*, Chapter 28, says: 'Ceaseless crying exhausts the ye fluids; when the ye fluids are exhausted the jing essence cannot irrigate (the eyes); failure of jing essence to irrigate the eyes will lead to blindness.'[44]

From the opposite point of view, shen controls (as in Porkert's 'configurative force') the activity and continued production of qi, blood, jing, and jin and ye fluids. This is done primarily through the sovereign influence of the Heart on all the other zang-fu (which Maciocia translates as 'Internal Organs'). If the Heart shen is peaceful, their functioning is normal and the supply of basic substances is unimpeded. If the Heart shen is upset, as we can see clinically in emotionally disturbed patients, there may be a series of disruptions both to the functioning of the zang-fu and in the production and activity of the qi, blood, jing, and jin and ye fluids.

More specifically, normal shen activity exerts a direct control upon body fluids, again through the activity of the Heart. This is explained in the Twenty-eighth Chapter of the *Ling Shu*: 'Sadness, worry, depression and melancholy disturb the peaceful activity of the Heart, which in turn disturbs the functioning of the Five Zang and Six Fu, which itself in turn affects the channels, so that the fluid pathways (ye dao) of the eyes, nose, and mouth open, and tears and nasal mucous pour out.'

The eyes are a major gathering point of the channels, while nose and mouth are major qi passageways.

It is a matter of common experience that fear or shock can produce spontaneous perspiration, urination, and tears.

Classical Essay

The Thirty-sixth Chapter of the *Ling Shu* differentiates the jin fluids and the ye fluids, while also discussing the influence of weather, temperature and emotions on the different processes of fluid excretion, and certain basic principles of the pathology behind fluid obstruction. It is also the source of the quote, expanded upon in the next chapter, attributing special types of fluids to the Five Zang. It is translated below in its entirety:

THE Emperor addressed this question to Qi Bo, saying:
'Water and foods enter through the mouth and are transported to the Stomach and Intestines. After digestion, the fluid portion is differentiated into five types, all of which undergo different methods of excretion from the body. When the weather is cold, for example, or the clothing is thin, the fluids are excreted via the urine or return to qi. When the weather is hot, or the clothing heavy, they become sweat. On the other hand, sadness causes the qi to rise with crying, and the fluids come out as tears; while in still another case, with heat in the middle Jiao, the Stomach relaxes [its downward tendency], qi rebels upward, and the fluids become saliva (tuo). Pathogenic qi can block the flow of normal qi internally, which can lead to fluids obstruction and finally bloating (shui zhang).
'All of this we know, but one would like to know the reasoning behind it.'
Qi Bo replied:
'Fluid and foods both enter through the mouth, and the essence derived from the Five Flavors are separately distributed to their respective zang-organ or one of the Four Seas (i.e. the Sea of Blood, Sea of Qi, Sea of Marrow, and Sea of Food and Fluids) in order to nourish the whole body. Jin and ye each go their separate ways. [That which accompanies] the clear qi that issues through the San Jiao to warm the tissues and flesh, and suffuse the skin, is the jin. That which flows deep into the zang-fu and their orifices, and nourishes the brain and marrow, without being spread and dispersed, is called the ye.[45]
'On hot summery days, or with thick clothing, the subcutaneous tissues [respond to this increase of yang and] open, so sweating occurs. When cold occupies the spaces between the muscles, the jin and ye fluids accumulate, impair yang qi flow, and pain results. In cold weather the surface tissues close, and neither qi nor the usually excreted waste fluids can move outward, and so this water descends into the Urinary Bladder, gathers until qi transformation occurs, and then is excreted as urine.
'The Heart is the ruler of the Five Zang and Six Fu, and controls all the activity of these organs. The hearing of the ears, the sight of the eyes, all are in the service of the Heart. The Lungs command the Hundred Channels, and help the Heart maintain rhythmic circulation, and so assume functions resembling those of a Prime Minister; the Liver controls planning and decision making, like a General; the Spleen rules the muscles, like a bodyguard; and the Kidneys maintain the bones, the framework of the body, and therefore are responsible for the exterior (Shen wei zhi zhu wai). Now as we know, the eyes collect the qi of all the channels of the zang-fu, and this includes the jin and ye fluids as well.
'But when sorrow takes hold of the Heart, its largest vessel (xin xi, the channel through which the Heart connects with the other zang-fu) spasms, and the Lung qi follows it, rising. As the Lung qi rises, the fluids also rush upwards. Of course, this unnatural situation of spasm and rising cannot last, and so repeated rising and falling of the Heart and Lungs occur, and sobbing results, with tightened throat, tears and running nose, and even coughing.

'Heat in the middle Jiao will cause the digestion of food to speed up, and the Stomach to empty more quickly than usual. [But if there are intestinal parasites, these] parasites will then move up and down between the Stomach and Intestines, looking for food. When the Stomach empties, the Intestines will fill; the Stomach then relaxes and its qi rebels upward, followed by fluids, which become [excessive] saliva (tuo).[46]

'The jin and ye fluids from the Five Grains can combine harmoniously and form a thick paste-like substance, which can seep into the spaces of the bones, and nourish and strengthen the brain and marrow, and also flow downward to the groin (yin gu).

'If yin and yang are not in harmony [so that yang qi cannot restrain jing], then this fluid (ye) spills out through the lower yin orifice, which lessens not only the jing, but also the marrow. Once this passes a certain degree, deficiency results, deficiency that causes pain in the lumbar and back as well as aching in the shins.

'If the qi pathway (qi dao) connecting yin and yang is interrupted, the Four Seas are closed off, qi transformation cannot occur, and San Jiao can neither distribute refined fluids nor drain away residue. As a consequence, food and fluids accumulate in the Stomach and Intestines. The food may be able to pass through the ileum (hui chang) to the Colon, the water however has no recourse but to settle in the lower Jiao. It is unable to pass into the Urinary Bladder, and without any means of escape, simply gathers, finally causing distention in the lower Jiao.[47]

'The foregoing is the description of jin and ye fluids' five differentiations, in both normal and abnormal situations.'[48]

NOTES

1. Some may object, saying 'What about jing-essence? or shen?' But jing-essence, while it can be moved, is not active: it is primarily stored potential which must be transformed into one of the above media before it can act; while shen is the final manifestation of the harmonious activity of the whole organism.
2. Since we are discussing *fluid* metabolism, the activity of the Spleen on the solid foods is not mentioned.
3. Zhou Xue-Hai, in the *Du Yi Sui Bi* ('Random Notes while Reading Medicine', 1898), comments on this, saying:

   It has been said that when reading books, one must know the breaks in continuity, the start and finish [of sentences], the extensions [of meaning], the singular [utterance] and the repetitions. Here, in this passage, all these apply.

   The sentence 'Imbibed fluids enter the Stomach' should be considered a single paragraph.

   The statements 'The essential qi of these fluids [is carried] to the Spleen. The Spleen then transports this qi, returning upward to the Lungs' are another section.

   The two sentences 'opening and regulating of the fluid pathways' and 'fluids are transported downward to the Urinary Bladder' refer to both the Lungs and the Stomach, not only to the Lungs. The water passageway goes via the San Jiao, from the Stomach, to descend to the Urinary Bladder; it does not actually rise to the Lungs and then descend. But it must borrow Lung qi to remain open and regulated, and thus the words 'open and regulate' refer to the Lungs, while the words 'fluid pathways' refer to the Stomach.

   The meaning of 'water essence' is the essential qi of water, which refers to the Lungs and the fluid pathways, not to the Urinary Bladder. Lungs receive essence from the Spleen, and distribute it; [but] when that which is left over from the absorption of essence [by the Spleen] returns to travel along the San Jiao, it is distributed along the way [rather than stored as 'jing'] and thus it is not, in the end, called 'jing' (essence), but is still called 'water essence' (shui jing).

   'The Five Channels' mean the channels of the Five Zang organs. The water essence moves from the channels of the Five Zang organs to circulate around the entire body, and this happens all at the same time, there is no first and last implied [by mentioning the 'Four Directions' and the 'Five Channels']. The 'Discussion of Bi' (Chapter 43 of the *Su Wen*) says: 'The essential qi of food and fluids is harmonized and regulated in the Five Zang organs, and seeps into the Six Fu organs, and only then can it enter the vessels (mai).' Is this a true rendering?

   If it is, then the four paragraphs in the section above fit together in a marvelously coherent way.

[But] Zhang Yin-An (a respected Qing dynasty commentator on the *Nei Jing*) says that this fluid distribution issues from the Urinary Bladder, because he reads the two sentences 'transported downward to the Urinary Bladder', and 'the essential qi [of the fluids] spread outward in the four directions' as connected, which would make the jing qi of the body become putrid [as urine]. Is this true, or not? *Du Yi Sui Bi* ('Random Notes while Reading Medicine'), 1898, by Zhou Xue-Hai; Jiangsu Science and Technology Press, 1983, pp. 68-69.

This commentary explicitly describes the difficulties in dealing with ancient texts. If this is true within the single language—Chinese—then one can begin to appreciate the difficulty of encompassing the whole meaning of such a passage in translation *between* languages. This is especially true when each copy of a text had to be copied out by hand, and so were written 'telegram style', with a lot left to the individual teacher-student relationship to clarify. Thus here, in this short example, is demonstrated the reason why we are unlikely to ever have the definitive translation of the *Nei Jing* into English. The best a translator can do is to be thorough in checking parallel passages and commentaries, and supplying these to the reader. As far as possible, this has been done throughout this book.

One of the most interesting ideas in this comment is the point Zhou Xue-Hai makes about the fluid pathways not actually reaching the Lungs but simply borrowing the Lung qi for their movement. The original *Nei Jing* text is indeed somewhat ambiguous about this (an ambiguity I have tried to maintain in the above translation by saying, as the original text does, 'returning upward to the Lungs' (shang gui yu Fei), instead of the more usual translation 'Spleen carries the essential qi of fluids up to the Lungs'. Looked at from this point of view, many of the Classical references are found to be equivocal, for example the *Ling Shu* quote which says 'when this place (i.e. the middle Jiao) receives the qi, it secretes the waste and steams the jin and ye fluids, transforming the subtle essence (jing wei), lifting and pouring it into the Lung channel; then it is transformed into blood, to nourish the whole body...'. This certainly suggests that fluid essence is carried upward with essential qi, but it could be read as saying only that the essential qi of foods is carried upwards. On the other hand, Li Dong-Yuan is quite explicit on this point, in the *Pi Wei Lun* ('Discussion of Spleen and Stomach'): 'Food and drink enter the Stomach, yang qi moves upward, fluids (jin-ye) and qi enter the Heart and pour into the Lungs, filling out the skin, and dispersing through the Hundred Vessels.' (Quoted in *Pi Wei Lun Zuan Yao*, 'A Compilation of Essential Discussions on the Spleen and Stomach', Shaanxi College of TCM, Shaanxi Science and Technology Press, 1986, p. 12)

And yet Zhou Xue-Hai himself provides what may be the final answer, saying in another context:

Chao Jing-Chu says: 'Although jin-fluids are categorized as yin, they still cannot separate from yang qi'. The *Nei Jing* mentions that [that which] steams the skin, fills the body, and moistens the hair [and skin] like the saturation from foggy mist, is called qi. The saturation from foggy mist which makes everything wet, is this not the jin-fluids in the midst of qi? Test it by blowing out the moist breath from the mouth: this proves that qi and jin-fluids cannot be separated. If the qi is separated from the jin-fluids, then its yang nature becomes overbearing: which is termed 'excessive qi then becomes fire'. *Du Yi Sui Bi* ('Random Notes while Reading Medicine'), 1898, by Zhou Xue–Hai, p. 13.

4. According to Zhou Xue-Hai in the *Du Yi Sui Bi* ('Random Notes while Reading Medicine'), 1898, p. 185. See Chapter 4 for a more complete explanation.
5. In the *Lei Jing* ('Systematic Categorization of the *Nei Jing*'), Chapter 3, Section 3, which is an explanation of the *Ling Shu*, Chapter 2, it says:

[The *Ling Shu*, Chapter 2, says:] 'Shao Yang belongs to the Kidneys, the Kidneys link upwards to the Lungs, and thus control two organs'. The Shao Yang here means San Jiao, the main channel of which rises toward Heaven, and disperses in the chest. The Kidney channel also links with the Lungs above. The lower shu-point of the San Jiao belongs to Urinary Bladder (i.e. its lower He-sea point Wei Yang Bl-39), and the Urinary Bladder is linked with the Kidneys, therefore the San Jiao also belongs to the Kidneys. Thus the San Jiao is the Repository in the midst of the Waters (San Jiao wei zhong du zhi fu 三焦为中渎之府), and Urinary Bladder is the repository of the jin and ye fluids: Kidneys, as the Water zang-organ, command the water repositories. The logic is natural... when the *Ling Shu*, Chapter 47, says: 'Kidneys combine with the San Jiao and Urinary Bladder', this is what is meant.

Lei Jing ('Systematic Categorization of the *Nei Jing*'), 1624, by Zhang Jing-Yue; People's Health Publishing, 1982, p. 35.
6. The term 'you men' 幽门—the pylorus, the lower opening of the stomach—is used as early as the *Nan Jing*, in the Forty-fourth Difficulty.
7. *Zhong Yi Li Dai Yi Lun Xuan* ('Selected Medical Essays by Traditional Chinese Doctors of Past Generations'), 1983, p. 97.
8. *Yi Guan* ('Key Link of Medicine'), 1687, by Zhao Xian-Ke; published by the People's Health Press, 1959, p. 95.
9. This frequently quoted statement is almost never found in context, which may be of interest to those who like to know the origin of things:

THE Emperor asked: 'What causes hot hands and feet (re jue 热厥)?'

Qi Bo answered: 'When people drink alcohol, it first enters the Stomach; but the liquid's strong yang heating nature soon rises to the surface causing the surface collaterals to fill, which leaves the channels inside relatively deficient. This is what is called channel yin deficiency with yang excess. Now Spleen mainly helps the Stomach move its fluids. Spleen is yin, while Stomach is yang, and if yin is deficient, then yang will predominate, which in this case will cause a disharmony of the Stomach qi, and the end result is a failure of the essence of food and fluids to nourish the four limbs.

If this person indulges in sexual behavior while thus habitually overeating and consuming alcohol, not only will the Spleen and Stomach be harmed, but the Kidneys will suffer injury as well. Spleen will be unable to help Stomach distribute fluids; further alcohol on top of this causes a struggle between the qi of the alcohol and the qi of food, which leads to an accumulation of heat in the center which will be spread around the body as distribution proceeds. Internal heat will generate darkish urine. The situation internally is now one of excess yang and deficient yin; if more alcohol with its violently heating nature is taken in, the Kidney yin will be further damaged, yang qi will be in unopposed supremacy, the heat will spread to the limits of the body, and the hands and feet will feel hot'.

10. *Yi Xue Zhong Zhong Shen Xi Lu* ('Records of Heart-felt Experiences in Medicine with Reference to the West'), 1918-34, Zhang Xi-Chun; Hebei People's Publishing, 1974, p. 234.

11. Quoted in *Pi Wei Lun Zuan Yao* ('A Compilation of Essential Discussions on the Spleen and Stomach'), Shaanxi College of TCM, Shaanxi Science and Technology Press, 1986, p. 29. The Four Masters in the title are Qi Bo, Huang Di, Qin Yue-Ren, and Zhang Zhong-Jing. Huang Yuan-Yu felt that, since the time of the Four Masters, only Sun Si–Miao had been loyal to their original bequest. Perhaps this attitude was colored by the fact that as a youth Huang lost the sight in his left eye due to malpractice: after which he studied medicine himself.

12. The Emperor in China faced South because he could be compared to the Pole Star. Ho Peng-Yoke, in his modern *Li, Qi and Shu: An Introduction to Science and Civilization in China* (Hong Kong University Press, 1985) says, on page twelve: 'The movement of the stars round a fixed North Pole had perhaps impressed the Chinese much more than it had any other civilization in the world. Confucius compared a virtuous ruler to the Northern Asterism, which sits at its place with the myriad stars going round and paying homage to it.' In the Northern hemisphere, too, the sun moves through the Southern half of the sky. Yet if there was any doubt that assuming a posture of facing South was intended to understand

this concept of yin-yang ascending and descending qualitites of qi, it should be quickly dispelled by the statement on page four of the *Lei Jing Tu Yi* quoting the philosopher Shao Yong who says: 'The head is round, like the Heavens, the feet are square and tread the Earth, facing South and the back to the North, on the left is the East, on the right the West, standing straight in the middle between the two: thus undeviatingly (zheng) occupying the position of zi (midnight) and wu (noon).' *Lei Jing Tu Yi* ('Illustrated Wing to the Systematic Categorization of the *Nei Jing*'), 1624, by Zhang Jing–Yue; Peoples' Health Publishing, Beijing, 1982, p. 4.

13. The *Su Wen*, Chapter 52, says: 'Liver produces (sheng) on the left, Lungs store (cang) on the right'.

14. Thus it will be seen that this diagram with the Earth in the middle is intended to illustrate the quality of energy which characterizes each zang-organ. Many students of TCM become confused when trying to relate this diagram with other Five Phase diagrams intended to show the physiological relationships between the zang-organs within the body.

Manfred Porkert gives a relatively detailed account of this aspect of Earth in his *Theoretical Foundations of Chinese Medicine*, MIT Press, 1974, pp. 49-50, but even he, surprisingly, has trouble with the attributions of 'left' to yang and 'right' to yin, saying it 'is probably due, according to Granet, to early ritualization of certain manual functions'. *ibid.* p. 24.

Finally, chapter five of the *Su Wen* says: 'Left and right are the pathway of yin and yang' to which Zhang Jing-Yue remarks: 'Yang left and ascends, yin right and descends'. *Lei Jing*, p 20.

15. *Yi Bian* ('Fundamentals of Medicine'), 1751, by He Meng-Yao; Shanghai Science and Technology Press, 1982, p. 4.

16. Quoted in *Pi Wei Lun Zuan Yao* ('A Compilation of Essential Discussions on the Spleen and Stomach', Shaanxi College of TCM, Shaanxi Science and Technology Press, 1986, p. 6.

17. *Yi Bian* ('Fundamentals of Medicine'), 1751, by He Meng-Yao; Shanghai Science and Technology Press, 1982, p. 9.

18. *Du Yi Sui Bi* ('Random Notes while Reading Medicine'), 1898, by Zhou Xue-Hai; Jiangsu Science and Technology Press, 1983, pp. 16-17.

19. One example of this disordered movement is ben tun qi, the 'running piglet qi', *cf.* the following essay.

20. Here, Ba Wei Wan (literally 'Eight Flavors Pill') refers to Jin Gui Shen Qi Wan ('Kidney Qi Pill from the Golden Cabinet', *Formulas and Strategies*, p. 275).

21. From *Yi Jia Mi Ao* ('Secrets of the Physicians') by Zhou Shen-Zai, a Ming dynasty doctor; quoted in the *Zhong Yi Li Dai Yi Lun Xuan* ('Selected Medical Essays by Traditional Chinese Doctors of Past Generations'), 1983, p. 75.

22. *Sheng Ji Zong Lu*, in two volumes, ordered by Zhao Ji, 1112 AD (Southern Song Dynasty); Beijing People's Health Publishing, 1992, vol. 1, p. 1154.

23. If this is considered 'reading too much into the text', consider the following from *Du Yi Sui Bi* ('Random Notes while Reading Medicine'), 1898, p. 5, by Zhou Xue-Hai: ' ...Openly traveling the interior and exterior, corresponding to the crevices of the surface and interior (cou li) and influencing the half-interior half-exterior portion of the whole body, is the Shao Yang San Jiao's qi: (with two other previously discussed types of qi) these are the three divisions of the movement of constitutional (xian tian) yuan qi.'

24. *Yi Yuan* ('Origin of Medicine'), 1861, by Shi Shou-Tang; Jiangsu Science and Technology Press, 1983, p. 22.

25. 'Bie shi' 別使. In his translation of the *Nan Jing*, Unschuld translates this as 'special envoy', taking 'bie' in its meaning of 'te bie' (special) and 'shi' as in 'te shi' (special envoy).

In fact 'bie' 別, in ancient medical literature, is used predominantly in the original meaning of 'separate' (the structure of the character is that of a knife separating a knuckle-bone), to part, to leave, to differentiate, or distinguish; although it does have the secondary common meanings of other, or another.

The next word in the combination, 'shi' in ancient medical literature, can mean 1. to send a command, to make or allow (someone to do something); 2. a transmitter of commands or messages, an envoy; 3. one who exercises authority; 4. a use or effect, or to use or create or enable an effect; and 5. to comply with, to obey. It is formed of 'a man' who is 'holding a stylus': i.e. an officer of government who 'makes things happen', thus to cause or to make, or one who carries an order or message in order to 'make things happen', therefore 'bie shi' is better translated 'one who makes separation happen' rather than 'the special envoy'.

Thus the meaning of 'San Jiao zhe, yuan qi shi bie shi' 三焦者, 原气之別使 should be understood as 'The function of the San Jiao is to make the yuan qi separate' into its different uses around the body. This takes 'zhe' 者 as 'the function of', 'bie' as 'separate', and 'shi' as 'to make or cause an effect', the idea being that the San Jiao separates the originally undifferentiated yuan qi and directs it into different channels and organs to perform its various functions. Then the next sentence makes sense: 'It is responsible for the passage of the three qi through the Five Zang and Six Fu'.

This understanding also makes the supporting quote from the Thirty-eighth Difficult Issue very clear: 'It is like this. The San Jiao can be called the reason why there are six fu, as this is where the yuan qi is separated: it supports all of the qi.'

In his translation of this supporting quote, Unschuld has had to ignore one character, and insert another here, in order to avoid giving the character 'bie' the meaning of 'separate'. Here (*Nan Jing*, the Classic of Difficult Issues, p. 395) he does not translate 'bie' as 'special', as he did above, but as

'additional'; he has ignored the character 'yan' 焉 which is either a question indicator or means 'here' or 'in this place'; and he has had to insert the English word 'source', which not only has no basis in the original text but also suddenly makes yuan qi appear from a new 'source': the San Jiao (which, by definition as a fu organ, can only pass things on, not originate anything).

If we now go back to the Sixty-sixth Difficult Issue, we can check to see if this idea of 'San Jiao as the separator of the yuan qi' is consistent with the understanding of the later commentators.

Ye Lin, in his *Nan Jing Zheng Yi* ('The Correct Meaning of the *Nan Jing*', 1895), is quite clear about this in part of his commentary to the Sixty-sixth Difficulty; which strangely Unschuld omits, although he does quote him in other passages (as Yeh Lin), Ye says

> The root of San Jiao is in Ming Men between the Kidneys, the source of people's life, the basis of the twelve channels: all are linked at this place. The Tian Yang (yang of heaven) inspired through the nose, passes the Lungs to reach the Heart, and leads Heart fire—following the tendons of the backbone—to enter the Kidney channel ('xi' 系, also used for the internal connection between a zang organ and its sense organ) and reach Ming Men, to vaporize the Water of the Urinary Bladder and transform qi to rise. The San Jiao presides over ministerial fire, and is the director of separation (bie shi) of the yuan qi in the Kidneys. The movement of the nutritive qi and protective qi in the twelve channels is all directed (shi) by the San Jiao.

From the *Nan Jing Zheng Yi* ('The Correct Meaning of the *Nan Jing*', 1895), by Ye Lin; Shanghai Science and Technology Press (no date supplied), punctuation added by Wu Kao Pan, p. 117.

Finally, the defining statement from Xu Da-Chun (Hsu Ta-ch'un in Unschuld's text) is most unequivocal, as he says: 'gen ben yuan qi, fen xing zhu jing, gu yue bie shi' 根本原气, 分行诸经, 故曰別使 which means 'The fundamental yuan qi is separated to travel in each and every channel, thus the term 'bie shi'.' From the *Ba Shi Yi Nan Jing Ji Jie* ('Collected Explanations of the Classic of Eighty-One Difficulties') edited by Guo Ai-Chun and Guo Hong-Tu. Tianjin, Tianjin Science and Technology Press, 1984, p. 123.

(Thanks to Dan Bensky for the location of this quote!)

26. *Zhong Yi Fang Ji Yu Zhi Fa* ('TCM Formulas and Treatment Methods'), from the Chengdu TCM College, Sichuan Science and Technology Press, 1984, p. 298).

27. Quoted in *Zhong Yi Ji Chu Li Lun Xiang Jie* ('Detailed Explanation of TCM Basic Theory'), Fujian Science and Technology Press, 1981, pp. 55-56.

28. In the *Tai Su* version of the same passage, however, it says 'to link the Heart and Lungs', suggesting that 'vessels' in the *Ling Shu* may have been a mistake, especially as 'Lungs' fits the sense of the sentence better.

   While we are discussing clarifications: a similar quote from the 'Spiritual Axis', on p. 84 of Maciocia's *Foundations of Chinese Medicine*, says 'Big Qi gathers together without moving to accumulate in the chest'. While the original Chinese does indeed say 'without moving' (bu xing), the meaning is that it does not disperse but instead is gathered in the upper sea of qi. Hence Maciocia's use of 'Gathering Qi' is further substantiated.

29. *Lei Jing* ('Systematic Categorization of the *Nei Jing*'), 1624, Zhang Jing-Yue; People's Health Publishing, Beijing, 1982, p. 30.

30. One excellent acupuncture point to restore Small Intestine fluid separation is Shui Fen (CV-9), located directly above the point at which this separation occurs. Indeed, the term 'Shui Fen' means 'Water Separation': it was named for this function. If it is combined with Lie Que (LU-7), the opening point for the Ren channel, three actions are achieved with two points: the Ren channel is opened, so that Shui Fen (CV-9) is better empowered; the Lungs' function of regulating fluid pathways is brought into play; and the rhythmic descent of Lung qi is enhanced, which will assist the descending action of Stomach qi, and thus re-establish the separating function of Small Intestine qi transformation.

31. *Yi Xue Jian Neng*, page one in the chapter entitled 'Methods of Diagnosis', quoted in *Zhong Yi Ming Yan Lu* ('Records of Famous Sayings in TCM'), Guangdong Science and Technology Press, 1986, p. 77.

32. Quoted in *Zhong Yi Ji Chu Li Lun Xiang Jie* ('Detailed Explanation of TCM Basic Theory'), Fujian Science and Technology Press, 1981, p. 122.

33. *Zhong Zang Jing Wu Jie* ('Vernacular Translation of the Treasury Classic', People's Health Publishing, 1990, p. 57.

34. This is not to say that other aspects of the Large Intestine functioning have not been discussed in traditional Chinese medicine. For a single example, Tang Rong-Chuan says:

   The ability of the Large Intestine to pass [stool] depends completely on the qi. Qi is controlled by the Lungs, and it is not only the Large Intestine which depends upon this sending action of the Lung qi, urination also requires its transforming movement: this is the ability of the rhythmic control of Lung Metal. But the qi transformation of the Large Intestine is also related to its connection with the Metal pathway (i.e. the Lung channel), thus those treating disease [of the Colon] usually treat the Lungs. Large Intestine's position of residence in the lower Jiao also connects it to control by the Kidneys, so the *Nei Jing* says: 'The Kidneys open into the two yin orifices of the lower body', and they also say: 'Kidneys are the floodgate of the Stomach'. Therefore Kidney yin must be full and sufficient for the Large Intestine to be plump and moist. The Jue Yin Liver channel also encircles the rectum, and the Intestine and the uterus both reside next to each other, thus the Liver channel and the Intestine also have a relationship. So in terms of illness, there may be descent of weak central qi allowing damp-heat to pour in; there may be Lung channel heat transferred to the Large Intestine; there may be Kidney channel yin deficiency unable to moisten the bowel; and there may be Liver channel blood-heat seeping into the Large Intestine, all are based upon the connections between the bowel and other organs. Even though the disease has come from elsewhere, though, once it is in the Intestine it cannot return to the other organs; the Intestine must be treated first to eradicate the branch, and then afterwards the other organs should be treated to clear the origin, and there will then be no other relapses.

   From the *Xue Zheng Lun* ('Discussion of Blood Syndromes', 1884) by Tang Rong-Chuan; People's Health Publishing, 1986, pp. 135-136.

35. See the chapter on edema for a more complete discussion of this passage.

36. *Lei Jing* ('Systematic Categorization of the *Nei Jing*'), 1624, Zhang Jing-Yue; People's Health Publishing, Beijing, 1982, p. 30.

37. 'Water', capitalized, in this book refers to the Water of the Five Phases.

38. *Lei Jing* ('Systematic Categorization of the *Nei Jing*'), 1624, Zhang Jing-Yue; People's Health Publishing, Beijing, 1982, p. 84.

39. From the *Shang Han Lun* ('Discussion of Cold-Induced Disorders'): 'Treatment of Taiyang Syndrome, No. 6'.

40. *ibid.*, clause 87 (according to the numbering in the New World Press English edition).

41. *Mai Jing* ('Pulse Classic'), 1984, People's Health Publishing, p. 605.

42. In this case, the excess water will not 'swell the volume of blood and result in a heavier menses' because the fluids here are pathological, being untransformed water and damp building up from Spleen deficiency. In the previous case discussed in the *Mai Jing*, the heavy menses resulted from normal already-transformed fluids unable to move in their channels and instead pouring into the Chong and Ren to swell the volume of blood. The point that pathological agents cannot act as physiological substances may be repeated throughout this book to the stage of risking tedium, but the risk is necessitated by the widespread lack of representation on this point in the English literature of TCM to date.

43. There is an amusing epilogue to the story. The Western gynecologist, apparently, was most im-

pressed, although he would not admit it to our patient. According to one of his staff members (who came in for a consultation about nine months after the event), they had apparently been laying bets around the office that the herbs would not work!

44. The heart-rending truth of this has been demonstrated by the 'medical puzzle' of the Cambodian widows, relocated in California, who had cried themselves blind due to the loss of their families under Pol Pot.

45. Zhang Jing-Yue, in the *Lei Jing* annotation of this chapter, notes:

> Here is the difference between jin and ye. Zong (gathering) qi collects in the upper Jiao, ying (nutritive) qi issues from the middle Jiao, wei (defensive) qi issues from the lower Jiao. That which reaches the surface is the qi of yang, therefore the qi that comes out of the San Jiao to warm the tissues and flesh, and suffuse the skin, is jin; jin belongs to yang.
>
> That which nourishes internally is the qi of yin, therefore that which circulates within the blood vessels, and is not dispersed outward, and also flows into the zang-fu and benefits the jing marrow, is ye; ye belongs to yin.' *Lei Jing* ('Systematic Categorization of the *Nei Jing*'), 1624, Zhang Jing-Yue; People's Health Publishing, Beijing, 1982, p. 541.

46. Zhang Jing-Yue notes:

> In the 23rd Chapter of the *Su Wen* it states that tuo-type saliva belongs to the Kidneys, yet here it says the Stomach. It is correct that both the Kidneys and the Stomach influence tuo; because the tuo that results from obstructed Earth is from the Stomach, while the tuo that results from flooding fluids is from the Kidneys. *Lei Jing*, p. 542.

47. Zhang Jing-Yue remarks:

> The treatment of this problem requires attention to the root cause: the obstruction of qi. One must re-establish qi transformation. Try imagining a flood: if the rays of the sun are unable to reach the waters, the water's yin-congealing nature would never be dispersed, and the mire would never dry out. If one can grasp this, then understanding of the Way of the qi transformation between yin and yang will follow. *loc. cit.*

48. Zhang Jing-Yue explains: 'When yin and yang are in harmony, the Five Fluids will co-exist normally with the jing internally, until called upon to moisten and nourish the sense organs or other structures; if yin and yang are in disharmony, even the jing will follow the abnormal loss of fluids to the exterior, and lead to further deficiency.' *loc. cit.*

Fluids of the Five Zang organs

2

PHYSIOLOGY

Under normal physiological conditions, the body fluids will supply the needs of the various organs and tissues in the body. Each of these organs and tissues, because of their diverse activities and energetic qualities, will subject the fluids to a different transformational process, and each process will result in a different metabolic product. This product will, again, be excreted from the body by a distinct route.

The *Ling Shu,* Chapter 36, says:

> After food and fluids enter the mouth and are transported into and through the Stomach and Intestines, it is differentiated into five fluids (ye). When the weather is cold, or the clothing is thin, [the turbid aspect] becomes urine and [the subtle aspect] becomes qi [again, which circulates back into the body]; when the weather is hot, or the clothing thick, it becomes sweat; when there is sorrow, the qi [of the Five Zang] collects, [rises], and becomes tears; when there is heat in the middle Jiao, the [normal downward movement of the] Stomach relaxes, and [rising upward] produces [excessive] saliva.

Again, in the *Su Wen,* Chapter 23, it says: 'The fluid transformation of the Five Zang [is as follows]: in the Heart, sweat; in the Lungs, nasal mucus; in the Liver, tears; in the Spleen, watery saliva (xian); in the Kidneys, mucoid saliva (tuo).'

Physiology of the Five Fluids

Sweat is the fluid of the Heart

Sweat is transformed from the jin fluids by the steaming action of heat, and jin-fluids are the main fluid component of the blood (see Chapter 1). Because the blood is ruled by the Heart, so it is said that 'sweat is the fluid of the Heart'. If Heart yang is deficient, profuse sweating can result; likewise Heart yin deficiency can lead to nightsweats. These examples are not as tenuous as may first appear. The qi and blood flows around the surface of the body are mainly controlled by the Lungs (associated with skin and protective qi) and the Heart (associated with blood and nutritive qi). Internal disharmony or external pathogenic influence can affect the delicate balance between yin and yang here, deflecting or depleting yang (protective qi) so that yin (nutritive qi) lacks control, flows out as sweat, and is lost.

This is described by the Qing dynasty physician Zhang Zhi-Cong (1644-1722) in his *Lu Shan Tang Lei Bian* ('Catalogued Differentiations from Lu Shan Hall', 1670)[1]: 'Now sweat has two sources: one comes from blood that suffuses the hot flesh, the fluid (ye) in this blood transforms and becomes sweat, which is the sweat of the surface; the other comes from the Yang Ming Stomach fu-organ, and this is the sweat of [pathogenic] water-fluid (shui-ye).'[2]

The transformation and steaming-outward action of the yang qi, in terms of sweat, is very closely related to the activity of the Heart shen. As Heart shen is yang, it can exert a controlling influence on the process.

In the *Ling Shu*, Chapter 28, it says:

Sorrow, worry and anxiety will agitate the Heart. If the Heart is agitated, the Five Zang and Six Fu will be shaken, which will in turn affect the eyes (zong mai, literally 'the confluence of the vessels'). If the eyes are affected the fluid pathways will open, and tears and nasal mucus will come forth.

A disturbed shen will disturb all of the qi within the body, however, and thus affect the fluid pathways (ye dao). It is a matter of everyday experience that emotional disturbance will lead to sweating, especially in those areas most closely related to the Heart: the armpits (Ji Quan H-1) and the palms (Shao Fu H-8 and Lao Gong P-8)

However, both physiologically and pathologically, the process of sweating is much more complicated than can be subsumed under the simple saying 'sweat is the fluid of the Heart'. These mechanisms are examined more closely in Chapter 3.

Tears are the fluid of the Liver

Liver opens into the eyes, and tears flow out of the eyes, so it can be said that 'tears are the fluid of the Liver'. When Liver yin or Liver blood is deficient, the eyes lack lubrication and so feel dry, gritty, tired and difficult to move. Excessive lacrimation, on the other hand, can indicate yin deficiency taken one step further, so that fire flares up and tears are forced out. These tears will be hot, however, and can occur anytime. These type of tears are different from the tears that point to Liver and Kidney deficiency. This

is a deficiency of both yin and yang, and the fluid of the eyes becomes uncontrolled, causing frequent lacrimation, especially in the cold. These tears will be cold, and they will be accompanied by other (rather severe) symptoms of Liver and Kidney deficiency of both yin and yang. The fact that exogenous pathogens can take advantage of deficiency in the Liver channel, invade, and also contribute to lacrimation disorders certainly does complicate differentiation and treatment, but serves to underscore the point that Liver and tears are related (see the detailed differentiations below).

Watery saliva (xian) is the fluid of the Spleen

The Spleen opens into the mouth, and therefore saliva can be said to be the fluid of the Spleen. Dry mouth can result from a Spleen yin deficiency, among other things; while excessive salivation can result from xu-cold in the Spleen and Stomach (as well as Kidney yang deficiency: see below).

Mucoid saliva (tuo) is the fluid of the Kidneys

These two types of saliva are distinguished in the *Zhong Yi Da Zi Dian* ('The Comprehensive Dictionary of Traditional Chinese Medicine'), which says 'Xian ... is relatively thin, and mainly moistens the oral cavity, while tuo is relatively thick, and primarily helps digestion.' Kidneys have a claim upon the latter due to the branch of the Kidney channel which reaches the root of the tongue at Lian Quan (Ren 23), and again the quote mentioned above from the *Su Wen*, Chapter 23: 'The fluids produced from the Five Zang are: sweat from the Heart, nasal mucus from the Lungs, tears from the Liver, thin saliva from the Spleen, and thick saliva from the Kidneys. These are called the Five Fluids.' In the *Lei Jing* ('Systematic Categorization of the Nei Jing', 1624) Zhang Jing-Yue comments about tuo and the Kidneys: 'Tuo is produced from beneath the tongue: the Foot Shao Yin Kidney channel ascends along the throat to bracket the root of the tongue.'[3]

Excessive mucoid saliva (tuo) is a deficiency condition related closely to Spleen and Kidneys. Excess damp from Spleen deficiency can cause profuse mucoid saliva, and will be associated with typical symptoms like epigastric and abdominal fullness, loose stool and so on. The pulse will be weak, floating and thready, the tongue pale and large, with a white greasy coat. Kidney yang deficiency can allow pathogenic water to ascend, causing a welling-up of saliva, but here there will also be vertigo and a fainting feeling, palpitations and shortness of breath, all worsened with exertion. If more severe, there will be palpitations below the navel, which is diagnostic. The pulse will be wiry and slippery, the tongue coat white and glossy.

It is important to note that excessive mucoid saliva is always a result of deficiency, either of the Kidneys, or the Spleen, or both.

Nasal mucus is the fluid of the Lungs

This normal mucus moistens the nose and the air that enters the Lungs. Both Lung yin deficiency and exogenous parching (zao) wind-heat affecting the Lungs share dryness of the nasal cavity as a symptom, while excessive secretion of nasal mucus is a frequent and well-known sign of Lung pathology, showing that Lungs' spreading and descending function is impaired, and that the normal nasal mucus, instead of simply moistening the nasal cavity, is beginning to accumulate.

Summary

The above are examples of jin and ye fluids in action. Supplied from the essence of food and fluids in the middle Jiao and distributed around the body by the San Jiao, they attach themselves to whatever zang-fu sphere of activity may require them. These fluids can be observed either carrying out the normal functions of that position, or involved in pathology affecting that sphere of activity.

As guides to diagnosis, though, the above examples are only indicators of a line of possible questioning, and should not be considered conclusive or decisive on their own. For instance, in the 'dry nose' example that seems to point so clearly to a Lung pathology, it is equally possible that Stomach heat is the culprit, flaring up the Stomach channel that brackets the nose. A few more questions, however, can quickly determine which is which, as the Lung pathology will be associated with respiratory symptoms, while the Stomach will of course be linked with digestive symptoms.[4]

Likewise sweat, while 'the fluid of the Heart', is also closely related in its metabolism to Lungs, Stomach, and Kidney functioning (see Chapter 3).

CLINICAL DIFFERENTIATION AND TREATMENT[5]

This section will introduce examples of the pathological mechanisms affecting the 'Five Fluids of the Zang', their differentiation and possible treatment. It will not cover zang or fu organ yin deficiencies as such, or complete disciplines such as ophthalmology; rather it is intended to indicate the clinical applications which observation of the external manifestations of the Five Fluids can provide.

Differentiation of pathological lacrimation

Tears or crying from emotional upset is normal. But tears can also be the result of pathological wind-heat or wind-cold invasion, or shi-fire in the Liver and Gall Bladder channels, or fire forcing the movement of water, all of which are discussed below. The following differentiation does not cover lacrimation resulting from opthalmological disease only.

Common symptom patterns

Liver channel wind-cold lacrimation. Cold tears appear on exposure to wind. This is called 'leng lei' (cold tears) in Chinese, and is often seen in older patients who are blood deficient. The main manifestations will be watery eyes in the wind, emaciation, pallid face, pale lips and nails, pale tongue body, and thready pulse. If the deficiency involves yang, they will have chills and cold limbs, a white moist tongue coat, and a deep slow pulse.

Liver channel wind-heat lacrimation. Hot tears appear on exposure to wind. This is called 're lei' (hot tears) in Chinese. The main manifestations will be hot watery eyes in the wind but despite the tears the eyes will feel gritty and red, with a dry mouth and nose, dizziness and tinnitus. The tongue body will be red, the tongue coat thin white and the pulse wiry, or possibly thready and rapid.

Dual deficiency of Kidney and Liver lacrimation. Cold tears (leng lei) appear randomly. The main manifestations will be frequently watering eyes, worse in cold temperatures. At first the lacrimation will stop by itself without the appearance of any other symptoms, but gradually the condition will worsen with more frequent tears, accompanied by dizziness, faintness, blurry vision, tinnitus, loss of hearing, insomnia, spermatorrhea, lower backache and weak knees. The pulse will be thready and weak and the tongue coat white.

Yin deficiency with fire flaring lacrimation. Hot tears (re lei) appearing randomly. The main manifestations will include frequent hot lacrimation during the daytime but dryness of the eyes at night, associated with blurry vision, a fainting feeling, red tongue body, tongue coat thin white or thin yellow, and a thready rapid pulse.

Differentiation and treatment

Liver channel xu-cold lacrimation. This is usually a result of Liver blood deficiency so that it is unable to rise and nourish the eyes. The deficiency is coupled with an exogenous wind-cold pathogen taking advantage of the weakened area and invading. The pathogenic cold lodges in the optical orifice and obstructs—as is its nature—but on further exposure to external wind (and the pathogenic wind's own yang-dispersing nature), the tears begin to flow. The *Sheng Ji Zong Lu* ('Comprehensive Recording of the Sages' Benefits', 1117) in its chapter on lacrimation from wind, remarks: 'Liver opens into the eyes, and Liver's fluid is tears. When the Liver qi (here, its function) is weak, pathogenic wind will take advantage of this [and invade], so that the fluid of the Liver lacks control and frequently flows out. Upon encountering wind, it becomes worse.'

This symptom is often found in older people with Liver deficiency, and soon a vicious circle can develop: the more tears are lost, the more the Liver fluids are damaged. In the end it becomes very difficult to treat. The approach to treatment is to begin to nourish blood and expel cold, using the formula Yang Xue Qu Han Yin ('Nourish the Blood and Drive Out Cold Decoction')[6]:

Formulas

Yang Xue Qu Han Yin ('Nourish the Blood and Drive Out Cold Decoction')

Gou Qi Zi	Lycii Chinensis, Fructus
Ju Hua	Chrysanthemi Morifolii, Flos
Dang Gui	Angelica Polymorpha, Radix
Bai Shao	Paeoniae Lactiflora, Radix
Chuan Xiong	Ligustici Wallichii, Radix
Cang Zhu	Atractylodis, Rhizoma
Bai Zhu	Atractylodis Macrocephalae, Rhizoma
Fu Ling	Poriae Cocos, Sclerotium
Du Huo	Duhuo, Radix
Xi Xin	Asari cum Radice, Herba
Rou Gui	Cinnamomi Cassiae, Cortex
Fu Pen Zi	Rubi, Fructus

Source text: *Yan Ke Quan Jing* ('Complete Mirror of Ophthalmology')

If the cold watery eyes are chronic, with loss of visual clarity, Gou Qi Zi Jiu ('Lycium Berry Wine') can be used, which is simply rice wine in which *Gou Qi Zi* (Lycii Chinensis, Fructus) have been soaked.

Liver channel wind-heat lacrimation. This is predominantly caused by Liver channel pent-up heat, with a further exposure to pathogenic wind, so that the two yang pathogens combine, struggle, and bring on an external manifestation: a rushing upward to the eyes, so that exposure to further wind elicits the shedding of hot tears.

If the struggle of wind and heat should lead to a build-up of fire, there will be red gritty eyes, dry parched mouth and nose, vertigo and tinnitus. All of these symptoms are markedly different from the Liver deficiency wind-cold discussed above.

Treatment in a mild case should be to cool the Liver and expel wind, with a prescription made up of herbs appropriate for the individual patient, selected from formulas such as Ling Yang Jiao San ('Antelope Horn Powder') and Bai Jiang Can San ('White Bombyx Powder').

If the condition is more severe, the treatment must be to lift and disperse exogenous pathogenic yang while simultaneously nourishing yin and bringing down fire. In this case, the formula should be Sheng Yang Jiang Huo Tang ('Lift Yang and Bring Down Fire Decoction') with appropriate adjustments. Long Dan Xie Gan Tang ('Gentiana Longdancao Decoction to Drain the Liver') plus *Xia Ku Cao* (Prunellae Vulgaris, Spica) and *Qing Xiang Zi* (Celosiae Argenteae, Semen) can also be used.

Formulas

Ling Yang Jiao San ('Antelope Horn Powder')

Ling Yang Jiao	15 g	Antelopis, Cornu
Ju Hua	3 g	Chrysanthemi Morifolii, Flos
Chao Shan Zhi Zi	15 g	Fried Gardeniae Jasminoidis, Fructus
Huang Qin	15 g	Scutellariae Baicalensis, Radix
Hu Huang Lian	9 g	Picrorrhizae, Rhizoma
Xuan Shen	15 g	Scrophulariae Ningpoensis, Radix
Qiang Huo	15 g	Notopterygii, Rhizoma et Radix
Xi Xin	3 g	Asari cum Radice, Herba
Gua Lou Ren	15 g	Trichosanthes, Semen
Che Qian Zi	15 g	Plantaginis, Semen

The antelope horn is finely powdered by filing, the other ingredients are finely powdered in the normal way, then combined. Six grams are taken after meals, washed down with a decoction of *Zhu Ye* (Lophatheri Gracilis, Herba).

Source text: *Shen Shi Yao Han* ('Scrutiny of the Precious Jade Case', 1644)[7]

Bai Jiang Can San ('White Bombyx Powder')

Jiang Can	Bombyx Batryticatus
Sang Ye	Mori Albae, Folium
Jing Jie	Schizonepetae Tenuifoliae, Herba et Flos
Mu Zei Cao	Equiseti Hiemalis, Herba
Xuan Fu Hua	Inulae, Flos
Xi Xin	Asari cum Radice, Herba
Gan Cao	Glycyrrhizae Uralensis, Radix

Source text: *Shen Shi Yao Han* ('Scrutiny of the Precious Jade Case', 1644)

Sheng Yang Jiang Huo Tang ('Lift Yang and Bring Down Fire Decoction')

Sang Shen Zi	Mori Albae, Fructus
Ju Hua	Chrysanthemi Morifolii, Flos
Huang Bo	Phellodendri, Cortex
Zhi Mu	Anemarrhenae Asphodeloidis, Radix
Xuan Shen	Scrophulariae Ningpoensis, Radix
Tian Men Dong	Asparagi Cochinchinensis, Tuber
Sheng Di	Rehmannia Glutinosae, Radix

Mu Zei Cao	Equiseti Hiemalis, Herba
Jing Jie	Schizonepetae Tenuifoliae, Herba et Flos
Fang Feng	Ledebouriellae Sesloidis, Radix
Xi Xin	Asari cum Radice, Herba

Source text: *Yan Ke Quan Jing* ('Complete Mirror of Ophthalmology')

Long Dan Xie Gan Tang ('Gentiana Longdancao Decoction to Drain the Liver')

Long Dan Cao	Gentianae Scabrae, Radix
Huang Qin	Scutellariae Baicalensis, Radix
Shan Zhi Zi	Gardeniae Jasminoidis, Fructus
Mu Tong	Mutong, Caulis
Che Qian Zi	Plantaginis, Semen
Ze Xie	Alismatis Plantago-aquaticae, Rhizoma
Chai Hu	Bupleuri, Radix
Sheng Di	Rehmannia Glutinosae, Radix
Dang Gui	Angelica Polymorpha, Radix
Gan Cao	Glycyrrhizae Uralensis, Radix

Source text: *Yi Fang Ji Jie* ('Analytic Collection of Medical Formulas', 1682) [*Formulas and Strategies*, p. 96]

Dual deficiency of Kidneys and Liver lacrimation. This is frequently a result of excessive sexual activity weakening the jing-essence and blood, but can also occur from continual emotional crying exhausting the yin fluids. Once Kidney and Liver yin is damaged, the yang can also be reduced, which is what happens in this case, and the lacrimal fluids become erratic, causing frequent watery eyes with cold tears. This will be worse in the cold. Other clinical manifestations will include dry gritty eyes and blurry vision, and further Kidney yin and yang deficiency symptoms such as dizziness and vertigo, aching and weakness of the lower back and legs, insomnia and spermatorrhea. This condition is similar to the Liver channel xu-cold described above but is more severe, as there not only are two zang-organs involved but also a combined yin and yang deficiency. So it is truly 'dual'. Treatment requires warming Liver and Kidneys, and nourishing jing-essence and blood, with formulas like Ju Jing Wan ('Chrysanthemum Eye Pills') plus *Wu Wei Zi* (Schisandrae Chinensis, Fructus) and *Tong Ji Li* (Astragali, Semen), or Gan Shen Shuang Bu Wan ('Liver Kidney Dual Tonification Pills'). These can be combined with She Xiang San ('Musk Powder') which is sniffed into the nostrils.

Formulas

Ju Jing Wan ('Chrysanthemum Eye Pills')

Ju Hua	120 g	Chrysanthemi Morifolii, Flos
Gou Qi Zi	90 g	Lycii Chinensis, Fructus
Rou Cong Rong	60 g	Cistanches, Herba
Ba Ji Tian	30 g	Morindae Officianalis, Radix

Powder finely and make into small pills with honey, 9 g per dose, to be taken on an empty stomach before meals with warm wine or salty water.

Source text: *Shen Shi Yao Han* ('Scrutiny of the Precious Jade Case', 1644)

Gan Shen Shuang Bu Wan ('Liver Kidney Dual Tonification Pills')

Dang Gui	Angelica Polymorpha, Radix
Chuan Xiong	Ligustici Wallichii, Radix
Shan Zhu Yu	Corni Officinalis, Fructus
Ba Ji Tian	Morindae Officianalis, Radix
Gou Qi Zi	Lycii Chinensis, Fructus
Fu Ling	Poriae Cocos, Sclerotium
Shi Hu	Dendrobii, Herba
Fang Feng	Ledebouriellae Sesloidis, Radix
Xi Xin	Asari cum Radice, Herba
Sheng Jiang	Zingiberis Officinalis Recens, Rhizoma
Gan Cao	Glycyrrhizae Uralensis, Radix

Source text: *Yan Ke Quan Jing* ('Complete Mirror of Ophthalmology')

She Xiang San ('Musk Powder')

She Xiang	Moschus Moschiferi, Secretio
Xiang Fu	Cyperi Rotundi, Rhizoma
Cang Zhu	Atractylodis, Rhizoma
Chuan Jiao	Zanthoxyli Bungeani, Fructus

Source text: *Shen Shi Yao Han* ('Scrutiny of the Precious Jade Case', 1644)

Yin deficiency with fire flaring lacrimation. This is usually a consequence of Liver and Kidney yin deficiency, so that Water is unable to control Fire. This xu-fire (i.e. relatively excess yang which is itself the result of a weak yin) flares upward and forces out hot tears. Wang Ken-Tang, in his *Zheng Zhi Zhun Sheng* ('Standards of Patterns and Treatments', 1602) says:

> When the yin fluids of the Kidneys, Liver and Gall Bladder are exhausted and the yin jing-essence depleted [and unable to reach the orifices], and there is stress and worry with excessive concentration upon problems, this will incite the fire and damage the juices (zhi, literally 'juices'), weakening the blood and the paste-like fluids (i.e. the ye-fluids). People who cry immoderately often get this.

Clinical manifestations include frequent hot lacrimation occurring randomly but especially frequent during the day, while the eyes will be dry and gritty at night, with dizziness and blurry vision, and other yin deficiency symptoms such as thready rapid pulse and little or no tongue coat, which differentiate this syndrome from the excess type wind-heat in the Liver channel condition, which will have more of a tongue coat and a stronger wiry pulse. Treatment requires tonification of the Liver and Kidneys in order to bring yang back into yin, with a formula like Jiao Xia Wan ('Zanthoxyli and Rehmannia Pills').

If there is deficiency, but also some pathogenic activity from Liver and Gall Bladder fire, then Jia Wei Dang Gui Yin Zi ('Augmented Dang Gui Decoction') should be used.

Formulas

Jiao Xia Wan ('Zanthoxyli and Rehmannia Pills')[8]

Shou Di	Rehmanniae Glutinosae Conquitae, Radix
Sheng Di	Rehmannia Glutinosae, Radix
Chuan Jiao	Zanthoxyli Bungeani, Fructus (removing the seed and the closed fruits, and lightly fried).

Grind equal amounts of the above herbs into fine powder, then make into small honey pills. One dose is fifty pills, to be taken on an empty stomach and swallowed with salt water.

Source text: *Shen Shi Yao Han* ('Scrutiny of the Precious Jade Case', 1644)

Jia Wei Dang Gui Yin Zi ('Augmented Dang Gui Decoction')

Dang Gui	Angelica Polymorpha, Radix
Ren Shen	Ginseng, Radix
Chai Hu	Bupleuri, Radix
Huang Qin	Scutellariae Baicalensis, Radix
Bai Shao	Paeoniae Lactiflora, Radix
Da Huang	Rhei, Rhizoma
Zhi Mu	Anemarrhenae Asphodeloidis, Radix
Huang Bo	Phellodendri, Cortex
Sheng Di	Rehmannia Glutinosae, Radix
Gan Cao	Glycyrrhizae Uralensis, Radix
Hua Shi	Talc

Source text: *Yan Ke Quan Jing* ('Complete Mirror of Ophthalmology')

Summary

The first step in differentiating the various symptom patterns in excess lacrimation is to determine whether the tears are hot or cold. Hot tears are from fire, cold tears are from cold. The next step is to identify the precipitating factor.

If hot tears were brought on by wind, then the condition is that of pent-up heat in the Liver channel being stirred by pathogenic wind. If the hot tears were to occur randomly it will be an internal problem, and the condition will likely be that of Kidney and Liver yin deficiency, where Water is failing to control Fire, and this deficiency-based fire is flaring upward and 'steaming' out the tears.

If cold tears were brought on by wind, the condition is Liver blood unable to nourish the eyes, which then cannot withstand the exogenous pathogenic wind attack. If the cold tears were to occur randomly, then internal reasons are the cause: in this case a deficiency of Liver and Kidneys again but involving yang as well as yin. Yang is unable to control the fluids, which well up and the tears appear.

Excessive mucoid saliva (duo tuo)

This is either a subjective sensation of excessive salivary excretion or—when severe—a repeated involuntary expectoration of the excessive saliva. In the *Sheng Ji Zong Lu* ('Comprehensive Recording of the Sages' Benefits', 1117) and the *Tai Ping Hui Min He Ji Ju Fang* ('Imperial Grace Formulary of the Tai Ping Era', 1078-85), the condition is called 'excessive mucoid saliva from Kidney deficiency' (Shen xu duo tuo).

Common symptom patterns

Excessive mucoid saliva from Kidney deficiency. Profuse sticky saliva, vertigo, palpitations, dizziness and shortness of breath, all exacerbated by exertion. If the flooding water is more severe, there will be palpitations below the navel, which is an important differentiating sign. The pulse will be wiry and slippery, the tongue body pale, and the tongue coat white and slippery.

Excessive mucoid saliva from Spleen and Stomach deficient cold. Profuse sticky saliva, epigastric and abdominal distention with a sensation of a solid obstruction just below the diaphragm (pi), loss of taste sensation, lassitude, reluctance to speak much due to tiredness, sallow complexion and loose stool. The pulse will be weak, floating and thready, the tongue pale and large, with a white greasy coat. The pulse will be soft, languid and 'ru' (floating thready and weak).

Differentiation

Excessive mucoid saliva from Kidney deficiency versus that from Spleen and Stomach deficient cold. Kidney deficiency allowing pathogenic water to flood is caused by a weakness of the Kidney yang. The weakness may be constitutional or the result of protracted illness. Kidneys rule water and the fluid of the Kidneys is mucoid saliva; if yang is deficient then the transformation of fluids in the lower Jiao would suffer, fluids would fail to be eliminated via the urine, and then the resulting pathogenic fluids would well up and produce excessive salivary excretion. Profuse mucoid saliva from Spleen and Stomach deficiency, on the other hand, usually results from over-consumption of cold or raw foods, or incorrect treatment with cold herbs or medicines, or again from protracted illness that has damaged the Spleen yang. Spleen yang fails to transform, and is unable to transport the fluids effectively, so that they rebel upward and cause profuse sticky saliva. Here again the yang qi cannot transform fluids, but the location is limited to the middle Jiao rather than affecting the lower Jiao as with the Kidney yang deficiency.

This middle Jiao yang deficiency allows cold to develop and then, because of the relative preponderance of yin, contraction and accumulation of the fluids lead to a feeling of obstructed fullness in the epigastric area known as 'pi' 痞.[9] The important points in identifying the middle Jiao as the source of the profuse saliva are the Spleen symptoms of sallow face and epigastric fullness, the digestive symptoms of loss of taste, poor appetite, loose stool and finally the qi deficiency symptoms of reluctance to speak and tiredness.

In the lower Jiao, because the Kidney yang cannot support the steaming transformation of fluids in the Urinary Bladder, the output of urine is reduced, followed by a severe build-up of pathogenic fluids in the lower body. This can cause a palpitating sensation below the umbilicus, and, if the fluids rush up into the chest, heart palpitations and vertigo as well. Weak Kidney yang, further blocked by the pathogenic water, is unable to grasp qi, so that there is shortness of breath. The important points in identifying the Kidneys as the source of the profuse saliva are the palpitations, vertigo and shortness of breath, all worsened by exertion, and the reduced urination.

Treatment of the Spleen yang deficiency allowing cold fluids to accumulate requires warming of the middle Jiao to restore its transforming and transporting function, using a combination of formulas such as Li Zhong Tang ('Regulate the Middle Decoction') and He Li Le Wan ('Terminalia Pill').

Treatment of the Kidney yang deficiency allowing water to flood and produce excessive mucoid saliva is to warm Kidney yang and promote transformation of fluids in the Urinary Bladder and thus encourage urination. An appropriate formula is Ji Sheng Shen Qi Wan ('Kidney Qi Pill from *Formulas to Aid the Living*').

Formulas

Li Zhong Tang ('Regulate the Middle Decoction')

Ren Shen	Ginseng, Radix
Gan Jiang	Zingiberis Officianalis, Rhizoma
Bai Zhu	Atractylodis Macrocephalae, Rhizoma
Zhi Gan Cao	Honey-fried Glycyrrhizae Uralensis, Radix

Source text: *Shang Han Lun* ('Discussion of Cold-Induced Disorders', *c*. 210AD) [*Formulas and Strategies*, p. 219]

He Li Le Wan ('Terminalia Pill')

He Zi	Terminaliae Chebulae, Fructus (coated in flour and baked)
Fu Zi	Aconiti Carmichaeli Praeparata, Radix
Rou Dou Kou	Myristicae Fragranticis, Semen (coated in flour and baked)
Mu Xiang	Saussureae seu Vladimiriae, Radix (not baked)
Wu Zhu Yu	Evodiae Rutacarpae, Fructus (soaked in water then fried)
Long Gu	Draconis, Os (raw)
Fu Ling	Poriae Cocos, Sclerotium
Bi Ba	Piperis Longi, Fructus

Finely powder 15 g each of the above and make into small pills with ginger juice. Seventy pills per dose, taken on an empty stomach with thin rice soup.

Source text: *Ji Sheng Fang* ('Formulas to Aid the Living', 1253)

Ji Sheng Shen Qi Wan ('Kidney Qi Pill from *Formulas to Aid the Living*')

Fu Zi	Aconiti Carmichaeli Praeparata, Radix
Rou Gui	Cinnamomi Cassiae, Cortex
Shou Di	Rehmanniae Glutinosae Conquitae, Radix
Shan Zhu Yu	Corni Officinalis, Fructus
Shan Yao	Dioscoreae Oppositae, Radix
Mu Dan Pi	Moutan Radicis, Cortex
Fu Ling	Poriae Cocos, Sclerotium
Ze Xie	Alismatis Plantago-aquaticae, Rhizoma
Che Qian Zi	Plantaginis, Semen
Chuan Niu Xi	Cyathulae, Radix

Source text: *Ji Sheng Fang* ('Formulas to Aid the Living', 1253) [*Formulas and Strategies*, p. 278]

Summary

Excessive mucoid salivation can result from yang deficiency either in the middle Jiao or the lower Jiao. In the middle Jiao, the Spleen loses control of transformation and transportation, and pathogenic fluids ascend instead of being carried downward.

In the lower Jiao, the Kidney yang fails to support the Urinary Bladder function of separating out clear from murky fluids, and the latter accumulate and flood, inundating the lower body and finally welling up as profuse saliva.

In both cases, the origin is deficiency of yang; accompanying symptoms will help to sort out the primary location of the deficiency.

Differentiation of drooling (xian xia)

Watery saliva (xian) runs from the corners of the mouth. In the *Nei Jing* this is called 'xian xia' (saliva dropping).

Common symptom patterns

In children xian xia often indicates Stomach heat from parasitic accumulation.

In adults there are four causes of drooling. The first is wind-stroke into the collaterals, which will be associated with continuous drooling, deviation of the eyes and mouth, or even paraplegia. The tongue will have a white coat, and the pulse will be floating and wiry.

The second is wind-phlegm welling upwards: the sound of phlegm in the throat will be obvious, and the symptoms more serious, with affected speech, vertigo or even coma. The tongue coat will be thick and greasy, and the pulse wiry and slippery.

The third cause of drooling in adults is a weakness of Spleen qi unable to control fluids, so that clear watery fluids run from the corners of the mouth. This will be associated with other Spleen qi deficiency signs.

The fourth cause is Spleen and Stomach heat steaming upwards. This heat can result from constitutional smoldering heat, or from habitual consumption of rich or spicy foods, either of which can result in a steaming upward of Spleen and Stomach heat, or even Heart and Stomach fire rising and forcing Lian Quan (Ren 23) to secrete fluids into the mouth. The drooling here will be associated with oral cavity pain or ulceration, dryness, bitter taste, constipation, dark urine, anxiety, red tongue tip or prickles. The tongue coat will be yellow and may be greasy, the pulse will be slippery and rapid.

Differentiation

Spleen and Stomach heat steaming upwards versus weak Spleen qi. While both these belong to the Spleen, they differ in etiology and pathology.

Spleen and Stomach heat is an excess condition, where the heat is forcing the saliva out; the *Ling Shu*, Chapter 28, says 'In the Stomach there is heat … therefore drooling [occurs]'. There is usually ulceration of the tongue, gums and lips, with prickles on the tip and sides of the tongue, and other signs of Stomach and Intestinal excess heat such as constipation and dark urine, and the rising heat may disturb the Heart, leading to insomnia and irritability. The mouth is often dry because the excessive saliva is not the result of harmonious physiological processes but rather pathological, and so can not be expected to perform normal physiological functions such as moistening. The pulse and tongue are distinctive: reddish tongue tip, with a yellow coat that could be greasy (i.e. if the heat has started to dry normal fluids into damp), and a rapid slippery pulse. The treatment requires cooling and clearing of Spleen and Stomach excess heat with formulas such as Qing Wei San ('Cooling Stomach Powder') and/or Xie Huang San ('Drain the Yellow Powder'), adjusted appropriately for the individual patient.

Spleen weakness failing to control fluids is very different in almost all symptoms except the drooling. It is often seen in children. The saliva itself is clear and thin, and the drooling continues all day, even wetting the collar and the front of the clothes. The face is pale, the spirit listless, and other familiar Spleen qi deficiency signs such as abdominal bloating with loose stool will be evident. Treatment here requires tonification of Spleen qi, warming the Center and containing the fluids. The best formula is a combination of Liu Jun Zi Tang ('Six-Gentlemen Decoction') and Gan Cao Gan Jiang Tang ('Licorice and Ginger Decoction'), with suitable adjustments for the patient.

A word of warning, however: in cases of weak Spleen qi failing to control fluids, one must not recklessly attack the excess fluids and try to eliminate them with phlegm-cutting or fluid-eliminating herbs, as this will simply further weaken the Spleen. Although the fluids are pathological in origin, the proper approach is to tonify the qi of the Center to transform, as this is treating the root of the problem.

Formulas

Qing Wei San ('Cooling Stomach Powder')

Huang Lian	Coptidis, Rhizoma
Sheng Ma	Cimicifugae, Rhizoma
Mu Dan Pi	Moutan Radicis, Cortex
Sheng Di	Rehmannia Glutinosae, Radix
Dang Gui	Angelica Polymorpha, Radix

Source text: *Lan Shi Mi Cang* ('Secrets from the Orchid Chamber', 1336) [*Formulas and Strategies*, p. 93]

Xie Huang San ('Drain the Yellow Powder')

Shi Gao	Gypsum
Shan Zhi Zi	Gardeniae Jasminoidis, Fructus
Fang Feng	Ledebouriellae Sesloidis, Radix
Huo Xiang	Agastaches seu Pogostemi, Herba
Gan Cao	Glycyrrhizae Uralensis, Radix

Source text: *Xiao Er Yao Zheng Zhi Jue* ('Craft of Medicinal Treatment for Childhood Disease Patterns', 1119) [*Formulas and Strategies*, p. 92]

Liu Jun Zi Tang ('Six Gentlemen Decoction')

Ren Shen	Ginseng, Radix
Bai Zhu	Atractylodis Macrocephalae, Rhizoma
Fu Ling	Poriae Cocos, Sclerotium
Ban Xia	Pinelliae Ternata, Rhizoma
Chen Pi	Citri Reticulatae, Pericarpium
Gan Cao	Glycyrrhizae Uralensis, Radix

Source text: *Yi Xue Zheng Chuan* ('True Lineage of Medicine', 1515) [*Formulas and Strategies*, p. 238]

Gan Cao Gan Jiang Tang ('Licorice and Ginger Decoction')

Gan Cao	Glycyrrhizae Uralensis, Radix
Gan Jiang	Zingiberis Officianalis, Rhizoma

Source text: *Jin Gui Yao Lue* ('Essentials from the Golden Cabinet', 210AD) [*Formulas and Strategies*, p. 225]

Wind-stroke into the collaterals versus wind-phlegm welling upwards. Both conditions are related to pathogenic wind, and both have deviation of the eye and mouth. But the former is a light attack into the collaterals by exogenous wind during (perhaps temporary) weakness in the hand and foot Yang Ming channels. This obstructs the normal flow within these channels so that, on the one hand, the mouth is no longer able to close completely, while on the other, the fluids are not restrained and so drooling occurs.

The latter condition of wind-phlegm welling upwards is usually seen in stroke or epilepsy, and results from internal wind combining with phlegm to rush upwards and disturb the head.

Analysis of the symptoms will show that drooling from wind-stroke into the collaterals is a relatively minor condition, with only the deviated mouth and eye that are typical of facial paralysis. Drooling from wind-phlegm welling upwards, however, is a more severe condition. It can affect the tongue so that speech is disturbed; there will also be numbness of the limbs, and other symptoms such as affected consciousness or even coma. Phlegm will be evident from its sound in the throat, its appearance as a thick tongue coat, and the wiry rolling pulse.

The wind-stroke into the collaterals is minor and relatively easy to treat by expelling wind and opening the collaterals; once the mouth has regained its control the drooling will stop. The best formula is Qian Zheng San ('Lead to Symmetry Powder') plus *Chan Tui* (Cicadae, Periostracum), *Jing Jie* (Schizonepetae Tenuifoliae, Herba et Flos), *Fang Feng* (Ledebouriellae Sesloidis, Radix), *Man Jing Zi* (Viticis, Fructus) and *Gou Teng* (Uncariae Cum Uncis, Ramulus).

Treatment of wind-phlegm welling upwards, though, requires further differentiation of xu and shi, hot and cold. For those cases which are deficient or cold, the treatment principle should be to tonify qi and cut phlegm, extinguish wind and open the collaterals, using Liu Jun Zi Tang ('Six Gentlemen Decoction') plus *Tian Ma* (Gastrodiae Elatae, Rhizoma), *Qin Jiao* (Gentianae Macrophyllae, Radix) and ginger juice.

For those phlegm cases which are also hot, the principle of treatment is to cool heat, cut phlegm, regulate the qi flow and open the collaterals. The best formula is Dao Tan Tang ('Guide Out Phlegm Decoction') plus *Shan Zhi Zi* (Gardeniae Jasminoidis, Fructus), *Huang Lian* (Coptidis, Rhizoma) and *Zhu Li* (Bambusae, Succus).

Formulas

Qian Zheng San ('Lead to Symmetry Powder')

Bai Fu ZI	Typhonii Gigantei, Rhizoma seu Aconiti Coreani, Radix)

| Jiang Can | Bombyx Batryticatus |
| Quan Xie | Buthus Martensi |

Source text: *Yang Shi Jia Zang Fang* ('Collected Formulas of the Yang Family', 1178) [*Formulas and Strategies*, p. 399]

Liu Jun Zi Tang ('Six Gentlemen Decoction')
    See above. *Formulas and Strategies*, p. 238]
Dao Tan Tang ('Guide Out Phlegm Decoction')

Ju Hong	Citri Erythrocarpae, Pericarpium
Ban Xia	Pinelliae Ternata, Rhizoma
Fu Ling	Poriae Cocos, Sclerotium
Gan Cao	Glycyrrhizae Uralensis, Radix
Zhi Shi	Citri seu Ponciri Immaturis, Fructus
Dan Nan Xing	Arisaemae cum Felle Bovis, Pulvis

Source text: *Ji Sheng Fang* ('Formulas to Aid the Living', 1253) [*Formulas and Strategies*, p. 448]

A note in the *Zhen Ben Tu Shu Ji Cheng* ('Pearl Volume Library Collection', *c.* 1725) summarizes the physiology, pathology and treatment of this condition succinctly, saying:

> Although Spleen opens into the mouth, still jin and ye fluids come from the Kidneys. The [yang] qi of Foot Shao Yin rises and meets Yang Ming; Earth and Water combine, and only after [this combining] can they transform food and fluid essence. If qi does not rise to meet [Yang Ming], then instead pathogenic water will rise along the Ren channel to the point Lian Quan (Ren 23), and cause drooling.
>
> Simply tonify Foot Shao Yin to assist the lower Jiao's living qi to rise up, and the Ren channel, being strong below, will have its upper point Lian Quan open. Then xian (saliva) will descend internally, and not descend externally (i.e. out of the mouth)!'

Excessive nasal mucus

Healthy people have a small amount of nasal mucus, which functions to moisten the nasal passages and also to clear away extraneous material. Excessive nasal mucus or frequent runny nose, however, is pathological. Exogenous invasions often include runny nose, and in this case clear thin mucus is wind-cold, while thick yellow mucus is wind-heat. On the other hand, if there is pathogenic drying (zao) heat in the Lung channel there will be little or even no nasal mucus at all.

Long term or recurring watery nasal mucus is an indication of Lung and Spleen cold from yang deficiency. Blood in the mucus shows Lung heat, or Liver fire affecting the Lungs. Chronic dryness of the nasal passages is a symptom of severe damage to Lung yin, and should not be ignored.

Differentiation is usually based on the nature of the mucus, which traditionally is of several types: 'clear mucus', 'white sticky mucus', 'sticky pus-like mucus', 'yellow pus-like mucus', 'pus and blood mucus' and 'odorous mucus'.

Common symptom patterns

Wind-cold nasal mucus. Profuse clear mucus, with blocked nose and repeated sneezing, accompanied by chills and fever, headache, cough, mild sore throat, no sweating, pale red tongue body, thin white tongue coat, and floating tight pulse.

Wind-heat nasal mucus. Profuse thick yellow mucus, with reddish swollen painful nostrils if severe, and blocked nose, accompanied by headache, fever, chills, more severe sore throat, cough and sweating, reddish tongue, white tongue coat, and floating rapid pulse.

Damp-heat nasal mucus. Profuse sticky murky odorous yellow mucus, which even flows down the throat if severe. A completely blocked nose so that the sense of smell is affected, accompanied by heavy head, headache, stuffy chest, poor appetite, bitter taste and a sticky feeling in the mouth. No thirst, yellow urine, red tongue with a greasy yellow coat, and a slippery rapid or thin floating and rapid pulse.

Drying-heat (zao) nasal mucus. Scanty sticky yellow mucus that may include blood or pus or both. A blocked dry painful nasal passages, accompanied by headache, chest and epigastric distention and fullness. A dry throat, bitter taste, thirst for cold drinks, dry stool, yellow urine, red tongue with a dry yellow tongue coat, and a thready rapid pulse.

Qi (or yang) deficient nasal mucus. Clear watery mucus, that may become white, sticky and chronic. Alternatively the mucus may change from clear to yellow and back again, or even be light yellow with an odor; the nose will be blocked. The condition may arise from exposure to cold, or from exposure to a variety of allergenic substances, and may be accompanied by tiredness, shortness of breath, reluctance to talk, and possibly poor appetite, epigastric fullness and loose stool. The tongue body will be flabby and pale, the tongue coat thin and the pulse languid and weak.

Kidney deficient nasal mucus. Chronic scanty thin clear mucus that becomes profuse upon exposure to cold, and may turn from clear to yellow and back again. The nose will be blocked causing impaired sense of smell, and may be accompanied by lower backache, weak legs, pale tongue with a white coat, and a deep thready and weak pulse, especially at the chi (proximal) position.

Differentiation

Wind-cold nasal mucus versus wind-heat nasal mucus. Both conditions are caused by an exogenous pathogen invading the Lungs, so that Lungs lose their spreading and descending action, and the pathogen is allowed to obstruct the nasal passages. Thus both conditions are accompanied by surface symptoms. The differentiation is between cold and heat. Careful attention to the color and consistency of the nasal mucus, as well as the accompanying symptoms, should make differentiation relatively easy.

Exogenous wind-cold is one pathogenic factor. The nasal mucus is clear and thin, and the surface symptoms are all of the cold type: chills and fever, no sweating, mild sore throat, pale red tongue, floating tight pulse, accompanied by cough and headache.

The alternate pathogenic factor is exogenous wind-heat. Mucus is profuse, thick and yellow and surface symptoms of the hot type: fever and chills, sweating, more severe sore throat, red tongue with yellow coat, floating rapid pulse, accompanied by cough and headache.

Treatment of wind-cold requires the use of pungent warm surface openers to expel wind and disperse cold, using a formula like Cong Shi Tang ('Scallion and Prepared Soybean Decoction') with additions.

Treatment of wind-heat requires the use of pungent cool surface openers to expel wind and clear heat while opening the orifice, with the best formula being Cang Er Zi San ('Xanthium Powder') with additions.

Formulas

Cong Chi Tang ('Scallion and Prepared Soybean Decoction')

Cong Bai	Allii Fistulosi, Herba
Dan Dou Chi	Sojae Preaparatum, Semen

Source text: *Zhou Hou Bei Ji Fang*, ('Emergency Formulas to Keep Up One's Sleeve', 341AD) [*Formulas and Strategies*, p. 32]

Cang Er Zi San ('Xanthium Powder')

Cang Er Zi	Xanthii, Fructus
Xin Yi Hua	Magnoliae Liliflorae, Flos
Bai Zhi	Angelicae, Radix
Bai He	Lilii, Bulbus

Source text: *Ji Sheng Fang* ('Formulas to Aid the Living', 1253) [*Formulas and Strategies*, p. 51]

Damp-heat nasal mucus versus drying-heat nasal mucus. Both of these conditions from heat but one is internal damp-heat, the other exogenous drying (zao) heat.

The damp-heat nasal mucus is caused by the damp-heat pathogen injuring the Spleen and Stomach transformation and transportation, with damp-heat building up and obstructing the nasal passages. Therefore the mucus is profuse, deep yellow or yellowish-green, murky and odorous. Accompanying symptoms will be those of damp-heat obstruction: heavy painful head, epigastric fullness and poor appetite, bitter taste and a greasy or sticky feeling in the mouth, lack of normal thirst, yellowish urine, red tongue body and yellow greasy tongue coat. The pulse will be either slippery and rapid, or thin weak floating (i.e. a 'ru' pulse) and rapid.

Drying-heat nasal mucus results from an exogenous hot zao ('parching') pathogen affecting the upper body and drying the nasal orifice, so that the mucus is yellow, scanty, and sticky, and may contain traces of blood and even pus if the pathogen has injured the collaterals. The nasal passages will feel dry and even painful. Accompanying symptoms will be those of drying-heat damaging the jin and ye fluids: thirst for cold liquids, headache, fullness in the chest, dry throat with bitter taste in the mouth, dry stool, yellow urine, red tongue with dry thin yellow coating, and thready rapid pulse, which may be floating and weak at the Lung position.

The two conditions are not difficult to differentiate if attention is paid to the amount and nature of the nasal mucus, the thirst (or lack of), the thickness and moisture of the tongue coat, and finally the pulse.

Treatment for the damp-heat nasal mucus involves cooling heat, removing damp and opening the orifices. If the damp is worse than the heat, one should promote damp expulsion while cooling heat, by adding cooling herbs to Si Ling San ('Four Ingredient Powder with Poria'). If the heat is worse than the damp, cooling should be the main approach, adding herbs to eliminate damp: Huang Qin Hua Shi Tang ('Scutellaria and Talcum Decoction') can be used.

Treatment of drying-heat nasal mucus calls for clearing the drying pathogen and draining fire. If the dryness is worse than the heat, one should moisten with Qing Zao Jiu Fei Tang ('Eliminate Dryness and Rescue the Lungs Decoction'); if the heat is worse than the dryness, drain and clear fire with Liang Ge San ('Cooling the Diaphragm Powder').

Formulas

Si Ling San ('Four Ingredient Powder with Poria')

Zhu Ling	Polypori Umbellati, Sclerotium
Fu Ling	Poriae Cocos, Sclerotium
Bai Zhu	Atractylodis Macrocephalae, Rhizoma
Ze Xie	Alismatis Plantago-aquaticae, Rhizoma

Source text: *Ming Yi Zhi Zhang* ('Displays of Enlightened Physicians', 16th Century) [*Formulas and Strategies*, p. 176]

Huang Qin Hua Shi Tang ('Scutellaria and Talcum Decoction')

Huang Qin	Scutellariae Baicalensis, Radix
Hua Shi	Talc
Fu Ling Pi	Poriae Cocos, Cortex
Da Fu Pi	Arecae Catechu, Pericarpium
Bai Dou Kou	Amomi Cardamomi, Fructus
Tong Cao	Tetrapanacis Papyriferi, Medulla
Zhu Ling	Polypori Umbellati, Sclerotium

Source text: *Wen Bing Tiao Bian* ('Systematic Differentiation of Warm Diseases', 1798) [*Formulas and Strategies*, p. 187]

Qing Zao Jiu Fei Tang ('Eliminate Dryness and Rescue the Lungs Decoction')

Sang Ye	Mori Albae, Folium
Shi Gao	Gypsum
Mai Men Dong	Ophiopogonis Japonici, Tuber
E Jiao	Asini, Gelatinum
Hei Zhi Ma	Sesami Indici, Semen
Xing Ren	Pruni Armeniacae, Semen
Pi Pa Ye	Eriobotryae Japonicae, Folium
Ren Shen	Ginseng, Radix
Gan Cao	Glycyrrhizae Uralensis, Radix

Source text: *Yi Men Fa Lu* ('Precepts for Physicians', 1658) [*Formulas and Strategies*, p. 160]

Liang Ge San ('Cooling the Diaphragm Powder')

Da Huang	Rhei, Rhizoma
Mang Xiao	Mirabilitum
Gan Cao	Glycyrrhizae Uralensis, Radix
Huang Qin	Scutellariae Baicalensis, Radix
Shan Zhi Zi	Gardeniae Jasminoidis, Fructus
Lian Qiao	Forsythiae Suspensae, Fructus
Bo He	Menthae, Herba

Source text: *Tai Ping Hui Min He Ji Ju Fang* ('Imperial Grace Formulary of the Tai Ping Era', 1078-85) [*Formulas and Strategies*, p. 119]

Qi deficiency nasal mucus versus Kidney deficiency nasal mucus. Both of these conditions are deficiency states, but the former is lighter, in the qi level, while the latter is deeper, in the Kidneys.

Qi deficiency unable to contain Lung fluids leads to profuse nasal mucus, and will be accompanied by other symptoms of qi deficiency. Kidney deficiency, however, results in a double condition. On the one hand, fluids in the lower Jiao are not being transformed through Kidney yang and therefore are not being recycled up through the Lungs, which leads to the scanty amount of mucus. On the other hand, the weak Kidneys lose consolidation and so the nasal mucus runs chronically, and worsens with cold. There will also be other Kidney deficiency symptoms.

Again, qi deficiency can involve the Lungs only, or both Spleen and Lungs. In the first case, the protective qi will be weak with susceptibility to exogenous pathogenic invasions that occur repeatedly, and the nasal mucus will be watery and clear, with other Lung qi deficiency symptoms such as weak voice, shortness of breath and lack of energy. Here the treatment should be to benefit the Lungs while consolidating the surface, and one can use Yu Ping Feng San ('Jade Screen Powder') plus Cang Er Zi San ('Xanthium Powder').

In the second case, the Lungs and Spleen are both weak, so that Spleen damp is actually carried up and obstructs the functioning of the Lungs, leading to a constant thick stickier mucus that can change from white to yellow if the mucus obstruction has led to local heat. Spleen deficiency symptoms such as epigastric fullness and loose stool will be found with the other Lung qi deficiency indications noted above. The tongue here will be flabby and pale, the pulse languid (huan) and weak. Treatment calls for tonifying Lungs, supporting the Spleen, and benefiting qi, with a formula like Bu Zhong Yi Qi Tang.

If this deficiency situation is complicated by the Spleen damp accumulating and turning hot, and then producing damp-heat, so that a combined excess-deficiency condition results, the mucus will be thick, yellow and syrup-like, with an odor. Treatment in this case still needs qi tonification based upon Bu Zhong Yi Qi Tang ('Tonify the Middle and Augment the Qi Decoction') but herbs to transform damp and open the nasal orifice must also be used, such as *Bai Zhi* (Angelicae, Radix), *Huo Xiang* (Agastaches seu Pogostemi, Herba), *Xia Ku Cao* (Prunellae Vulgaris, Spica), *Cang Er Zi* (Xanthii, Fructus) and *Xin Yi Hua* (Magnoliae Liliflorae, Flos).

Kidney deficiency nasal mucus, like that from Lung deficiency, can change: being either scanty and then increasing with exposure to cold, or sometimes yellow and sometimes white, but always chronic. The differentiating point here is the presence of Kidney deficiency symptoms like lower backache, weak knees, and deep weak Kidney position on the pulse. Treatment requires restoring Kidney fluid control while assisting Lungs with formulas like Cang Er Zi Tang ('Xanthium Powder') and either Zhen Wu Tang ('True Warrior Decoction') or Shen Qi Wan ('Kidney Qi Pill from *Formulas to Aid the Living*').

Formulas

Yu Ping Feng San ('Jade Screen Powder')

Huang Qi	Astragali, Radix

Bai Zhu	Atractylodis Macrocephalae, Rhizoma
Fang Feng	Ledebouriellae Sesloidis, Radix

Source text: *Dan Xi Xin Fa* ('Teachings of Dan Xi', 1481) [*Formulas and Strategies*, p. 352]

Cang Er Zi San ('Xanthium Powder')

Cang Er Zi	Xanthii, Fructus
Xin Yi Hua	Magnoliae Liliflorae, Flos
Bai Zhi	Angelicae, Radix
Bo He	Menthae, Herba

Source text: *Ji Sheng Fang* ('Formulas to Aid the Living', 1253) [*Formulas and Strategies*, p. 51]

Bu Zhong Yi Qi Tang ('Tonify the Middle and Augment the Qi Decoction')

Huang Qi	Astragali, Radix
Ren Shen	Ginseng, Radix
Bai Zhu	Atractylodis Macrocephalae, Rhizoma
Dang Gui	Angelica Polymorpha, Radix
Chen Pi	Citri Reticulatae, Pericarpium
Sheng Ma	Cimicifugae, Rhizoma
Chai Hu	Bupleuri, Radix
Zhi Gan Cao	Honey-fried Glycyrrhizae Uralensis, Radix

Source text: *Pi Wei Lun* ('Discussion of the Spleen and Stomach', 1249) [*Formulas and Strategies*, p. 241]

Zhen Wu Tang ('True Warrior Decoction')

Fu Zi	Aconiti Carmichaeli Praeparata, Radix
Bai Zhu	Atractylodis Macrocephalae, Rhizoma
Fu Ling	Poriae Cocos, Sclerotium
Bai Shao	Paeoniae Lactiflora, Radix
Sheng Jiang	Zingiberis Officinalis Recens, Rhizoma

Source text: *Shang Han Lun* ('Discussion of Cold-Induced Disorders'), 210AD [*Formulas and Strategies*, p. 197]

Shen Qi Wan ('Kidney Qi Pill from *Formulas to Aid the Living*')

Fu Zi	Aconiti Carmichaeli Praeparata, Radix
Rou Gui	Cinnamomi Cassiae, Cortex

Shou Di	Rehmanniae Glutinosae Conquitae, Radix
Shan Zhu Yu	Corni Officinalis, Fructus
Shan Yao	Dioscoreae Oppositae, Radix
Mu Dan Pi	Moutan Radicis, Cortex
Fu Ling	Poriae Cocos, Sclerotium
Ze Xie	Alismatis Plantago-aquaticae, Rhizoma
Che Qian Zi	Plantaginis, Semen
Chuan Niu Xi	Cyathulae, Radix

Source text: *Ji Sheng Fang* ('Formulas to Aid the Living', 1253) [*Formulas and Strategies*, p. 278]

Summary

When treating nasal mucus, the emphasis in clinic should be to differentiate surface or interior, hot and cold, deficiency and excess.

As a rule of thumb, surface conditions will show headache, chills and fever. Clear thin mucus will be cold, while thick sticky yellow mucus will usually be heat. Yellow purulent odorous mucus will be damp-heat, and scanty mucus with traces of blood will be drying-heat. All of these are excess.

Of the deficiency conditions, qi deficiency will be accompanied by tiredness and shortness of breath, or Spleen symptoms such as poor appetite and loose stool, while Kidney deficiency will have symptoms like lower backache and weak legs.

In most cases the nature of the nasal mucus itself will already have given a clear indication of the source of the problem.

NOTES

1. Zhang Zhi-Cong taught at Lu Shan Hall, where his motto was 'first investigate that which is difficult, then one can be relaxed about that which is simple'. The book is a collection of the 'Differentiations of True and False' in TCM theory which formed the substance of his lectures.
2. *Lu Shan Tang Lei Bian* ('Catalogued Differentiations from Lu Shan Hall'), 1670, by Zhang Zhi-Cong; Jiangsu Science and Technology Press, 1982, p. 34.

The quote continues 'Thus with the sweat of the surface (biao han), one can only use mild diaphoresis, for fear that blood-fluids (xue-ye) will be damaged and the yang qi will collapse [from being carried out with the sweat]; but if it is sweat from [pathogenic] water-fluids, there is no harm in it dripping out like water [because this will reduce the pathogen].'
3. *Lei Jing* ('Systematic Categorization of the *Nei Jing*'), 1624, by Zhang Jing-Yue; People's Health Publishing, 1982, p. 460.
4. Dr Dan Bensky comments that this is an over-simplification, saying: Often respiratory symptoms are primarily Stomach problems as in Mai Men Dong Tang ('Ophiopogonis Decoction', *Formulas and Strategies*, p. 165) without any clear Stomach symptoms (but very clear Stomach signs). (Personal communication.) This is true: Mai Den Dong Tang is an elegant and apropos example of the finesse possible in TCM diagnostics and treatments. My point, however, was not so subtle, being simply that a single symptom or sign by itself will not indicate a whole condition—one must seek further for corroborating evidence, especially in one's early stages of clinical practice.
5. The following differentiations and treatments are based upon the *Zhong Yi Zheng Zhuang Jian Bie Zhen Duan Xue* ('Diagnostic Studies of Symptom Differentiation in Chinese Medicine'), Peoples' Health Publishing, Beijing, 1985.
6. Throughout this book, formulas which are fully described in Bensky and Barolet's *Formulas and Strategies* (Eastland Press, 1990) are referenced as to the page number of the 1990 edition; readers who require information concerning weights of individual ingredients can find them there. In other formulas not included in *Formulas and Strategies*, every effort has been made to access the original text or a reliable source for the original weights. In some cases, unfortunately, this has not been possible.
7. The *Shen Shi Yao Han* ('Scrutiny of the Precious Jade Case') is also known as the *Yan Ke Da Quan* ('A Complete Work on Ophthalmology'), and is a seven volume opus listing one hundred and eight kinds of eye troubles and their treatments, published in 1644 by Fu Yun-Ke.
8. The unusual character 'xia', written with a grass radical with the character 'xia' ('below') underneath, is an ancient term for Rehmannia.
9. This is a symptom of Spleen obstruction defined as a sensation of obstructed fullness but without pain. The *Nan Jing* ('Classic of Difficulties') in the Fifty-sixth Difficulty, when describing 'the Five Accumulations', says: 'Spleen accumulation is termed 'pi''. 痞.

Sweat 3

The fluids of the body interact with all of the organs and tissues, qi and blood, supporting them and in turn being transformed by their functioning. Depending upon the location of this interaction, and the needs of the body, the fluids can be changed into a number of different forms before being either conserved or excreted from the body. The route of excretion will, again, depend upon the type of metabolic product which has resulted from the interaction.

The two products of this metabolism most obviously connected to the state of the fluids in the body are sweat and urine, and in fact each will vary in amount according to the condition of the other.

Clinically, attention to the processes of urination and sweating, together with the degree of thirst, will provide a reliable indication of fluid status within the body.

In this chapter we will investigate sweat, its physiology, pathology, differentiation and treatment. Urine will be covered in Chapter 4.

PHYSIOLOGY

Under normal physiological conditions, perspiration is occurring constantly, albeit imperceptibly, until heat or activity increases the amount of fluid being lost. The sweat itself, which is the fluid discharged through the pores to the surface of the body, has its source in the body fluids, which are in turn derived from the essence of fluids and food (shui gu jing wei), as discussed in Chapter 1.

The *Su Wen*, Chapter 33, states: 'All of the sweat discharged from the body is produced from food.' And again: 'Sweat is essential qi (i.e. from food and fluids).'

In the *Ling Shu*, Chapter 36, it describes the following physiological process:

When the weather is hot, or the clothing thick, the surface tissues open and thus sweating occurs...

When the weather is cold, the surface tissues close, the qi and damp (i.e. the jin-ye) cannot move, the water (i.e. fluids) descends into the Urinary Bladder, and [the turbid aspect] becomes urine while [the subtle aspect] becomes qi [again, through the normal process of qi transformation, and this qi circulates back into the body].

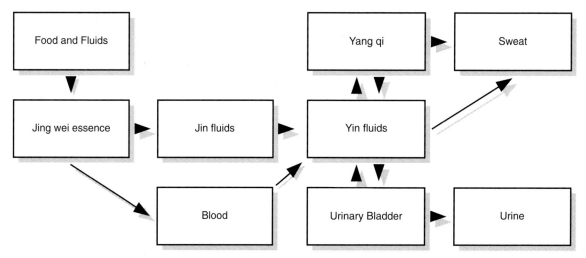

Fig. 3.1 Sweat production

Figure 3.1 illustrates that sweat is derived from the essence of food and fluids, and sweat is the fluid discharged from the pores through the action of the yang qi upon the yin fluids.

'Yang qi' here includes a number of levels, including the transforming action of yang qi upon the fluids at each stage in the process of fluid metabolism. The most direct action, however, is that exerted by the 'wei yang', the protective yang qi which 'warms the surface tissues ... and controls opening and closing'.

The term 'yin fluids', which generally implies all of the physiological fluids within the body, in this context refers primarily to the jin portion of the fluids, as described below by Zhang Jing-Yue, in the *Lei Jing* section on zang xiang (internal organ theory):

Now jin is the clear portion of ye, while ye is the murky portion of jin. Jin is classed as yang because it travels the surface and becomes sweat, ye is classed as yin because it pours into the bones and supplements the brain and marrow.[1]

Under certain circumstances, though, fluid can be pulled from the blood itself to become sweat. This is described by the Qing dynasty physician Zhang Zhi-Cong in his *Lu Shan Tang Lei Bian* ('Catalogued Differentiations from Lu Shan Hall', 1670):

This sweat has two sources: one comes from the blood that suffuses the hot flesh, the fluid

(ye) in this blood transforms and becomes sweat, which is the sweat of the surface; the other comes from the Yang Ming Wei-Fu (Stomach), and this is the sweat of [pathogenic] water-fluid (shui-ye).[2]

A similar quote from the well-known Qing Dynasty commentator on the *Su Wen*, Zhang Yin-An, says: 'Sweat has two sources: one is the essence of food and fluids, another the essence stored in the Kidneys.'

The 'Kidney essence' referred to here means the blood, as Zhang notes in the continuation of this quotation: 'The sweat from blood originates in the Kidneys. If the pathogen is in the flesh, the sweat from food and fluids will expel it. If the pathogen has moved into the bones, the sweat from the Kidney essence will expel it.'[3]

In the *Su Wen*, Chapter 5, there is a famous quotation: 'The sweat from yang (i.e. the surface) is like the rain from heaven and earth.'

This is explained by Zhang Yin-An as follows:

The 'sweat of yang' is so called because it issues from the surface. The sweat is derived from yin fluids, but depends upon the expansion of yang qi. This is why [elsewhere in the Classics] it says: 'yang added to yin is called sweat'. Rain is the yin damp of earth which has been acted upon by the active transformation of the heavens. Thus it can be used as a model of human sweat.[4]

The whole procedure of yin fluids being transformed by yang qi and steamed out through the surface has a balancing effect upon the yin and yang within the body. First, fluids are expelled with the process, which lessens the overall yin; second, a certain amount of yang heat is dispersed by this activity, which reduces the level of yang.

Thus, in the quotation above which opened this section on sweat physiology, the *Ling Shu* says 'When the weather is hot, or the clothing thick', these conditions are such as to increase the level of yang heat in the body to unbalanced proportions. Sweating in this case is able to drain away excessive yang heat, and bring yin and yang back into harmony. Likewise, 'when the weather is cold' the surface tissues close to prevent any further loss of yang heat through sweating, and thus yin and yang within the body, and the yin and yang of the body within its environment, are both maintained in a harmonious state.

PATHOLOGY

The most fundamental mechanism of sweat pathology is disharmony between the yang qi and the yin fluids. Because this occurs at the surface of the body, it is often referred to as a disharmony between the protective (yang) qi and the nutritive (yin) qi.

Chao Yuan-Fang, the Sui Dynasty author of the *Zhu Bing Yuan Hou Lun* (610 AD) remarks: 'Nutritive [in fact] means the blood, protective [in fact] means the qi',[5] which is meant as a statement of functional relationship, rather than a statement of true equivalence.

The disharmony can result from pathogenic interference, in which case it is an excess (shi) condition, or it can arise through deficiency (xu). In the former case, treatment will involve identification and removal of the pathogen, after which the normal physiological mechanisms of the body will naturally re-establish harmony, and the sweating will become normal and appropriate.

In the latter condition, the nature—and source—of the deficiency must be recognised, and treatment instituted to correct the normal functioning of the system involved so as to ensure a regular provision of the deficient substance or energy. Once this is accomplished, sweating will again become normal.

Many of the early sections of the *Shang Han Lun* ('Discussion of Cold-induced Disorders'), which discuss the diagnosis and treatment of Tai Yang conditions, deal with the mechanisms of pathogenic interference in the sweating process. Wind-cold, for example, invades with a double-pronged effect on the exterior: the wind, which is a yang pathogen with a moving dispersing nature, first scatters the protective yang qi. The pores, which then lack the controlling influence of the protective qi, open in response to the pathogenic wind's dispersal, allowing pathogenic cold to invade. Once the cold has entered the surface tissues, its yin-contracting nature asserts itself, and the pores clamp tightly shut, preventing both the normal circulation of the protective yang qi and the normal process of perspiration.

The effects of this closure can be easily understood in terms of the normal yin-yang balancing action of sweating discussed above: the struggle between the pathogenic cold and the protective qi leads to heat but the heat-reducing action of the sweating has been lost, and so heat builds up at the surface leading to fever, i.e. an excessive imbalance of yang. The protective yang qi, unable to circulate properly, cannot warm the surface tissues, and this gives rise to chills.[6]

At the same time, the sealing of the pores gives exogenous wind-cold a characteristic lack of perspiration which serves to help differentiate it from other exterior pathogenic symptom patterns.

Warm disease (wen bing) provides a counter example.[7] In acute febrile disease, the sweating which occurs in the early stages of a warm disease is the result of the organism seeking to protect itself by expelling the damaging pathogenic factor. This is also a means of eliminating the excessive yang heat. The body's goal is to 'resolve through sweating', a process which we try to encourage if treatment is provided.

However, because the warm pathogen is a toxic yang heat type of pathogen, it can easily damage the jin-fluids and harry the blood. Sweat, jin-fluids and blood are three different manifestations from the same source: they all originate in the food and fluids.

Therefore when the disease reaches the middle and late stages, the physiological heat ('shao huo', literally 'small fire'), originally intended to expel the pathogen, struggles with the intense pathological heat, and the combination of the two yang energies results in a fiery accumulation of extreme heat ('zhuang huo', literally 'vigorous fire'). The physiological heat in this situation cannot eject the pathogenic heat but instead involuntarily works with it to push sweat out of the surface tissues. This causes the surface tissues to open, and profuse sweat to discharge, resulting in fever that is not diminished by perspiration. The end result is intense heat damaging the jin-fluids. This very damage to the fluids prevents the heat from being controlled, so that it becomes fire, and the outcome is a major disruption of yin and yang harmony within the body.

This pathological process can have two disastrous consequences. The first is that fluids are lost by being discharged externally while also being dried internally, which reduces the fluid content of the blood, concentrating and thickening it. As the *Ling Shu*, Chapter 18, observes 'those with loss of blood, do not [bring on] sweat; those with loss of sweat, do not [cause them to] bleed.'

In this way, on the exterior the skin is burning, even to the extent that there may be no fluids available for distribution, so that the skin becomes crinkled and rough without sweat[8], while in the interior the directing guidance of the Heart and brain are affected by the slow circulation of the condensed blood. The Heart fluids themselves may possibly suffer damage, which enables the toxic pathogenic heat to take advantage of this weakness and plunge deep into the body, directly causing disturbed consciousness and coma. At the same time, fire can desiccate the Kidney and Liver yin, so that fluids become insufficient for sweating or nourishment of the tendons, and internal wind can be generated as a result. The *Ling Shu* Chapter 30 refers to this when it says: 'Those with collapse of fluids will have limitation of the movement of the joints.'

The second disastrous consequence of the yin-yang imbalance caused by the warm disease pathogen is the result of the opened surface being uncontrolled by the protective yang, which is engaged in the struggle with the pathogen. Because the surface is open, this will lead to loss not only of fluids but also more yang which is carried out with the fluids. At this point both the yang and the

yin are exhausted, and 'sweating of collapse' (tuo han) occurs, so that great oily beads of sweat like pearls are exuded from the skin. This can also happen if the yang is severely depleted externally, allowing qi to be dispersed and the jin-fluids to become spent, and the yin can no longer be held internally. The yin follows the yang collapse, and the 'sweating of collapse' appears as a constant dripping perspiration.

Although yin and yang each control different aspects of the process of sweating, the above result is the product of a yin-yang disharmony so severe that separation of the two is imminent.

As described above, sweating in the course of a warm disease is a primary indication of the relative status of both 'heat' and 'jin-fluids'. Thus, by observing the presence, amount and nature of the perspiration, we have a practical means to analyse the pathological mechanism and differentiate the individual symptoms.

Lack of sweating

In warm disease, because a patient may present at different stages in the disease, we have three possible situations:

Early-stage lack of sweat. The accompanying symptoms are fever and chills. This indicates that the pathogen is obstructing the surface tissues, the pores are blocked, and the protective qi cannot circulate to perform its normal function.

Middle-stage lack of sweat. The accompanying symptoms are restlessness (fan zao), high fever and scarlet tongue. This suggests that heat has entered the ying (nutritive qi) level, ying yin (the moistening yin aspect of the nutritive qi) is being scorched, and the fluids are so reduced that sweating cannot take place.

Late-stage lack of sweat. The accompanying symptoms will be cold limbs, thready pulse and rough skin. This indicates exhausted fluids with internal deficiency of both yin and yang, and hence inability to provide either the fluids for sweating, or the yang warmth to transform them into sweat.

Sweating

The amount, location and nature of the perspiration will vary depending, again, upon the stage of the warm disease. They can be typified as follows:

Early-stage spontaneous perspiration. Two possible sets of symptoms are as follows. First, generalized intermittent mild sweating, accompanied by surface symptoms such as fever, headache, dizziness, thirst and floating rapid pulse. This is a pathogen attacking the wei (protective qi) level and being opposed by the physiological yang heat. The surface opens occasionally to throw off the excess heat generated.

A second set of accompanying symptoms are frequent clammy skin with sticky odorous sweat, accompanied by epigastric fullness, a sensation of heaviness in the body, a low grade fever, and a white greasy tongue coat. These signs point to damp-heat infiltrating the Yang Ming and Tai Yin levels of the surface, with heat steaming the damp. The sticky thick sweat is a special characteristic of damp-heat.

Middle-stage profuse sweat. This condition may manifest itself by generalized profuse steaming sweat, accompanied by high fever and insatiable thirst. This is a pathogen in the qi level strongly opposed by an as-yet-unweakened protective yang. The sweat is forced out by the struggle.

Alternatively, middle-stage signs may be profuse sweat found only on the head or forehead, accompanied by fever, jaundiced skin, scanty urine and thirst. This is internally pent-up heat combining with damp, the sweat being expressed through the Yang Ming channel (which traverses the forehead).

Late-stage profuse sweat. This late-stage condition may manifest itself in three various sets of symptoms. First, oily sweat quickly replaced if wiped away, accompanied by fever and urgent pulse. This is jin-fluid exhaustion and weakened yang, with qi unable to control the pores so that yang is flowing out with the draining yin.

Second, cold continuous sweat, with chilly limbs, lack of energy, and indistinct pulse. In this case the yang exhaustion precedes the yin loss, so that yin is unable to hold itself internally because of the lack of yang consolidation.

A third form of late-stage profuse sweat is trembling sweat, which in warm disease is usually seen in the stage where the pathogen has entered the qi level. It has a characteristic manifestation: a sudden cold commencing from the back and trembling of the whole body, accompanied by chilled limbs, bluish nails, a superficially soft weak pulse which however is still rooted (i.e. it can be felt harmoniously at both the deep level and also the Kidney positions), followed by a high fever and localized sweating that temporarily relieves the fever and settles the pulse. This is the zheng qi (i.e. all of the activated qi of the body but especially the protective qi) gathering to oppose the strength of the pathogen, engaging it and expelling the pathogen through the sweat. Once the surface and the interior have been cleared of pathogenic influence, the qi is restored to harmony, and the prognosis is good.

If, along with the trembling sweat, the pulse is deep, weak and indistinct, the sweat that accompanies the trembling is not complete or even fails to appear, and then the body becomes feverish and restless with an urgent pulse, there is a severe deficiency of qi and fluids unable to evict the pathogen. The pathogenic heat instead plunges deeper into the body, and the prognosis is grave.

To summarize the above points: fever and sweating are closely interwoven. In the progressive course of a warm disease, the strength of both the zheng qi and the pathogenic qi, and thus the severity of the illness, can be gauged by the actual appearance of the sweat, as well as its normality or abnormality.

TREATMENT

Principle of treatment

Because abnormal sweating is the result of disharmony between the yin fluids and the yang qi at the surface, treatment should be based upon elimination of the cause of that disharmony. This in turn depends upon accurate identification of the cause.

In the case of abnormal sweating from an exogenous pathogenic attack, it will require, first, identification of the nature of the pathogen, and then expulsion of the pathogen with the means appropriate to that nature. Wind-cold, for example, will require pungent-warm surface opening herbs, while wind-heat will need pungent-cooling surface openers. Summerheat, on the other hand, by its very nature will damage the qi and fluids, so treatment must not only aim at clearing the summerheat but also at replenishing the qi and fluids. An exogenous pathogen which has moved internally into the mid-stage of Shao Yang will require the use of a harmonizing formula such as Xiao Chai Hu Tang ('Minor Bupleurum Decoction').

An internal pathogen causing sweating again necessitates the elimination of the pathogen, for example intense excess (shi) heat calls for the use of bitter-cold herbs to cool and drain away the pathogen. Damp is less straightforward to manage, because of its propensity to combine with other pathogens, and because it can accumulate in different levels and areas of the body. (See the chapter on the treatment of damp, or the individual sections on sweating below.)

Deficiency, perhaps even more than the pathogenic influences described above, demands accurate differentiation of exactly what substance or activity in the body is functioning below par. Careful note should be taken of the numerous commentators throughout the ages who have stressed, for example, that yin deficiency need not be the sole cause of nightsweats, or qi deficiency the sole cause of spontaneous perspiration, and that all of the presenting symptoms of a patient must be considered and explained as a whole, before treatment is initiated.

It is in the area of sweating from deficiency, however, that the technique of 'constriction' plays its greatest role. The deficiency is replenished using, say, warm herbs for yang deficiency, or cool moistening herbs for yin deficiency; but in conjunction with these, certain astringent herbs which have the ability to 'constrict the sweat' (lian han) are employed.

Ma Huang Gen (Ephedrae, Radix), *Fu Xiao Mai* (Tritici Aestivi Levis, Semen), and *Nuo Dao Gen* (Oryzae Glutinosae, Radix et Rhizoma) are herbs of this type, and are often combined with *Mu Li* (Ostreae, Concha) and *Long Gu* (Draconis, Os) to improve results.

If the protective qi on the exterior is weak, surface strengthening qi tonics should be used as well, such as *Huang Qi* (Astragali, Radix), *Bai Zhu* (Atractylodes Macrocephalae, Rhizoma) and *Fang Feng* (Ledebouriellae Sesloidis, Radix).

Many sour herbs can be used to constrict fluid loss from sweating. For example *Suan Zao Ren* (Ziziphi Spinosae, Semen) can be combined with *Ren Shen* (Ginseng, Radix) and *Fu Ling* (Poriae Cocos, Sclerotium), which is especially effective for nightsweats accompanied by symptoms of Heart deficiency such as forgetfulness.

Wu Bei Zi (Rhi Chinensis, Galla) can be ground into a powder, moistened, applied to the umbilicus, and covered with a bandage to treat either spontaneous perspiration or nightsweats. Similarly, *Shan Zhu Yu* (Corni Officinalis, Fructus) may be combined with *Wu Wei Zi* (Schisandrae Chinensis, Fructus) and *Ren Shen* (Ginseng, Radix) to treat profuse perspiration with qi and yin collapse.

In many cases, though, where the problem is more severe or complicated, such simplified approaches will not be sufficient. Yin deficiency with fire flaring, for example, where the fire is forcing the fluids out, will not respond to simply constricting the surface to stop the loss of fluids. Herbs to nourish the yin while cooling the heat must be used together, such as in the formula Dang Gui Liu Huang Tang ('Dang Gui and Six-Yellow Decoction', *Formulas and Strategies,* p. 354).

It is even more important to note that 'constriction' to stop perspiration should not be used in cases resulting from an excess pathogen, except in the end stages of the treatment when the pathogen has already been eliminated, otherwise the process of pathogenic removal through the surface may itself be hindered.

As a general comment on the differing approaches used to treat exogenous pathogenic sweating in wind-cold (shang han) and in warm disease, the *Wen Bing Tiao Bian* ('Systematic Differentiation of Warm Diseases', 1798) by the Qing Dynasty physician Wu Ju-Tong has this to say:

> If the yin essence is abundant, but the yang qi is weak, the sweat cannot come out in a natural way, and this can be dangerous.[9]
>
> If the yang qi is abundant, but the yin essence weak, the sweat can indeed come out, but the yang's unbalanced expansion will be such that yin fluids are damaged. If diaphoresis is used at this point, convulsions can result [from extreme exhaustion of yin essence], and again the condition becomes serious. If external application of heat (literally 'fumigating and scorching') is used in an attempt to force the sweat out, but it does not [because of the damage to the fluids already done by the internal yang plus the external heat], the situation becomes grave.
>
> So in those cases where a patient is deficient in yang qi but abundant in yin essence, and they

have been invaded by a cold contracting pathogen, the yang qi will be even less able to expel the sweat [because the yang qi is blocked by the cold pathogenic constriction]. In these cases pungent-warm and rapidly acting herbs should be used to encourage the yang qi [to expel the pathogen]. This is [Zhang] Zhong-Jing's treatment of Shang Han (injury from cold). The book *Shang Han Lun* is, from start to finish, based upon recovering the yang qi.

In those cases where the yin essence is weak however, and the yang qi abundant, and the patient has been invaded by a warm pathogen, this warm pathogen will exert a rising and an expanding effect. Whether the patient is sweating or not, the things to use are pungent-cooling [herbs] to stop [or prevent] the loss of sweat [while expelling the pathogen], and sweet-cool and sweet-moistening [herbs] to cultivate the yin essence. This is the method of this book (i.e. the *Wen Bing Tiao Bian*, in contradistinction to the *Shang Han Lun*) to treat warm disease. This book, from start to finish, is based upon the protection of yin essence.

So in Shang Han, sweating [as a treatment] cannot be done without; while in warm disease, sweating should be avoided. This is the greatest difference between the two. Yet since the Tang dynasty, despite the large number of commentaries on this, people still insist on using Shang Han treatments on warm disease, with disastrous consequences for their warm disease patients, more's the pity. Is this the scourge of fate? or humanity?[10]

DIFFERENTIATION AND TREATMENT OF ABNORMAL SWEATING

The following sections examine specific abnormalities of perspiration, their differentiation and treatment.

Lack of perspiration (wu han)

This refers to a lack of perspiration in conditions under which perspiration would normally occur. In general, a healthy person's yang qi is most open and flowing in spring and summer, so that qi and blood move toward the surface, and this is when

sweating is most appropriate. In autumn and winter the qi and blood tend toward the interior, so perspiration is reduced or absent. These are normal conditions.

Pathologically, however, there are cases where sweating should occur but does not, such as when a pathogen invades the surface tissues and disrupts the normal opening and closing of the pores. The following section describes the differentiation and treatment of this pathology.

Common symptom patterns

Wind-cold exterior excess. Lack of perspiration, chills and fever, aching body and head, blocked nose, raspy voice, sneezing and runny nose, itchy throat and cough, thin white tongue coat, floating tight pulse.

Exterior cold with simultaneous interior heat. Lack of perspiration, fever and chills, restless aching of the limbs, blocked nose, sore throat, insatiable thirst, cough with yellow phlegm, constipation and dark yellow urine, tongue coat white or thin yellow, pulse floating and rapid.

Cold-damp fettering the exterior. Lack of perspiration, heaviness and distention of the head as if wrapped up, heaviness of the limbs, aching joints, chills with slight fever, worse in the late afternoon, white greasy tongue coat, floating tight and possibly slow pulse.

Differentiation and treatment

Wind-cold exterior excess versus exterior cold with simultaneous interior heat causing lack of sweating. Both conditions have wind-cold on the surface but the latter also has symptoms of internal heat.

Wind-cold invades the surface and, because cold is a yin pathogen with a contracting nature, it easily damages yang qi and fetters the surface tissues so that the yang-natured protective qi is unable to perform its functions. One of the most important of these is to control the opening and closing of pores, which now remain closed due to cold constriction, and perspiration is unable to occur.

The *Shang Han Ming Li Lun* ('Clarification of the Theory of Cold-induced Disorders', 1156) describes this process clearly:

The cold pathogen strikes the channel, the surface tissues become dense, the jin-ye percolates to the interior, and therefore no sweating can take place.

The most important differentiating point is that, in conjunction with the lack of normal perspiration, there are also symptoms of wind-cold fettering the exterior (i.e. chills and fever, aching of the body and head, thin white tongue coat, and floating tight pulse). The treatment here is to use pungent-warm surface openers to resolve the exterior and promote perspiration. The formula used should be Ma Huang Tang ('Ephedra Decoction').

Lack of perspiration from exterior cold with interior heat results from either constitutional internal Heat, or pent-up Lung heat then suffering a further exposure to wind-cold which ties up the surface, so that the internal heat does not have even the normal surface cooling mechanisms to dissipate it, and it builds up inside. Colloquially this is known as 'cold enveloping heat'.

A different path to the same end arises when both the defensive qi and the pathogen are forceful in attack and defense, so that a heated battle takes place below a thoroughly locked up surface.

The important differentiating point here is the combined presence of two types of symptoms: both pathogenic cold tying up the exterior (lack of perspiration, chills and fever, aching), and internal heat (restless feelings of heat and agitation in the chest, thirst, sore throat, yellow tongue coat).

Treatment calls for dispersal of wind-cold combined with the clearing of internal heat. In mild cases use Cong Bai Jie Geng Tang ('Scallion and Platycoden Decoction'); with more severe wind-cold, use Da Qing Long Tang ('Major Bluegreen Dragon Decoction').

Formulas

Ma Huang Tang ('Ephedra Decoction')

Ma Huang	Ephedrae, Herba
Gui Zhi	Cinnamomi Cassiae, Ramulus
Xing Ren	Pruni Armeniacae, Semen
Gan Cao	Glycyrrhizae Uralensis, Radix

Source text: *Shang Han Lun* ('Discussion of Cold-induced Disorders', *c.* 210AD) [*Formulas and Strategies*, p. 33]

Cong Bai Jie Geng Tang ('Scallion and Platycoden Decoction')

Cong Bai	Allii Fistulosi, Herba
Dan Dou Chi	Sojae Praeparatum, Semen
Jie Geng	Platycodi Grandiflori, Radix
Shan Zhi Zi	Gardeniae Jasminoidis, Fructus
Bo He	Menthae, Herba
Lian Qiao	Forsythiae Suspensae, Fructus
Dan Zhu Ye	Lophatheri Gracilis, Herba

Source text: *Tong Su Shang Han Lun* ('Popular Guide to the Discussion of Cold-induced Disorders') [*Formulas and Strategies*, p. 33]

Da Qing Long Tang ('Major Bluegreen Dragon Decoction')

Ma Huang	Ephedrae, Herba
Xing Ren	Pruni Armeniacae, Semen
Gui Zhi	Cinnamomi Cassiae, Ramulus
Zhi Gan Cao	Glycyrrhizae Uralensis, Radix
Shi Gao	Gypsum
Sheng Jiang	Zingiberis Officinalis Recens, Rhizoma
Da Zao	Zizyphi Jujubae, Fructus

Source text: *Shang Han Lun* ('Discussion of Cold-induced Disorders', *c.* 210AD) [*Formulas and Strategies*, p.34]

Cold-damp fettering the exterior causing lack of sweating. This condition of cold-damp obstruction in the surface tissues is a result of exposure to pathogenic wind while sweating, or prolonged residence in a damp-cold environment, or injury from foggy moist weather conditions while weak.

Pathogenic cold is contracting, while damp's nature is sticky and obstructive. The flow of yang qi through the surface tissues can become blocked by either pathogen on its own; in combination they are particularly deleterious: the yang qi cannot carry out its warming controlling functions, the pores fail to open as they should, and lack of perspiration is the result.

The *Jin Gui Yao Lue* describes the situation in Chapter 2 ('On Convulsions, Damp, and Heatstroke'):

The patient's whole body aches, there is fever which is worse in the late afternoon; this is called wind-damp. This disease comes about through injury from wind while sweating, or through long-term desire for cold.

Important differentiating points are: lack of perspiration, with symptoms of cold-damp obstructing the exterior (head distension as if wrapped in something, heavy limbs, chills, fever worse in the late afternoon). The main method of treatment is to disperse cold and expel damp, using formulas like Ma Xing Yi Gan Tang or Qiang Huo Sheng Shi Tang.

Formulas

Ma Xing Yi Gan Tang ('Ephedra, Apricot Kernel, Coicis and Licorice Decoction')

Ma Huang	Ephedrae, Herba
Xing Ren	Pruni Armeniacae, Semen
Yi Yi Ren	Coicis Lachryma-jobi, Semen
Gan Cao	Glycyrrhizae Uralensis, Radix

Source text: *Jin Gui Yao Lue* ('Essentials from the Golden Cabinet', *c.* 210 AD) [*Formulas and Strategies,* p. 35]

Qiang Huo Sheng Shi Tang ('Notopterygium Decoction to Overcome Dampness')

Qiang Huo	Notopterygii, Rhizoma et Radix
Du Huo	Duhuo, Radix
Gao Ben	Ligustici Sinensis, Radix
Fang Feng	Ledebouriellae Sesloidis, Radix
Chuan Xiong	Ligustici Wallichii, Radix
Man Jing Zi	Viticis, Fructus
Zhi Gan Cao	Glycyrrhizae Uralensis, Radix

Source text: *Nei Wai Shang Bian Huo Lun* ('Clarifying Doubts about Injury from Internal and External Causes', 1247) [*Formulas and Strategies,* p. 203]

Modern work in the area of obstructed sweating

Dr. Gong Wen-De et al. have reported their work on eighty-five cases of obstructed perspiration seen at their hospital in Shanghai during the years 1985-1990:[11]

> In TCM literature, we only find spontaneous perspiration and nightsweats mentioned, never lack of perspiration [sic]; even though in the *Shang Han Lun* 'no sweating' is mentioned as a symptom, it is really only a temporary manifestation of an exogenous wind-cold invasion, which is different from lack of perspiration stemming from the sweat glands themselves.

When Dr. Gong first started treating obstructed perspiration, he began by using warming and opening protective yang, moving blood and harmonizing nutritive qi, and the results were not too bad. But as more cases began to come up, it became apparent that the results were not completely satisfactory.

After analysis of the presenting symptoms, he felt that although the immediate cause of the obstructed perspiration was, as traditionally dictated, a disharmony of the nutritive and protective qi, still this was not the primary underlying cause. Dr. Gong pointed out that harmony between nutritive and protective qi is based upon the healthy functioning of the zang-fu, especially the production, lifting and distribution of the Spleen and Kidney yang qi, assisted by the simultaneous driving force of the Heart qi and the spreading and dispersal (xuan fa) of the Lung qi, as well as the movement (shu xie) of the Liver and the Gall Bladder which allows the Shao Yang pivot (between the interior and exterior, and also between yang-opening and yin-closing) to be properly coordinated.[12]

So the five basic mechanisms as determined by Dr. Gong are as follows:

Protective yang unaroused. Treat by warming and opening the protective yang, moving blood and harmonizing nutritive qi.

Formula

Gui Zhi	Cinnamomi Cassiae, Ramulus
Ma Huang	Ephedrae, Herba
Fu Zi	Aconiti Carmichaeli Praeparata, Radix
Xi Xin	Asari cum Radice, Herba
Bai Zhi	Angelicae, Radix
Dan Shen	Salviae Miltiorrhizae, Radix
Chi Shao	Paeoniae Rubra, Radix
Tao Ren	Persicae, Semen
Hong Hua	Carthami Tinctorii, Flos
Gan Cao	Glycyrrhizae Uralensis, Radix
Sheng Jiang	Zingiberis Officinalis Recens, Rhizoma
Hong Zao	Zizyphi Jujubae, Fructus

Green Scallion Stalks

Amounts: Gui Zhi, Chi Shao, Tao Ren, Hong Hua all 10 g; Dan Shen 30 g; Ma Huang prepared with honey, prepared Fu Zi and Bai Zhi all 5 g; prepared Xi Xin, baked Gan Cao each 3 g; Sheng Jiang 2 slices; *green scallion stalks 5*; and *red dates 5*.

Liver qi blockage. The pivot of Shao Yang has lost its opening aspect, and Heart qi is affected, leading to inability of the nutritive and protective qi to move properly. Sweat, which is the fluid of the Heart, is therefore also controlled by Shao Yang's pivotal opening function. So symptoms of disharmony here will be mood swings, unilateral headaches, irregular menses and wiry pulse.

Treat by opening (shu) Liver and moving blood, and opening (tong) and harmonizing nutritive and protective qi.

Formula

Chai Hu	Bupleuri, Radix
Chuan Xiong	Ligustici Wallichii, Radix
Xiang Fu	Cyperi Rotundi, Rhizoma
Zhi Ke	Citri seu Ponciri, Fructus
Dan Shen	Salviae Miltiorrhizae, Radix
Tao Ren	Persicae, Semen
Hong Hua	Carthami Tinctorii, Flos
Yuan Zhi	Polygalae Tenuifoliae, Radix
Shi Chang Pu	Acori Graminei, Rhizoma
Bo He	Menthae, Herba
Gan Cao	Glycyrrhizae Uralensis, Radix

Amounts: Xiang Fu, Bo He (add at end of cooking), Zhi Ke, Chuan Xiong, Yuan Zhi all 5 g. Chai Hu, Shi Chang Pu, Gan Cao (baked without honey) all 3 g; Dan Shen 30 g; Tao Ren, Hong Hua both 10 g.

Heat from Liver and Gall Bladder stasis. It should be remembered that excessive sweating can also result from Liver and Gall Bladder imbalance because of the influence that the Shao Yang pivot function has on the nutritive and protective qi, again by impeding the Heart qi. Typical symptoms will be bitter taste, tight chest, anxiety and anger, with rapid pulse, and greasy yellow tongue coat.

Treatment is to cool and clear Liver and Gall Bladder, open (kai tong) Heart qi, move blood and harmonize nutritive qi.

Formula

Qin Lian Wen Dan Tang ('Warm the Gall Bladder Decoction with Scutellaria and Coptis').

Huang Qin	Scutellariae Baicalensis, Radix
Huang Lian	Coptidis, Rhizoma
Zhu Ru	Bambusae in Taeniis, Caulis
Zhi Shi	Citri seu Ponciri Immaturis, Fructus
Chen Pi	Citri Reticulatae, Pericarpium
Fu Ling	Poriae Cocos, Sclerotium
Chai Hu	Bupleuri, Radix
Yuan Zhi	Polygalae Tenuifoliae, Radix
Shi Chang Pu	Acori Graminei, Rhizoma
Dan Shen	Salviae Miltiorrhizae, Radix
Tao Ren	Persicae, Semen
Hong Hua	Carthami Tinctorii, Flos
Bo He	Menthae, Herba
Gan Cao	Glycyrrhizae Uralensis, Radix

Amounts: Huang Qin, Huang Lian, Zhi Shi, Zhu Ru, Chen Pi, Bo He (add at end of cooking), Yuan Zhi, each 5 g; Chai Hu, Shi Chang Pu, Gan Cao (raw), each 3 g; Dan Shen 30 g, Tao Ren, Hong Hua, Fu Ling each 10 g.

Spleen deficiency Gan accumulation. This is a pediatric condition, manifesting as sallow complexion, emaciation, abdominal distention and fullness, thready slippery pulse, pale tongue, and a greasy tongue coat.

Sweat as a fluid does depend on nutritive and protective qi but Spleen transformation as the source of this qi is crucial. Here, however, the whole condition is severe, not just the lack of sweat, which is simply a manifestation.

Treatment requires benefiting qi, strengthening Spleen, breaking up accumulated food obstruction, and promoting production of nutritive and protective qi.

Formula

Huang Qi	Astragali, Radix
Tai Zi Shen	Pseudostellariae Heterophyllae, Radix
Bai Zhu	Atractylodis Macrocephalae, Rhizoma
Fu Ling	Poriae Cocos, Sclerotium
Mu Xiang	Saussureae seu Vladimiriae, Radix
Zhi Shi	Citri seu Ponciri Immaturis, Fructus
Bing Lang	Arecae Catechu, Semen
Dan Shen	Salviae Miltiorrhizae, Radix

Chi Shao	Paeoniae Rubra, Radix
Di Bie Chong	Eupolyphagae seu Opisthoplatiae
Lai Fu Zi	Raphani Sativi, Semen
Shan Zha	Crataegi, Fructus
Gu Ya	Oryza Sativae Germinatus, Fructus
Mai Ya	Hordei Vulgaris Germinantus, Fructus
Ji Nei Jin	Corneum Gigeraiae Galli, Endithelium
Gan Cao	Glycyrrhizae Uralensis, Radix
Hong Zao	Zizyphi Jujubae, Fructus
Jing Mi	polished round-grained non-glutinous rice

Amounts: Huang Qi (baked), Tai Zi Shen, Bai Zhu, Fu Ling, Lai Fu Zi, Shan Zha, Gu Ya, Mai Ya, Di Bie Chong, Dan Shen, Chi Shao all 10 g; Mu Xiang, Zhi Shi, Gan Cao (baked) all 3 g; Bing Lang, Ji Nei Jin (cooked), all 5 g; Hong Zao 7; Jing Mi (bag) 30 g.

Spleen and Kidney yang deficiency. This is constitutional, originating in childhood or persisting for over twenty years, with weak build, poor energy, sensitivity to cold, pale face, flabby tender tongue with tooth marks and deep thready weak pulse.

The distribution of nutritive and protective qi over the surface (and also therefore the control of the secretion of sweat) depends not only upon the lifting transformation and transportation of the Spleen but perhaps even more on the force from the steaming of Kidney yang.

Treatment is to warm and tonify Spleen and Kidneys, lift transportive yang, move blood, and harmonize nutritive qi.

Formula

Huang Qi	Astragali, Radix
Dang Shen	Codonopsis Pilosulae, Radix
Bai Zhu	Atractylodis Macrocephalae, Rhizoma
Shou Di	Rehmanniae Glutinosae Conquitae, Radix
Shan Zhu Yu	Corni Officinalis, Fructus
Rou Cong Rong	Cistanches, Herba
Ba Ji Tian	Morindae Officianalis, Radix
Gui Zhi	Cinnamomi Cassiae, Ramulus
Bai Shao	Paeoniae Lactiflora, Radix
Chi Shao	Paeoniae Rubra, Radix
Dan Shen	Salviae Miltiorrhizae, Radix
Tao Ren	Persicae, Semen
Hong Hua	Carthami Tinctorii, Flos
Chai Hu	Bupleuri, Radix
Sheng Ma	Cimicifugae, Rhizoma
Gan Cao	Glycyrrhizae Uralensis, Radix
Sheng Jiang	Zingiberis Officinalis Recens, Rhizoma
Hong Zao	Zizyphi Jujubae, Fructus

Green scallion stalks

Amounts: Huang Qi (raw), Dan Shen each 30 g; Dang Shen, Bai Zhu, Shou Di, Shan Zhu Yu, Ba Ji Tian, Rou Cong Rong, Tao Ren, Hong Hua, Gui Zhi, Chi Shao, Bai Shao, all 10 g; Sheng Ma (baked), Chai Hu, Gan Cao (baked without honey), each 3 g; Sheng Jiang 2 slices; *green scallion stalks* 5; *red dates* 7.

In Dr. Gong's analysis of the eighty-five cases seen, heat from Liver and Gall Bladder stasis and Spleen and Kidney yang deficiency were the most common of the above conditions, the next being unaroused protective yang and Liver qi blockage, while the children's Gan disorder was least often seen.

The basic approach was to treat each patient according to their underlying condition, while adding blood movers in order to open and harmonize the blocked nutritive qi and regulate the distribution of protective qi.

From a Western point of view the effect was to produce an improvement in the circulation through the superficial capillary system, so that the sweat glands regained their normal functioning.

Summary

Obstructed perspiration can occur as a result of either exogenous or endogenous conditions. For this reason simply using diaphoretic formulas to bring on sweating is not only simple-minded but can be dangerous, as the zheng qi can easily be damaged in this way. Differentiation is essential, not only of internal or external, but also of hot or cold, excess or deficiency.

Spontaneous perspiration (zi han)

This refers to perspiration which is not the result of physical exertion, hot weather, heavy clothing, or the consumption of diaphoretics.

This section only discusses generalized spontaneous perspiration; other sections follow which delineate the differentiation and treatment of localized sweating (such as 'Sweating on the Head', 'Sweating of the Hands and Feet', etc.).

Common symptom patterns

Nutritive and protective qi disharmony. Sweating with aversion to wind, generalized aching, alternating chills and hot flushing, thin white tongue coat, soft (huan, usually translated 'languid' but here meaning 'not tight') pulse.

Wind-damp injuring the exterior. Intermittent perspiration in small amounts, aversion to wind and cold, numbness and heaviness of the limbs, scanty urination, thin white tongue coat, floating languid or slippery thin floating and weak pulse.

Heat accumulated in Yang Ming. Frequent and relatively copious sweating, high fever, red face, insatiable thirst and drinking, dry yellow tongue coat, large strong tidal (hong) pulse.

Summerheat injuring qi and yin. Frequent and relatively copious sweating, insatiable thirst and drinking, sensation of fullness in the chest and diaphragm, reddish tongue body, dry yellow tongue coat, pulse large and tidal but forceless.

Qi deficiency. Frequent sweating worse with movement, occasional chilliness, shortness of breath, soft voice, tiredness and lethargy, pale face, poor resistance with frequent colds, pale tongue body, thin white tongue coat, languid weak pulse.

Yang deficiency. Sweating worse with movement, cold body and limbs, poor appetite, abdominal distention, loose stool, pale sallow face, pale tongue body, white tongue coat, weak pulse.

Differentiation of patterns

Spontaneous perspiration from nutritive and protective qi disharmony. Nutritive and protective qi can be disharmonious if either part is weak in relation to the other, for example, during a wind invasion of the exterior. Wind is a yang pathogen with a moving nature. During a wind invasion the protective qi, which is also yang in nature, builds up at the surface in order to battle the pathogen. This, however, leads to an imbalance between it and the nutritive qi, so that the protective qi's rising, warming, moving and dispersing nature predominates, and fever, sweating, headache and floating soft pulse result. This warming dispersal of the protective qi is reduced by loss of protective qi during the sweating, and the cooling, descending and contracting nature of nutritive qi temporarily prevails, leading to chills.

Another type of disharmony is described in Clause 53 of the *Shang Han Lun* which states:

> Illness with frequent spontaneous perspiration demonstrates an as yet undamaged nutritive qi. Although it is 'as yet undamaged', it is not in harmony with the protective qi. Because the nutritive qi travels within the vessels, and the protective qi travels outside them, diaphoresis will harmonize the two, and the illness will be cured. Use *Gui Zhi Tang*.

This clause describes a condition wherein the nutritive qi is relatively unaffected (because there is still fluid to perspire) but the protective qi is weak and unable to consolidate the surface. The single symptom is spontaneous perspiration. This situation can be treated with Gui Zhi Tang ('Cinnamon Twig Decoction') to harmonize the nutritive and protective qi, but a more modern approach would be to strengthen the protective qi with a formula like Yu Ping Feng San ('Jade Screen Powder', *Formulas and Strategies*, p. 352), as described in the qi deficiency section below.

The purpose of the above discussion is to point out the importance of spontaneous perspiration as an indication of disharmony between the nutritive qi and the protective qi, regardless of whether the disharmony stems from external pathogenic attack or from internal weakness.

Formula

Gui Zhi Tang ('Cinnamon Twig Decoction')

Gui Zhi	Cinnamomi Cassiae, Ramulus
Bai Shao	Paeoniae Lactiflora, Radix
Sheng Jiang	Zingiberis Officinalis Recens, Rhizoma
Da Zao	Zizyphi Jujubae, Fructus
Gan Cao	Glycyrrhizae Uralensis, Radix

Source text: *Shang Han Lun* ('Discussion of Cold-Induced Disorders', 210AD) [*Formulas and Strategies*, p. 35]

Spontaneous perspiration from wind-damp injuring the exterior. In most cases this type of sweating occurs in bi-syndrome ('painful obstruction') patients (those with arthritis, rheumatism and so on) who have 'caught cold'; in TCM terms it is pathogenic wind and damp combined. One pathogen is yang, so is dispersing, the other is yin, heavy and obstructing; each affects the other so that the pores open sporadically and sweating is intermittent. The pores are uncontrolled because the pathogens prevent the normal flow of protective qi and, if wind, which by nature is spreading and dispersing, temporarily predominates between the pathogens, the pores will open and perspiration flows out. But because damp is heavy and obstructing, the amount of the sweat is curtailed and the pores soon close again. The lack of normal protective qi flow also explains the aversion to wind and cold felt by the patient, and likewise the numbness resulting from failure of the surface tissues, and then gradually the channels and collaterals, to be nourished by normal qi and blood because of the pathogenic obstruction of damp. The heaviness of the limbs reflects both the decreased ability to move without sufficient qi and blood supply, and most importantly the heavy nature of the sinking damp.

Damp, again, most easily dams up the pathway for fluids, that is, the San Jiao fluid metabolism functioning. This damming may lead to scanty urination.

If the wind is predominant and the condition is mainly in the surface tissues, the pulse will reflect this, being floating and languid (fu, huan).

If, though, the damp is predominant and the condition has entered the channels and collaterals rather than only the surface, the pulse will be slippery and 'ru' (thin, floating and forceless). The floating aspect of the ru pulse is a result of the wind component but the oppressive effect of the damp pathogen on the qi and blood prevents their full strength from reaching the surface, resulting in a thready weak pulse.

The thin white tongue coat shows wind-damp on the surface that has not yet become hot.

The treatment should be to expel wind and remove damp, tonify qi and consolidate the surface, using a formula such as Fang Ji Huang Qi Tang with appropriate additions.

Formula

Fang Ji Huang Qi Tang ('Stephania and Astragalus Decoction')

Huang Qi	Astragali, Radix
Han Fang Ji	Stephaniae Tetrandrae, Radix
Bai Zhu	Atractylodis Macrocephalae, Rhizoma
Gan Cao	Glycyrrhizae Uralensis, Radix
Sheng Jiang	Zingiberis Officinalis Recens, Rhizoma
Da Zao	Zizyphi Jujubae, Fructus

Source text: *Jin Gui Yao Lue* ('Essentials from the Golden Cabinet', *c*. 210AD) [*Formulas and Strategies*, p.179]

Spontaneous perspiration from heat accumulated in Yang Ming versus spontaneous perspiration from Summerheat injuring qi and yin. Both conditions are spontaneous perspiration from heat, and symptom-wise are very similar. But they differ in two things: the causative pathogen and the season of occurrence.

The first is an exogenous wind-cold pathogen that has moved into the interior—into Yang Ming, the deepest of the yang levels in the *Shang Han Lun* 'six channel' system—and turned hot. This type of pathogenic transformation is not limited to summertime. The second condition is caused by the Summerheat (shu) pathogen, which by nature is very damaging to the qi and yin, and of course most common in summertime.

The important differentiating points for the Yang Ming heat are the high fever, profuse sweating, insatiable thirst and the large strong pulse. (Often known as the 'four greats' in the *Shang Han Lun* literature, as all four symptoms are extreme.) Treatment is to cool heat and drain away fire, using a formula like Bai Hu Tang ('White Tiger Decoction'):

For Summerheat, the important differentiating points are the season and the patient's recent history (i.e. any exposure to excessive and oppressive heat), as well as the combination of both excess and deficiency symptoms: the excess symptoms are the Summerheat manifestations of fever and sweating, while the deficiency symptoms are those of damage to qi and yin: thirst, red tongue and, especially,the large pulse, (because there is excessive heat, as in the Yang Ming situation) that in fact is forceless (because the qi and yin fluids have been damaged).

Treatment is to clear Summerheat and drain heat, replenish qi, and produce jin-ye, using Master Wang's Qing Shu Yi Qi Tang ('Master Wang's Decoction to Clear Summerheat and Augment the Qi').

Formulas

Bai Hu Tang ('White Tiger Decoction')

Shi Gao	Gypsum
Zhi Mu	Anemarrhenae Asphodeloidis, Radix
Jing Mi	Oryza Sativae, semen
Gan Cao	Glycyrrhizae Uralensis, Radix

Source text: *Shang Han Lun* ('Discussion of Cold-Induced Disorders', 210AD) [*Formulas and Strategies*, p. 70]

Wang Shi Qing Shu Yi Qi Tang ('Master Wang's Decoction to Clear Summerheat and Augment the Qi')

Xi Yang Shen	Panacis Quinquefolii, Radix
Xi Gua Pi	Pericarpium Citrulli Vulgaris
Lian Geng	Nelumbinis Nuciferae, Ramulus
Shi Hu	Dendrobii, Herba
Mai Men Dong	Ophiopogonis Japonici, Tuber
Dan Zhu Ye	Lophatheri Gracilis, Herba
Zhi Mu	Anemarrhenae Asphodeloidis, Radix
Huang Lian	Coptidis, Rhizoma
Gan Cao	Glycyrrhizae Uralensis, Radix
Jing Mi	Oryza Sativae, semen

Source text: *Wen Re Jing Wei* ('Warp and Woof of Warm-febrile Diseases', 1852) [*Formulas and Strategies*, pp. 106-107]

Spontaneous perspiration from qi deficiency versus yang deficiency spontaneous perspiration. Both are deficiency conditions, and share certain symptoms such as worsening with exertion. However, the origin and pathological mechanism in each case differ.

Spontaneous perspiration from qi deficiency is based on Heart and Lung dysfunction. This is so because while sweat is the fluid of the Heart, Lungs also rule the qi of the whole body, and the skin and pores. Because, in Chinese medicine, the zang-fu are not considered separate from their external manifestations (so that, for example, Heart is blood and pulse and spirit; Lungs are qi and skin; Kidneys are bone and marrow and hearing; and so on), a local disharmony of two factors can be seen as a zang-fu disharmony, and so treatment is based on re-establishing the balanced functioning of those zang-fu. In this sense the 'disharmony of the nutritive and protective qi' discussed previously in the first section is a local manifestation of what may be, or may turn into, a larger problem. The decisive point as to whether to deal with the situation as a local problem, or as a sign of a larger imbalance, is the presence or absence of generalized symptoms.

In this case, because the Heart and Lung qi is weak, the surface is unconsolidated and the jin-ye is allowed to leak away in the form of sweat. The important differentiating points identifying qi—as opposed to yang—deficiency are spontaneous perspiration worsening on the slightest movement, sensitivity to wind and cold temperatures even at the best of times, frequent colds, plus other common qi deficiency symptoms. The pulse will be languid (huan, here meaning somewhat slow), slippery, and weak. The treatment requires tonification of qi, consolidation of the exterior, and stopping perspiration, using a combination of the two formulas Yu Ping Feng San ('Jade Screen Powder') and Bu Zhong Yi Qi Tang ('Tonify the Middle and Augment the Qi Decoction').

Spontaneous perspiration from yang deficiency is more deep-set, being rooted in deficiency of the Spleen and Kidneys. Spleen is the source of qi and blood, while Kidneys (in this context) function mainly as a treasury, storing true yin and housing original yang. On the surface, the local mechanism producing the spontaneous perspiration is the same as the previous example: protective qi (also commonly known as protective yang) cannot control the opening and closing of the pores. However the source of this weakness is no longer located in the Heart and Lungs but deeper, in the Kidneys and Spleen. Therefore the accompanying symptoms will be different: more obvious chills, loose stool, poor appetite, lower backache, weak legs and so on. Treatment, too, must be altered in two ways: not only should the protective qi be immediately strengthened with a formula like Bu Zhong Yi

Qi Tang ('Tonify the Middle and Augment the Qi Decoction') but the yang of the Kidneys (which will then support Spleen yang) must be enhanced to achieve long-term results. Jin Gui Shen Qi Wan ('Kidney Pill from the Golden Cabinet') is a good formula for this. The second alteration is to add some astringent surface consolidating herbs such as prepared *Long Gu* (Draconis, Os) and *Mu Li* (Ostreae, Concha), and sour yin-contractors like *Wu Wei Zi* (Schisandrae Chinensis, Fructus). This will support the weakened Kidneys' ability to contain and store, as well as closing the pores.

Formulas

Yu Ping Feng San ('Jade Screen Powder')

Huang Qi	Astragali, Radix
Bai Zhu	Atractylodis Macrocephalae, Rhizoma
Fang Feng	Ledebouriellae Sesloidis, Radix

Source text: *Dan Xi Xin Fa* ('Teachings of Dan Xi', 1481) [*Formulas and Strategies*, p. 352]

Bu Zhong Yi Qi Tang ('Tonify the Middle and Augment the Qi Decoction')

Huang Qi	Astragali, Radix
Ren Shen	Ginseng, Radix
Bai Zhu	Atractylodis Macrocephalae, Rhizoma
Dang Gui	Angelica Polymorpha, Radix
Chen Pi	Citri Reticulatae, Pericarpium
Sheng Ma	Cimicifugae, Rhizoma
Chai Hu	Bupleuri, Radix
Gan Cao	Glycyrrhizae Uralensis, Radix

Source Text: *Pi Wei Lun* ('Discussion of the Spleen and Stomach', 1249) [*Formulas and Strategies*, p. 241]

Jin Gui Shen Qi Wan ('Kidney Pill from the *Golden Cabinet*')

Shou Di	Rehmanniae Glutinosae Conquitae, Radix
Shan Zhu Yu	Corni Officinalis, Fructus
Shan Yao	Dioscoreae Oppositae, Radix
Fu Zi	Aconiti Carmichaeli Praeparata, Radix
Gui Zhi	Cinnamomi Cassiae, Ramulus
Ze Xie	Alismatis Plantago-aquaticae, Rhizoma
Fu Ling	Poriae Cocos, Sclerotium
Mu Dan Pi	Moutan Radicis, Cortex

Source text: *Jin Gui Yao Lue* ('Essentials from the Golden Cabinet', *c.* 210AD) [*Formulas and Strategies*, p. 275]

Summary

As we have demonstrated above, the temptation to immediately assume spontaneous perspiration to be qi or yang deficiency should be avoided. As the *Shang Han Ming Li Lun* ('Clarification of the Theory of Cold-induced Disorders', 1156) points out: 'Spontaneous perspiration ... in each individual case has differences of yin and yang symptoms, so one should not say that spontaneous perspiration must be from yang deficiency.' (In relation to this, see also Zhang Jing–Yue's comments at the end of this chapter.)

The first steps in clinical differentiation should be to decide whether the case is one of exterior invasion or interior disharmony. Exterior invasions are primarily excess, while interior conditions are usually deficient. Deficiency is the most commonly seen cause, while mixed deficiency and excess conditions are also quite common.

Nightsweats (dao han)

Nightsweats are defined as perspiration which occurs during sleep but ceases upon awakening.

Common symptom patterns

Heart blood insufficiency. Frequent nightsweats, with palpitations, insomnia, pallor, shortness of breath, tiredness and exhaustion, pale tongue thin tongue coat, xu pulse (big, floating and weak).

Yin deficiency and interior heat. Frequent nightsweats, hot flushes in the afternoon, malar flush, five-hearts heat, thin body type, in women irregular menstruation, in men spermatorrhea, red tongue body with little coat, pulse thready and rapid.

Spleen deficiency with damp obstruction. Frequent nightsweats, headache as if wrapped up, heaviness of the limbs and general lethargy, poor appetite, greasy feeling in the mouth, thin white greasy tongue coat, pale tongue body, languid ru (thready, floating, and weak) pulse.

Mid-stage pathogenic invasion. Nightsweats of recent onset, alternating chills and fever, tightness in the chest and flanks, bitter taste, nausea, tongue coat thin white or thin yellow, wiry slippery or wiry rapid pulse.

Differentiation

Nightsweats from heart blood insufficiency versus nightsweats from yin deficiency and interior heat. Both are deficiency patterns but in the latter the deficient heat manifestations are very obvious. Nightsweats from Heart blood insufficiency result from consumption damage (lao shang) to the blood. 'Heart storage: internally the blood, externally the sweat'. If Heart blood is damaged, its fluid—sweat—instead of being stored by the Heart will follow the now un-rooted qi of the Heart as it floats outward, and will be lost through the exterior. Therefore the frequent nightsweats will be accompanied by palpitations, insomnia and other symptoms of qi and blood deficiency such as pallor, tiredness and lethargy, pale tongue body, and a pulse that is floating and big (showing un-rooted qi) but weak upon pressure.

Treatment requires tonification of the blood, nourishment of the Heart, and constraint of the perspiration, using a formula like Gui Pi Tang ('Restore the Spleen Decoction') plus other herbs such as *Mu Li* (Ostreae, Concha), *Long Gu* (Draconis, Os), and *Wu Wei Zi* (Schisandrae Chinensis, Fructus).

Nightsweats from yin deficiency and interior heat result from damage to the yin fluids or even the Kidney jing, allowing yang heat to become unbalanced by yin. Deficient heat flares, and yin is unable to constrain its fluids, leading to frequent nightsweats and other yin deficiency symptoms such as malar flush, five-hearts heat and hot flushes in the late afternoon and evening. In women, this easily causes menstrual irregularity, especially early periods or inter-menstrual bleeding; in men, excessive sexual desire coupled with impotence or spermatorrhea of various kinds can result. Damage to the yin and jing eventually leads to emaciation.

The tongue body will be red with little coat, and the pulse will be rapid and thready: these are standard yin xu signs.

Treatment must be to nourish yin, bring down fire, and constrain perspiration. Dang Gui Liu Huang Tang ('Dang Gui and Six-Yellow Decoction') can be used, plus *Nuo Dao Gen* (Oryzae Glutinosae, Radix et Rhizoma) and *Fu Xiao Mai* (Tritici Aestivi Levis, Semen).

Formulas

Gui Pi Tang ('Restore the Spleen Decoction')

Ren Shen	Ginseng, Radix
Huang Qi	Astragali, Radix
Bai Zhu	Atractylodis Macrocephalae, Rhizoma
Fu Ling	Poriae Cocos, Sclerotium
Suan Zao Ren	Ziziphi Spinosae, Semen
Long Yan Rou	Euphoriae Longanae, Arillus
Mu Xiang	Saussureae seu Vladimiriae, Radix
Dang Gui	Angelica Polymorpha, Radix
Yuan Zhi	Polygalae Tenuifoliae, Radix
Gan Cao	Glycyrrhizae Uralensis, Radix
Sheng Jiang	Zingiberis Officinalis Recens, Rhizoma
Da Zao	Zizyphi Jujubae, Fructus

Source text: *Ji Sheng Fang* ('Formulas to Aid the Living', 1253) [*Formulas and Strategies*, p. 255]

Dang Gui Liu Huang Tang ('Dang Gui and Six-Yellow Decoction')

Dang Gui	Angelica Polymorpha, Radix
Sheng Di	Rehmannia Glutinosae, Radix
Shou Di	Rehmanniae Glutinosae Conquitae, Radix
Huang Lian	Coptidis, Rhizoma
Huang Qin	Scutellariae Baicalensis, Radix
Huang Bo	Phellodendri, Cortex
Huang Qi	Astragali, Radix

Source text: *Lan Shi Mi Cang* ('Secrets from the Orchid Chamber', 1336) [*Formulas and Strategies*, p. 354]

Nightsweats from Spleen deficiency with damp obstruction versus nightsweats from mid-stage pathogenic invasion. Both are excess conditions. Nightsweats from Spleen deficiency with damp obstruction usually result from over-consumption of hard-to-digest substances, such as cold or raw foods or rich greasy foods and alcohol; or from poor eating habits like repeated fasting then over-eating. All of these practices damage Spleen and Stomach and bring about disruption in the digestive and distributive capabilities of these two organs, allowing murky damp to build up and obstruct the normal ascent and descent of qi. Damp being a yin-natured pathogen, as the yang activity of the day decreases, damp obstruction to the flow of protective qi through the surface tissues increases. During sleep, when the main portion of the protective qi moves internally, the remainder is insufficient to control the pores which open and sweating occurs. If pathogenic heat accumulates as a result of the damp obstruction, this only exacerbates the problem.[13]

The accompanying symptoms are characteristic of damp: headache with the sensation of the head being wrapped up, lethargy of the body and limbs, anorexia, greasy sensation in the mouth, pale tongue body with a thin white greasy tongue coat, and a languid thready floating and weak (huan, ru) pulse.

Treatment aims at transforming damp, harmonizing the center, and promoting normal qi flow around the body. A good formula to use for this would be Huo Po Xia Ling Tang ('Agastache, Magnolia Bark, Pinellia, and Poria Decoction'), eliminating the *Xing Ren* (Pruni Armeniacae, Semen), *Zhu Ling* (Polypori Umbellati, Sclerotium), *Dan Dou Chi* (Sojae Praeparatum, Semen), and *Ze Xie* (Alismatis Plantago-aquaticae, Rhizoma), while adding *Nuo Dao Gen* (Oryzae Glutinosae, Radix et Rhizoma), *Cang Zhu* (Atractylodis, Rhizoma) and *Chen Pi* (Citri Reticulatae, Pericarpium).

Nightsweats from mid-stage pathogenic invasion are usually seen in the early- to mid-stage of a febrile disease, so history is probably the most crucial differentiating point here.

In the course of an exogenous pathogenic invasion of the surface, if the pathogen is not expelled from the exterior, it tends to move internally into Shao Yang and become jammed half-internally and half-externally, neither able to move inward nor able to move out. The conflict leads to alternating chills and fever as the pathogenic struggle

with the by-now-weakened zheng qi waxes and wanes, and as the protective qi on the surface is further reduced by its normal emphasis on interior movement during sleep, the struggle with the pathogen causes nightsweats by forcing fluids outwards through the poorly controlled pores. Symptoms of interference in the Shao Yang channel appear: fullness of the flanks, tightness in the chest, bitter taste in the mouth, nausea; wiry rapid pulse and thin yellow tongue coat are standard for Shao Yang Syndrome.

Treatment is to harmonize Shao Yang with Xiao Chai Hu Tang ('Minor Bupleurum Decoction'), removing *Dang Shen* (Codonopsis Pilosulae, Radix) and *Da Zao* (Zizyphi Jujubae, Fructus), and adding *Huang Lian* (Coptidis, Rhizoma).

Formulas

Huo Po Xia Ling Tang ('Agastache, Magnolia Bark, Pinellia and Poria Decoction')

Huo Xiang	Agastaches seu Pogostemi, Herba
Ban Xia	Pinelliae Ternata, Rhizoma
Chi Fu Ling	Poriae, Cocos Rubrae, Sclerotium
Xing Ren	Pruni Armeniacae, Semen
Yi Yi Ren	Coicis Lachryma-jobi, Semen
Bai Dou Kou	Amomi Cardamomi, Fructus
Zhu Ling	Polypori Umbellati, Sclerotium
Dan Dou Chi	Sojae Praeparatum, Semen
Ze Xie	Alismatis Plantago-aquaticae, Rhizoma
Hou Po	Magnoliae Officianalis, Cortex

Source text: *Yi Yuan* ('Origin of Medicine', 1861) [*Formulas and Strategies*, p. 187]

Xiao Chai Hu Tang ('Minor Bupleurum Decoction')

Chai Hu	Bupleuri, Radix
Huang Qin	Scutellariae Baicalensis, Radix
Ban Xia	Pinelliae Ternata, Rhizoma
Dang Shen	Codonopsis Pilosulae, Radix
Sheng Jiang	Zingiberis Officinalis Recens, Rhizoma
Gan Cao	Glycyrrhizae Uralensis, Radix
Da Zao	Zizyphi Jujubae, Fructus

Source text: *Shang Han Lun* ('Discussion of Cold-Induced Disorders', 210AD) [*Formulas and Strategies*, p. 136]

Summary

In the *Jing Yue Quan Shu* ('Complete Works of Jing Yue', 1624), the careful differentiation of night-sweats is emphasized:

> 'Nightsweats have both yin and yang syndromes, and it should not be said that nightsweats are only from yin deficiency.'

So the first thing is to determine whether the cause is endogenous or exogenous. If endogenous, it will usually be from a deficiency condition; if exogenous, it will usually be the result of pathogenic excess. Deficiency is the most common cause; however, mixed xu and shi conditions occur, as well as dual deficiencies such as qi and yin both deficient. Treatment of nightsweats without clear differentiation yields particularly poor results.

Yellow sweat (huang han)

Yellow sweat is the condition wherein the sweat itself turns yellow and stains the clothes. Historically, the *Jin Gui Yao Lue* ('Golden Cabinet') included a description of 'yellow sweat' as a syndrome in its chapter on edema; later yellow sweat was almost always classed with jaundice, and especially the yang type of jaundice: yang huang.

The two conditions are not completely the same, however, as yellow sweat as a symptom can occur without any other part of the body going yellow.

This section will deal with this latter type of condition: yellow sweat not in the context of jaundice but as an individual symptom on its own.[14]

Common symptom patterns

Yellow sweat from nutritive and protective qi congestion. Yellowish watery sweat, hot flushing, heaviness and swelling of the body, crawling feeling of the skin, thirst, difficult urination, white tongue coat, deep pulse.

Yellow sweat from pent-up damp-heat. Yellowish sweat, hot flushing, slight swelling of the body, pain in the flanks, poor appetite, bitter taste in the mouth, darkish urine, yellow greasy tongue coat, wiry slippery pulse.

Differentiation

Yellow sweat from nutritive and protective qi congestion. There are two factors responsible for

the production of yellow sweat here. The first is an already existing heat condition in the body leading to sweating. The second factor is a subsequent exposure to wet weather, or cold baths, causing the surface tissues to close down tightly and restrict the flow of nutritive and protective qi as well as obstructing local fluid circulation. The protective qi is weak while the nutritive qi is blocked so that the 'heat and the water clash', the accumulating fluids are affected by the heat, and so become yellow.

These factors also lead to the accompanying symptoms of generalized swelling of the surface tissues and consequently lethargy and heaviness, and the crawling feeling of the skin.

The impeded flow of qi and fluids means that, in the upper body, normal fluids cannot rise to moisten the mouth and throat so thirst occurs; while in the lower body, the Urinary Bladder qi transformation is affected and the urination becomes difficult.

Treatment should aim at removing obstruction and opening the flow of qi, while harmonizing the nutritive and protective qi, with a formula like Huang Qi Shao Yao Gui Zhi Ku Jiu Tang.

Formula

Huang Qi Shao Yao Gui Zhi Ku Jiu Tang ('Astragalus, Peony, Cinnamon and Vinegar Decoction')

Huang Qi	15 g	Astragali, Radix
Bai Shao	9 g	Paeoniae Lactiflora, Radix
Gui Zhi	9 g	Cinnamomi Cassiae, Ramulus

The above three herbs should be mixed with *Vinegar* 200 g. and 1.4 litres of water, and boiled down to 600 ml. One dose is 200 ml. If a sensation of restlessness in the chest occurs after taking the decoction, the patient should be encouraged to continue, as the sensation will pass in several days.

Source text: *Jin Gui Yao Lue* ('Essentials from the Golden Cabinet', *c.* 210AD)

Yellow sweat from pent-up damp-heat. Most often this is a result of exogenous damp-heat but it can also come about through long-term internal damp retarding the flow of qi and so gradually turning hot. The two pathogens, one being yin and the other yang, clash with each other and intensify the severity of the condition, the damp becoming thicker and more obstructive. The heat, now even less able to escape and be dissipated, grows more intense. The damp and the heat first affect the organs most sensitive to damp: the Earth organs. Steaming from the damp-heat, the fluids moving through the Earth level (the flesh) become yellowish, the color of earth. These factors finally produce yellowish sweat, bitter taste in the mouth, pain in the flanks, loss of appetite and darkish urine, with a yellow tongue coat and wiry slippery pulse, all of which are manifestations of damp-heat. The treatment calls for cooling heat while removing damp. Yu Ping Feng San ('Jade Screen Powder'), suitably altered, can be used for this, adding such herbs as *Pei Lan* (Eupatorii Fortunei, Herba) and *Sha Ren* (Amomi, Fructus et Semen) as fragrant damp-dispersers, *Huang Qin* (Scutellariae Baicalensis, Radix), *Shan Zhi Zi* (Gardeniae Jasminoidis, Fructus), and *Huang Lian* (Coptidis, Rhizoma) as bitter-cold draining and cooling for both the damp and the heat, and finally *Chai Hu* (Bupleuri, Radix) and *Zhi Shi* (Citri seu Ponciri Immaturis, Fructus) to restore normal flow of qi, and so break up the condensed damp and heat.

Formula

Yu Ping Feng San ('Jade Screen Powder')

Huang Qi	Astragali, Radix
Bai Zhu	Atractylodis Macrocephalae, Rhizoma
Fang Feng	Ledebouriellae Sesloidis, Radix

Source text: *Dan Xi Xin Fa* ('Teachings of Dan Xi', 1481) [*Formulas and Strategies*, p. 352]

Summary

Of the two conditions described above, one is the result of constricted exterior from going into cold water while sweating, and the other from damp-heat steaming the Spleen and Stomach. One is completely a local surface problem, the other systemic, involving even the zang-fu. The first requires harmonization of the nutritive and protective qi in order to restore normal fluid movement and eliminate accumulated damp. The second needs to both clear damp-heat and open nutritive and protective qi flow. Once the damp-heat goes, so will the yellow sweat.

Perspiration partially obstructed (ban shen han, hemihidrosis)

This refers to sweating occurring only on one side of the body. Its first classical reference appears in the *Su Wen* Chapter 3: 'Partially obstructed secretion of sweat causes partial dehydration.' The condition usually is seen in wind-stroke or in some patients with weakened zang-fu functions.

The following differentiation only applies to perspiration obstruction on the left or right of the body. Upper and lower body perspiration will fall into the categories following this one.

Common symptom patterns

Qi and blood deficiency. Perspiration only occurring on one half of the body, shortness of breath, weak voice, tiredness and lethargy, facial pallor, lack of shine on the skin, dizziness, numbness of the hands and feet, pale tongue body, thready weak pulse.

Cold-damp obstruction. Perspiration only occurring on one half of the body, stiffness and pain of the tendons with limited movement of the limbs, a sensation of heaviness in the body, and even difficulty in turning the trunk, tongue coat white and greasy, pulse floating thin and weak (i.e. a 'ru' pulse) and possibly slow.

Nutritive and protective qi disharmony. Perspiration only occurring on one half of the body, fever, aversion to wind, headache, tongue coat white and moist, pulse floating soft and weak.

Differentiation

Hemihidrosis from qi and blood deficiency. Usually a result of over-exertion, or subsequent to a long illness or heavy bleeding, any of which can lead to qi and blood injury and deficiency so that they cannot circulate evenly throughout the body, and sweating therefore can only take place on one side of the body because of the lack of qi to consolidate the surface. The *Zhong Yi Lin Chuang Zheng Bei Yao* ('TCM Synopsis of Clinical Syndromes') says: 'When perspiration only appears on half the body, whether left or right, the most common cause is unconsolidated qi and blood.'

Essential points in differentiation are the qi deficiency symptoms, plus the numbness of the hands and feet, facial pallor and lack of lustre to the skin, all of which demonstrate the inability of the qi and blood to reach the limbs and the surface. The pale tongue body and thready weak pulse confirm this. It should be noted that the side of the body with sweating is the side which lacks the normal consolidation of the qi and blood, whereas hemihidrosis from cold-damp invasion is the opposite, having the surface of that side obstructed by the pathogens and therefore unable to perspire.

Treatment is aimed at restoring the ability to consolidate the surface, with a formula such as Ren Shen Yang Ying Tang.

Formula

Ren Shen Yang Ying Tang ('Ginseng Decoction to Nourish the Nutritive Qi')

Bai Shao	Paeoniae Lactiflora, Radix
Dang Gui	Angelica Polymorpha, Radix
Chen Pi	Citri Reticulatae, Pericarpium
Huang Qi	Astragali, Radix
Rou Gui	Cinnamomi Cassiae, Cortex
Ren Shen	Ginseng, Radix
Bai Zhu	Atractylodis Macrocephalae, Rhizoma
Gan Cao	Glycyrrhizae Uralensis, Radix
Shou Di	Rehmanniae Glutinosae Conquitae, Radix
Wu Wei Zi	Schisandrae Chinensis, Fructus
Fu Ling	Poriae Cocos, Sclerotium
Yuan Zhi	Polygalae Tenuifoliae, Radix
Sheng Jiang	Zingiberis Officinalis Recens, Rhizoma
Da Zao	Zizyphi Jujubae, Fructus

Source text: *Tai Ping Hui Min He Ji Ju Fang* ('Imperial Grace Formulary of the Tai Ping Era', 1078-85) [*Formulas and Strategies*, p. 260]

Hemihidrosis from cold-damp obstruction. When cold and damp invade the body, they obstruct the channels and collaterals. This can happen uniformly throughout the body, or be paramount in certain areas, as in this case where the channels of one side are affected more than the other, so that qi and blood flow is unable to reach certain areas. These areas suffer disruption of the normal functioning of the pores, and lack of sweating on that side of the body results.

Essential points in differentiation are the pain, stiffness and limited movement of the limbs, plus the heaviness and lethargy, all of which are worse in the morning because of the preponderance of yin qi throughout the night compounding the two yin pathogens cold and damp. Qi and blood deficiency, by way of contrast, tends to be better in the morning because the rest during the night has allowed them to be restored. The tongue coat being white and greasy confirms the diagnosis.

Treatment should be directed towards the expulsion of damp and warming the channels and collaterals to encourage blood flow, with either Juan Bi Tang ('Remove Painful Obstruction Decoction from *Medical Revelations*') plus *Xi Xin* (Asari cum Radice, Herba) and *Zhi Chuan Wu* (Aconiti Carmicheali Praeparata, Radix) or Xiao Huo Luo Dan ('Minor Invigorate the Collaterals Special Pill').

Formulas

Juan Bi Tang ('Remove Painful Obstruction Decoction from *Medical Revelations*')

Qiang Huo	Notopterygii, Rhizoma et Radix
Du Huo	Duhuo, Radix
Qin Jiao	Gentianae Macrophyllae, Radix
Sang Zhi	Mori Albae, Ramulus
Hai Feng Teng	Piperis, Caulis
Dang Gui	Angelica Polymorpha, Radix
Chuan Xiong	Ligustici Wallichii, Radix
Ru Xiang	Olibanum, Gummi
Mu Xiang	Saussureae seu Vladimiriae, Radix
Gui Zhi	Cinnamomi Cassiae, Ramulus
Gan Cao	Glycyrrhizae Uralensis, Radix

Source text: *Yi Xue Xin Wu* ('Medical Revelations', 1732) [*Formulas and Strategies*, p. 204]

Xiao Huo Luo Dan ('Minor Invigorate the Collaterals Special Pill')

Zhi Chuan Wu	Aconiti Carmicheali Praeparata, Radix
Zhi Cao Wu	Aconiti Kusnezoffii Praeparata, Radix
Dan Nan Xing	Arisaemae cum Felle Bovis, Pulvis
Mo Yao	Myrrha
Ru Xiang	Olibanum, Gummi
Di Long	Lumbricus

Source text: *Tai Ping Hui Min He Ji Ju Fang* ('Imperial Grace Formulary of the Tai Ping Era', 1078-85) [*Formulas and Strategies*, p. 398]

Nutritive and protective qi disharmony. As seen in previous sections, nutritive and protective qi disharmony can be an effect of either exogenous wind invasion, or interior exhaustion. The former is more common in cases of hemihidrosis. In either situation, protective qi is unable to properly control the pores, and spontaneous perspiration occurs on the affected side of the body. Most patients will have symptoms of wind invasion: headache, aversion to wind, fever, soft floating pulse (i.e. 'huan fu pulse').

Treatment requires restoration of nutritive and protective qi harmony, with a formula like Gui Zhi Tang.

Formula

Gui Zhi Tang ('Cinnamon Twig Decoction')

Gui Zhi	Cinnamomi Cassiae, Ramulus
Bai Shao	Paeoniae Lactiflora, Radix
Sheng Jiang	Zingiberis Officinalis Recens, Rhizoma
Da Zao	Zizyphi Jujubae, Fructus
Gan Cao	Glycyrrhizae Uralensis, Radix

Source text: *Shang Han Lun* ('Discussion of Cold-Induced Disorders', 210AD) [*Formulas and Strategies*, p. 35]

Summary

Hemihidrosis is always a result of disruption to the even flow of qi and blood to both sides of the body. The mechanism can be either through pathogenic obstruction or through shortage of qi and blood.

In older patients, though, this condition may be an early sign of susceptibility to wind-stroke, and therefore early and appropriate treatment is essential, as well as instructions to avoid over-exertion in order to maintain sufficient qi and blood.

Perspiration from the head (tou han)

Perspiring only from the head is in some people a normal condition, for example while eating or, with children, during sleep. In conjunction with general symptoms however it is a sign of pathology.

Common symptom patterns

Damp-heat. Perspiration only from the head, difficult urination that is scanty and yellow, jaundice, bitter taste, chills, hot flushing, tongue coat yellow and greasy, pulse thin floating weak (i.e. 'ru' pulse) and rapid.

Insufficient yang qi. Perspiration only from the head, facial pallor, cold limbs, shortness of breath, chills, tiredness, pale flabby tongue body, weak forceless pulse.

Differentiation

Damp-heat causing perspiration from the head. Pathogenic damp, either invading from the exterior or building up inside, can easily become hot through the obstruction of the normal qi flow. If the damp is primarily distributed throughout the surface tissues, this heat will be prevented from dissipating outwards, will build up inside, and finally push upwards towards the head: the place where damp, being heavy and sinking, is likely to be least concentrated. The heat then forces out what can be very profuse quantities of sweat. This common pathological mechanism was recognized as early as the second century A.D., and is described in the *Shang Han Lun*.

Damp stasis in the surface tissues will, of course, also hamper protective and nutritive qi flow, leading to chills and possibly aching joints, and provide a further source of heat as the protective qi struggles with the pathogen. Further evidence of damp accumulation can be found in the dysfunction of the Urinary Bladder which, clogged by damp, can no longer separate fine from murky fluids, and urine becomes difficult.

If the condition worsens, and damp-heat steams the Liver and Gall Bladder, the bile can be forced out to the surface and to the eyes, leading to jaundice in these areas and bitter taste in the mouth.

Yellow greasy tongue coat and rapid ru pulse (floating thready and weak) are typical manifestations of equal measures of damp and heat.

Treatment should clear heat and remove damp, with a formula such as Yin Chen Wu Ling San.

Formula

Yin Chen Wu Ling San ('Artemesia Yinchenhao and Five-Ingredient Powder with Poria')

Yin Chen Hao	Artemesiae Capillaris, Herba
Ze Xie	Alismatis Plantago-aquaticae, Rhizoma
Fu Ling	Poriae Cocos, Sclerotium
Zhu Ling	Polypori Umbellati, Sclerotium
Bai Zhu	Atractylodis Macrocephalae, Rhizoma
Gui Zhi	Cinnamomi Cassiae, Ramulus

Source text: *Jin Gui Yao Lue* ('Essentials from the Golden Cabinet', *c.* 210AD) [*Formulas and Strategies*, p. 176]

If the damp and heat are unequally proportioned, the treatment must be adjusted accordingly to account for the difference. Strategies for this can be found in the section on damp-heat.

Insufficient yang qi causing perspiration from the head. This develops from deficiency, especially following an illness or giving birth, or in old age. The yang qi is weak and can no longer consolidate the surface, especially at the head to which it is unable to rise. Inability of the qi to lead blood upwards causes facial pallor, which can also ensue from the natural weakening of the blood when yang qi is deficient, and the coldness of the limbs in the context of all the other yang qi deficiency signs is a consequence of the failure of yang warmth to reach the extremities.

The pale tender tongue and the forceless pulse clinch the diagnosis.

Treatment aims at warming yang and aiding qi, consolidating the exterior and constraining sweat, with a formula like Qi Fu Tang plus *Ren Shen* (Ginseng, Radix), *Long Gu* (Draconis, Os), and *Mu Li* (Ostreae, Concha).

Formula

Qi Fu Tang ('Astragalus and Aconitum Decoction')

Huang Qi	Astragali, Radix
Fu Zi	Aconiti Carmichaeli Praeparata, Radix
Sheng Jiang	Zingiberis Officinalis Recens, Rhizoma

Source text: *Lei Zheng Zhi Cai* ('Tailored Treatments Arranged According to Pattern')

Summary

Clinically, the above two causes are the most common. It should be noted, however, that sweating only from the head can arise as a symptom in other syndromes, such as guan-ge ('block and repulsion'), shui jie xiong ('water binding the chest') and Shao Yang syndrome, as well as in geriatric asthma and the extreme stage of yang collapse. These possibilities should be kept in mind during differentiation.

Sweating on the chest (xiong han)

This is also known as 'heart sweating' (xin han), from the location in the center of the chest.

Common symptom patterns

Heart and Spleen qi deficiency. Chest sweating, pale face, lassitude, palpitations, forgetfulness, poor appetite, loose stool, pale tender tongue, weak languid pulse.

Heart and Kidney Yin deficiency. Chest sweating, insomnia, restlessness, palpitations, forgetfulness, tinnitus, dizziness, dry throat and tongue, lower backache and weak legs, excessive dreaming, spermatorrhea, hot flushes, 'steaming bones', scanty dark urine, red tongue with little coat, thready rapid pulse.

Differentiation

Sweating on the chest from Heart and Spleen qi deficiency compared with that from Heart and Kidney yin deficiency. Both are deficiency conditions, but the two differ in etiology and pathological mechanism. Heart and Spleen qi deficiency, leading to sweating on the chest, results from excessive thinking or worry, overwork and irregular eating patterns, all of which can injure the qi of the Spleen and Heart, so that the yang of the chest is not aroused, the local protective qi fails to consolidate the surface, and the jin-ye seeps out. All the symptoms point to deficiency, and the pale face and tongue, plus the latter's tenderness and the weak languid pulse, indicate that the deficiency is that of qi, rather than yin.

Treatment, therefore, should be to tonify Heart and Spleen, consolidate the surface, and stop sweating. Gui Pi Tang ('Restore the Spleen Decoction') can be used, adding *Long Gu* (Draconis, Os) and *Mu Li* (Ostreae, Concha).

The Heart and Kidney yin deficiency which is causing sweating on the chest can be either constitutional, or the result of a long illness or blood loss, or again from excessive worry. Because of the imbalance of relative strengths, yin cannot constrict yang, and this, plus the internal heat generated by the relatively excessive yang, pushes the fluids out leading to sweating. This appears first in the region of the Fire zang-organ itself—the Heart. The accompanying symptoms are the usual yin deficiency with xu-fire flaring indications.

Treatment of xu-fire requires tonification of the Heart and Kidneys to redress the imbalance of yin and yang, and so cool heat. A combination of Tian Wang Bu Xin Dan ('Emperor of Heaven's Special Pill to Tonify the Heart') with Liu Wei Di Huang Wan ('Six-Ingredient Pill with Rehmannia') plus appropriate additions is best.

Formulas

Gui Pi Tang ('Restore the Spleen Decoction')

Ren Shen	Ginseng, Radix
Huang Qi	Astragali, Radix
Bai Zhu	Atractylodis Macrocephalae, Rhizoma
Fu Ling	Poriae Cocos, Sclerotium
Suan Zao Ren	Ziziphi Spinosae, Semen
Long Yan Rou	Euphoriae Longanae, Arillus
Mu Xiang	Saussureae seu Vladimiriae, Radix
Dang Gui	Angelica Polymorpha, Radix
Yuan Zhi	Polygalae Tenuifoliae, Radix
Gan Cao	Glycyrrhizae Uralensis, Radix
Sheng Jiang	Zingiberis Officinalis Recens, Rhizoma
Da Zao	Zizyphi Jujubae, Fructus

Source text: *Ji Sheng Fang* ('Formulas to Aid the Living', 1253) [*Formulas and Strategies*, p. 255]

Tian Wang Bu Xin Dan ('Emperor of Heaven's Special Pill to Tonify the Heart')

Sheng Di	Rehmannia Glutinosae, Radix
Ren Shen	Ginseng, Radix
Tian Men Dong	Asparagi Cochinchinensis, Tuber
Mai Men Dong	Ophiopogonis Japonici, Tuber
Xuan Shen	Scrophulariae Ningpoensis, Radix
Dan Shen	Salviae Miltiorrhizae, Radix
Fu Ling	Poriae Cocos, Sclerotium
Yuan Zhi	Polygalae Tenuifoliae, Radix
Dang Gui	Angelica Polymorpha, Radix
Wu Wei Zi	Schisandrae Chinensis, Fructus
Bo Zi Ren	Biotae Orientalis, Semen
Suan Zao Ren	Ziziphi Spinosae, Semen
Jie Geng	Platycodi Grandiflori, Radix
Zhu Sha	Cinnabaris

Source text: *She Sheng Mi Pou* ('Secret Investigations into Obtaining Health', 1638) [*Formulas and Strategies*, p. 378]

Liu Wei Di Huang Wan ('Six-Ingredient Pill with Rehmannia')

Shou Di	Rehmanniae Glutinosae Conquitae, Radix
Shan Zhu Yu	Corni Officinalis, Fructus
Shan Yao	Dioscoreae Oppositae, Radix
Fu Ling	Poriae Cocos, Sclerotium
Mu Dan Pi	Moutan Radicis, Cortex
Ze Xie	Alismatis Plantago-aquaticae, Rhizoma

Source text: *Xiao Er Yao Zheng Zhi Jue* ('Craft of Medicinal Treatment for Childhood Disease Patterns', 1119) [*Formulas and Strategies*, p. 263]

Classical comments

The *Zhang Shi Yi Tong* ('Comprehensive Medicine According to Master Zhang', 1695) says: 'No other place has sweating, but only the cardiac region of the chest; this is thinking damaging the Heart. Since the problem is in the Heart, the name is 'Heart Sweat'. Gui Pi Tang with doubled *Huang Qi*.'

The *Lei Zheng Zhi Cai* ('Tailored Treatments Arranged According to Pattern') section on 'Sweat Symptoms' says: 'Sweat around the heart is a result of thinking and worry injuring the Spleen.'

Sweating from the hands and feet (shou zu han chu)

The first mention of this symptom is found in the *Shang Han Ming Li Lun* ('Clarification of the Theory of Cold-induced Disorders', 1156), which also says:

'The Stomach rules the four limbs. Sweating from the hands and feet is a Yang Ming symptom.'

However, because it is not a major symptom of the Yang Ming stage of exogenous disease, and will not always occur in that context, Yang Ming etiology will not be covered in this section.

Common symptom patterns

Spleen and Stomach damp-heat. Sweaty hands and feet, stuffy chest and fullness in the epigastrium, no desire for food, heaviness and lethargy, scanty dark urine, yellow greasy tongue coat, pulse ru and rapid, or ru and slippery.

Spleen and Stomach qi deficiency. Sweaty hands and feet, tiredness and lack of energy, shortness of breath and weak voice, cold limbs, poor appetite, loose stool, pale tongue with a white coat, weak forceless pulse.

Spleen and Stomach yin deficiency. Sweaty hands and feet, dry throat and mouth worsening after sleep, poor appetite with a feeling of hunger but no desire to eat, possible dry retching or hiccups, irregular bowel motions. Red tongue with little coat, pulse thready and rapid.

Differentiation

Sweating on the hands and feet from Spleen and Stomach damp-heat. Stomach function is to accept food, while Spleen rules the limbs and controls digestion and distribution of the essential material derived from the food and fluids held by the Stomach.

If the Spleen is injured through overwork or any other reason so that distribution breaks down, or pathogenic damp invades the Spleen and Stomach, then damp will build up and, if obstructed, can turn to heat. Damp holds the heat within and prevents it from being normally dispersed, while heat acts on the damp, causing a 'steaming' effect that allows the normal fluids within the Stomach to be forced outward toward the extremities, resulting in sweating of the hands and feet. Thus the *Shang Han Ming Li Lun* ('Clarification of the Theory of Cold-induced Disorders', 1156) says: 'The reason for sweating on the hands and feet is heat accumulated in the Stomach. This is the 'lateral arrival of the jin-ye'.

Damp pathogen obstruction in the middle disturbs digestive functioning and causes loss of desire for food, stuffy fullness of the chest and epigastrium, and finally heaviness and lethargy. Damp, being heavy itself, usually sinks into the lower Jiao, carrying heat with it, and builds up in the Urinary Bladder so that urine becomes scanty and dark. The portion of damp which is steamed upwards by the heat forms the yellow greasy tongue coat. Rapid and ru (floating thin and weak) pulse is the standard for damp-heat conditions, from the damp oppression of normal qi and blood.

Treatment is to cool heat, parch damp, and harmonize digestion. One can choose or combine Lian Pu Yin and Wei Ling Tang, with appropriate alterations.

Formulas

Lian Po Yin ('Coptis and Magnolia Bark Decoction')

Huang Lian	Coptidis, Rhizoma
Hou Po	Magnoliae Officianalis, Cortex
Shan Zhi Zi	Gardeniae Jasminoidis, Fructus
Dan Dou Chi	Sojae Praeparatum, Semen
Shi Chang Pu	Acori Graminei, Rhizoma
Ban Xia	Pinelliae Ternata, Rhizoma
Lu Gen	Phragmitis Communis, Rhizoma

Source text: *Huo Luan Lun* ('Discussion of Sudden Turmoil Disorders', 1862) [*Formulas and Strategies*, p. 189]

Wei Ling Tang ('Calm the Stomach and Poria Decoction')

Cang Zhu	Atractylodis, Rhizoma
Hou Po	Magnoliae Officianalis, Cortex
Chen Pi	Citri Reticulatae, Pericarpium
Gan Cao	Glycyrrhizae Uralensis, Radix
Sheng Jiang	Zingiberis Officinalis Recens, Rhizoma
Da Zao	Zizyphi Jujubae, Fructus
Ze Xie	Alismatis Plantago-aquaticae, Rhizoma

Fu Ling	Poriae Cocos, Sclerotium
Zhu Ling	Polypori Umbellati, Sclerotium
Bai Zhu	Atractylodis Macrocephalae, Rhizoma
Gui Zhi	Cinnamomi Cassiae, Ramulus

Source text: *Dan Xi Xin Fa* ('Teachings of Dan Xi', 1481) [*Formulas and Strategies*, p. 176]

Sweating on the hands and feet from Spleen and Stomach qi deficiency versus that from Spleen and Stomach yin deficiency. Both are deficiency conditions but the pathological mechanisms are different. Spleen and Stomach qi deficiency results from irregular eating, excessive worry or overwork, and Spleen transportation functions incorrectly so that jin-ye is transported outward toward the limbs, causing sweating of the hands and feet. Differentiation will be made by the accompanying qi deficiency symptoms; chilled limbs indicate that weakness of Spleen qi is beginning to involve Spleen yang. Treatment must be to tonify Spleen qi with a formula like Shen Ling Bai Zhu San ('Ginseng, Poria, and Atractylodes Macrocephala Powder'), adjusted as required.

Spleen and Stomach yin deficiency usually results from either a febrile pathogen damaging yin, or habitual consumption of pungent-hot or rich foods which build up into stagnant heat that overcomes yin. Once yin is damaged, normal yang becomes excessive relative to the weakened yin, and internal xu heat is generated which disturbs the remaining yin fluids, forcing them to flow outwards towards the limbs, causing sweating from the hands and feet. Spleen and Stomach yin deficiency symptoms are also a result of disturbance from this internal heat, such as dryness of the throat and mouth which is more obvious after sleeping. Also because of the disruption to Stomach's ability to hold and warm the food from the lack of yin fluids, there is a sensation of hunger but no desire to eat, and this may worsen into dry retching or hiccups. Bowels will also react, the motions becoming irregular. Red tongue with little coat, thready rapid pulse, these are the standard indications for yin deficiency with fire flaring.

Treatment should be to moisten and nourish Stomach yin with a formula like Sha Shen Mai Men Dong Tang ('Glehnia and Ophiopogonis De-

coction') and appropriate additions such as *Wu Wei Zi* (Schisandrae Chinensis, Fructus).

Formulas

Shen Ling Bai Zhu San ('Ginseng, Poria, and Atractylodes Macrocephala Powder')

Dang Shen	Codonopsis Pilosulae, Radix
Bai Zhu	Atractylodis Macrocephalae, Rhizoma
Fu Ling	Poriae Cocos, Sclerotium
Gan Cao	Glycyrrhizae Uralensis, Radix
Shan Yao	Dioscoreae Oppositae, Radix
Bai Bian Dou	Dolichos Lablab, Semen
Lian Zi	Nelumbinis Nuciferae, Semen
Yi Yi Ren	Coicis Lachryma-jobi, Semen
Sha Ren	Amomi, Fructus et Semen
Jie Geng	Platycodi Grandiflori, Radix

Source text: *Tai Ping Hui Min He Ji Ju Fang* ('Imperial Grace Formulary of the Tai Ping Era', 1078-85) [*Formulas and Strategies*, p. 239]

Sha Shen Mai Men Dong Tang ('Glehnia and Ophiopogonis Decoction')

Sha Shen	Glehniae Littoralis, Radix
Mai Men Dong	Ophiopogonis Japonici, Tuber
Yu Zhu	Polygonati Odorati, Rhizoma
Sang Ye	Mori Albae, Folium
Tian Hua Fen	Trichosanthis, Radix
Bai Bian Dou	Dolichos Lablab, Semen
Gan Cao	Glycyrrhizae Uralensis, Radix

Source text: *Wen Bing Tiao Bian* ('Systematic Differentiation of Warm Diseases', 1798) [*Formulas and Strategies*, p. 161]

Summary

Of the three most common causes of sweating from the hands and feet, damp-heat and deficiency of either qi or yin, the deficiencies are the most often seen. If the qi deficiency is prolonged, the lack of qi will weaken the blood, so that treatment will need to address not only the qi but will also have to tonify blood.

Classical comments

Zhang Shi Yi Tong ('Comprehensive Medicine According to Master Zhang', 1695): 'Hands and feet sweating ... if hot, use Er Chen Tang plus *Huang Lian* and *Bai Shao*; if cold, use Li Zhong Tang plus *Wu Mei*; if weak, use Shi Quan Da Bu Wan, removing *Chuan Xiong*, but adding *Wu Wei Zi*.'

Underarm sweating (ye xia han)

This refers to continual moisture, or even continual dripping sweat from the armpits, so that the ribs are wet. In fact the condition in a number of texts is actually referred to as 'sweating of the ribs'.

Common symptom patterns

Liver deficiency internal heat. Underarm perspiration but without offensive odor, restlessness, excessive dreaming and difficulty sleeping, easily startled, dizziness, lack of strength, facial pallor, hot flushes after noon or five-hearts heat, dry throat and mouth, red tongue with little coat, pulse wiry thready rapid.

Liver and Gall Bladder damp-heat. Underarm perspiration, but with an offensive odor, stuffy chest, loss of appetite, bitter taste and sticky sensation in the mouth, thirst without desire to drink, sensation of heaviness, lethargy, scanty dark yellow urine, yellow greasy tongue coat, wiry rapid pulse.

Differentiation

Underarm sweating from Liver deficiency internal heat versus that from Liver and Gall Bladder damp-heat. Both conditions have heat manifestations, and both involve the Liver but differ in pathological mechanism. Liver and Gall Bladder control the region under the arms, through channel distribution, and it is along the channel pathway that the sweating mostly occurs. Either deficiency of Liver yin and blood, or obstructive damp-heat, can interfere with Liver movement, and disrupt normal traffic through the channels, so that fluids seep out as sweat. Thus Shen Jin-Ao, in his *Za Bing Yuan Liu Xi Zhu* ('Wondrous Lantern for Peering into the

Origin and Development of Miscellaneous Diseases', 1773), in its section on 'Origins of Sweating' says: 'When a pathogen is in the exterior, the surface tissues (cou li) fail to close, and sweat exudes from the jing luo.'

Liver becomes deficient in blood and yin either after illness, or following a period of overwork, or even excessive thinking and desire damaging the jing and blood, so that weak Liver yin, on the one hand, cannot ensure the patency of Liver qi, while on the other, internal xu-heat resulting from an imbalanced relative excess of yang building up forces the fluids outwards. Since the source of the heat is the Liver, the first area to manifest the sweating is the course of the Liver channel above the zang itself, as heat tends to rise.

Important points in differentiating underarm sweating from Liver deficiency internal heat are the lack of offensive odor, and the presence of Liver deficiency and internal heat signs, such as restless insomnia, dreaming, jumpiness, thirst, five-hearts heat and hot flushes.

Treatment should be to nourish yin, soften the Liver, and cool heat. Liu Wei Di Huang Wan ('Six-Ingredient Pill with Rehmannia') combined with Yi Guan Jian ('Linking Decoction') should be used internally, while externally Mu Fan Dan ('Ostreae, Alum and Minium Pill') can be rubbed underneath the arms.

Underarm sweating from Liver and Gall Bladder damp-heat results from the obstruction to the channels by the damp-heat which has accumulated internally in the Liver and Gall Bladder. As the *Za Bing Yuan Liu Xi Zhu* ('Wondrous Lantern for Peering into the Origin and Development of Miscellaneous Diseases', 1773) in its section on sweat notes: 'Sweating under both arms ... that has continued for a long time without clearing up is the flow of damp-heat.'

The important differentiating points are the odor of the perspiration and the signs of the damp-heat accumulating in the Liver and Gall Bladder: fullness in the chest, loss of appetite, bitter taste and greasy sticky sensation in the mouth, thirst but no desire to drink, exhaustion with a feeling of heaviness, scanty dark urine, yellow greasy tongue coat and a wiry rapid pulse.

Treatment requires cooling heat and promoting the expulsion of damp. Long Dan Xie Gan Tang

('Gentiana Longdancao Decoction to Drain the Liver') with alterations can be used internally, while externally Mu Fan Dan can be rubbed underneath the arms.

Formulas

Liu Wei Di Huang Wan ('Six-Ingredient Pill with Rehmannia')

Shou Di	Rehmanniae Glutinosae Conquitae, Radix
Shan Zhu Yu	Corni Officinalis, Fructus
Shan Yao	Dioscoreae Oppositae, Radix
Fu Ling	Poriae Cocos, Sclerotium
Mu Dan Pi	Moutan Radicis, Cortex
Ze Xie	Alismatis Plantago-aquaticae, Rhizoma

Source text: *Xiao Er Yao Zheng Zhi Jue* ('Craft of Medicinal Treatment for Childhood Disease Patterns', 1119) [*Formulas and Strategies*, p. 263]

Yi Guan Jian ('Linking Decoction')

Sheng Di	Rehmannia Glutinosae, Radix
Gou Qi Zi	Lycii Chinensis, Fructus
Sha Shen	Glehniae Littoralis, Radix
Mai Men Dong	Ophiopogonis Japonici, Tuber
Dang Gui	Angelica Polymorpha, Radix
Chuan Lian Zi	Meliae Toosendan, Fructus

Source text: *Xu Ming Yi Lei An* ('Continuation of Famous Physicians' Cases Organized by Categories', 1770) [*Formulas and Strategies*, p. 271]

Mu Fan Dan ('Ostreae, Alum and Minium Pill')

Mu Li	Ostreae, Concha
Ku Fan	Alum
Huang Dan	Minium

Source text: *Lei Zheng Zhi Cai* ('Tailored Treatments Arranged According to Pattern')

Long Dan Xie Gan Tang ('Gentiana Longdancao Decoction to Drain the Liver')

Long Dan Cao	Gentianae Scabrae, Radix
Huang Qin	Scutellariae Baicalensis, Radix
Shan Zhi Zi	Gardeniae Jasminoidis, Fructus
Mu Tong	Mutong, Caulis
Che Qian Zi	Plantaginis, Semen
Ze Xie	Alismatis Plantago-aquaticae, Rhizoma
Chai Hu	Bupleuri, Radix
Sheng Di	Rehmannia Glutinosae, Radix
Dang Gui	Angelica Polymorpha, Radix
Gan Cao	Glycyrrhizae Uralensis, Radix

Source text: *Yi Fang Ji Jie* ('Analytic Collection of Medical Formulas', 1682) [*Formulas and Strategies*, p. 96]

Classical comments

Za Bing Yuan Liu Xi Zhu: 'Further movement and draining is forbidden when treating sweating from Liver deficiency. Bai Shao Tang should be used... *Suan Zao Ren* and *Shan Yao* should be used for sweat from the Liver.'

Lei Zheng Zhi Cai: 'When Shao Yang has heat involved ... there may be underarm sweat or flank sweating. It should be realized that if, at the time when yin and yang alternate, there is leakage at the place where yin and yang alternate, then this is yin-yang disharmony at the mid-stage level between interior and exterior. Xiao Chai Hu Tang and Xiao Yao San should be combined.'

Formulas

Xiao Chai Hu Tang ('Minor Bupleurum Decoction')

Chai Hu	Bupleuri, Radix
Huang Qin	Scutellariae Baicalensis, Radix
Ban Xia	Pinelliae Ternata, Rhizoma
Dang Shen	Codonopsis Pilosulae, Radix
Sheng Jiang	Zingiberis Officinalis Recens, Rhizoma
Gan Cao	Glycyrrhizae Uralensis, Radix
Da Zao	Zizyphi Jujubae, Fructus

Source text: *Shang Han Lun* ('Discussion of Cold-Induced Disorders', 210AD) [*Formulas and Strategies*, p. 136]

Xiao Yao San ('Rambling Powder')

Chai Hu	Bupleuri, Radix
Dang Gui	Angelica Polymorpha, Radix
Bai Shao	Paeoniae Lactiflora, Radix

Bai Zhu	Atractylodis Macrocephalae, Rhizoma
Fu Ling	Poriae Cocos, Sclerotium
Bo He	Menthae, Herba
Gan Cao	Glycyrrhizae Uralensis, Radix

Source text: *Tai Ping Hui Min He Ji Ju Fang* ('Imperial Grace Formulary of the Tai Ping Era', 1078-85) [*Formulas and Strategies*, p. 147]

SWEAT AND ACUPUNCTURE

The acupuncture treatment of sweating will, of course, also require accurate differentiation of the underlying cause of the imbalance, and the appropriate choice of points and manipulation to restore harmony within the affected channels.

The use of the two points He Gu (LI-4) and Fu Liu (KI-7) to promote or reduce sweating is noted in many of the ancient texts and 'Songs of Acupuncture'.

The *Yu Long Fu* ('Jade Dragon Verses') says, for example: 'Lack of sweat from shang han (cold-injury) attack, Fu Liu (KI-7) should be reduced. Shang han with sweating, select He Gu (LI-4).'

The *Yu Long Ge* ('Song of the Jade Dragon') says, similarly: 'Lack of sweat from shang han, reduce Fu Liu (KI-7); profuse sweat use He Gu (LI-4) to constrict.'

The *Zhou Hou Ge* ('Songs from the *Zhen Jiu Ju Ying*') notes: 'Lack of sweat when there should be sweating, reduce He Gu (LI-4); spontaneous perspiration with jaundice, rely on Fu Liu (KI-7).'

Zhen Jiu Da Cheng ('The Great Compendium of Acupuncture') states: 'Profuse sweat, first reduce He Gu (LI-4), then tonify Fu Liu (KI-7); scant sweat first tonify He Gu (LI-4) and then reduce Fu Liu (KI-7).'

The *Yi Xue Gang Mu* ('Outline of Medicine') says: 'Shang han with sweat unable to escape, needle He Gu (LI-4) and Fu Liu (KI-7), reducing both.'

The *Shi Si Jing Yao Xue Zhu Zhi Ge* ('Song of the Main Indications of the Important Points on the Fourteen Channels') points out: 'Fu Liu (KI-7)...must be quickly reduced if perspiration is absent in shang han, [so that even if] the six pulses are all deep and hidden, this will spread [and restore the zheng qi by eliminating the influence of the pathogen deep within the body].[15]

The *Yi Xue Ru Men* ('Introduction to Medicine') has the following detailed recommendations:

The method of sweating [as a treatment] in shang han: needle He Gu (LI-4) shallowly (literally 'two fen'), and, using the 9x9 method, twist it several tens of times, males twist left, females twist right; once the sweat begins, then use reducing method, when the sweat stops and the body feels warm, remove the needle. If the sweat does not stop, needle Yin Shi (ST-33) and tonify He Gu (LI-4).[16]

Obviously there are a number of contradictions between the various recommendations quoted above. Some say to tonify He Gu (LI-4) for lack of sweat in exterior-cold (shang han) conditions while others say to reduce, and the same for Fu Liu (KI-7), and again contradictions appear if there is sweating.

Looking at the point physiology may provide a rational basis for deciding which approach makes more sense.

He Gu (LI-4) is generally conceded to be an important point for the control of sweating, being known as a 'han xue'—a 'sweat point'.

It is the yuan-source point of the Hand Yang Ming Large Intestine channel, which because of its connection to the Stomach (Yang Ming) channel contains a full measure of qi and blood, and therefore He Gu (LI-4) shares with Zu San Li (ST-36) the distinction of being a major tonification point for both qi and blood. The ability of blood to move continuously through the mai (vessels) depends, besides the Heart functioning, upon the qi which leads it and restores it. 'Blood relies upon qi for production, and also relies upon qi for movement.'[17]

If blood is deficient, tonifying He Gu (LI-4) can supplement the blood through enhancing the qi. 'The material blood cannot produce itself, it is produced through the immaterial qi.'[18]

On the other hand, reducing He Gu (LI-4) can assist qi movement in case of obstruction and, by moving the qi, also encourage the movement of blood and so diminish blood stagnation.

When He Gu's powerful ability to tonify and remove obstruction in both the qi and the blood is considered in the light of its connection with the Lungs (i.e. it is the Yuan-source point on the yang channel interiorly-exteriorly connected with the

Lungs—which rule the skin), then the importance of He Gu (LI-4) as a point for controlling sweat should become clear.

Considering the factors mentioned above, it would appear most correct to reduce He Gu (LI-4) in the case of exterior wind-cold blocking the surface with lack of sweating, in order to remove obstruction in the flow of protective qi, thereby opening the exterior and expelling the pathogen with the sweat in a manner similar to Ma Huang Tang ('Ephedra Decoction').

In the opposite case, where exogenous wind has dispersed the protective qi so that the pores are uncontrolled and abnormal sweating is taking place, tonification of He Gu (LI-4) will bolster the available qi for protection. This will allow both expulsion of the pathogen and recovery of authority over the functioning of the pores, and so stop the sweating.

Fu Liu (KI-7) is the Metal point on the Kidney channel, which makes it the mother point (Metal produces Water) of the Kidneys. Its effect is primarily tonification of Kidney yin (moistening, sinking, contracting). The action of Fu Liu (KI-7) in sweating disorders is mainly that of either restoring yin-fluids lost through sweating, or supplementing Kidney yin in order to control flaring fire from deficient yin.

In the first case, sweating may be occurring because of exogenous wind on the exterior disturbing pore control, as described above. Here, tonification of He Gu (LI-4) to enhance protective qi may be combined with tonification of Fu Liu (KI-7) to restore basic fluids, weakened by the continuous perspiration. This resembles the action of Gui Zhi Tang ('Cinnamon Decoction') in which *Gui Zhi* (Cinnamomi Cassiae, Ramulus), acting to warm the surface and expel the pathogen, is combined with *Bai Shao* (Paeoniae Lactiflora, Radix), which is sour contracting and fluid restoring.

The second case, that of fire flaring from lack of yin to control yang, leading to nightsweats, is best treated by strengthening Kidney yin through tonifying Fu Liu (KI-7), while cooling and clearing Heart fire by reducing Yin Xi (HT-6), the xi-cleft point on the Heart channel. The action of xi-cleft points is to constrict, stop pain, and stop bleeding. Here, the required action is, of course, constriction.[19]

Classical essays

1. Sweat is transformed from the body's fluids

The following is from the *Zhi Yi Lu* ('Investigation into Matters of Doubt', 1687), by Zhang Jing-Yue.

Most books of prescriptions say that blood and sweat are 'of two names, but of one type'. Because of this, [Zhu] Dan Xi formed his doctrine of 'Internally it is blood, externally it is sweat', as if blood is sweat and sweat is blood! Does he not know the origin of the two, and that one cannot talk of the two as being in the same category?

The Classic says: 'The Heart rules blood, blood is produced in the Heart.'[20]

The Classics also say: 'Kidneys control the Five Fluids, [that which] enters the Heart becomes blood'. And again it says: 'Sweat, the fluid of the Heart.'[21]

This says sweat is 'the fluid of the Heart', it does not say 'the blood of the Heart'.

Blood is produced in the Heart, is controlled by the Spleen, and is stored in the Liver, but its origin is the essential qi of foods and fluids received in the middle Jiao, then transformed to extract the liquid (zhi), which is finally harmonized with the Five Zang and distributed throughout the Six Fu, in order to nourish and develop the whole body.

But as to sweat, it is the fluid of the body which, if the surface tissues are open [so that] the skin cannot protect the exterior, and pathogenic wind, summerheat, damp, or heat disrupts it, will emanate like steam and overflow as sweat.

This sweat is transformed through the body's yang qi, hence the saying 'Yang added to yin is called sweat.'[22]

We should say 'internally it is qi, externally it is sweat'. We can talk about qi here, but cannot class [sweat] with blood.

Do they mean to say that the exterior sweat can be mixed up with the interior blood?!

In the body, there are nasal mucus, tears, watery saliva (xian), mucoid saliva (tuo), stool, and urine, all of which are transformed from a single Water, and excreted from the nine orifices. Thus that which the nose excretes is called nasal mucus, that which the eyes excrete is called tears, that which the mouth excretes is called saliva, that which the lower orifices excrete is called stool and urine, and that which the skin excretes is then called sweat.

If sweat can be classed with blood, then surely nasal mucus, tears, saliva, stool, and urine can also be categorized in the same way?!2[23]

2. Spontaneous perspiration and nightsweats

The following is part of the introduction to the treatment of spontaneous perspiration and nightsweats found in the *Jing Yue Quan Shu* ('Complete Works of Jing-Yue', 1624).

The single symptom of sweating can be divided into spontaneous perspiration and nightsweats. Spontaneous perspiration breaks out at any time, and is worse with exertion. Nightsweats occur in the midst of sleep, can be all over the body, and gradually diminish with awakening.

All the ancient precepts say: spontaneous perspiration is yang deficiency, the surface tissues are not consolidated, and this is under the control of the protective qi. The protective qi consolidates the exterior of a person's body, and if it does not consolidate, then the exterior is open, spontaneous perspiration occurs, and the jin-ye are drained away. The treatment should be to strengthen the exterior and tonify the yang.

Nightsweats are from yin deficiency: if yin is weak, yang will certainly encroach upon it. Thus yang steaming the yin level will lead to heat in the blood, heat in the blood will lead to fluids (ye) being forced out, and this becomes nightsweats. The treatment should be to cool the heat and tonify the yin.

This is the standard approach, and as such cannot be ignored.

All this notwithstanding, as I see it, spontaneous perspiration also has [cases of] yin deficiency, nightsweats also have [cases of] yang deficiency. If you come across high fever from internal injury, for example, the vast majority will have spontaneous perspiration. Thus whether this is fire in the Stomach from food or drink, or the deficient fire of exhaustion arising from the Spleen, or excessive alcohol or sex leading to fire in the Kidneys, all of these can make people sweat spontaneously. In these cases, if this is not called yang excess with yin deficiency, what is it?

Again, a person's sleep and wakefulness is after all a result of the movement of protective qi into and out of [the interior]. Protective qi is yang qi, and when a person sleeps, then protective qi moves into the yin levels. At this time, if yang qi is not deficient externally, what is it?

Therefore spontaneous perspiration and nightsweats each have yin and yang patterns, and it will not do to say that spontaneous perspiration must be yang deficiency, nightsweats must be yin deficiency.

Having established that yin and yang may have different [results], how are they to be differentiated?

I say: simply check if the patient has fire or not, then whether it is yin or is yang can be seen naturally. This is so because in those cases of sweating with prevailing fire, the yin deficiency can be known from the incineration of yin by the fire; in those cases of sweating without fire, the deficiency of yang can be known from the inability to consolidate the surface.

For those who know these two things, the essentials of sweating will have no other [hidden] meanings, and the general methods of treatment can also be deduced.[24]

NOTES

1. *Lei Jing* ('Systematic Categorization of the *Nei Jing*'), 1624, by Zhang Jing-Yue; People's Health Publishing, 1982, p. 84.
2. *Lu Shan Tang Lei Bian* ('Catalogued Differentiations from Lu Shan Hall'), 1670, Zhang Zhi-Cong; Jiangsu Science and Technology Press, 1982, p. 34. For the continuation of this quote, see note 2 in Chapter 2.
3. Zhang Yin-An, *Huang Di Nei Jing Su Wen Ji Zhu* ('Collected Annotations to the *Huang Di Nei Jing Su Wen*') Chapter 33, Shanghai Science and Technology Press, 1959, from note p. 131.
4. *ibid.* Chapter 5, p. 27.
5. *Zhu Bing Yuan Hou Lun Jiao Shi*, People's Health Publishing, 1982, Vol. 2, p. 871.
6. Beginning students often ask 'Well, why are there chills when there is so much heat at the surface?' The answer is that the surface heat is pathological heat, which cannot perform the functions of normal physiological heat within the body. Anyone who has had a fever, with simultaneous chills, can feel the difference once it has been drawn to their attention.
7. This discussion of sweating in warm disease is based on that in the *Wen Bing Shu Ping* ('Review of Warm Disease'), edited by Guo Qian-Heng, *Shanxi* Science and Technology Press, 1987, pp. 97-100.
8. The importance of differentiating this lack of sweating from the previously mentioned case of wind-cold attack cannot be over-emphasized. Luckily, the history and the accompanying symptoms are such that differentiation is not difficult.
9. For example, an exogenous cold pathogenic invasion not expelled in its initial stages can move into the interior, further damaging yang qi, and eventually leading to serious illness.
10. *Wen Bing Tiao Bian Bai Hua Jie* ('Vernacular Explanation of the Systematic Differentiation of Warm Diseases'), from the chapter 'Discussion of Sweat', Zhejiang TCM College, published by People's Health Publishing, 1978, p. 185.
11. Extracted from Dr. Gong Wen-De *et al.*, 'Differentiation and Treatment of 85 cases of Obstructed Perspiration' (in Chinese), Journal of Traditional Chinese Medicine, 1991, Vol. 32, no. 8, pp. 22-24.
12. Thus Tang Rong-Chuan (1862-1918) in the *Xue Zheng Lun* ('Discussion of Blood Syndromes', 1884)

says: 'in terms of interior and exterior, the qi of Shao Yang moves internally through the San Jiao and externally through the surface tissues (cou li), becoming the pivotal mechanism for the nutritive and protective qi'. *Xue Zheng Lun*, People's Health Publishing, 1986, p. 30.
13. It may be asked why the damp itself does not block the pores. It can do so, as will be seen in the section to follow on sweating from the head, but this does not inevitably happen. The effects of a pathogen on an individual patient will depend on a myriad of factors, including constitution, habitual activity, diet and past history.
14. See also Chapter 5 for more information on yellow sweat.
15. 'Fu Liu ... shang han wu han ji xie zi, liu mai chen fu ji ke shen'. In shang han, the pulses should be tight and floating if the problem is only on the surface. The deep hidden pulses here show that the pathogen has influenced the deep interior, a dangerous situation requiring Fu Liu (KI-7) to be 'quickly reduced', expelling the pathogen from the Kidney channel and allowing the zheng qi to restore itself—and therefore the pulse. From the *Zhen Jiu Ge Fu Jiao Shi* ('Comparative Explanations of the Songs of Acupuncture'), Shanxi Science and Educational Press, 1987, p. 171.
16. Li Chan, *Yi Xue Ru Men* ('Introduction to Medicine', 1575) Jiangxi Science and Technology Press, 1988, p. 226.
17. xue lai qi sheng, you lai qi xing.
18. you xing zhi xue bu neng zi sheng, sheng yu wu xing zhi qi.
19. Further suggestions for acupuncture treatment of the individual symptoms discussed above may be found in the 'Journal of Chinese Medicine', (UK), January, 1992, Number 38, pp. 30-33. This article—to my great chagrin!—used the same source material as that from which the 'Differentiation' section above is taken: the popular modern work *Zhong Yi Zheng Zhuang Jian Bie Zhen Duan Xue* ('Diagnostic Studies of Symptom Differentiation in Chinese Medicine'), People's Health Publishing, 1985, pp. 19-30.
20. *Su Wen*, Chapter 44, 'On Atrophy Syndrome' says: 'The Heart controls the blood and Mai—vessels and

pulse—of the body.' The *Su Wen*, Chapter 5, says: 'The Heart produces the blood.'

21. *Su Wen*, Chapter 23, says: 'The fluids transformed through the Five Zang: for the Heart it is sweat, for the Lungs it is nasal mucus, for the Liver it is tears, for the Spleen it is watery saliva (xian), and for the Kidneys it is mucoid saliva (tuo). These are called the Five Fluids.'

22. From the *Su Wen*, Chapter 7.

23. *Zhi Yi Lun* ('Investigation into Matters of Doubt', 1687), by Zhang Jing–Yue; Jiangsu Science and Technology Press, 1981, pp. 27-28.

24. *Jing Yue Quan Shu* ('Complete Works of Jing Yue'), 1624, by Zhang Jing-Yue; Shanghai Science and Technology Press, 1991, pp. 214-215.

Urination 4

The excretion of urine is directly controlled by the Urinary Bladder but is also closely related to the functioning of the Kidneys' qi transformation, the transport and transformation of the Spleen, the regular spread and descent of the Lung qi, and the maintenance of open fluid pathways by the San Jiao. The urination will also reflect the state of the fluids within the body.

Under normal circumstances, the frequency and amount of urine excreted by a healthy person will vary according to the amount of fluid intake, the temperature, the amount of perspiration, the consumption (or not) of diuretic beverages and food, and the person's age. Pathological situations such as deficiency of jin and ye fluids or disturbed qi transformation allowing pathological water to accumulate will lead to abnormalities in the frequency, amount and sensations of urination.

PHYSIOLOGY

The basic mechanisms of fluid metabolism have already been covered. This short section will expand upon several important concepts not covered previously which are directly involved in Urinary Bladder physiology and pathology.

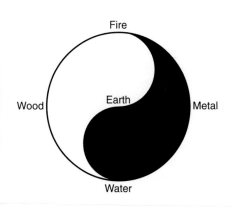

Fig. 4.1

Mingmen

The Urinary Bladder, the lowest organ in the body, is the yang organ of the Water phase, with all the qualities and attributes of that phase, with one additional property: as the yang aspect of Water, it is the place where the warming yuan qi issues from the Kidneys to be spread around the body by the San Jiao.[1]

The meaning and implications of this can be understood by a look at Figure 4.1.

As yin enters the phase of Water, it reaches its ultimate influence but maintains within itself the seed of yang. That seed is the Mingmen fire, the 'fire contained within water' symbolized by the trigram Kan (The Abysmal, Water ☵) a yang line between two yin lines. This fire is also known as 'long-lei zhi huo': Dragon-thunder fire.[2]

At the extreme of yin, yang is born, moving (up and to the left) out of Water and growing into Wood's Shao Yang[3], finally manifesting (like the sun rising in the East) as Fire, the energy of the South, noon, and Summer. This is symbolized by the trigram Li (The Clinging, the Sun ☲) a yin line between two yang lines. Thus Zhao Xian-Ke says 'Fire is yang outside but yin inside'.

This process of yang growth is matched within the body by the circulation of yang-natured yuan qi, moving out of Mingmen, through the yang Water organ (Urinary Bladder), into Wood's Shao Yang San Jiao to be carried upward throughout the body, and finally linking with Fire—the Heart. After yang Fire reaches its extreme (e.g. at noon or high Summer, or any other situation where yang has reached a peak), then yin begins its gradual descent through Metal, settling, slowing and contracting, to reach completion in Water.[4]

Zhang Jing-Yue has this (among much else) to say about Mingmen:

Mingmen is the Sea of Jing-essence and Blood; Spleen and Stomach are the Sea of Food and Fluids; these two form the basis of the Five Zang and Six Fu. Mingmen is the root of yuan (source) qi, and the residence of water and fire. Without it, the yin qi of the Five Zang cannot be nourished; without it, the yang qi of the Five Zang cannot expand ...

Mingmen has fire as a symbol; this refers to the original yang (yuan yang 元陽), which is the fire that produces things ... But how could it all come back to Mingmen? [People] do not know that the Fire in the midst of Water is none other than the First True Qi of Heaven, stored in the midst of Kan ☵. This qi rises from below, connecting to the Stomach qi of later heaven to produce transformation, and thus sustains the basis of the production of life (sheng sheng zhi ben). Thus the glory of a bloom stems from its root, the functioning of a stove-pot from the firewood [beneath it] ...

The life-giving qi of Mingmen is the eternal movement of the Original [yang, symbolized by the trigram] Qian (The Creative, Heaven ☰) without creation there is cessation. Now yang controls movement, yin controls stillness; yang controls ascent, yin controls descent. Only through movement and rising can yang obtain the quality of creating (sheng qi); only through stillness and descending can yin obtain the quality of dying off (si qi). Thus the qi of Original Qian begins below but flourishes above: through rising it moves toward life; the qi of Original [yin, symbolized by the trigram] Kun (The Receptive, Earth, ☷) begins above but reaches completion below: through descending it moves toward death. Therefore yang is produced from the midst of zi 子, and first rises then descends; yin is produced from the midst of wu 午, and first descends then rises ...

Mingmen has a doorway which is the gate of consolidation for the whole body (wei yi shen gong gu zhi guan ye). The Classics say: 'The reason that the granary cannot store is that the doorway is not fastened[5]. The reason that the stream of water cannot be stopped is that the Urinary Bladder cannot store. Those which can maintain, live; those which lose the ability to maintain, die.' And again: 'The Kidneys are the floodgate of the Stomach; if the floodgate cannot move smoothly, the water will accumulate and gather with its kind'.[6] And yet again: 'The North is black, and relates to the Kidneys, which open into the two lower orifices'.[7] From these we can see that the master of the door of the North is the Kidneys, but the governing command of the Kidneys is in Mingmen. Now Mingmen is the axis of the North Pole,[8] holding the rod [of authority] in control over yin and yang; if yin and yang are in harmony then exiting and entering are in order, if yin and yang are diseased then opening and closing are in disarray. Thus there are those with urinary obstruction from exhaustion of yin and parched water: dried and withered, it cannot flow; there are those with unstoppable leakage and draining from yang deficiency and failed fire: holding in and containing have lost control. Once yin jing-essence is exhausted, without strengthening water it will be unable to flow; once yang qi is deficient, without assisting fire it will not be able to consolidate. This is the standard method. But jing-essence without qi cannot move, just as qi without water cannot transform, and in this there is also the subtle employment of 'separable' and 'inseparable' which is within the ken of the wise, but which cannot be completely expressed with paper and ink.[9]

Kidney qi consolidation

Kidney qi is derived from the steaming action of Kidney yang on the Kidney yin, and thus Kidney qi deficiency is based upon deficiency of either Kidney yang or Kidney yin, and symptoms of Kidney qi deficiency will usually be accompanied by symptoms of Kidney yin or Kidney yang weakness.

Lack of Kidney qi consolidation (Shen qi bu gu) is based upon Kidney qi deficiency. The functions of Kidney qi are to nourish and support the tendons and bones, especially those of the lower back and the knees. This is the reason that Kidney deficiency will often manifest weakness and aching of these areas: there is lack of normal nourishment. Because Kidney qi is the 'True qi' (zhen qi) underlying all of the qi processes in the body, when Kidney qi is weak there will usually be symptoms of generalized qi deficiency as well, such as tiredness and lack of spirit, pale face, pale tongue, and deep weak pulse.

Urinary Bladder's consolidation—its ability to hold in urine—depends primarily upon the Kidney qi. If the Kidney qi becomes weak, the Urinary Bladder consolidation will lack support and this will be reflected in frequent or uncontrolled urination. Nocturia or enuresis can reflect a borderline Kidney qi deficiency: normally controlled during the day when yang qi is at its best, the weakening of yang qi at night with the preponderance of yin influence overcomes the ability of the Kidney qi to assist Urinary Bladder control, and urination becomes frequent or incontinent. The *Zhu Bing Yuan Hou Lun* ('General Treatise on the Etiology and Symptomatology of Disease', 610 AD) describes the process in the context of enuresis (niao chuang):

When a person during sleep voids urine without realizing, this is the result of a constitution which is relatively predominant in yin and relatively deficient in yang; the qi of both the Kidney and Urinary Bladder is then cold and unable to effect a warming controlling influence on the water [in the Urinary Bladder], thus urine becomes profuse or even incontinent. Urinary Bladder is Foot Tai Yang and is the fu-organ of the Kidneys; Kidneys are Foot Shao Yin, and are the zang-organ [responsible for storage] connected to the Urinary Bladder; both control water.

In terms of a person's yin and yang, the normal order of circulation for the yang [-natured protective (wei) qi] is to move through the yang levels [during the day], but as the sun sets, the [protective] qi enters the [Foot Shao Yin channel] yin levels, and by the middle of the night this meeting of [yin and yang] qi allows one to sleep.

Now urine is the residue from the body's fluids (shui ye zhi yu) which has entered the Urinary Bladder, from which it will be expelled as urine. At night during sleep the yang qi is weak and subdued (衰伏 shuai fu); it is unable to exert control over [the night-time's predominant] yin. Thus the yin qi, unbalanced by yang energy, is overbearing, and water descends without control causing enuresis.[10]

Weakness of Kidney qi does not only cause incontinence of urine but can also lead to lack of force in the expulsion of urine, so that the contents of the Urinary Bladder are not completely expelled and terminal dribbling occurs.

Lack of Kidney qi consolidation can also affect the storage of Kidney jing-essence, so that jing leaks out into the urine causing spermaturia.[11]

PATHOLOGY

Abnormalities in the amount of urine

Increased amount. There are two primary mechanisms involved in this condition. The first mechanism is pathogenic cold obstructing the qi mechanism so that fluids are not transformed and instead pour down into the Urinary Bladder, where the cold interferes with the ability of the Urinary Bladder to transform and the Kidneys to gather and store, leading to profuse output of urine.

The second mechanism is Kidney yang failing to support Urinary Bladder qi transformation of fluids already received from the other areas of the body. Fluids from which reusable qi has not been recovered accumulate in the Urinary Bladder, and the weakened Kidneys, which rule the lower orifices, are unable to maintain consolidation and thus urine becomes profuse.

These two mechanisms are similar in that both involve cold but differ in the role that deficiency plays. The cold in the first mechanism can be shi-cold (excess cold) resulting either from exogenous invasion or intake of cold food and fluids, or it can be xu-cold developed as a result of general yang deficiency in the body. In either situation, it is the excessive influence of the cold which interferes with the fluid metabolism. In the second mechanism, deficiency is primary: the yang qi of the Kidneys does not support Urinary Bladder's separation of reusable qi from the fluids it is holding.

Decreased amount. Decreased amount of urine can result from either reduced fluid levels in the body or failure of these fluids to undergo qi transformation in the Urinary Bladder.

In the first situation, there may have been increased perspiration so that fluids are eliminated through the skin rather than through the urine, or vomiting or diarrhea causing loss of fluids, or lack of fluid intake, or internal pathogenic heat (excess or deficient heat) may have dried the fluids.

In the second situation, impaired qi transformation of fluids from yang qi deficiency can result in fluids not reaching the Urinary Bladder to be eliminated (or failing to be transformed after they have reached the Urinary Bladder), but instead these fluids flood outward to the surface and cause edema.

Abnormalities in frequency

Increased frequency. Damp-heat or cold-damp in the Urinary Bladder are the two most common excess conditions leading to frequency of urination, due to interference of the pathogenic damp in the qi transformation of the Urinary Bladder. Liver qi blockage, however, can also be involved because obstruction at the intersection of the Liver channel directly above the Urinary Bladder will influence qi flow throughout the whole area.

Many types of deficiency can result in increased urinary frequency, such as Kidney yin deficiency leading to internal heat which then forces fluids out of the Urinary Bladder; or Kidney yang deficiency both failing to support Urinary Bladder qi transformation and failing to consolidate the lower orifice so that untransformed fluids build-up and demand frequent elimination; or Lung and Spleen qi deficiency allowing large amounts of untransformed fluid to pour down into the Urinary Bladder which, overwhelmed, has no choice but to expel the fluids as urine.

Nocturia and incontinence are more extreme examples of increased frequency. Nocturia usually results from yang deficiency, either solely of the Kidneys, or of both the Kidneys and the Spleen, so that during the night when yang is at its weakest, yang fails to maintain consolidation and urine is uncontrolled. Incontinence can result from the same mechanisms as the above, or involve Lung and Spleen qi deficiency, or pent-up heat in the Urinary Bladder, or Kidney yin deficiency with internal heat. Incontinence in the sequelae of wind-stroke is a sign of general disruption to qi flow throughout the whole body.

Decreased frequency. The mechanisms for decreased frequency of urination are generally the same as those discussed under decreased amount of urination, unless there is hesitancy or dribbling, or the urination is partially or completely obstructed. Hesitancy or dribbling can result from Urinary Bladder damp-heat, or cold in the Urinary Bladder, or Spleen qi deficiency.

In damp-heat, the mechanism producing dribbling is as follows: the damp prevents complete expulsion of the urine, while the expanding nature of the pathogenic heat prevents complete closure of the lower orifice, resulting in dribbling.

In the latter two cases, the mechanisms are similar to those discussed in the previous sections: cold in the Urinary Bladder results from insufficient Kidney yang, which cannot consolidate the lower orifice; deficient Spleen qi fails to rise, but instead descends, so that the lack of lifting ascent by the middle Jiao qi plays a role similar to that of any prolapse, and urine continues to dribble out.

Partial or complete obstruction of urination is called 'long bi' 癃闭 (see the detailed differentiation section), and can result from both excess or deficiency mechanisms. The excess mechanisms include Urinary Bladder damp-heat, Lung qi obstruction, Liver qi blockage, and stagnant blood in the Urinary Bladder. The deficiency mechanisms involve middle Jiao Spleen qi deficiency and lower Jiao Kidney yang deficiency. (For detailed mechanisms of the pathologies involved see the differentiation section.)

Abnormalities in the sensations of urination

Burning urination. A burning sensation with urination can result from Urinary Bladder damp-heat, Heart fire passing into the Small Intestine, Liver qi blockage producing fire, or Kidney yin deficiency with internal xu-heat.

Painful urination. Pain with urination can be the result of burning, and so can be caused by any of the factors discussed above; or it can be the result of stagnant blood or stones in the Urinary Bladder, or Liver qi obstruction, any of which will cause sensations of strangulating pain or stabbing pricking pain in the urethra.

Difficult urination. The mechanisms producing sensations of difficulty in urination are the same as those described under decreased amount and frequency of urination in the sections above.

DIFFERENTIATION OF URINARY SYMPTOMS

This section will cover the differentiation and treatment of darkish urine, cloudy urine, clear profuse urine, difficult urination, anuria, frequent urination, dribbling after urination, incontinence, nocturia, enuresis, painful urination, hematuria, and spermaturia.

Darkish urine

This means urine that is yellow, dark yellow, or even brown. It does not include differentiation of hematuria, which will be covered in a separate section. It also does not cover darkish urine from normal physiological causes, such as that resulting from insufficient fluid intake in hot weather when the sweating is profuse or that resulting from drug or vitamin therapy; although these of course must be considered in clinical differentiation.

Common symptom patterns

Pent-up heat in the Heart channel. Scanty darkish urine difficult to pass, with sensations of heat and pain in the urethra, fever, reddish complexion, with typical Heart fire symptoms such as restless feelings of agitation in the chest (xin fan), insomnia, disturbing dreams and, when severe, even clouded consciousness and delirium. The tongue will be red with prickles at the tip, the tongue coat very yellow or even brownish yellow, and the pulse will be rapid.

Excess (shi) heat in the Stomach and Intestines. Scanty darkish urine; as well as characteristic symptoms of shi-heat in the Stomach and Intestines such as dry mouth, intense thirst, bad breath, constipation, abdominal distension and tenderness, red tongue with a dry yellow coat, and a slippery rapid or deep strong rapid pulse.

Damp-heat in the Liver and Gall Bladder. Recent onset of scanty darkish or even dark reddish urine, and yellowish discoloration of the eyes and skin; as well as characteristic symptoms of Liver and Gall Bladder damp-heat such as bitter taste in the mouth, poor appetite, nausea, vomiting, and pain in the flanks. There may also be a yellow tinge to the eyes, or fever, or alternating chills and fever. The tongue will be red with a greasy yellow coat, and the pulse will be wiry and rapid.

Obstructed cold-damp. Gradual onset of darkish tea-colored yellow urine, but not scanty, and yellowish discoloration of the eyes and skin; as well as characteristic symptoms of cold-damp such as lassitude, heavy limbs, sensitivity to cold, poor appetite, abdominal distension, loose unformed stool, pale tongue with a greasy white coat, and a languid ru (thready floating weak) pulse.

Urinary Bladder damp-heat. Scanty yellow or reddish urine, usually with frequency, urgency, or difficulty of urination and lower abdominal pain or distension; plus characteristic symptoms of damp-heat such as bitter taste in the mouth, dry mouth and throat but without much desire to drink. The tongue will be red with a yellow coat, the pulse will be slippery and rapid.

Yin deficient internal heat. Scanty yellow urine with sensations of burning or difficulty, and characteristic symptoms of yin deficiency such as nightsweats, vertigo, tinnitus, dry throat but easily quenched thirst, hot flushes worse in the afternoon or evening, heat in the palms, soles and center of the chest, aching of the lower back and knees, spermatorrhea, red tongue with little or no coat, and thready rapid pulse.

Summertime damp-heat. Darkish urine after exposure to hot summer weather, low-grade fever, spontaneous perspiration, insatiable thirst, nausea, epigastric fullness, loose-yet-incomplete stool, floating yet weak and expanded pulse, and a thin white and slightly greasy tongue coat.

Exogenous wind-heat invading the Lungs. Darkish urine associated with recent cough producing thick yellow phlegm, fever, chills, dry sore throat, red tongue tip with a thin yellow coat, and a floating rapid pulse.

Differentiation

Pent-up heat in the Heart channel versus excess heat in the Stomach and Intestines. Both are internal shi-heat conditions. Pent-up heat in the Heart channel results from either emotional imbalance or excessive consumption of spicy pungent heating foods. The heat in the Heart is then transferred into the Small Intestine where it interferes with the Small Intestine separation of clear fluids from the murky waste passed down from the Stomach, and the urine becomes scanty and dark.

Excess heat in the Stomach and Intestines can also result from over-consumption of heating spicy foods, or alternatively from the invasion of an exogenous pathogen which has descended into the Yang Ming level and then produced heat.

Pent-up heat in the Heart channel will produce characteristic symptoms indicating its pathogenesis: restless feelings of agitation in the chest (xin fan), irritability and insomnia; the tongue will be red at the tip which may even have raised prickles, and the urine will be hot, difficult and scanty as well as dark because of the failure of the Small Intestine's separation function. The treatment requires cooling Heart heat and draining that heat which has moved into the Small Intestine out through the urine, using a formula such as Dao Chi San ('Guide Out the Red Powder'). If there is confusion or other signs of unclear consciousness then, besides cooling heat, the Heart orifice must

also be opened, using Qing Gong Tang ('Clear the Palace Decoction') to wash down the pills of An Gong Niu Huang Wan ('Calm the Palace Pill with Cattle Gallstone').

With excess heat in the Stomach and Intestines, the focus of intensity should be determined: whether the heat is more severe in the Stomach or in the Intestines. If worse in the Stomach, then there will be symptoms such as bad breath, mouth ulcers, toothache and hot discomfort in the epigastric area. If worse in the Intestines, the symptoms will be those of accumulated pathogenic heat which has linked with the stool, parching it and leading to severe constipation with abdominal fullness, distension and tenderness. If the heat is in the Stomach, then the treatment requires the cooling of Stomach heat with Qing Wei San ('Cool the Stomach Powder'). If the heat is in the Intestines and has linked with the stool causing constipation, then either Da Cheng Qi Tang ('Major Order the Qi Decoction') or Xiao Cheng Qi Tang ('Minor Order the Qi Decoction') should be used.

Formulas

Dao Chi San ('Guide Out the Red Powder')

Sheng Di	Rehmannia Glutinosae, Radix
Mu Tong	Mutong, Caulis
Dan Zhu Ye	Lophatheri Gracilis, Herba
Gan Cao	Glycyrrhizae Uralensis, Radix

Source text: *Xiao Er Yao Zheng Zhi Jue* ('Craft of Medicinal Treatment for Childhood Disease Patterns', 1119) [*Formulas and Strategies*, p. 95]

Qing Gong Tang ('Clear the Palace Decoction')

Xi Jiao	Rhinoceri, Cornu
Sheng Di	Rehmannia Glutinosae, Radix
Xuan Shen	Scrophulariae Ningpoensis, Radix
Zhu Ye	Lophatheri Gracilis, Herba
Jin Yin Hua	Lonicerae Japonicae, Flos
Lian Qiao	Forsythiae Suspensae, Fructus
Huang Lian	Coptidis, Rhizoma
Dan Shen	Salviae Miltiorrhizae, Radix
Mai Men Dong	Ophiopogonis Japonici, Tuber

Source text: *Wen Bing Tiao Bian* ('Systematic Differentiation of Warm Diseases', 1798)

An Gong Niu Huang Wan ('Calm the Palace Pill with Cattle Gallstone')

Niu Huang	Bovis, Calculus
Xi Jiao	Rhinoceri, Cornu
She Xiang	Moschus Moschiferi, Secretio
Huang Lian	Coptidis, Rhizoma
Huang Qin	Scutellariae Baicalensis, Radix
Shan Zhi Zi	Gardeniae Jasminoidis, Fructus
Xiong Huang	Realgar
Bing Pian	Borneol
Yu Jin	Curcumae, Tuber
Zhu Sha	Cinnabaris
Zhen Zhu	Margarita

Source text: *Wen Bing Tiao Bian* ('Systematic Differentiation of Warm Diseases', 1798) [*Formulas and Strategies*, p. 416]

Qing Wei San ('Cool the Stomach Powder')

Huang Lian	Coptidis, Rhizoma
Sheng Ma	Cimicifugae, Rhizoma
Mu Dan Pi	Moutan Radicis, Cortex
Sheng Di	Rehmannia Glutinosae, Radix
Dang Gui	Angelica Polymorpha, Radix

Source text: *Lan Shi Mi Cang* ('Secrets from the Orchid Chamber', 1336) [*Formulas and Strategies*, p. 93]

Da Cheng Qi Tang ('Major Order the Qi Decoction')

Da Huang	Rhei, Rhizoma
Mang Xiao	Mirabilitum
Zhi Shi	Citri seu Ponciri Immaturis, Fructus
Hou Po	Magnoliae Officinalis, Cortex

Source text: *Shang Han Lun* ('Discussion of Cold-Induced Disorders', c. 210AD) [*Formulas and Strategies*, p. 115]

Xiao Cheng Qi Tang ('Minor Order the Qi Decoction')

Da Huang	Rhei, Rhizoma
Hou Po	Magnoliae Officinalis, Cortex
Zhi Shi	Citri seu Ponciri Immaturis, Fructus

Source text: *Shang Han Lun* ('Discussion of Cold-Induced Disorders', c. 210AD) [*Formulas and Strategies*, p. 117]

Damp-heat in the Liver and Gall Bladder versus obstructed cold-damp. Both are internal damp conditions causing darkish urine and also yellowing of the eyes and skin, but the former is a yang syndrome while the latter is a yin syndrome. Both are actually the result of the mechanisms leading to yin and yang type jaundice, first completely described in the *Shang Han Lun* ('Discussion of Cold-Induced Disorders').[12] The yellowness of the eyes, skin and urine in the yang syndrome will be brighter than those of the yin syndrome, and the urine will be scanty in the yang syndrome, while unaffected in the yin type.

Damp-heat in the Liver and Gall Bladder can result either from damp-heat directly affecting the Liver and Gall Bladder, or from Spleen and Stomach damp-heat spreading over into the Liver and Gall Bladder. In either case, the damp and heat obstruct the normal flow of qi so that movement along the fluid pathways is interrupted, and the two pathogens also descend directly into the Urinary Bladder and interfere with its functioning, the damp obstructing urinary excretion and the heat drying and concentrating the fluids, so that the urine becomes scanty and dark. It is the effect of the heat which lends a bright orange tinge to the yellowishness of the urine, eyes and skin.

In the yin syndrome of obstructed cold-damp, which may be the result of either direct invasion of cold then linking with endogenous damp, or yang deficiency leading to cold-damp accumulation, the mechanism is that of damage to Spleen yang and obstruction of the activity of qi, so that long-term damp accumulation results. Damp is Earth, and thus thorough inundation with pathogenic damp can lead to the eyes, skin, and urine taking on the color of Earth: yellow. But because of the influence of cold, this yellow will not be as bright as the color in the Liver and Gall Bladder condition described above.

In the first condition, all the symptoms will be those of heat in the Liver and Gall Bladder: bitter taste and dryness in the mouth, alternating chills and fever, pain and distension in the ribs and flanks. The condition will be of sudden onset and short duration, and should be treated by cooling Liver and Gall Bladder, while eliminating damp and draining heat, with a formula such as Long Dan Xie Gan Tang ('Gentiana Longdancao Decoction to Drain the Liver').

In the second condition, all the symptoms will be those of cold-damp damaging Spleen yang: chills, lassitude, heavy limbs, poor appetite, abdominal distension, and loose stool. The condition will not be of recent onset but rather long-term and insidious, and the treatment requires warming of Spleen yang to transform damp with a formula such as Yin Chen Zhu Fu Tang ('Artemesia Yinchenhao, Atractylodes, and Prepared Aconite Decoction').

Formulas

Long Dan Xie Gan Tang ('Gentiana Longdancao Decoction to Drain the Liver')

Long Dan Cao	Gentianae Scabrae, Radix
Huang Qin	Scutellariae Baicalensis, Radix
Shan Zhi Zi	Gardeniae Jasminoidis, Fructus
Mu Tong	Mutong, Caulis
Che Qian Zi	Plantaginis, Semen
Ze Xie	Alismatis Plantago-aquaticae, Rhizoma
Chai Hu	Bupleuri, Radix
Sheng Di	Rehmannia Glutinosae, Radix
Dang Gui	Angelica Polymorpha, Radix
Gan Cao	Glycyrrhizae Uralensis, Radix

Source text: *Yi Fang Ji Jie* ('Analytic Collection of Medical Formulas', 1682) [*Formulas and Strategies*, p. 96]

Yin Chen Zhu Fu Tang ('Artemesia Yinchenhao, Atractylodes, and Prepared Aconite Decoction')

Yin Chen Hao	Artemesiae Capillaris, Herba
Bai Zhu	Atractylodis Macrocephalae, Rhizoma
Gan Jiang	Zingiberis Officianalis, Rhizoma
Fu Zi	Aconiti Carmichaeli Praeparata, Radix
Rou Gui	Cinnamomi Cassiae, Cortex
Zhi Gan Cao	Honey-fried Glycyrrhizae Uralensis, Radix

Source text: *Yi Xue Xin Wu* ('Medical Revelations', 1732) [*Formulas and Strategies*, p. 190]

Urinary Bladder damp-heat versus yin deficient internal heat: causing darkish urine. Both of these are lower Jiao pathologies, and both involve heat. But the heat is of different origin and of different nature in each.

Urinary Bladder damp-heat can result from long-term accumulation of pathogenic damp in the Urinary Bladder leading to build-up of heat, or the consumption of heating food and drink. This is excess heat.

Yin deficient internal heat can result from constitutional weakness of yin, long-term illness, excessive sexual activity, or again over-consumption of heating food and drink which over a long period of time has damaged the yin fluids in the body. This is by definition xu-heat.

Urinary Bladder damp-heat will have characteristic symptoms of damp-heat such as bitter taste in the mouth, dry throat but without much desire to drink. The tongue will be red with a yellow coat, the pulse will be slippery and rapid.

Yin deficient internal heat will have characteristic symptoms of yin deficiency such as vertigo, tinnitus, dry throat, hot flushes worse in the afternoon or evening, heat in the palms, soles and center of the chest, aching of the lower back and knees, spermatorrhea, red tongue with little or no coat, and thready rapid pulse.

The important points in differentiation will be that in the Urinary Bladder damp-heat condition, the onset is rapid and the urination will be frequent, urgent and painful, and the lower abdomen will hurt; while in the darkish urine from deficient heat, the urine may be dark and scanty but will only be slightly hot, the condition will be chronic, and the other yin deficiency symptoms should be apparent.

Treatment of the Urinary Bladder damp-heat condition requires cooling of the heat and expulsion of the damp through the urine, using a formula like Ba Zheng San ('Eight-Herb Powder for Rectification').

Treatment of the yin deficiency with internal heat requires nourishment of yin while bringing down flaring fire, with a formula like Zhi Bai Di Huang Wan ('Anemarrhena, Phellodendron, and Rehmannia Pill').

Formulas

Ba Zheng San ('Eight-Herb Powder for Rectification')

Mu Tong	Mutong, Caulis
Hua Shi	Talc
Che Qian Zi	Plantaginis, Semen

Qu Mai	Dianthi, Herba
Bian Xu	Polygoni Avicularis, Herba
Shan Zhi Zi	Gardeniae Jasminoidis, Fructus
Zhi Da Huang	Rhei, Rhizoma (treated)
Deng Xin Cao	Junci Effusi, Medulla
Gan Cao	Glycyrrhizae Uralensis, Radix

Source text: *Tai Ping Hui Min He Ji Ju Fang* ('Imperial Grace Formulary of the Tai Ping Era', 1078-85) [*Formulas and Strategies*, p. 192]

Zhi Bai Di Huang Wan ('Anemarrhena, Phellodendron, and Rehmannia Pill')

Zhi Mu	Anemarrhenae Asphodeloidis, Radix
Huang Bo	Phellodendri, Cortex
Sheng Di	Rehmannia Glutinosae, Radix
Shan Zhu Yu	Corni Officinalis, Fructus
Shan Yao	Dioscoreae Oppositae, Radix
Fu Ling	Poriae Cocos, Sclerotium
Mu Dan Pi	Moutan Radicis, Cortex
Ze Xie	Alismatis Plantago-aquaticae, Rhizoma

Source text: *Zheng Yin Mai Zhi* ('Pattern, Cause, Pulse, and Treatment', 1702) [*Formulas and Strategies*, p. 265]

Summertime damp-heat versus exogenous wind-heat invading the Lungs causing darkish urine. There are two exogenous conditions that can also cause darkish urine, which should also be considered in addition to the less seasonal internal syndromes presented above. The first is summertime damp-heat (shu shi), which most easily invades either the Lung channel or the Yang Ming Stomach channel, and damages both the qi and the body fluids. Summerheat can affect the fluids, and thus lead to darkish urine, in a number of ways but the two most common are by causing sweating which reduces the fluids, and by binding the Lungs so that the fluid pathways lose the regulating effect of Lung qi. According to Zhang Jing-Yue, there are eight characteristic symptoms of Summerheat: 'a xu pulse (floating, big, slow, and soft), spontaneous perspiration, fever, cold sensations on the back, an oily-looking face, a restless feeling of agitation in the chest (xin fan), insatiable thirst, slightly chilled hands and feet, and a feeling of heaviness in the body'. Other authors (such as Cheng Guo-Peng in his *Yi Xue Xin Wu*, 'Medical Revelations', 1732)

have virtually identical lists which however include darkish urine as a typical symptom of Summerheat. Other possible symptoms include nausea, sensations of stuffiness in the chest, thirst, dyspnea, epigastric fullness, and loose-yet-incomplete stool, with a thin white slightly greasy tongue coat. Summerheat leading to darkish urine should be treated by cooling heat, transforming damp, and harmonizing the middle Jiao with a formula such as Lian Po Yin ('Coptis and Magnolia Bark Decoction').

Similarly, exogenous wind-heat invading the Lungs, interfering with the Lung function of regulating the fluid pathways and allowing heat to damage the body fluids, can also lead to darkish urine.[13] The presenting symptoms, though, will be quite distinctive: the darkish urine will be associated with a relatively recent cough producing thick yellow phlegm, fever, mild chills, dry sore throat, thirst for cold drinks, red tongue tip with a thin yellow coat, and a floating rapid pulse, especially noticeable at the right distal (cun) position.

Exogenous wind-heat invading the Lungs and interfering with fluids should be treated by cooling heat and promoting urination with a formula like Qing Zao Jiu Fei Tang ('Eliminate Dryness and Rescue the Lungs Decoction').

Formulas

Lian Po Yin ('Coptis and Magnolia Bark Decoction')

Huang Lian	Coptidis, Rhizoma
Hou Po	Magnoliae Officinalis, Cortex
Shan Zhi Zi	Gardeniae Jasminoidis, Fructus
Dan Dou Chi	Sojae Praeparatum, Semen
Shi Chang Pu	Acori Graminei, Rhizoma
Ban Xia	Pinelliae Ternata, Rhizoma
Lu Gen	Phragmitis Communis, Rhizoma

Source text: *Huo Luan Lun* ('Discussion of Sudden Turmoil Disorders', 1862) [*Formulas and Strategies*, p. 189]

Qing Zao Jiu Fei Tang ('Eliminate Dryness and Rescue the Lungs Decoction')

Sang Ye	Mori Albae, Folium
Shi Gao	Gypsum
Mai Men Dong	Ophiopogonis Japonici, Tuber
E Jiao	Asini, Gelatinum

Hei Zhi Ma	Sesami Indici, Semen
Xing Ren	Pruni Armeniacae, Semen
Mi Zhi Pi Pa Ye	Honey-fried Eriobotryae
	Japonicae, Folium
Ren Shen	Ginseng, Radix
Gan Cao	Glycyrrhizae Uralensis, Radix

Source text: *Yi Men Fa Lu* ('Precepts for Physicians', 1658) [*Formulas and Strategies*, p. 160]

Summary

Darkish urine is a common clinical symptom seen in many conditions. Although it is rarely a presenting symptom, careful consideration and differentiation of its mechanism can be very useful for determining the underlying cause of the illness. For example, with internal heat conditions the degree of darkness of the urine can assist in determining the severity of the heat involved. Again, if the darkish urine is seen with a jaundiced appearance, then if the urine is scanty and hot this will show that the condition is that of yang type jaundice, while the urine in yin type jaundice will be neither hot nor scanty. The exogenous conditions will be characterized by either their seasonal relationship, as in Summerheat, or by the relatively recent onset of the problem. In the latter two cases, however, darkish urine is unlikely to be the presenting symptom, which is why these are placed last in the categories above.

Cloudy urine

This refers to urine that is turbid and unclear, but not painful when passed. The category also includes urine which appears clear at first but precipitates a sediment when allowed to sit for a time.

Although painful urination is occasionally cloudy as well, the two conditions are different: in the former, pain is the predominant characteristic, while in cloudy urine there will be no—or only slight—pain. This should be kept in mind when selecting categories of differentiations.

Hematuria and spermaturia will also be considered separately in subsequent sections.

Common symptom patterns

Lower Jiao damp-heat. Whitish cloudy urine resembling water in which rice has been washed,

occasionally containing a slippery greasy substance; or dark yellow cloudy urine; usually with scantiness, frequency and a burning sensation. There may be occasional mild pain. There will also be characteristic symptoms of damp-heat: sensations of fullness in the chest and epigastric area, dry mouth without much desire to drink, red tongue with greasy yellow coat, and a rapid slippery or rapid soft (ru) pulse.

Kidney yin deficiency. Whitish cloudy urine in small amounts, with characteristic symptoms of yin deficiency such as tinnitus, deafness, vertigo, dry throat, malar flush, nightsweats and hot flushes, aching and weakness of the lower back and knees, dry stool, red tongue with little coat, and a thready rapid pulse.

Kidney yang deficiency. Cloudy, frequent and profuse urination, with typical symptoms of Kidney yang deficiency such as tiredness, pale face, cold limbs, sexual dysfunction, cold aching of the lower back and knees, pale flabby tongue body with a white tongue coat, and a deep weak pulse.

Spleen qi deficient and unable to rise. Long-term cloudy urine, or urinary sediment, with dribbling afterwards, and other typical symptoms of Spleen qi deficiency such as sallow complexion, lack of energy, poor appetite, dragging feeling in the lower abdomen, loose stool, pale tongue with a white coat, and a weak forceless pulse.

Dual deficiency of Spleen and Kidneys. Cloudy, frequent and profuse urination, with symptoms of both Spleen and Kidney deficiency such as dizziness, tinnitus, sallow face, poor appetite, shortness of breath, emaciation, cold limbs, sore lower back and knees, pale tongue with a white slippery coat, and a languid weak pulse.

Blood stagnation in the lower abdomen. Cloudy, painful and possibly obstructed urine, with characteristic symptoms of blood stagnation in the lower abdomen including stabbing pain and distension both worsening with pressure, with darkish areas or purple spots on the tongue; in women, dark and clotted menstrual blood and menstrual irregularity.

Differentiation

Lower Jiao damp-heat versus Kidney yin deficiency causing cloudy urine. Both of these conditions are caused by accumulated heat in the Urinary Bladder interfering with qi transformation but the former is excess heat while the latter is deficient heat.

Lower Jiao damp-heat causing cloudy urine can result from either exogenous damp-heat invasion or excessive consumption of rich sweet foods or excessive consumption of alcohol. The latter will produce damp in the middle Jiao which then creates heat; the two pathogens then link and pour downward into the Urinary Bladder. (See the chapter on damp-heat for detailed description of these and other possible mechanisms.) The damp and heat interfere with the Urinary Bladder qi transformation, and thus separation of clear and murky fluids; if damp is predominant then the urine will be white and cloudy, resembling water in which rice has been washed; if the heat is acting upon the damp so that it thickens, the urine will occasionally contain a slippery greasy substance; while if the heat is predominant then the urine will be dark yellow and cloudy, and there may be occasional mild pain. There will also be characteristic symptoms of damp-heat: sensations of fullness in the chest and epigastric area, dry mouth without much desire to drink, red tongue with greasy yellow coat, and a rapid slippery or rapid soft (ru) pulse. Treatment requires separation of the two pathogens by expelling damp and cooling heat, so that Urinary Bladder qi transformation can be restored to normal, using a formula such as Bei Xie Fen Qing Yin ('Dioscorea Hypoglauca Decoction to Separate the Clear from Medical Revelations').

Kidney yin deficiency causing cloudy urine can result from constitutional yin deficiency, or from febrile disease damaging yin, either of which can allow internal pathogenic heat to build-up and disrupt Urinary Bladder qi transformation, so that excessively turbid urine is expelled before proper separation of clear and murky can take place; in some cases the cloudiness may be seminal fluid forced by the heat out of the weak and unconsolidated Kidneys (see the section on spermatorrhea). The urine will be scanty due to the deficiency of yin fluids which has given rise to the condition, and there will be other characteristic symptoms of yin deficiency with xu-fire flaring such as feelings of restless agitation in the chest, insomnia, tinnitus, vertigo, dry throat, malar flush, nightsweats and hot flushes, aching and weakness of the lower back and knees, dry stool, red tongue with little coat, and a thready rapid pulse. Cooling is not appropriate for xu-heat; instead the treatment requires tonification of the yin fluids to control the unbalanced yang, with a formula like Zhi Bai Di Huang Wan ('Anemarrhena, Phellodendron, and Rehmannia Pill') with Bei Xie (Dioscoreae, Rhizoma) added to contribute its special ability to expel damp and promote the separation of clear and murky fluids.

Formulas

Bei Xie Fen Qing Yin ('Dioscorea Hypoglauca Decoction to Separate the Clear from *Medical Revelations*')

Bei Xie	Dioscoreae, Rhizoma
Huang Bo	Phellodendri, Cortex
Shi Chang Pu	Acori Graminei, Rhizoma
Fu Ling	Poriae Cocos, Sclerotium
Bai Zhu	Atractylodis Macrocephalae, Rhizoma
Dan Shen	Salviae Miltiorrhizae, Radix
Che Qian Zi	Plantaginis, Semen

Source text: *Yi Xue Xin Wu* ('Medical Revelations', 1732) [*Formulas & Strategies*, p. 210]

Zhi Bai Di Huang Wan ('Anemarrhena, Phellodendron, and Rehmannia Pill') [*Formulas & Strategies*, p. 265]
(See above)

Kidney yang deficiency versus Spleen qi weak and descending causing cloudy urine. Both are deficient cold conditions which manifest frequent profuse urination. The former, however, is based on deficiency of Kidney yang, which fails to support Urinary Bladder qi transformation so that urine is profuse, frequent and cloudy. The cloudiness may appear because of three reasons: one, the excessive untransformed fluids may give rise to damp in the Urinary Bladder; two, the weak yang may allow yin cold to predominate locally and concentrate the damp so that it becomes visible as murkiness; three, as in the Kidney yin deficiency condition, the cloudiness may reflect the presence of seminal fluid, (which Zhang Jing-Yue and others call 'bai jing'—'failed jing').[14]

The latter Spleen qi weakness can also allow jing-essence to leak out through the urine. This jing-essence is not that of the Kidneys, however, but the jing-essence acquired from food and fluids, which rather than being carried up to the Lungs instead drops into the Urinary Bladder. This condition can be caused by any factors which damage the Spleen or the qi, such as overwork, worry, or irregular eating. Of course, the excessive damp which can be formed under such conditions is even more likely to descend (due to its yin nature), and will contribute to the cloudiness. If it is primarily the jing-essence from food and fluids, the urine will initially appear relatively clear but if allowed to sit will precipitate a sediment; otherwise the cloudy urine reflects pathogenic damp from untransformed food and fluids. Both conditions will be exacerbated with exertion.

Kidney yang deficiency will manifest the characteristic symptoms such as lethargy, tinnitus, pale face with perhaps darkened areas under the eyes, cold limbs, sexual dysfunction, cold aching of the lower back and knees, pale flabby tongue body with a white tongue coat, and a deep weak pulse. Treatment requires warming of the yang coupled with consolidation of the Kidneys, with a formula such as You Gui Wan ('Restore the Right [Kidney] Pill') plus *Bu Gu Zhi* (Psoraleae Corylifoliae, Fructus) and *Wu Wei Zi* (Schisandrae Chinensis, Fructus) to increase both warmth and consolidation.

Weak and descending Spleen qi will manifest characteristic Spleen symptoms such as sallow complexion, lack of energy, poor appetite and loose stool containing undigested food, as well as symptoms of failure of Spleen qi to rise, such as a dragging feeling in the lower abdomen or even prolapse of various internal organs or the rectum, poor concentration and dry mouth and lips. There will be pale tongue with a white coat and a weak forceless pulse. The treatment requires the restoration of Spleen qi ascent with a formula such as Bao Yuan Tang ('Preserve the Basal Decoction') plus *Qian Shi* (Euryales Ferox, Semen) and *Sheng Ma* (Cimicifugae, Rhizoma) to improve Urinary Bladder consolidation and the ascent of Spleen qi. Bu Zhong Yi Qi Tang ('Tonify the Middle and Augment the Qi Decoction') with appropriate alterations can also be used.

Formulas

You Gui Wan ('Restore the Right [Kidney] Pill')

Fu Zi	Aconiti Carmichaeli Praeparata, Radix
Rou Gui	Cinnamomi Cassiae, Cortex
Lu Jiao Jiao	Cervi Colla Cornu
Shou Di	Rehmanniae Glutinosae Conquitae, Radix
Shan Zhu Yu	Corni Officinalis, Fructus
Shan Yao	Dioscoreae Oppositae, Radix
Gou Qi Zi	Lycii Chinensis, Fructus
Tu Si Zi	Cuscutae, Semen
Du Zhong	Eucommiae Ulmoidis, Cortex
Dang Gui	Angelica Polymorpha, Radix

Source text: *Jing Yue Quan Shu* ('Complete Works of Jing Yue', 1624) [*Formulas & Strategies*, p. 278]

Bao Yuan Tang ('Preserve the Basal Decoction')

Huang Qi	Astragali, Radix
Ren Shen	Ginseng, Radix
Zhi Gan Cao	Honey-fried Glycyrrhizae Uralensis, Radix
Rou Gui	Cinnamomi Cassiae, Cortex
Glutinous rice	

Source text: *Jing Yue Quan Shu* ('Complete Works of Jing Yue', 1624) [*Formulas & Strategies*, p. 239]

Bu Zhong Yi Qi Tang ('Tonify the Middle and Augment the Qi Decoction')

Huang Qi	Astragali, Radix
Ren Shen	Ginseng, Radix
Bai Zhu	Atractylodis Macrocephalae, Rhizoma
Zhi Gan Cao	Honey-fried Glycyrrhizae Uralensis, Radix
Dang Gui	Angelica Polymorpha, Radix
Chen Pi	Citri Reticulatae, Pericarpium
Sheng Ma	Cimicifugae, Rhizoma
Chai Hu	Bupleuri, Radix

Source text: *Pi Wei Lun* ('Discussion of the Spleen and Stomach', 1249) [*Formulas & Strategies*, p. 241]

Dual deficiency of Spleen and Kidneys causing cloudy urine. Spleen qi failing to rise coupled with failure of the Kidneys to both support the Urinary Bladder and consolidate the lower orifice is a severe development of the two conditions described above.

In addition to the cloudy, frequent and profuse urination, there will be symptoms of both Spleen and Kidney deficiency such as dizziness, tinnitus, sallow face, poor appetite, shortness of breath, emaciation, cold limbs, sore lower back and knees, pale tongue with a white slippery coat, and a languid weak pulse. Treatment requires attention to both Spleen and the Kidneys, using a combination of formulas such as Bu Zhong Yi Qi Tang ('Tonify the Middle and Augment the Qi Decoction') and Wu Bi Shan Yao Wan ('Incomparable Dioscorea Pill'). You Gui Wan ('Restore the Right [Kidney] Pill') would also be effective as a substitute for the latter.

Formulas

Bu Zhong Yi Qi Tang ('Tonify the Middle and Augment the Qi Decoction') [*Formulas & Strategies*, p. 241]
(See above)

Wu Bi Shan Yao Wan ('Incomparable Dioscorea Pill')

Shan Yao	Dioscoreae Oppositae, Radix
Rou Cong Rong	Cistanches, Herba
Shou Di	Rehmanniae Glutinosae Conquitae, Radix
Shan Zhu Yu	Corni Officinalis, Fructus
Fu Shen	Poriae Cocos Paradicis, Sclerotium
Tu Si Zi	Cuscutae, Semen
Wu Wei Zi	Schisandrae Chinensis, Fructus
Chi Shi Zhi	Halloysitum Rubrum
Ba Ji Tian	Morindae Officinalis, Radix
Ze Xie	Alismatis Plantago-aquaticae, Rhizoma
Du Zhong	Eucommiae Ulmoidis, Cortex
Niu Xi	Achyranthis Bidentatae, Radix

Source text: *Tai Ping Hui Min He Ji Ju Fang* ('Imperial Grace Formulary of the Tai Ping Era', 1078-85)

You Gui Wan ('Restore the Right [Kidney] Pill') [*Formulas & Strategies*, p. 278]
(See above)

Blood stagnation in the lower abdomen. Lower abdominal blood stagnation can also cause cloudy urine by interfering with Urinary Bladder qi transformation. Often in this case the urine will not only be cloudy but painful, and possibly obstructed as well, and may contain blood so that its color becomes cloudy and dark purple. There will also be symptoms of lower abdominal blood stagnation such as stabbing pain and distension, with darkish areas or purple spots on the tongue, and menstrual irregularity in women and possible prostatic disturbance in men. The treatment requires the warming of yang qi to promote the removal of stagnant blood with a formula such as Shao Fu Zhu Yu Tang ('Drive Out Blood Stasis in the Lower Abdomen Decoction') with the addition of *Qu Mai* (Dianthi, Herba), *Mu Tong* (Mutong, Caulis) and *Jin Qian Cao* (Jinqiancao, Herba) to drain Urinary Bladder obstruction.

Formula

Shao Fu Zhu Yu Tang ('Drive Out Blood Stasis in the Lower Abdomen Decoction')

Xiao Hui Xiang	Foeniculi Vulgaris, Fructus
Gan Jiang	Zingiberis Officinalis, Rhizoma
Yan Hu Suo	Corydalis Yanhusuo, Rhizoma
Dang Gui	Angelica Polymorpha, Radix
Chuan Xiong	Ligustici Wallichii, Radix
Mo Yao	Myrrha
Rou Gui	Cinnamomi Cassiae, Cortex
Chi Shao	Paeoniae Rubra, Radix
Pu Huang	Typhae, Pollen
Wu Ling Zhi	Trogopterori seu pteromi, Excrementum

Source text: *Yi Lin Gai Cuo* ('Corrections of Errors Among Physicians', 1830) [*Formulas & Strategies*, p. 316]

Summary

Cloudy urine can result from either excess or deficiency. If from excess, the location of the problem will be in the Urinary Bladder, and the most common excess factor will be that of damp-heat, although blood stagnation can also be involved. In both of these excess conditions the urine will be concentrated and painful. The deficiency conditions result from weakness of the yang qi, either of the Spleen and Kidneys; the urine is rarely painful or concentrated, and indeed may be profuse.

Clear profuse urination

This condition is different from that of frequent urination, where the urine can be either clear or cloudy, and either profuse or scanty; however clear profuse urination as a condition will often include frequency as a symptom. Clinically, attention to the possibility of habitual consumption of diuretic beverages is necessary.

Common symptom patterns

Kidney yang deficiency. Clear, profuse and frequent urination with characteristic symptoms of Kidney yang insufficiency such as facial pallor, tiredness, soreness of the lower back and knees, coldness of the limbs and general sensitivity to cold, dizziness, tinnitus, pale tongue with a white coat, and a deep slow weak pulse, especially at the proximal (chi) position.

Internal yin cold predominating over yang. Clear profuse urination with obvious sensitivity to cold, lower abdominal cold pain which markedly improves with heat,[15] preference for warm food and drinks, cold limbs, loose stool, pale tongue with a white coat, and deep wiry pulse.

Differentiation

These two are both cold conditions but the former is xu-cold from deficiency of Kidney yang, while the latter is shi-cold due to a direct invasion of pathogenic cold, for example through over-consumption of cold food and drinks.

If Kidney yang is deficient, it is unable to either support the qi transformation of fluids held in the Urinary Bladder, or consolidate the lower orifice, and so the urine becomes profuse and clear. Because this is a result of weakness, there will also be signs of deficiency, such as tiredness and pale face, coupled with typical Kidney symptoms. The treatment involves warming Kidney yang and improving Kidney consolidation with a combination of formulas such as Suo Quan Wan ('Shut the Sluice Pill') and You Gui Wan ('Restore the Right [Kidney] Pill').

Internal yin cold predominating over yang and leading to clear profuse urination is an excess condition, and thus there will be few signs of deficiency but many symptoms of cold; the pulse is especially significant here, as the strength of the wiriness in the pulse will clearly reflect the vigor of the pathogen rather than the feebleness of a weak Kidney yang. The mechanism is that of cold interfering with qi transformation throughout the body so that fluids are not transformed but instead pour down into the Urinary Bladder, where again the cold acts to curtail the physiological consolidation by the Kidney yang, and causes urine to become profuse and clear.[16] The treatment requires warming the center and expelling the cold, with a formula based upon Li Zhong Wan ('Settle the Middle Pill'), adding *Yi Zhi Ren* (Alpiniae Oxyphyllae, Fructus), *Xiao Hui Xiang* (Foeniculi Vulgaris, Fructus), *Jiu Zi* (Alli Tuberosi, Semen), *Fu Pen Zi* (Rubi, Fructus) and *Wu Yao* (Linderae Strychnifoliae), Radix.

Formulas

Suo Quan Wan ('Shut the Sluice Pill')

Yi Zhi Ren	Alpiniae Oxyphyllae, Fructus
Wu Yao	Linderae Strychnifoliae, Radix
Shan Yao	Dioscoreae Oppositae, Radix

Source text: *Fu Ren Liang Fang* ('Fine Formulas for Women', 1237) [*Formulas & Strategies*, p. 363]

You Gui Wan ('Restore the Right [Kidney] Pill') [*Formulas & Strategies*, p. 278] (See above)

Li Zhong Wan ('Settle the Middle Pill')

Gan Jiang	Zingiberis Officianalis, Rhizoma
Ren Shen	Ginseng, Radix
Bai Zhu	Atractylodis Macrocephalae, Rhizoma
Gan Cao	Glycyrrhizae Uralensis, Radix

Source text: *Shang Han Lun* ('Discussion of Cold-Induced Disorders', c. 210AD) [*Formulas & Strategies*, p.219]

Difficult urination (xiao bian bu li)

This refers to reduced amount of urine which is also difficult to pass. In many texts this symptom is discussed under the heading 'obstructed urination' (xiao bian bu tong) but while the two symptoms can have similar etiologies, there are differences which make a separate discussion meaningful. Difficult urination has reduced amount as well as difficulty passing, and often is associated with edema,[17] while obstructed urine usually involves a full bladder which cannot be emptied (see the next section). 'Painful urination' (xiao bian teng tong) is also different from the above two conditions, although in some patients it may involve both as symptoms.

Common symptom patterns

Loss of Lung qi spread and descent. Difficult urination with edema of the eyelids followed by edema of the limbs and then generalized fluid retention, accompanied by aching heaviness of the limbs, chills and fever, cough, dyspnea, and possibly swollen sore throat, thin white tongue coat, and floating tight or floating rapid pulse.

Spleen yang deficiency. Scanty difficult urination, generalized edema which is most obvious below the waist, associated with characteristic symptoms of Spleen yang weakness such as lethargy, a sensation of cold heaviness in the limbs, sallow complexion, fullness of the epigastric area and the abdomen, poor appetite, loose stool, pale flabby moist tongue with a white slippery tongue coat, and a deep slow forceless pulse.

Kidney yang deficiency. Difficult urination with edema which is most obvious below the waist, dyspnea, cough with the sound of thin phlegm in the throat, palpitations, and characteristic symptoms of Kidney yang weakness such as chilled limbs and cold aching lower back, pale or darkish complexion, pale flabby tongue with a white slippery tongue coat, and a deep weak pulse especially forceless (or even absent) at the proximal (chi) position.

Internal obstruction by damp-heat. Scanty, dark and difficult urination with restless feelings of agitation in the chest (xin fan) and nausea, as well as other typical symptoms of damp-heat such as bitter sticky taste in the mouth, thirst without much desire to drink, poor appetite, abdominal distension, sticky difficult-to-pass stool (or alternating dry and loose stool), red tongue with a greasy yellow coat, and a rapid slippery or rapid soft (ru) pulse.

Qi blockage and damp obstruction. Difficult urination with bitter taste in the mouth and dry throat, discomfort in the flanks, belching, poor appetite with abdominal fullness after eating, sour regurgitation, red tongue with a thin yellow coat, and a wiry pulse.

Kidney and Liver yin deficiency. Scanty difficult urination with a dark yellow color, possibly with recurring edema, associated with typical symptoms of Kidney and Liver yin weakness such as tinnitus, vertigo, five-hearts heat, nightsweats, dry gritty red eyes, restless feelings of agitation in the chest, sore lower back and knees, red tongue with little coat, and a thready rapid pulse.

Differentiation

Loss of Lung qi spread and descent causing difficult urination. This condition is usually the result of a pathogenic wind invasion tying up the Lungs and disrupting their ability to preserve the regular movement of fluids through the fluid pathways. Symptoms will vary depending upon whether the pathogenic wind has combined with cold or with heat. In either case, however, the condition will be of sudden onset, and the edema will begin in the upper body and spread downwards.[18] (See p.126: wind-cold binding the Lungs and wind-heat disturbing the Lungs.) Treatment requires restoring the Lungs' spread and descent and opening the fluid pathways with a formula such as Yue Bi Jia Zhu Tang ('Maidservant from Yue Decoction plus Atractylodes').

Formulas

Yue Bi Jia Zhu Tang ('Maidservant from Yue Decoction plus Atractylodes')

Ma Huang	Ephedrae, Herba
Shi Gao	Gypsum
Sheng Jiang	Zingiberis Officinalis Recens, Rhizoma
Bai Zhu	Atractylodis Macrocephalae, Rhizoma
Gan Cao	Glycyrrhizae Uralensis, Radix
Da Zao	Zizyphi Jujubae, Fructus

Source text: *Jin Gui Yao Lue* ('Essentials from the Golden Cabinet', c. 210 AD) [*Formulas & Strategies*, p. 89]

Spleen yang deficiency versus Kidney yang deficiency causing difficult urination. Both of these conditions are the result of yang deficiency allowing pathogenic water and damp to accumulate internally, and the edema in both will be most marked below the waist.

The Spleen deficiency originates in the middle Jiao however, and thus will involve digestive symptoms, and the limbs will be more obviously affected because of the Spleen's affinity with the flesh (of which the limbs are primarily composed). The mechanism is also different from that of Kidney deficiency: in this case Spleen transformation is reduced so that pathogenic water and damp accumulate in the middle Jiao and spread out through the flesh instead of being carried downward to the Urinary Bladder for expulsion.

The Kidney deficiency originates in the lower Jiao, and is often the result of either constitutional factors or long term illness. In this case it is the qi transformation of the Urinary Bladder which is affected rather than that of the middle Jiao, so that untransformed fluids spread into the lower body and cause edema. The palpitations, dyspnea, cough and phlegm result from these fluids being carried upward through the San Jiao and the Kidney channel itself to assault the Lungs.[19]

Treatment in the case of Spleen yang deficiency requires warming Spleen to restore its normal transformation and transportation, plus promotion of fluid movement and urination, with a formula such as Shi Pi Yin ('Bolster the Spleen Decoction').

Treatment for Kidney yang deficiency requires tonification of the Kidneys, warming yang, promoting Urinary Bladder qi transformation, and assisting the expulsion of urine, with a formula such as Zhen Wu Tang ('True Warrior Decoction').

Formulas

Shi Pi Yin ('Bolster the Spleen Decoction')

Fu Zi	Aconiti Carmichaeli Praeparata, Radix
Gan Jiang	Zingiberis Officianalis, Rhizoma
Fu Ling	Poriae Cocos, Sclerotium
Bai Zhu	Atractylodis Macrocephalae, Rhizoma
Mu Gua	Chaenomelis Lagenariae, Fructus
Hou Po	Magnoliae Officinalis, Cortex
Mu Xiang	Saussureae seu Vladimiriae, Radix
Da Fu Pi	Arecae Catechu, Pericarpium
Cao Guo	Amomi Tsao-ko, Fructus
Gan Cao	Glycyrrhizae Uralensis, Radix

Source text: *Shi Yi De Xiao Fang* ('Effective Formulas from Generations of Physicians', 1345) [*Formulas & Strategies*, p. 199]

Zhen Wu Tang ('True Warrior Decoction')

Fu Zi	Aconiti Carmichaeli Praeparata, Radix
Bai Zhu	Atractylodis Macrocephalae, Rhizoma
Fu Ling	Poriae Cocos, Sclerotium
Bai Shao	Paeoniae Lactiflora, Radix
Sheng Jiang	Zingiberis Officinalis Recens, Rhizoma

Source text: *Shang Han Lun* ('Discussion of Cold-induced Disorders', c. 210AD) [*Formulas & Strategies*, p. 197]

Internal obstruction by damp-heat versus qi blockage and damp obstruction causing difficult urination. Both of these excess (shi) conditions involve heat, and both involve damp, but the origins and mechanisms are different in each case.

In the first condition, damp-heat is a combined pathogen that can result from either exogenous invasion, or from endogenous accumulation of damp which then creates heat, or from endogenous heat which then creates damp (see the chapter on damp-heat). This combined pathogen easily obstructs both the movement of fluids in the San Jiao and also the qi transformation in the Urinary Bladder, leading to difficult urination.

In the second condition, the qi blockage in the Liver channel is the primary mechanism, which then creates both heat from the obstruction of qi and damp from the obstruction of fluid movement. It is the qi blockage in the Liver channel which interferes with Urinary Bladder qi transformation, rather than the secondary damp and heat (see note 23).

The symptoms in the first condition are those of the primary pathogens: damp-heat obstructing the middle Jiao will cause nausea, epigastric fullness, poor appetite, thirst without desire to drink, and sticky loose stool or alternating constipation and loose stool.

The symptoms in the second section will be those of Liver qi blockage: tightness in the chest, anxiety and stress, sour regurgitation, burping and flatulence, abdominal distension, darkish color to the tongue body, and wiry pulse. If Liver overcomes the Spleen, the symptoms can resemble those of damp-heat in the middle Jiao: poor appetite, nausea and fullness; the differentiating points to look for will be the factors which make the symptoms worse, and the nature of the pulse and tongue.

Treatment of the damp-heat causing difficult urination requires cooling heat while eliminating damp and promoting urination with a formula like Ba Zheng San ('Eight-Herb Powder for Rectification').

Treatment of the Liver qi blockage leading to urinary difficulty requires restoring Liver qi movement, reducing damp, and promoting urination, with a combination of formulas such as Chai Hu Shu Gan San ('Bupleurum Powder to Spread the Liver') and Wei Ling Tang ('Calm the Stomach and Poria Decoction'.

Formulas

Ba Zheng San ('Eight-Herb Powder for Rectification')

Mu Tong	Mutong, Caulis
Hua Shi	Talc
Che Qian Zi	Plantaginis, Semen
Qu Mai	Dianthi, Herba
Bian Xu	Polygoni Avicularis, Herba
Shan Zhi Zi	Gardeniae Jasminoidis, Fructus
Zhi Da Huang	Treated Rhei, Rhizoma
Deng Xin Cao	Junci Effusi, Medulla
Gan Cao	Glycyrrhizae Uralensis, Radix

Source text: *Tai Ping Hui Min He Ji Ju Fang* ('Imperial Grace Formulary of the Tai Ping Era', 1078-85) [*Formulas & Strategies*, p. 192]

Chai Hu Shu Gan San ('Chai Hu Powder to Spread the Liver')

Chai Hu	Bupleuri, Radix
Bai Shao	Paeoniae Lactiflora, Radix
Chuan Xiong	Ligustici Wallichii, Radix
Xiang Fu	Cyperi Rotundi, Rhizoma
Zhi Ke	Citri seu Ponciri, Fructus
Chen Pi	Citri Reticulatae, Pericarpium
Gan Cao	Glycyrrhizae Uralensis, Radix

Source text: *Jing Yue Quan Shu* ('Complete Works of Jing Yue', 1624) [*Formulas & Strategies*, p. 146]

Wei Ling Tang ('Calm the Stomach and Poria Decoction')

Cang Zhu	Atractylodis, Rhizoma
Hou Po	Magnoliae Officianalis, Cortex
Chen Pi	Citri Reticulatae, Pericarpium
Gan Cao	Glycyrrhizae Uralensis, Radix
Sheng Jiang	Zingiberis Officinalis Recens, Rhizoma
Da Zao	Zizyphi Jujubae, Fructus
Ze Xie	Alismatis Plantago-aquaticae, Rhizoma
Fu Ling	Poriae Cocos, Sclerotium
Zhu Ling	Polypori Umbellati, Sclerotium
Bai Zhu	Atractylodis Macrocephalae, Rhizoma
Gui Zhi	Cinnamomi Cassiae, Ramulus

Source text: *Dan Xi Xin Fa* ('Teachings of Dan Xi', 1481) [*Formulas & Strategies*, p. 176]

Kidney and Liver yin deficiency causing difficult urination. In this condition the urine is difficult because of the lack of yin fluids, which also accounts for its scantiness; the urine is dark because of the drying action of the pathogenic xu-heat, which can also interfere with the Urinary Bladder transformation of fluids and lead to failure of those yin-fluids which remain to be transformed and excreted, and so cause recurring edema. Differentiation of this condition from the damp-heat will be based upon the associated symptoms of yin deficiency without any signs of damp, and especially upon the tongue's lack of a thick yellow coat, and the threadiness of the pulse.

Treatment requires nourishment of the yin-fluids of the Liver and Kidneys to control xu-heat, and the restoration of the Urinary Bladder qi transformation through diuresis, with a formula such as Ji Sheng Shen Qi Wan ('Kidney Qi Pill from *Formulas to Aid the Living*')

Formula

Ji Sheng Shen Qi Wan ('Kidney Qi Pill from *Formulas to Aid the Living*')

Shou Di	Rehmanniae Glutinosae Conquitae, Radix
Shan Zhu Yu	Corni Officinalis, Fructus
Shan Yao	Dioscoreae Oppositae, Radix

Fu Ling	Poriae Cocos, Sclerotium
Ze Xie	Alismatis Plantago-aquaticae, Rhizoma
Mu Dan Pi	Moutan Radicis, Cortex
Fu Zi	Aconiti Carmichaeli Praeparata, Radix
Rou Gui	Cinnamomi Cassiae, Cortex
Niu Xi	Achyranthis Bidentatae, Radix
Che Qian Zi	Plantaginis, Semen

Source text: *Ji Sheng Fang* ('Formulas to Aid the Living', Yan Yong–He, 1253) [*Formulas & Strategies*, p. 278]

Summary

The mechanisms causing difficult urination are closely related to the functioning of the three zang-organs the Lungs, Spleen and Kidneys. The excess mechanisms involved are usually those of exogenous wind, cold or damp-heat; while the most common deficient mechanism is that of yang deficiency, although Kidney and Liver yin deficiency is also seen occasionally.

If the difficult urination is the result of excessive sweating, vomiting or diarrhea damaging the body fluids, these conditions should be treated first, coupled with restoration of the yin-fluids.

Obstructed urination (xiao bian bu tong)

This refers to severe difficulty in passing urine which is present in the Urinary Bladder, so that only a few drops emerge. The difference between this condition and the previous one is that here urine has reached the Urinary Bladder but is unable to be passed. Again, in clinic this condition must be distinguished from painful urination, where the pain is the primary symptom; in obstructed urination, although some of the symptom patterns include pain, the primary symptom is the obstruction.

In the ancient, and some modern, texts, this is called 'long bi' 癃閉.

Common symptom patterns

Lower Jiao damp-heat. Obstructed flow of urine commonly associated with frequency, urgency and pain, with occasional burning upon the passage of urine. There will also be characteristic symptoms of damp-heat, such as bitter taste in the mouth, thirst without desire to drink much, difficult yet not dry stool, red tongue with a yellow greasy coat, and a deep rapid or soft (ru) rapid pulse.

Bound-up Lung qi. Obstructed flow of urine, associated with a sensation of tightness in the chest, cough, rough breathing, shortness of breath, constipation, red or pale red tongue with a white or thin yellow coat, and a soft (ru) rapid pulse.

Middle Jiao qi deficiency. Difficulty in the expulsion of urine, associated with characteristic symptoms of qi deficiency and digestive disorder, such as lethargy, tiredness, poor appetite, epigastric and abdominal distension and fullness, dragging sensation in the lower abdomen, loose stool, pale tongue with a thin white coat, and a deep weak pulse.

Kidney yang qi deficiency. Frequent urge yet forceless and difficult expulsion of urine, associated with characteristic symptoms of Kidney yang qi deficiency, such as lower backache, cold limbs, pale flabby tongue with a thin white coat, and a deep thready pulse which is soft at the proximal (chi) position.

Liver qi blockage. Obstructed flow of urine, or possibly flowing but not smoothly, with typical symptoms of Liver qi blockage such as mood swings, short temper, insomnia and disturbing dreams, distension in the flanks, bitter taste and sour regurgitation, red tongue with a thin yellow coat, and a wiry pulse.

Blood stagnation in the urinary pathways. Obstruction or periodic obstruction to the flow of urine, with sensations of lower abdominal fullness and pain, or even abdominal mass, purple tongue or purple areas on the tongue, with a white or thin yellow tongue coat, and a choppy (se) pulse.

Urinary tract stones or gravel. Sudden but intermittent urinary obstruction with scraping or cutting pain in the urethra, lessening when the urine flows smoothly, passage of small stones or gravel, and accompanied by symptoms of either Liver qi obstruction or damp-heat.

Differentiation

Lower Jiao damp-heat versus bound-up Lung qi causing urinary obstruction. Both of these are excess (shi) conditions, but the mechanism of the latter is located in the upper Jiao, while the focus of action of the damp-heat is in the lower Jiao.

Chao Yuan–Fang, in the *Zhu Bing Yuan Hou Lun* ('General Treatise on the Etiology and Symptomatology of Disease', 610 AD), says:

> The reason for urinary obstruction is heat in both the Urinary Bladder and the Kidneys. Kidneys control water, Urinary Bladder is the fu-organ of the jin and ye fluids, and these two channels stand in interior-exterior relationship with each other. When water moves from the Small Intestine, it enters the Bladder and becomes urine. But if the Kidneys and Urinary Bladder are hot, this heat enters the Bladder, and [because] the pathogenic hot qi is extreme, it knots and obstructs and thus urine is unable to flow.[20]

The dual pathogen damp-heat can obstruct the flow of urine in a number of ways beyond those mentioned in the quotation above. The most basic mechanism is that of qi obstruction: if the qi cannot move freely in the Urinary Bladder its qi transformation activity is greatly hampered, which is also the reason for the accompanying lower abdominal distension. This could also be expressed, although somewhat less obviously, as 'a local preponderance of yin in the Urinary Bladder': the pathogenic yin-natured damp, continually thickened by the pathogenic heat, congests the Urinary Bladder and prevails over the ability of the normal physiological yang qi to enter and perform the necessary function of qi transformation, so that fluids accumulate in the Urinary Bladder but are unable to be expelled. As the *Nei Jing* says: '[Only through] qi transformation can the fluids emerge'.

The damp-heat can also prevent the qi transformation more widely throughout the body, by obstructing the circulation of fluids and yuan qi in the San Jiao.[21]

The important points in differentiation will be the frequency, urgency and pain, with occasional burning sensation of the urine, as well as the presence of characteristic symptoms of damp-heat: bitter taste in the mouth, thirst without desire to drink much, difficult yet not dry stool, red tongue with a yellow greasy coat, and a deep rapid or soft (ru) rapid pulse.

Treatment requires cooling the heat and expelling the damp through encouraging diuresis with a formula such as Ba Zheng San ('Eight-Herb Powder for Rectification') or, if necessary, Shu Zao Yin Zi ('The Dispersing Chisel Decoction').

Bound-up Lung qi causing urinary obstruction is an upper Jiao pathology usually resulting from an exogenous invasion (see note 13). The differentiating points between this and Urinary Bladder obstruction are that Lung obstruction will not cause urinary burning and pain, and the yellowness of the urine is less. There will also be obvious Lung symptoms such as a sensation of tightness in the chest, cough, rough breathing, and shortness of breath, with possible constipation due to the failure of Lung qi to support rhythmic downward peristalsis, and a red or pale red tongue with a white or thin yellow coat, plus a soft (ru) rapid pulse.

In the early stages, something as simple as inciting a sneeze[22] can be used to open the flow of Lung qi but, if the blockage has continued for a time and produced heat, then a formula such as Qing Fei Yin ('Clear the Lungs Decoction') may need to be used.

Formulas

Ba Zheng San ('Eight-Herb Powder for Rectification', *Formulas & Strategies*, p. 192)
(See above)

Shu Zao Yin Zi ('Dispersing Chisel Decoction')

Shang Lu	Phytolaccae, Radix
Qiang Huo	Notopterygii, Rhizoma et Radix
Qin Jiao	Gentianae Macrophyllae, Radix
Bing Lang	Arecae Catechu, Semen
Da Fu Pi	Arecae Catechu, Pericarpium
Fu Ling Pi	Poriae Cocos, Cortex
Chuan Jiao	Zanthoxyli Bungeani, Fructus
Mu Tong	Mutong, Caulis
Ze Xie	Alismatis Plantago-aquaticae, Rhizoma
Chi Xiao Dou	Phaseoli Calcarati, Semen
Sheng Jiang Pi	Zingiberis Officinalis Recens, Cortex

Source text: *Ji Sheng Fang* ('Formulas to Aid the Living', 1253)

Qing Fei Yin ('Clear the Lungs Decoction')

Fu Ling	Poriae Cocos, Sclerotium
Huang Qin	Scutellariae Baicalensis, Radix
Sang Bai Pi	Mori Albae Radicis, Cortex
Mai Men Dong	Ophiopogonis Japonici, Tuber
Che Qian Zi	Plantaginis, Semen
Shan Zhi Zi	Gardeniae Jasminoidis, Fructus
Mu Tong	Mutong, Caulis

Source text: *Zheng Zhi Hui Bu* ('A Supplement to Diagnosis and Treatment', Qing dynasty)

Middle Jiao qi deficiency versus Kidney yang qi deficiency causing urinary obstruction. Both of these are deficient conditions, and the difficulty in urination stems from lack of force in expulsion.

The first can result from constitutional Spleen qi deficiency, or overexertion or irregular eating damaging the Spleen: its location is the middle Jiao. The mechanism can involve several aspects: the first is loss of fluids through the spontaneous perspiration often accompanying qi deficiency, so that fluids are lost through the surface and thus less fluids reach the Urinary Bladder; the second is poor Spleen transportation failing to maintain fluid circulation, so that fluids again fail to reach the Urinary Bladder (and indeed may congeal to become damp or phlegm); and the third is the general weakness of qi movement, which manifests as forceless expulsion of urine.

The latter is a lower Jiao deficient pathology resulting from old age, long-term illness or excessive reproductive activity injuring the Kidney yang, so that it cannot support the Urinary Bladder qi transformation of fluids and also fails to provide yang force for the expulsion of urine.

The important differentiating points are those which indicate the location of the weakness as being either in the middle or the lower Jiao. For example, with Spleen qi deficiency there will often be signs of abnormal Spleen transportation or middle Jiao qi failure to rise; the urinary blockage will vary depending upon the degree of tiredness of the patient: when they feel energetic the urine will flow with more strength, when tired it will cease. On the other hand, with Kidney yang deficiency there will be frequent urge to urinate, because of failing Kidney consolidation, but when the patient tries the flow will be forceless or absent altogether.

Treatment of the Spleen qi deficiency requires support of Spleen qi while assisting urinary output.

If Spleen transportation is obviously affected, with a build-up of damp or phlegm, Liu Jun Zi Tang ('Six-Gentlemen Decoction', *Formulas & Strategies*, p. 238) should be used with additions such as *Mu Tong* (Mutong, Caulis) and *Xiang Fu* (Cyperi Rotundi, Rhizoma); if qi fails to rise but instead pathologically descends, then one can use a formula such as Bu Zhong Yi Qi Tang ('Tonify the Middle and Augment the Qi Decoction'): as Zhu Dan-Xi remarked in another context 'When wishing descent (in this case, normal descent of urine), first lift'.

Treatment of the Kidney yang deficiency requires warming yang and supporting qi, tonifying Kidneys and promoting urination, with a formula such as Ji Sheng Shen Qi Wan ('Kidney Qi Pill from *Formulas to Aid the Living*').

Formulas

Liu Jun Zi Tang ('Six Gentlemen Decoction')

Ren Shen	Ginseng, Radix
Bai Zhu	Atractylodis Macrocephalae, Rhizoma
Fu Ling	Poriae Cocos, Sclerotium
Ban Xia	Pinelliae Ternata, Rhizoma
Chen Pi	Citri Reticulatae, Pericarpium
Gan Cao	Glycyrrhizae Uralensis, Radix

Source text: *Yi Xue Zheng Chuan* ('True Lineage of Medicine', 1515) [*Formulas & Strategies*, p. 238]

Bu Zhong Yi Qi Tang ('Tonify the Middle and Augment the Qi Decoction')

Huang Qi	Astragali, Radix
Ren Shen	Ginseng, Radix
Bai Zhu	Atractylodis Macrocephalae, Rhizoma
Dang Gui	Angelica Polymorpha, Radix
Chen Pi	Citri Reticulatae, Pericarpium
Sheng Ma	Cimicifugae, Rhizoma
Chai Hu	Bupleuri, Radix
Zhi Gan Cao	Honey-fried Glycyrrhizae Uralensis, Radix

Source text: *Pi Wei Lun* ('Discussion of the Spleen and Stomach', 1249) [*Formulas & Strategies*, p. 241]

Ji Sheng Shen Qi Wan ('Kidney Qi Pill from *Formulas to Aid the Living*', *Formulas & Strategies*, p. 278).
(See above)

Liver qi blockage causing urinary obstruction. This condition is usually a result of emotional factors upsetting the harmonious flow of Liver qi, which becomes obstructed and can either disturb San Jiao fluid pathway circulation or interfere with the Urinary Bladder qi transformation. The latter is not unusual, due to the intersection of the Liver channel with itself directly above the location of the Urinary Bladder. An obstruction here blocks movement of qi throughout the area, even to the extent that patients often mention aching in the tops of the thighs, as the qi flow through the Stomach, Spleen and Liver channels is impeded. The important points in differentiation are that the urinary obstruction worsens with stress and emotions, and that other symptoms of Liver qi blockage are present. In some cases, Liver qi blockage will lead to heat or to damp, or even to both, in which case it is important to differentiate this condition from that of damp-heat. In damp-heat, however, the symptoms will often be more localized in the lower Jiao, the urine will be burning and often cloudy, and the patient will report lethargy and other typical damp-heat symptoms. With Liver heat and damp, on the other hand, the symptoms will be more generalized, the damp symptoms will often be most obvious in the middle Jiao rather than the lower, and the patient will appear tense and anxious rather than tired and heavy. The tongue and pulse will also differ, presenting purple spots or general darkening with Liver qi blockage, while with damp-heat the tongue coat will be yellow, greasy and thicker at the base of the tongue.[23]

Treatment requires promotion of harmonious movement of Liver qi, while encouraging urination, with a combination of formulas such as Chen Xiang San ('Aquilariae Powder') and Chai Hu Shu Gan San ('Bupleurum Powder to Spread the Liver').

Formulas

Chen Xiang San ('Aquilariae Powder')

Chuan Xiong	Ligustici Wallichii, Radix
Shi Wei	Pyrrosiae, Folium
Hua Shi	Talc
Dang Gui	Angelica Polymorpha, Radix
Chen Pi	Citri Reticulatae, Pericarpium
Bai Shao	Paeoniae Lactiflora, Radix
Dong Kui Zi	Abutiloni seu Malvae, Semen

Wang Bu Liu Xing	Vaccariae Segetalis, Semen
Gan Cao	Glycyrrhizae Uralensis, Radix

Source text: *Jin Gui Yi* ('Supplement to the Golden Cabinet', 1768)

Chai Hu Shu Gan San ('Bupleurum Powder to Spread the Liver', *Formulas & Strategies*, p. 146) (See above)

Blood stagnation in the urinary pathways versus urinary tract stones or gravel causing urinary obstruction. Both are conditions of severe stagnation in the lower Jiao leading to painful obstructed urine. Blood stagnation can be the result of a number of factors, such as local injury from external trauma, qi blockage leading to stagnation in the flow of blood or heat drying the fluid portion of the blood so that it thickens and stagnates. Although different clinical manifestations will attend each of these factors, the end result of blood stagnation gives them all certain symptoms in common, such as fixed stabbing pain in the lower abdomen, darkish red or purple colored urine which may even contain clots, purple spots or areas of the tongue, and a choppy (se) pulse.

Stones or gravel in the urinary tract will also cause intense pain but more localized to the urethra, and more intermittent, as it will lessen when the urine flow is good. Stones or gravel can form as a result of the long-term influence of two factors: the first is damp-heat, the damp being dried by the heat until it thickens and then hardens into stones; the second is Liver qi blockage leading to heat which then moves into the Urinary Bladder and dries the Urinary Bladder fluids until they harden.

Treatment of lower Jiao blood stagnation requires the dispersal of stagnation and the movement of blood, with a formula such as Dai Di Dang Wan ('Substitute for "Resistance Decoction" Pill'). Alternatively, one could also use Yi Wei Niu Xi Gao ('Single Herb Achyranthes Syrup') plus *Tao Ren* (Persicae, Semen), as Shen Jin-Ao (1717-1776, author of *Shen Shi Zun Sheng Shu* 'Master Shen's Book for Revering Life', 1773) notes: 'In urinary obstruction from stagnant blood, *Niu Xi* (Achyranthis Bidentatae, Radix) and *Tao Ren* are the two most important herbs; when I have adopted this method, its use has been very effective'.

Treatment of stones and gravel causing urinary obstruction requires different formulas depending upon the etiology. If the problem results from Liver qi blockage, use Niao Lu Pai Shi Tang Yi Hao ('Urinary Tract Calculus-Expelling Decoction No. 1') plus *Yan Hu Suo* (Corydalis Yanhusuo, Rhizoma), *Xiang Fu* (Cyperi Rotundi, Rhizoma) and *Qing Pi* (Citri Reticulatae Viride, Pericarpium); if the problem results from damp-heat, use Niao Lu Pai Shi Tang Er Hao ('Urinary Tract Calculus-Expelling Decoction No. 2') plus *Pu Gong Ying* (Taraxaci Mongolici cum Radice, Herba) and *Zi Hua Di Ding* (Violae cum Radice, Herba).

Formulas

Dai Di Dang Wan ('Substitute for "Resistance Decoction" Pill')

Da Huang	Rhei, Rhizoma
Dang Gui Wei	Angelica Polymorpha, Radix
Sheng Di	Rehmannia Glutinosae, Radix
Chuan Shan Jia	Manitis Pentadactylae, Squama
Mang Xiao	Mirabilitum
Tao Ren	Persicae, Semen
Rou Gui	Cinnamomi Cassiae, Cortex

Source text: *Zheng Zhi Zhun Sheng* ('Standards of Patterns and Treatments', 1602)

Yi Wei Niu Xi Gao ('Single Herb Achyranthes Syrup')

Niu Xi	Achyranthis Bidentatae, Radix

Source text: *Zheng Zhi Zhun Sheng* ('Standards of Patterns and Treatments', 1602)

Niao Lu Pai Shi Tang Yi Hao ('Urinary Tract Calculus-Expelling Decoction No. 1')

Jin Qian Cao	30-60 g	Jinqiancao, Herba
Hai Jin Sha	10 g	Lygodii Japonici, Spora
Che Qian Zi	24 g	Plantaginis, Semen
Mu Tong	10 g	Mutong, Caulis
Hua Shi	15 g	Talc
Chi Shao	12 g	Paeoniae Rubra, Radix
Wu Yao	10 g	Linderae Strychnifoliae, Radix
Chuan Lian Zi	10 g	Meliae Toosendan, Fructus
Ji Nei Jin	10 g	Corneum Gigeraiae Galli, Endithelium
Gan Cao	3 g	Glycyrrhizae Uralensis, Radix

Source text: *Zhong Xi Yi Jie He Zhi Liao Chang Jian Wai Ke Ji Fu Zheng* ('Combined Chinese-Western Treatment of Acute Abdominal Conditions')[24]

Niao Lu Pai Shi Tang Er Hao ('Urinary Tract Calculus-Expelling Decoction No. 2')

Jin Qian Cao	45 g	Jinqiancao, Herba
Shi Wei	30 g	Pyrrosiae, Folium
Che Qian Zi	24 g	Plantaginis, Semen
Mu Tong	10 g	Mutong, Caulis
Bian Xu	24 g	Polygoni Avicularis, Herba
Qu Mai	15 g	Dianthi, Herba
Shan Zhi Zi	18 g	Gardeniae Jasminoidis, Fructus
Da Huang	12 g	Rhei, Rhizoma (add later)
Hua Shi	15 g	Talc
Gan Cao Xiao	10 g	Glycyrrhizae Uralensis, Radix
Niu Xi	15 g	Achyranthis Bidentatae, Radix
Zhi Shi	10 g	Citri seu Ponciri Immaturis, Fructus

Source text: *Zhong Xi Yi Jie He Zhi Liao Chang Jian Wai Ke Ji Fu Zheng* ('Combined Chinese-Western Treatment of Acute Abdominal Conditions')[25]

Classical comments

The *Bian Zheng Lu* ('Records of Syndrome Differentiation', 1687, by Chen Shi-Duo) contains the following interesting expansion on the pathological mechanism of 'Heart shifting fire to the Small Intestine':

> When people have obstructed urine which only dribbles without coming out [in a strong stream], and urgency with a blocked-up feeling [in the lower abdomen] so that they wish to die, with restlessness in the Heart and irritation in the mind, and thirst and continual drinking which only exacerbates the urgency, then doctors think that this is extreme heat in the Small Intestine. Who would guess that this is actually Heart fire flaring to an extreme degree? Heart and Small Intestine are internally-externally connected; extreme Small Intestine heat causing urinary obstruction (long bi) is nothing but heat in the Heart causing urinary obstruction. This is because the ability of the Small Intestine to open and close depends completely on the communication of the qi between the Heart and the Kidneys. In the present situation, Heart heat flares and so clear qi (qing qi) cannot interact with the Small Intestine—only a fierce heat which drives both (i.e. the Heart and Small Intestine). The Small Intestine [in this case] has

only yang and no yin, how could it transform? Since the Small Intestine cannot transform, how can the Urinary Bladder do the transforming for it? Not to mention that since the Heart and the Kidneys qi is unable to enter the Small Intestine, how could it enter the Urinary Bladder to transform the fluids held there? The method of treatment is to drain the fire in the midst of the Heart, while simultaneously promoting Urinary Bladder [urination]; then the qi of the Heart and the Kidneys will communicate, and the urination will likewise move freely.[26]

Frequent urination

This refers to an obvious increase in the frequency of urination, which when severe can occur up to every fifteen to twenty minutes during waking. This condition is different from both 'nocturia', which is frequency only at night, and 'clear profuse urination', which may be frequent but is always clear and profuse, whereas 'frequency' may be clear or dark, and profuse or scanty.

Common symptom patterns

Urinary Bladder damp-heat. Frequency, urgency, burning and pain with urination, which is scanty, yellow, and cloudy; accompanied by characteristic symptoms of Urinary Bladder damp-heat such as dry mouth with little desire to drink, sensations of lower abdominal fullness and distension, difficult-to-pass yet not dry stool, (or alternating dry and loose stool), red tongue with a greasy yellow coat, and a rapid slippery or rapid soft (ru) pulse.

Kidney yin deficiency. Frequent but scanty yellow urine with sensations of burning or difficulty, and characteristic symptoms of yin deficiency such as malar flush, insomnia, tinnitus, dry throat, hot flushes worse in the afternoon or evening, heat in the palms, soles and center of the chest, aching of the lower back and knees, spermatorrhea, red tongue with little or no coat, and thready rapid pulse.

Failing Kidney consolidation. Frequent clear and profuse urination, possibly with incontinence, associated with characteristic symptoms of Kidney yang deficiency such as weak aching lower back and knees, cold limbs, tinnitus, pale face, pale flabby tongue with a thin white coat, and a deep thready weak pulse, especially at the proximal (chi) position.

Lung and Spleen qi deficiency. Frequent, clear and profuse urination, with possible incontinence, worse with exertion, and accompanied by typical symptoms of qi deficiency of the Lungs and the Spleen, such as expectoration of clear thin mucus or excessive saliva, tiredness, shortness of breath, reluctance to speak much, sensitivity to cold, poor appetite, loose stool, pale lips and tongue, white tongue coat, and a large floating but forceless pulse.

Liver qi blockage. Frequency worsened by stress, and characterized by an unfinished feeling after voiding accompanied by typical symptoms of Liver qi blockage such as discomfort in the flanks and subcostal region, emotional tension and stress, anger, burping and flatulence, abdominal bloating, purplish tinge to the tongue body, and a wiry pulse.

Differentiation

Urinary Bladder damp-heat versus Kidney yin deficiency causing frequency. Both are lower Jiao pathologies, and both of these conditions manifest scanty dark urine. The former, however, is an excess condition involving pathogenic damp-heat pouring into the Urinary Bladder: the damp obstructing the normal qi transformative processes and the heat both drying the fluids and encouraging frequency; while the latter is a deficiency of the Kidneys leading to a loss of consolidation and the generation of xu-heat, both of which contribute to the frequency of urination.

Important points in differentiation are the excess type symptoms of the Urinary Bladder damp-heat: the urgency, burning and pain combined with the lower abdominal fullness and distension, and the dark yellowness of the urine. The urine in the Kidney yin deficiency condition is yellow as well but not as dark as the former, and both the accompanying symptoms and the pulse will indicate deficiency. The tongue coat in the Urinary Bladder damp-heat is yellow and greasy, while the tongue coat in Kidney yin deficiency is scanty or absent altogether.

Treatment of frequency from the Urinary Bladder damp-heat requires cooling heat and expelling damp, and thus separating these two pathogens, with the use of a formula such as Ba Zheng San ('Eight-Herb Powder for Rectification').

Kidney yin deficiency requires moistening rather than cooling tonification to control internal xu-fire, with a formula such as Zhi Bai Di Huang Wan ('Anemarrhena, Phellodendron, and Rehmannia Pill'), with suitable additions to improve Kidney consolidation such as *Wu Wei Zi* (Schisandrae Chinensis, Fructus), *Jin Ying Zi* (Rosae Laevigatae, Fructus), and increased dosages in the parent formula of *Shan Zhu Yu* (Corni Officinalis, Fructus) and *Shan Yao* (Dioscoreae Oppositae, Radix).

Formulas

Ba Zheng San ('Eight-Herb Powder for Rectification')

Mu Tong	Mutong, Caulis
Hua Shi	Talc
Che Qian Zi	Plantaginis, Semen
Qu Mai	Dianthi, Herba
Bian Xu	Polygoni Avicularis, Herba
Shan Zhi Zi	Gardeniae Jasminoidis, Fructus
Zhi Da Huang	Rhei, Rhizoma (treated)
Deng Xin Cao	Junci Effusi, Medulla
Gan Cao	Glycyrrhizae Uralensis, Radix

Source text: *Tai Ping Hui Min He Ji Ju Fang* ('Imperial Grace Formulary of the Tai Ping Era', 1078-85) [*Formulas & Strategies*, p. 192]

Zhi Bai Di Huang Wan ('Anemarrhena, Phellodendron, and Rehmannia Pill')

Zhi Mu	Anemarrhenae Asphodeloidis, Radix)
Huang Bo	Phellodendri, Cortex)
Sheng Di	Rehmannia Glutinosae, Radix)
Shan Zhu Yu	Corni Officinalis, Fructus)
Shan Yao	Dioscoreae Oppositae, Radix)
Fu Ling	Poriae Cocos, Sclerotium)
Mu Dan Pi	Moutan Radicis, Cortex)
Ze Xie	Alismatis Plantago-aquaticae, Rhizoma)

Source text: *Zheng Yin Mai Zhi* ('Pattern, Cause, Pulse, and Treatment', 1702) [*Formulas & Strategies*, p. 265]

Failing Kidney consolidation versus Lung and Spleen qi deficiency causing frequency. Both of these are deficiency conditions but the former is located in the lower Jiao, while the latter is located in the middle and upper Jiao. Both, too, have clear profuse urination as well as frequency.

The Kidney deficiency, however, will often involve yang deficiency symptoms, resulting from either constitutional factors, long illness or excessive reproductive activity, so that Kidneys lose their inherent yin-natured consolidation and also fail to support the qi transformation in the Urinary Bladder, each of which contributes to the frequency of urination. Lung and Spleen qi deficiency often results from over-exertion, excessive consumption of cold or raw foods, or exogenous cold invasion damaging yang qi. Once deficient, the qi can no longer lift properly and, lacking this support, the Urinary Bladder is unable to retain fluids. Added to this is the increased volume of fluids which impairment to the Spleen and Lung fluid functions generates: these fluids pour down into the Urinary Bladder and cause profuse clear urination, and also lead to the tell-tale expectoration of clear thin mucus as these fluids well upwards.

The important points in differentiation will be those which identify the location of the original problem as being either in the lower Jiao or alternatively in the middle and upper Jiao. Also, Kidney deficiency frequency will most often occur in older people with weak yang, or children whose physiological yang is not yet strong; while Lung and Spleen qi deficiency typically appears in over-worked middle age, and characteristically worsens with exertion.

Treatment of the Kidneys requires the warming of Kidney yang and support for Kidney consolidation with a formula such as You Gui Wan ('Restore the Right [Kidney] Pill'), with suitable additions such as *Fu Pen Zi* (Rubi, Fructus), *Sang Piao Xiao* (Mantidis, Ootheca) and *Bu Gu Zhi* (Psoraleae Corylifoliae, Fructus).

Treatment of Lung and Spleen qi deficiency requires warm tonification of the Lungs and Spleen, while assisting the rise of qi, with a formula such as Bu Zhong Yi Qi Tang ('Tonify the Middle and Augment the Qi Decoction') plus herbs to warm yang and support Lung and Spleen fluid transportation, such as *Gan Jiang* (Zingiberis Officianalis, Rhizoma) and *Yi Zhi Ren* (Alpiniae Oxyphyllae, Fructus) (which also consolidates the Urinary Bladder).

Formulas

You Gui Wan ('Restore the Right [Kidney] Pill')

Fu Zi	Aconiti Carmichaeli Praeparata, Radix
Rou Gui	Cinnamomi Cassiae, Cortex
Lu Jiao Jiao	Cervi Colla Cornu
Shou Di	Rehmanniae Glutinosae Conquitae, Radix
Shan Zhu Yu	Corni Officinalis, Fructus
Shan Yao	Dioscoreae Oppositae, Radix
Gou Qi Zi	Lycii Chinensis, Fructus
Tu Si Zi	Cuscutae, Semen
Du Zhong	Eucommiae Ulmoidis, Cortex
Dang Gui	Angelica Polymorpha, Radix

Source text: *Jing Yue Quan Shu* ('Complete Works of Jing Yue', 1624) [*Formulas & Strategies*, p. 278]

Bu Zhong Yi Qi Tang ('Tonify the Middle and Augment the Qi Decoction')

Huang Qi	Astragali, Radix
Ren Shen	Ginseng, Radix
Bai Zhu	Atractylodis Macrocephalae, Rhizoma
Zhi Gan Cao	Honey-fried Glycyrrhizae Uralensis, Radix
Dang Gui	Angelica Polymorpha, Radix
Chen Pi	Citri Reticulatae, Pericarpium
Sheng Ma	Cimicifugae, Rhizoma
Chai Hu	Bupleuri, Radix

Source text: *Pi Wei Lun* ('Discussion of the Spleen and Stomach', 1249) [*Formulas & Strategies*, p. 241]

Liver qi blockage causing frequency. This very common condition is relatively easy to identify, associated as it is with anxiety and other Liver symptoms. The difficulty occurs when it is combined with any of the other pathologies above. In that case one must differentiate the degree to which Liver qi blockage is contributing to the frequency, and this can be done by determining the degree to which the frequency is worsened by stress. Stress will inhibit the flow of qi in the Liver channel, which will in turn impede the circulation of normal qi throughout the lower Jiao, and thus exacerbate any other pathology occurring in the area.

Treatment requires freeing the flow of Liver qi (in addition, of course, to dealing with any other pathologies which may be involved) with a formula such as Xiao Yao San ('Rambling Powder') plus *Wu Yao* (Linderae Strychnifoliae, Radix).

Formula

Xiao Yao San ('Rambling Powder')

Chai Hu	Bupleuri, Radix
Dang Gui	Angelica Polymorpha, Radix
Bai Shao	Paeoniae Lactiflora, Radix
Bai Zhu	Atractylodis Macrocephalae, Rhizoma
Fu Ling	Poriae Cocos, Sclerotium
Bo He	Menthae, Herba
Gan Cao	Glycyrrhizae Uralensis, Radix

Source text: *Tai Ping Hui Min He Ji Ju Fang* ('Imperial Grace Formulary of the Tai Ping Era', 1078-85) [*Formulas & Strategies*, p. 147]

Summary

Frequency of urination can be divided into deficient and excess etiologies. The deficient conditions will usually involve qi or yang deficiency, which will have clear profuse urination, although Kidney yin deficiency is also possible, with scanty dark urination, which is however not as dark as that of the most common excess condition: damp-heat. Damp-heat will also manifest urgency, burning and pain. The other excess condition involves Liver qi blockage, with its characteristic unfinished feeling.

The three zang-organs most often implicated in frequency are the Kidneys, Spleen, and Lungs; these can be involved either singly or in combination.

Terminal dribbling

This refers to dribbling after otherwise complete voiding of urine. This condition is different from that of incontinence, in which the passage of urine is uncontrolled and of relatively greater volume. If drops of semen appear after voiding, this is categorized as 'spermaturia' and not dribbling.

Common symptom patterns

Kidney deficiency with cold in the Urinary Bladder. Frequent, clear and profuse urination with prolonged terminal dribbling, accompanied by symptoms of Kidney yang deficiency such as cold limbs, aching lower back and knees, sexual dysfunction, tiredness, pale tongue with a white coat, and a deep thready pulse, especially at the proximal (chi) position.

Middle Jiao qi deficiency. Intermittent dribbling, worsened during periods of tiredness, accompanied by symptoms of middle Jiao qi deficiency such as loose stool, poor appetite, dragging sensation in the lower abdomen, tiredness and lethargy, pale tongue with a white coat, languid (huan) and soft (ru) pulse, or a thready weak pulse.

Urinary Bladder damp-heat. Frequent, dark or cloudy urination with prolonged terminal dribbling and sensations of burning or pain in the urethra upon voiding, accompanied by typical symptoms of Urinary Bladder damp-heat, such as feelings of lower abdominal fullness and distension, with a red tongue, yellow greasy tongue coat, and a rapid soft (ru) pulse.

Differentiation

Kidney deficiency with cold in the Urinary Bladder versus middle Jiao qi deficiency causing dribbling. Both of these conditions are the result of deficiency but the locations of the deficiency differ: the former being in the lower Jiao while the latter is in the middle Jiao.

Kidney yang deficiency fails to consolidate the Urinary Bladder, and also fails to support Urinary Bladder qi transformation of fluids, so that the urine becomes frequent, clear, profuse and dribbles at the end.

Deficient middle Jiao qi fails to rise as it should but rather descends, and Urinary Bladder loses the lifting support of this qi. Dribbling occurs during times of tiredness and overwork especially when the qi is weakest.

The important points in differentiation will be the symptoms which identify the location of the deficiency. The age of the patient may also provide an important clue: Kidney yang deficient patients tend to be old, while those with middle Jiao qi deficiency tend to be middle-aged and over-worked.

Treatment of the Kidney yang deficiency with cold in the Urinary Bladder requires warm tonification of the Kidneys with support for Kidney consolidation, using a combination of formulas such

as Jin Gui Shen Qi Wan ('Kidney Qi Pill from the *Golden Cabinet*') and Sang Piao Xiao San ('Mantis Egg-Case Powder'); Tu Si Zi Wan ('Cuscuta Seed Pill') can also be used.

Treatment of the drooping middle Jiao qi requires lifting and tonification of qi with a formula such as Bu Zhong Yi Qi Tang ('Tonify the Middle and Augment the Qi Decoction').

Formulas

Jin Gui Shen Qi Wan ('Kidney Pill from the *Golden Cabinet*')

Shou Di	Rehmanniae Glutinosae Conquitae, Radix
Shan Zhu Yu	Corni Officinalis, Fructus
Shan Yao	Dioscoreae Oppositae, Radix
Fu Zi	Aconiti Carmichaeli Praeparata, Radix
Gui Zhi	Cinnamomi Cassiae, Ramulus
Ze Xie	Alismatis Plantago-aquaticae, Rhizoma
Fu Ling	Poriae Cocos, Sclerotium
Mu Dan Pi	Moutan Radicis, Cortex

Source text: *Jin Gui Yao Lue* ('Essentials from the Golden Cabinet', c. 210 AD) [*Formulas & Strategies*, p. 275]

Sang Piao Xiao San ('Mantis Egg-Case Powder')

Sang Piao Xiao	Mantidis, Ootheca
Long Gu	Draconis, Os
Ren Shen	Ginseng, Radix
Fu Shen	Poriae Cocos Paradicis, Sclerotium
Yuan Zhi	Polygalae Tenuifoliae, Radix
Shi Chang Pu	Acori Graminei, Rhizoma
Zhi Gui Ban	Honey-fried Testudinis, Plastrum
Dang Gui	Angelica Polymorpha, Radix

Source text: *Ben Cao Yan Yi* ('Extension of the Materia Medica', 1116) [*Formulas & Strategies*, p. 362]

Tu Si Zi Wan ('Cuscuta Seed Pill')

Tu Si Zi	Cuscutae, Semen
Lu Rong	Cervi Parvum, Cornu
Rou Cong Rong	Cistanches, Herba
Shan Yao	Dioscoreae Oppositae, Radix
Fu Zi	Aconiti Carmichaeli Praeparata, Radix

Wu Yao	Linderae Strychnifoliae, Radix
Wu Wei Zi	Schisandrae Chinensis, Fructus
Sang Piao Xiao	Mantidis, Ootheca
Yi Zhi Ren	Alpiniae Oxyphyllae, Fructus
Duan Mu Li	Calcined Ostreae, Concha
Ji Nei Jin	Corneum Gigeraiae Galli, Endithelium

Source text: *Ji Sheng Fang* ('Formulas to Aid the Living', 1253) [*Formulas and Strategies*, p. 280]

Bu Zhong Yi Qi Tang ('Tonify the Middle and Augment the Qi Decoction')

Huang Qi	Astragali, Radix
Ren Shen	Ginseng, Radix
Bai Zhu	Atractylodis Macrocephalae, Rhizoma
Dang Gui	Angelica Polymorpha, Radix
Chen Pi	Citri Reticulatae, Pericarpium
Sheng Ma	Cimicifugae, Rhizoma
Chai Hu	Bupleuri, Radix
Gan Cao	Glycyrrhizae Uralensis, Radix

Source text: *Pi Wei Lun* ('Discussion of the Spleen and Stomach', 1249) [*Formulas & Strategies*, p.241]

Urinary Bladder damp-heat causing dribbling. Pathogenic damp prevents normal qi transformation, while heat excites fluid movement and thus leads to terminal dribbling. The important points in differentiation will be those indicating the presence of these two pathogens, such as darkish color or cloudy consistency of the urine, and urgency, frequency, burning and pain upon voiding. Treatment requires cooling of the heat and elimination of the damp with a formula such as Ba Zheng San ('Eight-Herb Powder for Rectification').

Ba Zheng San ('Eight-Herb Powder for Rectification') [*Formulas & Strategies*, p. 192] (See above)

Summary

The first differentiation to make in terminal dribbling is that of excess or deficiency. The latter is the most common, and is characterized by frequent, clear and profuse urination, and also tends to be worse at night. Excess conditions will usually manifest not only frequency but also urgency, burning and pain.

If the dribbling is the result of either 'painful urination syndrome' (lin zheng) or external trauma, then treatment should be aimed at these factors, after the resolution of which the dribbling will clear of itself.

Urinary incontinence

This refers to lack of control over the process of urination, resulting in a loss of urine without warning. This may occur at night but when awake and clear-headed, which differentiates it from 'enuresis', as the latter occurs during sleep. Likewise 'terminal dribbling' refers to general control over urination, with only slight uncontrolled dribbling after otherwise complete voiding.

Incontinence during coma is not a prime presenting symptom, and thus is not included in the section. Treatment should be addressed to the major condition.

Common symptom patterns

Kidney yang deficiency. Urinary incontinence with clear profuse urination and other characteristic symptoms of Kidney yang deficiency such as tiredness and dispiritedness, pale face, cold limbs, weak and aching lower back and legs, sexual dysfunction such as impotence, spermatorrhea or infertility; pale flabby tongue with a thin white coat, and a deep thready and weak pulse.

Lung and Spleen qi deficiency. Incontinent, clear and frequent but not profuse urination, with typical symptoms of Lung and Spleen qi weakness such as cough, dyspnea, shortness of breath, tiredness, poor appetite with abdominal distension after eating, loose stool, pale tongue with a thin white coat, and a large but soft and weak pulse.

Urinary Bladder damp-heat. Relatively rapid onset of urinary incontinence with scanty, dark and only dribbling urine, pain and burning in the urethra with voiding, lower abdominal distension and discomfort, bitter taste and dry mouth, red tongue with a greasy yellow coat, and a wiry rapid pulse.

Liver and Kidney yin deficiency. Gradual onset of urinary incontinence with scanty yellow urine and characteristic symptoms of Liver and Kidney yin deficiency such as tinnitus, vertigo, malar flush, a sensation of dryness and grittiness in the eyes, aching weak lower back and legs, nightsweats, constipation with dry stool, thirst which is relatively easily quenched, red tongue and little or no coat, and a thready rapid and somewhat wiry pulse.

Differentiation

Kidney yang deficiency versus Lung and Spleen qi deficiency causing incontinence. Both of these are deficiency conditions but the former involves lack of yang warmth and is based in the lower Jiao, while the latter involves deficiency of the qi of both the Lungs and the Spleen and thus will manifest symptoms of both the middle and the upper Jiao.

Urinary incontinence from Kidney yang deficiency results from a loss of Kidney consolidation and lack of support for the Urinary Bladder qi transformation, so that urine is clear and profuse as well as incontinent. The condition is most common in older patients.

Lungs and Spleen qi deficiency can result from chronic cough injuring Lung qi, which then fails to regulate the movement of fluids; or constitutional weakness of Spleen qi failing to rise, and thus gradually involving the Lungs. There will be several ramifications from these combined deficiencies. The first is that fluids will often fail to reach the Urinary Bladder at all but instead flood outward and cause edema, and also scanty urine. The second is that the Urinary Bladder is not supported by the lifting of Spleen qi, and thus those fluids which do reach the Urinary Bladder cannot be held in properly and so incontinence occurs. This typically appears in middle-aged patients, and will be exacerbated with tiredness or during exogenous invasions involving the Lungs.

Treatment of the Kidney yang deficiency requires warm tonification of the Kidneys with a formula such as Gong Ti Wan ('Consolidate and Lift Pill') or Sang Piao Xiao San ('Mantis Egg-Case Powder').

Treatment of the Lung and Spleen qi deficiency requires warming of the Lungs and Spleen and restoration of the qi ascent, with a combination of formulas such as Bu Zhong Yi Qi Tang ('Tonify the Middle and Augment the Qi Decoction') and Gan Cao Gan Jiang Tang ('Licorice and Ginger Decoction') plus *Yi Zhi Ren* (Alpiniae Oxyphyllae, Fructus).

Formulas

Gong Ti Wan ('Consolidate and Lift Pill')

Shou Di	60 g	Rehmanniae Glutinosae Conquitae, Radix
Tu Si Zi	60 g	Cuscutae, Semen
Bai Zhu	60 g	Atractylodis Macrocephalae, Rhizoma
Wu Wei Zi	30 g	Schisandrae Chinensis, Fructus
Yi Zhi Ren	30 g	Alpiniae Oxyphyllae, Fructus
Bu Gu Zhi	30 g	Psoraleae Corylifoliae, Fructus
Fu Zi	30 g	Aconiti Carmichaeli Praeparata, Radix
Fu Ling	30 g	Poriae Cocos, Sclerotium
Jiu Zi	30 g	Alli Tuberosi, Semen

Source text: *Jing Yue Quan Shu* ('Complete Works of Jing Yue', 1624)

Grind the ingredients into a fine powder and make small pills with the paste of *Shan Yao* (Dioscoreae Oppositae, Radix). One dose is one hundred pills on an empty stomach taken with water or warm rice wine, two or three times per day. This formula can be used as a decoction with suitably reduced dosages.

Sang Piao Xiao San ('Mantis Egg-Case Powder') [*Formulas & Strategies*, p. 362]
(See above)

Bu Zhong Yi Qi Tang ('Tonify the Middle and Augment the Qi Decoction') [*Formulas & Strategies*, p. 241]
(See above)

Gan Cao Gan Jiang Tang ('Licorice and Ginger Decoction', *Formulas & Strategies*, p. 225)

Gan Jiang	Zingiberis Officianalis, Rhizoma)
Zhi Gan Cao	Honey-fried Glycyrrhizae Uralensis, Radix)

Source text: *Jin Gui Yao Lue* ('Essentials from the Golden Cabinet', c. 210 AD) [*Formulas & Strategies*, p. 225]

Urinary Bladder damp-heat versus Liver and Kidney yin deficiency causing incontinence. Both of these conditions involve heat but the former is excess heat while the latter is heat resulting from deficiency.

Urinary Bladder damp-heat can result from an exogenous invasion of pathogenic damp-heat through the lower orifice, or from the over-consumption of rich, spicy or otherwise heating foods or beverages. The damp blocks qi and so interferes with the Urinary Bladder qi transformation, the yang activity of the heat overwhelms the Urinary Bladder restraint, and thus causes urinary incontinence.

Kidney yin deficiency fails to control normal yang which flares uncontrolled into fire and tends to force urine out of the Urinary Bladder in a way similar to the above situation. Here however the Urinary Bladder restraint is even weaker due to the loss of Kidney consolidation from deficiency.

The Urinary Bladder damp-heat, because it is an excess condition, will usually have a rapid onset and the urine will be burning and painful as well as dark and scanty.

The Kidney and Liver yin deficiency will also have dark and scanty urine but without pain and little if any burning; the yellowness of the urine will also not be as dark as that of the damp-heat. One important indication that the condition is based in deficiency is the gradual onset: this, plus the accompanying—more generalized—symptoms of Liver and Kidney yin deficiency should assist differentiation.

Treatment of the Urinary Bladder damp-heat incontinence requires cooling of the heat coupled with expulsion of the damp, with a formula like Ba Zheng San ('Eight-Herb Powder for Rectification').

Treatment of the Liver and Kidney yin deficiency incontinence requires nourishing of the yin to control yang, so that the xu-fire is extinguished, and the Urinary Bladder restraint regained. This can be accomplished with a formula such as Da Bu Yin Wan ('Great Tonify the Yin Pill') plus *Shan Zhu Yu* (Corni Officinalis, Fructus), *Wu Wei Zi* (Schisandrae Chinensis, Fructus) and *Jin Ying Zi* (Rosae Laevigatae, Fructus).

Formulas

Ba Zheng San ('Eight-Herb Powder for Rectification') [*Formulas & Strategies*, p. 192] (See above)

Da Bu Yin Wan ('Great Tonify the Yin Pill')

Sheng Di	Rehmannia Glutinosae, Radix
Gui Ban	Testudinis, Plastrum
Huang Bo	Phellodendri, Cortex
Zhi Mu	Anemarrhenae Asphodeloidis, Radix

Source text: *Dan Xi Xin Fa* ('Teachings of Dan Xi', 1481) [*Formulas & Strategies*, p. 267]

Case history from Dr. Yi Pin Hai[27]

The patient, Deng, who was 32 years of age, presented in early summer, reporting that he had suffered from incontinence for over half a year, and had taken various medicines without success. He said that urine was urgent and uncontrollable both during the day and at night; he was dizzy and tired, the tongue body was pale, and all six pulses were thready and weak. Regarding this as Kidney yang deficiency with failure of consolidation, I gave him Suo Quan Wan ('Shut the Sluice Pill') with additions. He took ten packets and reported that his energy had begun to return and the urine had become slightly more controllable.

I thought: this patient must have engaged in excessive sexual activity which has damaged the jing-essence and blood so that Kidney qi has become deficient and unable to consolidate the lower source (xia yuan bu gu). The gateway has lost restraint (guan men shi yue, referring to the quote 'Kidneys are the gateway of the Stomach', see note eight in the chapter on edema), and caused urinary incontinence. Without warming the Kidneys and using binding astringents to assist the yang and increase the qi, there will be no chance of success.

So the prescription was designed thus:

Yi Zhi Ren	Alpiniae Oxyphyllae, Fructus
Wu Yao	Linderae Strychnifoliae, Radix
Shan Yao	Dioscoreae Oppositae, Radix
Gui Ban Jiao	Testudinis, Plastrum, Gelatinum
Lu Jiao Jiao	Cervi Colla Cornu
Sheng Long Gu	Draconis, Os
Duan Mu Li	Calcined Ostreae, Concha
Shan Zhu Yu	Corni Officinalis, Fructus
Wu Wei Zi	Schisandrae Chinensis, Fructus

[to assist consolidation]
to this was added

Gou Qi Zi	Lycii Chinensis, Fructus
Rou Cong Rong	Cistanches, Herba
Jin Ying Zi	Rosae Laevigatae, Fructus
Tu Si Zi	Cuscutae, Semen

[to tonify Kidney jing-essence].

The patient took one packet per day, and in just over a month he was cured.

Comment. The interesting thing about this case history is that Dr. Yi began with a straightforward consolidating prescription (Suo Quan Wan) but was not satisfied with the only slight improvement, which signalled to him that a deeper deficiency underlay the lack of consolidation. Working only at the relatively shallow level of strengthening consolidation was not enough, the underlying cause of the lack of Kidney qi must be resolved. Knowing that Kidney qi derives from the steaming action of Kidney yang on the Kidney yin, he designed a prescription to restore both, as well as further strengthening of the consolidating action of Kidney qi. The point is that Dr. Yi knew what his herbs should do, and could interpret the relative failure of his initial prescription, thus enabling him to adjust the approach. Such skill is the product of clinical experience, and is the reason that 'old' Chinese doctors are prized.

Nocturia (ye jian duo niao)

This refers to increased frequency and volume of urine at night. Usually this will be anything over two or three times per night, or urine output which exceeds one-fourth of the daytime volume; although in severe cases the night-time output can approach or exceed the daytime volume. Urine which is normal during the day and only increased at night is the special characteristic of this symptom, which distinguishes it from 'frequency'.

Common symptom patterns

Exhausted Kidney yang. Nocturia with frequency, terminal dribbling, or even incontinence or enuresis, accompanied by characteristic symptoms of Kidney yang deficiency such as cold lower backache, spermatorrhea, tinnitus, pale flabby tongue with a thin white coat, and a deep thready weak pulse.

Deficiency of both Spleen and Kidney yang. Frequent urination worsening at night, with cold limbs and general sensitivity to cold, lower backache, chronic loose stool possibly with undigested food, tiredness and lethargy, dizziness, tinnitus, pale flabby tongue with a white coat, and a deep weak pulse.

Differentiation

Exhausted Kidney yang causing nocturia. Old age, repeated or long-term illness, or even constitutional factors, can result in Kidney yang exhaustion, so that it has difficulty consolidating the Urinary Bladder and the lower orifice. At night, when the strength of yin is greatest, yang finally fails to maintain this consolidation and nocturia results. Treatment requires the warm tonification of Kidney yang and support for consolidation, with a formula such as Da Tu Si Zi Wan ('Great Cuscuta Seed Pill') adjusted for the necessities of the patient.

If the symptoms are less severe, as may be the case in younger patients or those with a shorter history of nocturia, then this can be termed 'Urinary Bladder qi deficiency' rather than 'Kidney yang exhaustion', and the treatment can focus on strengthening qi and consolidating the Urinary Bladder, with a formula such as Sang Piao Xiao San ('Mantis Egg-Case Powder').

Formulas

Da Tu Si Zi Wan ('Great Cuscuta Seed Pill')

Tu Si Zi	Cuscutae, Semen
Ze Xie	Alismatis Plantago-aquaticae, Rhizoma
Lu Rong	Cervi Parvum, Cornu
Long Gu	Draconis, Os
Rou Gui	Cinnamomi Cassiae, Cortex
Fu Zi	Aconiti Carmichaeli Praeparata, Radix
Shi Hu	Dendrobii, Herba
Shou Di	Rehmanniae Glutinosae Conquitae, Radix
Fu Ling	Poriae Cocos, Sclerotium
Chuan Duan	Dipsaci, Radix
Shan Zhu Yu	Corni Officinalis, Fructus
Rou Cong Rong	Cistanches, Herba
Fang Feng	Ledebouriellae Sesloidis, Radix
Du Zhong	Eucommiae Ulmoidis, Cortex
Niu Xi	Achyranthis Bidentatae, Radix
Bu Gu Zhi	Psoraleae Corylifoliae, Fructus
Chen Xiang	Aquilariae, Lignum
Ba Ji Tian	Morindae Officianalis, Radix
Xiao Hui Xiang	Foeniculi Vulgaris, Fructus
Wu Wei Zi	Schisandrae Chinensis, Fructus
Sang Piao Xiao	Mantidis, Ootheca
Chuan Xiong	Ligustici Wallichii, Radix
Fu Pen Zi	Rubi, Fructus
Bi Cheng Qie	Cucubae, Fructus

Source text: *Tai Ping Hui Min He Ji Ju Fang* ('Imperial Grace Formulary of the Tai Ping Era', 1078-85)

Sang Piao Xiao San ('Mantis Egg-Case Powder') [*Formulas & Strategies*, p. 362)
(See above)

Spleen and Kidney yang deficiency causing nocturia. This can result from either Kidney yang failing to support and warm Spleen yang, or conversely from an initial Spleen yang deficiency failing to produce 'later heaven' jing-essence (which would normally support the Kidney jing-essence) and Kidneys then gradually weaken. The mechanism producing the nocturia is similar to the above: weakened Kidney yang is overwhelmed by the strong yin influence at night and can no longer hold in urine. When Spleen is deficient as well, however, the Urinary Bladder also lacks the lifting support of Spleen qi, and so there may be frequency during the daytime too, typically worsened during periods of exhaustion.

The important differentiating points between this and sole deficiency of Kidney yang are that digestive symptoms, such as loose stool and poor appetite, appear in conjunction with the symptoms of lower Jiao yang deficiency. Differentiation is important because a treatment aimed solely at tonifying Kidney yang will only achieve partial results.

The correct approach is to tonify both the Kidneys and the Spleen, warming yang and consolidating the Urinary Bladder, with a combination of formulas such as Gu Pao Tang ('Consolidate the Bladder Decoction') and Suo Quan Wan ('Shut the Sluice Pill').

Formulas

Gu Pao Tang ('Consolidate the Bladder Decoction')

Huang Qi	Astragali, Radix
Tong Ji Li	Astragali, Semen
Shan Zhu Yu	Corni Officinalis, Fructus
Dang Gui	Angelica Polymorpha, Radix
Fu Shen	Poriae Cocos Paradicis, Sclerotium

Chong Wei Zi	Leonuri Heterophylli, Semen
Bai Shao	Paeoniae Lactiflora, Radix
Sheng Ma	Cimicifugae, Rhizoma
Yang Pao	Capra hircus (or Ovis aries), bladder

Source text: *Shen Shi Zun Sheng Shu* ('Master Shen's Book for Revering Life', 1773)

Suo Quan Wan ('Shut the Sluice Pill') [*Formulas & Strategies*, p. 363]
(See above)

Enuresis (yi niao)

This refers to urinary incontinence during sleep, commonly termed 'bed-wetting'; it is most often a pediatric condition. When it occurs in the course of an exogenous invasion, it is a sign of the pathogen moving deeper into the interior and becoming serious. In this case, however, it will not be the main symptom, and thus is not discussed in this section.

Common symptom patterns

Kidney yang deficiency. Enuresis and frequent, profuse and clear urination, accompanied by characteristic symptoms of Kidney yang insufficiency such as facial pallor, tiredness, soreness of the lower back and knees, coldness of the limbs and general sensitivity to cold, dizziness, tinnitus, pale tongue with a white coat, and a deep slow weak pulse, especially at the proximal (chi) position.

Kidney yin deficiency. Enuresis and frequent, scanty, dark and somewhat hot urine, accompanied by characteristic symptoms of yin deficiency such as tinnitus, deafness, vertigo, dry throat, malar flush, nightsweats and hot flushes, aching and weakness of the lower back and knees, dry stool, red tongue with little coat, and a thready rapid pulse.

Spleen qi weak and sinking. Enuresis when over-tired, accompanied by other symptoms of Spleen qi deficiency such as sallow complexion, lack of energy, poor appetite, abdominal distension after eating, dragging feeling in the lower abdomen, loose stool, pale tongue with a white coat, and a weak forceless pulse.

Lung qi deficiency. Enuresis when over-tired, often accompanied by chronic cough with profuse thin white mucus, pale flabby tongue with a white coat, and a thready languid pulse.

Differentiation

Kidney yang deficiency versus Kidney yin deficiency causing enuresis. Kidney yang deficiency leading to enuresis is often constitutional in origin but may also follow excessive sexual activity damaging the Kidney yang, or repeated exposure to cold on the soles of the feet draining Kidney yang warmth, or old age with exhaustion of the Kidneys, or be found in children whose Du and Ren channels have not yet matured to full functioning. Any of these reasons can reduce the ability of the Kidneys to support Urinary Bladder qi transformation, so that urine becomes clear and profuse, and the weakened Kidneys are unable to consolidate the Urinary Bladder, resulting in enuresis.

Kidney yin deficiency also leads to loss of consolidation but a complicating factor in this condition is the presence of yang heat uncontrolled by yin. This heat dries fluids so that urine becomes dark, scanty and somewhat hot, and the expanding yang heat tends to unsettle the Urinary Bladder fluids, leading to enuresis.

Treatment of Kidney yang deficiency enuresis requires warming and consolidating Kidneys with formulas such as Gong Ti Wan ('Consolidate and Lift Pill') or Sang Piao Xiao San ('Mantis Egg-Case Powder').

Treatment of Kidney yin deficiency requires nourishing yin to control yang with a formula such as Zhi Bai Di Huang Wan ('Anemarrhena, Phellodendron and Rehmannia Pill') with increased dosage of *Shan Zhu Yu* (Corni Officinalis, Fructus) and *Shan Yao* (Dioscoreae Oppositae, Radix), plus the addition of sour-astringent herbs such as *Wu Wei Zi* (Schisandrae Chinensis, Fructus) and *Jin Ying Zi* (Rosae Laevigatae, Fructus).

Formulas

Gong Ti Wan ('Consolidate and Lift Pill')
(See above)

Sang Piao Xiao San ('Mantis Egg-Case Powder')
[*Formulas & Strategies*, p. 362)
(See above)

Zhi Bai Di Huang Wan ('Amnemarrhena, Phellodendron and Rehmannia Pill') [*Formulas and Strategies*, p. 265]
(See above)

Spleen qi weak and sinking versus Lung qi deficiency causing enuresis. Both of these conditions are deficiencies of qi, and are often found in conjunction with each other. The deficient Spleen qi cannot lift, thus depriving Urinary Bladder of its support; the deficient Lung qi can no longer control the regularity of fluid passage, so that in the upper body fluids well upward and produce profuse thin mucus, while below the lack of fluid regulation causes enuresis.[28] Thus You Zai-Jing (d. 1749) comments: 'If Spleen and Lungs are deficient in qi, they cannot control the fluid pathways, resulting in the disease of incontinence; this is what the *Jin Gui Yao Lue* ('Essentials from the Golden Cabinet') termed "Upper deficiency unable to control below"'. Often the injury to the functioning of these two organs can be traced back to emotional causes: excessive concentration, worry or grief consuming the qi.

Treatment can be combined, or separate: if the Spleen is most implicated, formulas such as Gu Pao Tang ('Consolidate the Bladder Decoction') and Bu Zhong Yi Qi Tang ('Tonify the Middle and Augment the Qi Decoction') can be combined to restore and lift qi while consolidating the Urinary Bladder; if the Lungs are most involved, warming and tonifying Lungs with a formula such as Gan Cao Gan Jiang Tang ('Licorice and Ginger Decoction', *Formulas & Strategies*, p. 225) plus *Ren Shen* (Ginseng, Radix) is best.

Formulas

Gu Pao Tang ('Consolidate the Bladder Decoction')
(See above)

Bu Zhong Yi Qi Tang ('Tonify the Middle and Augment the Qi Decoction') [*Formulas & Strategies*, p. 241]
(See above)

Gan Cao Gan Jiang Tang ('Licorice and Ginger Decoction') [*Formulas & Strategies*, p. 225]
(See above)

Summary

The basic pathological mechanism involved in enuresis is lack of Urinary Bladder consolidation. But this consolidation is itself connected to the Urinary Bladder qi transformation, which in turn relies upon the proper functioning of each of the Five Zang: the warmth of the Heart (supporting Kidney yang), the regulation by the Lungs of the fluid pathways, the movement of Liver qi, the lifting of Spleen qi and most importantly the yang qi of the Kidneys and Du channel, which control 'kai he': opening and closing.

Painful urination

This refers to stabbing, burning, rough, or strangulation-like sensations in the urethra during voiding, with accompanying difficulty in urination. This is the key symptom in 'lin zheng'—painful urination syndrome, which is extensively discussed in Classical literature.

Painful urination, however, should be distinguished from difficult or obstructed urination. Difficult urination implies reduced volume of urination, and is not necessarily painful; obstructed urination refers to impeded passage of urine with little or no pain. The category of 'painful urination' is based on pain as the major presenting complaint, although some patients may also have difficult or obstructed urine.

If the urination is painful and also contains blood, this is usually considered under the classification 'painful urination', while blood in the urine without pain is classed as 'hematuria'. Similarly, cloudy urine with pain falls into the present category (as 'gao lin'—'cloudy painful urinary dysfunction'), while milky or greasy urine without pain is classed as 'cloudy urine'.

Common symptom patterns

Lower Jiao damp-heat. This is usually found in the three categories of painful urinary dysfunction called 'shi lin' (stone lin), 'xue lin' (blood lin) and 'gao lin' (cloudy lin). The urine is burning, rough and painful, with a dark reddish color, or possibly milky and cloudy. It may also contain gravel or stones and thus cause an unbearable strangulating pain, which can involve the lower abdomen, waist and lower back. There will also be characteristic lower Jiao damp-heat symptoms such as bitter taste in the mouth, thirst without much desire to drink, difficult-to-pass but not dry stool or alternating loose stool and constipation, red tongue body with a yellow or greasy yellow tongue coat, and a rapid slippery or wiry pulse.

Heart fire flaring. Hot, painful, scanty dark urine, with characteristic symptoms of Heart fire flaring such as red face, dry throat, thirst for cold drinks, ulceration of the mouth and tongue, sensations of restless heat in the chest, insomnia or disturbing dreams, crimson red tongue tip with a dry yellow coat, and a rapid pulse.

Lower Jiao blood stagnation. This belongs to the category of xue lin (blood lin). Stabbing or rough (se) pain with cloudy urine and hematuria. The urine color is dark purple and the urine itself may contain clots. There will also be characteristic symptoms of blood stagnation such as lower abdominal stabbing pain, purplish tinge to the lips, dry rough skin, darkish tongue color with purplish spots, and a deep thready choppy (se) pulse.

Liver qi blockage. Rough or stabbing pain with urination, accompanied by characteristic symptoms of Liver qi blockage such as distension of the flanks and subcostal areas, abdominal distension, burping and flatulence, headaches and dizziness, nausea, bitter taste in the mouth, bluish tinge to the tongue, thin yellow tongue coat, and a wiry pulse.

Kidney yin deficiency. This can be found in the deficiency categories of xue lin (blood lin) or gao lin (cloudy lin). Urine will be hot and painful, as well as cloudy or containing blood. There will also be characteristic symptoms of Kidney yin deficiency such as nightsweats, hot flushes, dizziness, tinnitus, dry throat, malar flush, lower backache and weak knees, reddish tongue with little coat, and a thready rapid pulse.

Differentiation

Lower Jiao damp-heat versus Heart fire flaring causing painful urination. Both are internal excess heat conditions, and both manifest scanty darkish urine. Lower Jiao damp-heat is usually a result of over-consumption of rich greasy foods or alcohol, which accumulate, ferment and create damp-heat which then sinks into the lower Jiao. It can also

result from an invasion of exogenous damp-heat. The general symptoms will be those of damp-heat: bitter taste in the mouth, thirst without desire to drink much, sensations of fullness in the chest and epigastric area, poor appetite, alternating constipation and loose stool or difficult-to-pass but not dry stool, thick yellow tongue coat especially at the back of the tongue, and a rapid slippery or rapid wiry pulse.

The nature of the pain from damp-heat will vary depending upon the category of lin (painful obstructed urination dysfunction) condition:

Blood lin: damp-heat pours into the Urinary Bladder, blood is affected by the heat and circulates erratically causing rough hot urine containing blood.

Cloudy lin: damp-heat pours downward and the damp interferes with the process of Urinary Bladder qi transformation so that clear and turbid are not separated properly, while the heat causes hot rough pain.

Stone lin: damp-heat pours downward and the heat gradually curdles and then congeals the damp until gravel or stones form.

Treatment for damp-heat involves a basic approach of separating pathogenic damp and heat, with specific adjustments according to the lin category involved.

For blood lin, the treatment should cool heat, remove damp, cool the blood and stop bleeding with a formula such as Xiao Ji Yin Zi ('Cephalanoplos Decoction').

For cloudy lin, the treatment should cool heat, remove damp, recover the clear and expel the murky with a formula such as Bei Xie Fen Qing Yin ('Dioscorea Hypoglauca Decoction to Separate the Clear from *Medical Revelations*').

For stone lin, the treatment should cool heat, remove damp, open the painful obstruction (lin) and expel stones, with a formula such as San Jin Tang ('Three Gold Decoction').

Heart fire flaring and descending into the Small Intestine channel will cause scanty, dark and painful burning urination, but the degree of pain will generally be somewhat less than that of the lin conditions described above. It will also be accompanied by other symptoms of Heart fire such as ulcerations of the mouth and tongue, palpitations, insomnia and a very red tongue tip. Treatment requires cooling the Heart and draining fire, with a combination of formulas such as Huang Lian Jie Du Tang ('Coptis Decoction to Relieve Toxicity') and Dao Chi San ('Guide Out the Red Powder').

Formulas

Xiao Ji Yin Zi ('Cephalanoplos Decoction')

Xiao Ji	Cephalanoplos Segeti, Herba
Ou Jie	Nelumbinis Nuciferae Rhizomatis, Nodus
Chao Pu	Huang Dry-fried Typhae, Pollen
Sheng Di	Rehmannia Glutinosae, Radix
Hua Shi	Talc
Mu Tong	Mutong, Caulis
Dan Zhu Ye	Lophatheri Gracilis, Herba
Shan Zhi Zi	Gardeniae Jasminoidis, Fructus
Dang Gui	Angelica Polymorpha, Radix
Gan Cao	Glycyrrhizae Uralensis, Radix

Source text: *Ji Sheng Fang* ('Formulas to Aid the Living', 1253) [*Formulas & Strategies*, p. 341]

Bei Xie Fen Qing Yin ('Dioscorea Hypoglauca Decoction to Separate the Clear from *Medical Revelations*')

Bei Xie	Dioscoreae, Rhizoma
Huang Bo	Phellodendri, Cortex
Shi Chang Pu	Acori Graminei, Rhizoma
Fu Ling	Poriae Cocos, Sclerotium
Bai Zhu	Atractylodis Macrocephalae, Rhizoma
Dan Shen	Salviae Miltiorrhizae, Radix
Che Qian Zi	Plantaginis, Semen

Source text: *Yi Xue Xin Wu* ('Medical Revelations', 1732) [*Formulas & Strategies*, p. 210]

San Jin Tang ('Three Gold Decoction')

Jin Qian Cao	Desmodii Styracifolii, Herba
Dong Kui Zi	Abutiloni seu Malvae, Semen
Hai Jin Sha	Lygodii Japonici, Spora
Shi Wei	Pyrrosiae, Folium
Qu Mai	Dianthi, Herba
Ji Nei Jin	Corneum Gigeraiae Galli, Endithelium

Source text: Shuguang Hospital of the Shanghai College of Traditional Chinese Medicine [*Formulas & Strategies*, p. 194]

Huang Lian Jie Du Tang ('Coptis Decoction to Relieve Toxicity')

Huang Lian	Coptidis, Rhizoma
Huang Qin	Scutellariae Baicalensis, Radix
Huang Bo	Phellodendri, Cortex
Shan Zhi Zi	Gardeniae Jasminoidis, Fructus

Source text: *Wai Tai Bi Yao* ('Arcane Essentials from the Imperial Library', 752) [*Formulas & Strategies*, p. 78]

Dao Chi San ('Guide Out the Red Powder')

Sheng Di	Rehmannia Glutinosae, Radix
Mu Tong	Mutong, Caulis
Dan Zhu Ye	Lophatheri Gracilis, Herba
Gan Cao Shao	Glycyrrhizae Uralensis, Radix tips

Source text: *Xiao Er Yao Zheng Zhi Jue* ('Craft of Medicinal Treatment for Childhood Disease Patterns', 1119) [*Formulas & Strategies*, p. 95)

Lower Jiao blood stagnation versus Liver qi blockage causing painful urination. Both are excess blockage conditions. The lower Jiao blood stagnation often results from trauma, qi deficiency failing to carry blood and allowing it to stagnate or pathogenic cold invading the lower Jiao and constricting blood to form stagnation. Once blood stagnation forms in the vessels, normal circulating blood cannot travel within them and instead extravasates to cause hematuria. The blood stagnation also interferes with the Urinary Bladder qi transformation so that voiding is painful but a special characteristic of this type of pain is the lack of a burning sensation: the pain is more stabbing or strangulating, and will be accompanied by other symptoms of blood stagnation as detailed above.

Liver qi blockage obstructs the flow of qi in the Liver channel and so produces heat, which then links with the obstructed qi in the lower Jiao (in this case) and interferes with the Urinary Bladder function, causing pain that is characteristically strangulating. This condition is most common in young or middle-aged patients with a recent history of stress.

Treatment of lower Jiao blood stagnation requires warming of the yang to transform the stagnation and open the painful obstruction (lin) with a formula such as Shao Fu Zhu Yu Tang ('Drive Out Blood Stasis in the Lower Abdomen

Decoction') plus *Jin Qian Cao* (Jinqiancao, Herba), *Qu Mai* (Dianthi, Herba) and *Mu Tong* (Mutong, Caulis).

Treatment of the Liver qi blockage requires restoring harmonious Liver qi flow and opening the painful obstruction with a formula such as Chen Xiang San ('Aquilariae Powder'). If Liver heat has become excessive, the treatment requires moving Liver qi and cooling heat to open the painful obstruction with a formula such as Jia Wei Xiao Yao San ('Augmented Rambling Powder') plus *Dong Kui Zi* (Abutiloni seu Malvae, Semen), *Che Qian Zi* (Plantaginis, Semen) and *Hai Jin Sha* (Lygodii Japonici, Spora).

Formulas

Shao Fu Zhu Yu Tang ('Drive Out Blood Stasis in the Lower Abdomen Decoction')

Xiao Hui Xiang	Foeniculi Vulgaris, Fructus
Gan Jiang	Zingiberis Officianalis, Rhizoma
Yan Hu Suo	Corydalis Yanhusuo, Rhizoma
Dang Gui	Angelica Polymorpha, Radix
Chuan Xiong	Ligustici Wallichii, Radix
Mo Yao	Myrrha
Rou Gui	Cinnamomi Cassiae, Cortex
Chi Shao	Paeoniae Rubra, Radix
Pu Huang	Typhae, Pollen
Wu Ling Zhi	Trogopterori seu pteromi, Excrementum

Source text: *Yi Lin Gai Cuo* ('Corrections of Errors Among Physicians', 1830) [*Formulas & Strategies*, p. 316]

Chen Xiang San ('Aquilariae Powder')

Chen Xiang	15 g	Aquilariae, Lignum
Shi Wei	15 g	Pyrrosiae, Folium
Hua Shi	15 g	Talc
Chao Dang Gui	15 g	Dry-fried Angelica Polymorpha, Radix
Chen Pi	0.3 g	Citri Reticulatae, Pericarpium
Bai Shao	1 g	Paeoniae Lactiflora, Radix
Chao Dong Kui Zi	1 g	Dry-fried Abutiloni seu Malvae, Semen
Wang Bu Liu Xing	15 g	Vaccariae Segetalis, Semen
Zhi Gan Cao	0.3 g	Honey-fried Glycyrrhizae Uralensis, Radix

Powder finely, take six grams before meals with barley tea.

Source text: *San Yin Ji Yi Bing Zheng Fang Lun* ('Discussion of Illnesses, Patterns, and Formulas Related to the Unification of the Three Etiologies', 1174).[29]

Jia Wei Xiao Yao San ('Augmented Rambling Powder')

Dang Gui	Angelica Polymorpha, Radix
Bai Shao	Paeoniae Lactiflora, Radix
Fu Ling	Poriae Cocos, Sclerotium
Bai Zhu	Atractylodis Macrocephalae, Rhizoma
Chai Hu	Bupleuri, Radix
Mu Dan Pi	Moutan Radicis, Cortex
Shan Zhi Zi	Gardeniae Jasminoidis, Fructus
Gan Cao	Glycyrrhizae Uralensis, Radix
Sheng Jiang	Zingiberis Officinalis Recens, Rhizoma
Bo He	Menthae, Herba

Source text: *Nei Ke Zhai Yao* ('Summary of Internal Medicine', mid-19th century) [*Formulas & Strategies*, p. 148]

Kidney yin deficiency causing painful urination. This condition can be the long-term result of other heat conditions mentioned in this section which have gone untreated and have damaged the yin-fluids, or a result of excessive reproductive activity, or possibly damage to the yin-fluids following febrile disease. Lack of yin allows yang heat to flare out of control; part of this heat affects the Urinary Bladder qi transformation function of separating clear and murky, which can result in cloudy urination (gao lin—cloudy lin). Uncontrolled yang heat can also cause the blood to circulate erratically, leave its channels and so enter the urine, leading to hematuria (xue lin—blood lin). Both of these painful urination conditions (lin) are the result of deficiency, and the pain experienced is relatively mild. If the flaring yang is extreme, the urine may feel somewhat hot, and there will also be other characteristic symptoms of xu-fire flaring such as hot flushes, nightsweats, dry throat, malar flush, dizziness and tinnitus. The tongue will be red with little or no coat, the pulse rapid and thready.

Treatment requires nourishing yin to control yang and bring down fire, with a formula such as Zhi Bai Di Huang Wan ('Anemarrhena, Phellodendron and Rehmannia Pill') plus *Yu Mi Xu* (Zeae Mays, Stylus), *Qian Shi* (Euryales Ferox, Semen) and *Wu Wei Zi* (Schisandrae Chinensis, Fructus).

Formula

Zhi Bai Di Huang Wan ('Anemarrhena, Phellodendron and Rehmannia Pill')

Zhi Mu	Anemarrhenae Asphodeloidis, Radix
Huang Bo	Phellodendri, Cortex
Sheng Di	Rehmannia Glutinosae, Radix
Shan Zhu Yu	Corni Officinalis, Fructus
Shan Yao	Dioscoreae Oppositae, Radix
Fu Ling	Poriae Cocos, Sclerotium
Mu Dan Pi	Moutan Radicis, Cortex
Ze Xie	Alismatis Plantago-aquaticae, Rhizoma

Source text: *Zheng Yin Mai Zhi* ('Pattern, Cause, Pulse, and Treatment', 1702) [*Formulas & Strategies*, p. 265]

Summary

The excess conditions in painful urination are more common than the deficiency conditions, and consequently the possibility of deficiency is frequently ignored. The *Jing Yue Quan Shu* ('Complete Works of Jing Yue', 1624), in its section on 'painful urinary dysfunction and cloudy urine' says:

> Painful urine (lin) in its early stages never results from anything but heat, and so there [seems to be] no need to differentiate. But there are those who take cool and cold [herbs] for an extended period of time and do not improve, and there are also those with a long history of painful urinary dysfunction whose pain and difficulty have stopped, but who still have cloudy urine. In these cases one must consider middle qi descending [causing] lack of Mingmen consolidation as a [possible] condition. Thus one must check the pulse and the other symptoms to differentiate hot or cold, excess or deficiency, so that one does not, in treatment, fall into error.[30]

The latter condition that Zhang Jing-Yue is describing is the deficiency component of 'qi lin'

(the excess component being the result of qi blockage as described above under 'Liver qi blockage'). This will be characterized by an urgent pressing sensation with the pain upon voiding, as well as the appearance of symptoms of Spleen qi deficiency and failure to rise. The treatment requires tonifying and encouraging the ascent of Spleen qi with a formula such as Bu Zhong Yi Qi Tang ('Tonify the Middle and Augment the Qi Decoction', *Formulas & Strategies*, p. 241).

Another situation which can arise in acute painful urinary dysfunction is the simultaneous appearance of chills and fever: in Western terms, an acute urinary tract infection. The Internal Medicine component of the *National Provisional Teaching Material for Higher Medical Education Institutions* (Quan Guo Gao Deng Yi Yao Yuan Xiao Shi Yong Jiao Cai) section on 'painful urinary dysfunction' points out a potential danger:

> In clinical practice, painful urinary dysfunction (lin) often has both chills and fever as well as painful and difficult urination appearing together. This is caused by the steaming of damp-heat and the struggle of the zheng qi with the pathogen, and is different from the usual fever of a surface condition (i.e. that caused by an exogenous invasion). One should not use a pungent-dispersing prescription as soon as fever and chills are seen, because lin conditions most often have both heat in the Urinary Bladder and also insufficiency of yin fluids. A pungent-dispersal which opens the surface, if used incorrectly, will not only not be able to eliminate the fever, but can instead damage the nutritive (ying qi) level [and its fluids], leading to a worsening of hematuria. If the painful urinary dysfunction is truly brought on by the exogenous invasion, there will be [other symptoms of exogenous invasion besides the] chills and fever, [such as] cough, runny nose, and so on. Then one can naturally use wind-expelling surface openers in conjunction [with herbs to remedy the painful urinary dysfunction] to treat both the interior and the exterior together.

Blood in the urine

The appearance of the urine can vary from pale with a slight reddish tinge, to fresh red or dark red; when the condition is severe there may even be passage of clots with the flow of urine.

There is a difference between 'blood in the urine' and 'blood lin' in the lin syndrome (painful urinary dysfunction): in simple 'blood in the urine' there is usually no pain, while 'lin' conditions by definition are painful.

Common symptom patterns

Urinary Bladder damp-heat. Scanty flow with fresh or darkish colored blood in the urine, or even clots, associated with pricking or stabbing pain or burning sensations, and other characteristic symptoms of Urinary Bladder damp-heat: lower abdominal fullness and discomfort, intermittent fever, bitter taste in the mouth, dry throat, red tongue with a thin yellow or thin greasy tongue coat, and a rapid pulse.

Liver and Gall Bladder damp-heat. Scanty darkish urine with blood, accompanied by typical Liver and Gall bladder damp-heat symptoms such as jaundice, fever, bitter taste in the mouth, thirst without desire to drink much, poor appetite, abdominal distension, nausea, painful flanks, red edges on the body of the tongue, yellow greasy tongue coat, and a wiry rapid pulse.

Heart-fire flaring. Deep red colored urine with a burning sensation, accompanied by characteristic symptoms of Heart-fire flaring, such as insomnia, palpitations, restless feelings of agitation in the chest, red face, dry throat and thirst for cold drinks, ulceration of the mouth and tongue, scarlet red tongue with a yellow coat, and a large (hong) rapid pulse.

Kidney yin deficiency. Fresh red colored blood in the urine, with typical symptoms of Kidney yin weakness such as nightsweats, insomnia, hot flushes in the afternoon and evening, malar flush, frequent thirst which is easily quenched, lower backache, dry stool, red tongue with little coat, and a thready rapid pulse.

Spleen and Kidney yang deficiency. Pale red urine, with characteristic symptoms of both Kidney and Spleen yang weakness, such as sallow complexion, tiredness, lack of stamina, tinnitus, poor appetite, sore weak lower back and knees, pale tongue with a thin white coat, and a languid pulse soft at the proximal (chi) position.

Blood stagnation. Dark purplish-colored cloudy urine with difficulty passing and mild pricking pain, occasionally containing clots. There will also be characteristic symptoms of blood stagnation such as stabbing pain fixed in location and often worse at night, generally darkened complexion or dark areas on the face, darkish or purplish areas of the tongue, and a thready choppy pulse.

Differentiation

Urinary Bladder damp-heat versus Liver and Gall Bladder damp-heat causing blood in the urine. Both are excess (shi) heat conditions, in which the heat is forcing the blood to circulate erratically so that is forced out of the vessels and manifests as blood in the urine. Urinary Bladder damp-heat is centered in the Urinary Bladder itself, and so there are less generalized symptoms and more local distension and fullness, and a sensation of burning with urination. Liver and Gall Bladder damp-heat must travel to enter the Urinary Bladder and cause blood in the urine, and thus the generalized symptoms around the body are correspondingly greater, such as jaundice, fever, bitter taste in the mouth, nausea and painful flanks. The red edges to the tongue and the wiry pulse are important signs to look for.

Treatment of Urinary Bladder damp-heat requires cooling heat, promoting urination, cooling the blood and preventing bleeding with a formula such as Xiao Ji Yin Zi ('Cephalanoplos Decoction').

Treatment of Liver and Gall Bladder damp-heat requires draining Liver and cooling Gall Bladder, cooling blood and stopping bleeding, using a formula such as Long Dan Xie Gan Tang ('Gentiana Longdancao Decoction to Drain the Liver') plus *Qian Cao Gen* (Rubiae Cordifoliae, Radix) and *Ce Bo Ye* (Biotae Orientalis, Cacumen).

Formulas

Xiao Ji Yin Zi ('Cephalanoplos Decoction') [*Formulas & Strategies*, p. 341]
(See above)

Long Dan Xie Gan Tang ('Gentiana Longdancao Decoction to Drain the Liver') [*Formulas & Strategies*, p. 96]
(See above)

Heart-fire flaring versus Kidney yin deficiency causing blood in the urine. Both are heat conditions with fire damaging the collaterals to cause bleeding but one is excess fire and the other is fire resulting from deficiency of yin.

Heart-fire flaring and causing hematuria is often caused by excessive mental or emotional activity so that Heart-fire flares and also moves into the Small Intestine, where it damages the collaterals and causes bleeding. The appearance of the urine is characterized by its crimson color, and the burning sensation will be marked.

Kidney yin deficiency allows ministerial fire to rampage out of control, and this too can injure the collaterals and lead to bleeding which is fresh or pale red in color, with a less obvious burning sensation.

The important points in differentiation are the relative degree of burning sensation and the accompanying symptoms: those of Heart-fire flaring in the first condition: palpitations, insomnia or restless sleep and dreaming, ulcerations of the mouth or the tongue, and red tongue tip; while in the second condition the accompanying symptoms will all be those of Kidney yin deficiency with xu-fire flaring: nightsweats, hot flushes, tinnitus, lower backache, thready rapid with a weak proximal (chi) position.

The treatment for Heart-fire flaring requires cooling the Heart and draining fire, cooling the blood and stopping bleeding with a formula such as Dao Chi San ('Guide Out the Red Powder') and appropriate additions such as *Pu Huang* (Typhae, Pollen), *Xiao Ji* (Cephalanoplos Segeti, Herba) and *Da Ji* (Cirsii Japonici, Herba).

Treatment for the Kidney yin deficiency with fire flaring requires nourishing yin to control flaring yang, relieving heat in the collaterals and stopping bleeding, with a formula such as Zhi Bai Di Huang Wan ('Anemarrhena, Phellodendron, and Rehmannia Pill') plus *Bai Mao Gen* (Imperatae Cylindricae, Rhizoma).

Formulas

Dao Chi San ('Guide Out the Red Powder') [*Formulas & Strategies*, p. 95]
(See above)

Zhi Bai Di Huang Wan ('Anemarrhena, Phellodendron, and Rehmannia Pill') [*Formulas & Strategies*, p. 265]
(See above)

Spleen and Kidney yang deficiency causing blood in the urine. This is a yang deficiency condition caused on the one hand by Spleen not controlling blood and on the other by Kidneys failing to hold in and store. Thus urination is frequent, clear and profuse, containing pale colored blood. The other important point in differentiating this from the other conditions causing hematuria will be the presence of symptoms of both Kidney and Spleen deficiency. Thus treatment requires tonification of both Spleen and Kidneys to increase the qi and consolidate, with a combination of formulas such as Bu Zhong Yi Qi Tang ('Tonify the Middle and Augment the Qi Decoction') and Wu Bi Shan Yao Wan ('Incomparable Dioscorea Pill'), plus herbs to stop bleeding such as *Pao Jiang* (baked Zingiberis Officinalis, Rhizoma), *Ou Jie* (Nelumbinis Nuciferae Rhizomatis, Nodus) and *Lu Jiao Shuang* (Cervi Degelatinatium, Cornu).

Formulas

Bu Zhong Yi Qi Tang ('Tonify the Middle and Augment the Qi Decoction') [*Formulas & Strategies*, p. 241]
(See above)

Wu Bi Shan Yao Wan ('Incomparable Dioscorea Pill')

Shan Yao	Dioscoreae Oppositae, Radix
Rou Cong Rong	Cistanches, Herba
Shou Di	Rehmanniae Glutinosae Conquitae, Radix
Shan Zhu Yu	Corni Officinalis, Fructus
Fu Shen	Poriae Cocos Paradicis, Sclerotium
Tu Si Zi	Cuscutae, Semen
Wu Wei Zi	Schisandrae Chinensis, Fructus
Chi Shi Zhi	Halloysitum Rubrum
Ba Ji Tian	Morindae Officianalis, Radix
Ze Xie	Alismatis Plantago-aquaticae, Rhizoma
Du Zhong	Eucommiae Ulmoidis, Cortex

Niu Xi   Achyranthis Bidentatae, Radix

Source text: *Tai Ping Hui Min He Ji Ju Fang* ('Imperial Grace Formulary of the Tai Ping Era', 1078-85)

Blood stagnation causing blood in the urine. This would usually be categorized as 'painful urination' of the 'blood lin' type, unless as in this situation the pain is minimal and the hematuria is the main presenting complaint.

Blood stagnation can be the result of qi deficiency failing to assist blood movement, or of cold slowing the circulation of blood until it stagnates. If the stagnation occurs in the Urinary Bladder, the blood cannot flow within the obstructed channels and extravasates into the urine.

Qi deficiency leading to blood stagnation is usually found in patients after a long illness or older patients with weak qi. Typical symptoms include tiredness, reluctance to speak, shortness of breath, and weak thready pulse combined with blood stagnation symptoms. Treatment requires tonifying qi to move and contain the blood, using a formula such as Bu Zhong Yi Qi Tang ('Tonify the Middle and Augment the Qi Decoction') plus *San Qi* (Pseudoginseng, Radix).

Cold causing blood stagnation can result from either exogenous cold invading the local area, or internal cold accumulation; typical symptoms include lower abdominal pain worse with cold and relieved by heat, lower abdominal mass, chilled purplish limbs, pale purplish tongue with a white coat, and a deep slow choppy pulse. In women, periods will often be late, clotted and painful. Treatment requires warming internal cold to remove stagnation with a formula such as Shao Fu Zhu Yu Tang ('Drive Out Blood Stasis in the Lower Abdomen Decoction') plus a relatively large amount of *Niu Xi* (Achyranthis Bidentatae, Radix).

Formulas

Bu Zhong Yi Qi Tang ('Tonify the Middle and Augment the Qi Decoction') [*Formulas & Strategies*, p. 241]
(See above)

Shao Fu Zhu Yu Tang ('Drive Out Blood Stasis in the Lower Abdomen Decoction') [*Formulas and Strategies*, p. 316]
(See above)

Summary

Attention to the color of the blood in the urine can provide a very useful aid to differentiation. For example if the blood is purplish red or fresh red this is usually excess heat, pale colored blood is usually qi deficiency, fresh red colored blood accompanied by steaming bones and nightsweats is usually heat from yin deficiency, and darkish purple colored blood is usually blood stagnation.

Spermaturia

This refers either to seminal fluid mixed with the urine, or to loss of seminal fluid after voiding of urine is complete. Although spermaturia can cause a cloudy appearance to the urine, in order to ensure proper treatment spermaturia must be differentiated from the more general condition of 'Cloudy Urine'.

Common symptom patterns

Damp-heat pent-up internally. Scanty dark or cloudy urine with difficulty voiding and occasional sensations of roughness or heat or pricking pain. After the passage of urine the urethral opening has a milky or pasty substance that leaks out uncontrollably, accompanied by sensations of itching or pain within the penis itself. There may also be spermatorrhea. The above symptoms will be accompanied by characteristic symptoms of damp-heat such as thirst and bitter taste in the mouth, sensations of fullness in the chest and epigastric area, moist and sticky but hard to pass stool, red tongue with a greasy yellow coat, and a rapid slippery pulse.

Yin deficiency with fire flaring. Scanty yellow and somewhat cloudy urine with a burning sensation, and possible dripping of a reddish turbid exudate from the urethral opening after urination. There will also be characteristic symptoms of yin deficiency with fire flaring such as restless sleep, nightsweats, hot flushes, malar flush with red lips, five-hearts-heat, thirst at night, vertigo, red tongue with little coat, and a thready rapid pulse.

Kidneys weak and failing to consolidate. Clear profuse and possibly frequent urination with threads of seminal fluid appearing after voiding, and no pain with urination. There will often be spermatorrhea and other characteristic symptoms of Kidney deficiency such as pale lusterless complexion, vertigo, tinnitus or poor hearing, aching of the lower back and knees, sensitivity to cold, chilled limbs, pale tongue with a thin white coat, and a deep thready pulse.

Differentiation

Damp-heat pent-up internally causing spermaturia. This is an internal excess heat condition characterized by relatively marked signs of cloudiness in the urine from the presence of 'failed' seminal fluids. It is usually the result of over-consumption of rich greasy foods which 'ferment' in the middle Jiao, creating damp-heat which then pours down into the lower Jiao and agitates the 'Chamber of Jing' (jing shi) so that jing-essence is driven out and into the urine, leading to cloudiness or a residual sticky exudate. The damp is obstructive, and this (combined with the yin-natured jing-essence which has been driven out and damaged by the heat) blocks the smooth flow of urine, causing difficulty. Pathogenic heat dries the fluids held in the Urinary Bladder so that urine becomes scanty, dark and hot. An important aid to differentiation, however, will be the presence of other generalized symptoms of damp-heat.

Treatment requires cooling heat and expelling damp in order to separate the two pathogens and prevent their mutual re-production. Only after this has been accomplished can one consider the use of consolidation to prevent the loss of jing-essence. The initial formula should be Bei Xie Fen Qing Yin ('Dioscorea Hypoglauca Decoction to Separate the Clear from *Medical Revelations*'). Consolidating herbs which can be added after damp and heat have been separated include *Sang Piao Xiao* (Mantidis, Ootheca), *Bai Shao* (Paeoniae Lactiflora, Radix), and *Rou Cong Rong* (Cistanches, Herba).

Formula

Bei Xie Fen Qing Yin ('Dioscorea Hypoglauca Decoction to Separate the Clear from *Medical Revelations*')

Bei Xie	Dioscoreae, Rhizoma
Huang Bo	Phellodendri, Cortex
Shi Chang Pu	Acori Graminei, Rhizoma
Fu Ling	Poriae Cocos, Sclerotium
Bai Zhu	Atractylodis Macrocephalae, Rhizoma
Dan Shen	Salviae Miltiorrhizae, Radix
Che Qian Zi	Plantaginis, Semen

Source text: *Yi Xue Xin Wu* ('Medical Revelations', 1732) [*Formulas & Strategies*, p. 210]

Yin deficiency with fire flaring causing spermaturia versus Kidneys weak and failing to consolidate causing spermaturia. Both of these are Kidney deficiency conditions. Deficiency of yin allows yang fire to flare and agitate the jing-essence, so that it moves out of its normal condition of storage and into the urine.

Kidney failure to consolidate is a result either of damage to the zheng qi through extended illness, or long-term spermatorrhea (from some other reason), so that injury to the yin-essence eventually involves the yang which then is even less able to contain the jing-essence.

Important points in differentiation are:

1. the accompanying symptoms of either yin deficiency with fire flaring or yang qi deficiency with chills
2. the nature of the urinary fluid, which will be scanty and yellow in yin deficiency but clear and profuse with yang qi deficiency
3. the texture of the lost seminal fluid itself, which will be thick and sticky with yin deficiency due to the drying of the heat but thin and thready with yang deficiency.

Treatment of the yin deficiency with fire flaring requires nourishing yin to control yang fire while assisting Kidney consolidation of jing-essence with formulas such as Zhi Bai Di Huang Wan ('Anemarrhena, Phellodendron and Rehmannia Pill') or San Cai Feng Sui Dan ('Three Powers Special Pill to Seal the Marrow'),[31] plus astringent consolidating herbs such as *Qian Shi* (Euryales Ferox, Semen) and *Jin Ying Zi* (Rosae Laevigatae, Fructus).

Treatment of the Kidney failure to consolidate requires tonification of Kidneys and support for consolidation with formulas such as Da Tu Si Zi Wan ('Great Cuscuta Seed Pill'), You Gui Wan ('Restore the Right [Kidney] Pill') or Jin Gui Shen Qi Wan ('Kidney Qi Pill from the Golden Cabinet').

Formulas

Zhi Bai Di Huang Wan ('Anemarrhena, Phellodendron, and Rehmannia Pill') [*Formulas & Strategies*, p. 265]
(See above]

San Cai Feng Sui Dan ('Three Powers Special Pill to Seal the Marrow')

Tian Men Dong	15 g	Asparagi Cochinchinensis, Tuber
Shou Di	15 g	Rehmanniae Glutinosae Conquitae, Radix
Ren Shen	15 g	Ginseng, Radix
Huang Bo	90 g	Phellodendri, Cortex
Sha Ren	45 g	Amomi, Fructus et Semen
Zhi Gan Cao	22.5 g	Honey-fried Glycyrrhizae Uralensis, Radix

Finely powder the above herbs and form into small pills with water. Fifty pills per dose, to be taken on an empty stomach with a decoction of *Rou Cong Rong* (Cistanches, Herba), 15 g of which has been soaked overnight in 300 ml. of wine, then brought to the boil three or four times and the dregs discarded.

Source text: *Yi Xue Fa Ming* ('Medical Innovations', Jin-Tarter Period)

Da Tu Si Zi Wan ('Great Cuscuta Seed Pill')

Tu Si Zi	Cuscutae, Semen
Ze Xie	Alismatis Plantago-aquaticae, Rhizoma
Lu Rong	Cervi Parvum, Cornu
Long Gu	Draconis, Os
Rou Gui	Cinnamomi Cassiae, Cortex
Fu Zi	Aconitii Carmicheli Praeparata, Radix
Shi Hu	Dendrobii, Herba
Shou Di	Rehmanniae Glutinosae Conquitae, Radix
Fu Ling	Poriae Cocos, Sclerotium
Chuan Duan	Dipsaci, Radix
Shan Zhu Yu	Corni Officinalis, Fructus
Rou Cong Rong	Cistanches, Herba
Fang Feng	Ledebouriellae Sesloidis, Radix
Du Zhong	Eucommiae Ulmoidis, Cortex
Niu Xi	Achyranthis Bidentatae, Radix

Bu Gu Zhi	Psoraleae Corylifoliae, Fructus
Chen Xiang	Aquilariae, Lignum
Ba Ji Tian	Morindae Officianalis, Radix
Xiao Hui Xiang	Foeniculi Vulgaris, Fructus
Wu Wei Zi	Schisandrae Chinensis, Fructus
Sang Piao Xiao	Mantidis, Ootheca
Chuan Xiong	Ligustici Wallichii, Radix
Fu Pen Zi	Rubi, Fructus
Bi Cheng Qie	Cucubae, Fructus

Source text: *Tai Ping Hui Min He Ji Ju Fang* ('Imperial Grace Formulary of the Tai Ping Era', 1078-85)

You Gui Wan ('Restore the Right [Kidney] Pill')

Fu Zi	Aconiti Carmichaeli Praeparata, Radix
Rou Gui	Cinnamomi Cassiae, Cortex
Lu Jiao Jiao	Cervi Colla Cornu
Shou Di	Rehmanniae Glutinosae Conquitae, Radix
Shan Zhu Yu	Corni Officinalis, Fructus
Shan Yao	Dioscoreae Oppositae, Radix
Gou Qi Zi	Lycii Chinensis, Fructus
Tu Si Zi	Cuscutae, Semen
Du Zhong	Eucommiae Ulmoidis, Cortex
Dang Gui	Angelica Polymorpha, Radix

Source text: *Jing Yue Quan Shu* ('Complete Works of Jing Yue', 1624) [*Formulas and Strategies*, p. 278]

Jin Gui Shen Qi Wan ('Kidney Pill from the *Golden Cabinet*')

Shou Di	Rehmanniae Glutinosae Conquitae, Radix
Shan Zhu Yu	Corni Officinalis, Fructus
Shan Yao	Dioscoreae Oppositae, Radix
Fu Zi	Aconiti Carmichaeli Praeparata, Radix
Gui Zhi	Cinnamomi Cassiae, Ramulus
Ze Xie	Alismatis Plantago-aquaticae, Rhizoma
Fu Ling	Poriae Cocos, Sclerotium
Mu Dan Pi	Moutan Radicis, Cortex

Source text: *Jin Gui Yao Lue* ('Essentials from the Golden Cabinet', *c.* 210 AD) [*Formulas & Strategies*, p. 275]

The etiological factors involved in the condition of spermaturia include both excess and deficiency but deficiency is the factor predominantly seen in clinic in China, while due to dietary and lifestyle circumstances in the West excess factors play a larger part, especially in middle-aged patients.

Classical Essay

The following essay 'Obstructed urination derives from weak Mingmen fire' is by Chen Shi–Duo from his *Bian Zheng Lu* ('Record of Differentiation of Syndromes', 1687).

Patients with obstructed urination so that the urine only dribbles out, and lower abdominal distension, and all this without pain or signs of upper Jiao restless anxiety, and no symptoms of stuffiness or disturbance in the chest (xiong zhong wu men luan), and no thirst or dry tongue: everyone often regards this as obstructed Urinary Bladder water—who would think that it is actually a result of weak Mingmen (Gate of Vitality) fire!

The Urinary Bladder is the Official in charge of Irrigation [where fluids are contained, and these fluids] can emerge when the qi in the Kidneys transforms [it]. This qi is the fire of Mingmen. When Mingmen fire is vigorous, the water in the Urinary Bladder can flow; if Mingmen fire is weak, then the water in the Urinary Bladder becomes obstructed.

Now it may be said: Frequent urination comes from weakness of Mingmen fire; if fire is weak then the urination should be profuse and frequent, how could it instead cause urinary obstruction?

[The questioner] does not know that Mingmen fire must have the mutual nourishing support of Kidney Water; if Water is strong only then will the Mingmen fire also be strong. If the fire is [overly] vigorous, then Water is powerless to control it. Fire without water may [appear to] be strong, in fact it is weak; Water without fire will seek for an open free flow but instead will become obstructed. Weak Mingmen fire leads to urinary frequency, when the weakness is extreme the frequency becomes extreme, when the frequency becomes extreme it instead becomes an extreme obstruction.

People see the obstruction and mistakenly imagine that it is Urinary Bladder [pathogenic] fire, and so use cold prescriptions which further damage Mingmen fire and consequently also reduce the Urinary Bladder qi: how could it transform the water? Then they change to using diuretic herbs: the more diuresis the more deficiency results.

The treatment method must be to assist Mingmen fire. But if one only assists Mingmen fire, the fear is that yang will flare and yin will be reduced. The fire must be tonified within water, then fire will be produced in the midst of the water, and then the water will flow freely from inside the fire!

The formula to use is Ba Wei Di Huang Tang ('Eight-Herb Rehmannia Decoction', here referring to Jin Gui Shen Qi Wan ('Kidney Qi Pill from the *Golden Cabinet*', *Formulas & Strategies*, p. 275). This is a marvellous formula for tonifying fire within water. If the fire is tonified in the midst of water, then there is no fear of fire raging; if water moves freely within the fire, then there is no worry that the stream of water will dry up. Even if the obstruction is prolonged and severe, the use of this formula will always achieve good results; even more is this the case in mild obstruction![32]

Incontinence

The following essay is taken from the *Jing Yue Quan Shu* ('Complete Works of Jing Yue', 1624) by Zhang Jing-Yue.

'Incontinence' has [three types of condition]: there is loss of control with voiding during sleep, there is incontinence from the lack of consolidation of the Gate of Qi (qi men) with frequency and loss of control, and there is collapse of qi in the upper body failing to control the lower body so that incontinence occurs without warning sensations—this [last] is a sign of extreme deficiency.

Thus all three conditions are the result of deficiency, but there are differences in degree. For example, incontinence during sleep is usually found in children [but] once the qi has become strong it will be able to consolidate; with perhaps a small amount of regulation it will clear up without doubt.

However if the spring of water does not stop, and the Urinary Bladder cannot consolidate, this is from qi deficiency. Now qi is the mother of water, the inability of water to be retained (xu) is from lack of ability of the qi to consolidate (gu). This is an ominous potent of [future] defeat. When severe the qi collapses and incontinence results, if there is lack of [warning] sensation, this is particularly severe. It is often found in patients with wind-stroke, or elderly patients with weak qi, or in those recovering from a serious illness. This is what [Zhang] Zhong–Jing referred to when he said 'lower Jiao is exhausted and the urine becomes incontinent'.[33]

Some ancient texts record that incontinence can be differentiated into those from heat and those from deficiency. Didn't they know that 'incontinence' (bu jin zhe) only refers to an excessive flow of urine? They all belong to deficient cold, how could there be a heat condition? If there is heat, and the urine is frequent, the symptom will be that of continuous dribbling, but the urine itself will not be flowing smoothly, and in many cases will also be painful and rough. Only in this case is there a heat condition, and in such a case there naturally is the 'painful urinary obstruction' approach to treatment: this is not referring to incontinence.

As to xu-cold being mistaken for heat, and the reckless use of fire-draining herbs: none of these patients survive.

When treating incontinence, the ancients always used consolidating herbs, for here consolidation is indicated. Consolidation (gu) however is but closing (gu) the door, which is the idea of treating the branch; this though is not the way to close off the source. What I mean is this: although the flow of urine is controlled by the Kidneys, the Kidneys themselves have an upward link to the Lungs. If the Lung qi lacks power, then the Kidney water, in the end, cannot be conserved (she).[34] Thus to treat water one must necessarily treat the qi, when treating the Kidneys one must necessarily treat the Lungs, using as primary herbs such things as *Ren Shen* (Ginseng, Radix), *Huang Qi* (Astragali, Radix), *Dang Gui* (Angelica Polymorpha, Radix), *Bai Zhu* (Atractylodis Macrocephalae, Rhizoma), *Rou Gui* (Cinnamomi Cassiae, Cortex), *Fu Zi* (Aconiti Carmichaeli Praeparata, Radix) and *Gan Jiang* (Zingiberis Officinalis, Rhizoma). After this one can use consolidating substances as an auxiliary approach. This is the only way of treating the root, so that the stream flows as it should. Otherwise one is vainly trying to stem the wild tide: there will be no benefit in the end. I have also created the formula called Gong Ti Wan ('Consolidate and Lift Pill', included in the incontinence section above) which is primarily designed for this condition no matter whether it involves Heart, Spleen, Lungs, or Kidneys.[35]

NOTES

1. According to Zhou Xue Hai in the *Du Yi Sui Bi* ('Random Notes while Reading Medicine'), 1898, p. 185.

   It should be remembered, when reading the following paragraphs discussing the Tai Ji illustration, that the subject under discussion is not anatomy but rather changes in qualities of energies.

   The intention of this description is highly practical: to be able to observe, predict and potentially alter these changes in energetic qualities. In order to do these things, a set of standard terms of measurement is required. The Tai Ji illustration, with the Five Phases embedded—Earth in the middle—actually forms a definition of the quality of energy of each term of measurement, as well as the usual relationship between these qualities, both macro- and micro-cosmically. This description goes far beyond yin yang and Five Phases, later adding the eight trigrams (which symbolize other aspects of these energetic qualities) and later still the 'Heavenly Stems and Earthly Branches', carrying the definition one step further, and still there is more beyond this (see the *I Ching*, Wilhelm/Baynes, London, Routledge & Kegan, 1971, pp. 270-271). These further levels are hinted at in the short discussion of Mingmen by adding the relevant trigrams in certain places. Thus Zhang Jing–Yue, after a long review of the relevance of *I Jing* ('Book of Changes') studies to medicine in the *Lei Jing Tu Yi* ('Illustrated Wing to the Systematic Categorization of the *Nei Jing*', 1624) concludes:

> The foregoing is why I say that the knowledge of medicine is contained in the *Changes*, whereas medicine is the use of the *Changes*. [One who is] studying medicine without studying the *Changes* is bound to say 'medical studies are not difficult, there is only "this" and no more': how would they know that [although] the eye sees, there is that which is unperceived, and that [although] the ear hears, there is that which is not apprehended. [Such people] cannot avoid ending in relative ignorance.
>
> [One who] knows the *Changes* without knowing medicine is bound to say 'the knowledge in the *Changes* is deep and dark, vague, uncertain and hard to use'. What is the difference [between such people and] one who fears the cold but, obtaining clothing, does not clothe himself, or one who fears hunger but, obtaining a stew, does not eat? It is a pity, but they have wasted this life.
>
> So it is that a physician cannot do without the *Changes*, and the *Changes* cannot do without medicine. If you can but avail yourself of it, then the changes of the *Changes*—which proceed from Heaven—can be put to a medical use: by you.'

Lei Jing Tu Yi ('Illustrated Wing to the Systematic Categorization of the *Nei Jing*'), 1624, by Zhang Jing-Yue; People's Health Publishing, 1982, p. 401.

2. 'The dragon is the symbol of the electrically-charged, dynamic, arousing force that manifests itself in the thunderstorm. In winter this energy withdraws into the earth; in the early summer it becomes active again, appearing in the sky as thunder and lightning. As a result the creative forces on earth begin to stir again.' *I Ching*, Wilhelm/Baynes, London, Routledge & Kegan, 1971, p. 7. The dragon symbolizes the yang energy rising out of the Kidneys, the thunder that yang energy rising from the Liver.

3. Which includes not only Gall Bladder but San Jiao as well (see Chapter One), and Liver, which shares this rising growing quality of yang energy.

4. See also *Forgotten Traditions of Ancient Chinese Medicine*, by Paul Unschuld, Paradigm Publications, 1990, p. 66; and also p. 81.

5. This quote, from the *Su Wen* Chapter 17, refers first to the bowels, which are 'unable to store' and become loose. Kidneys rule the two lower orifices, and are also the 'floodgates of the Stomach' (Wei zhi guan); in this context Kidney yang (Mingmen) is failing to support Spleen yang which causes diarrhea.

6. From the *Su Wen* Chapter 61. See note eight in the chapter on edema.

7. From the *Su Wen* Chapter 4, called 'True Words of the Golden Cabinet'.

8. See note 12 in Chapter 1 on the significance of the North Pole as the symbol of the Emperor.

9. This is not a 'cop-out': Zhang Jing–Yue expends reams of paper trying to express in as simple a way as possible the ramifications of the identity of cosmological alterations of yin and yang with those within the human body. The thoughtful reader may have already noted that he has hinted at the 'subtleties' involved with his choice of examples of pathology: urine failing to 'move'—movement being a yang activity—from exhausted yin; and leakage from deficient yang failing to hold in—stillness being a yin attribute. He is indicating the 'inseparable' interactions of the two qualities of energy, which nonetheless can be 'separated' for use by the skillful physician, and continues in the next paragraph to provide an example of how this can be done:

> Mingmen yin deficiency is manifested in the relative preponderance of pathological fire, which itself is due to the insufficiency of True Water. Thus its manifestations can be either insatiable thirst, or steaming bones, or coughing or spitting blood or in painful cloudy urination or spermatorrhea. Although these are understood to be fire symptoms, they are basically not comparable to those of pathogenic or excess heat. For the fire from excess heat comes on suddenly, and there must be some palpable reason; while the fire from xu-heat comes on slowly, and is necessarily the result of [gradually] accumulated damage. This excess heat and deficient heat are greatly different! In any treatment of fire, if it is fire from excess heat, one can use cold to overcome or water to break it, which is called 'those with heat should be cooled'. But the fire from deficient heat cannot be overcome with cold; this is called 'those with exhaustion should be warmed'. Why is this? It is because the reason for deficient fire is the lack of water, one need only tonify water to match fire and yin and yang will become even: the illness will naturally be cured. If one wants to eradicate fire to restore water, the already weakened water will not necessarily be restored, and the [physiological] fire will be eliminated as well—is this not defeating both yin and yang? Furthermore, bitter-cold herbs have absolutely no rising lifting life-giving qi, so if

one wants to replenish deficiency, this does not make sense. Therefore, my way of treating this is always to use sweet even-natured prescriptions aimed specifically at tonifying the True Yin. Although there may not be an immediate cure, naturally there is no [further] damage. After this I make an examination of what the patient can stand, and perhaps use a temporary cooling and clearing, or gradually add warming moistening herbs: one must make the life-giving qi (sheng qi) gradually come on, aiming for Spleen's return to health and then the fire will recede: the Lungs can be gradually moistened so that the cough will gradually settle. Only in this way will there be a gradual return of signs of health, and most will live. If one's only knowledge is that 'Zhi Mu (Anemarrhenae Asphodeloidis, Radix) and Huang Bo (Phellodendri, Cortex) are yin-tonifying herbs', then the Kidneys will become ever weaker, resulting in diarrhea and loss of appetite, and [this will] definitely speed the patient to an early grave.

Jing Yue Quan Shu ('Complete Works of Jing Yue'), 1624, by Zhang Jing-Yue; Shanghai Science and Technology Press, 1959, pp. 58-61.

10. Zhu Bing Yuan Hou Lun ('General Treatise on the Etiology and Symptomatology of Disease', 610 AD) by Chao Yuan–Fang; People's Health Publishing, 1982, p. 474.

11. As well as, of course, spermatorrhea; or, in women, the watery vaginal discharge characteristic of Kidney deficiency.

12. See the sections devoted to the 'Artemesia Yin-chenhao Decoctions' in the Shang Han Lun ('Discussion of Cold-Induced Disorders'); and also in Formulas & Strategies, pp. 189-190.

13. There are many exogenous pathogens which can invade the Lungs and cause such a disturbance but wind-heat is chosen as a kind of median representative because of the dual influence on the body fluids of a) interference with Lung fluid metabolism, and b) the direct effect of the heat on the fluids themselves. The choice of 'wind-heat' should not be construed as limiting the possible exogenous pathogenic influence on Lung fluid metabolism to wind-heat only, for indeed the list is long, including exogenous pathogenic cold, cold-damp, parching (zao) heat, and a further complication of these: internal pathogenic heat in the Lungs.

14. See footnote 29 in the Appendix on the development of phlegm theory in TCM for the implications of the term 'bai'. The 'others' mentioned here include Cheng Guo-Peng in the Yi Xue Xin Wu ('Medical Revelations', 1732), He Meng-Yao in the Yi Bian ('Fundamentals of Medicine', 1751) and Wang Ken-Tang in the Zheng Zhi Zhun Sheng ('Standards of Patterns and Treatments', 1602). The normally quiescent jing-essence has lost this attribute of stillness and gone 'bad' because of the inability of the weakened Kidneys to properly contain it, allowing it to leak away into the Urinary Bladder, and then into the urine. Li Zhong-Zi in the Yi Zong Bi Du ('Required Readings from the Masters of Medicine', 1637; Shanghai Science and Technology Press, 1957, p. 336) has a typical comment: 'The Heart is moved by desire, the Kidneys by sex or by forced celibacy, or by excessive consumption of sex tonics (literally 'perverse prescriptions'); corrupted (bai) jing leaks out, and becomes white turbid [urine]'. See the section on spermaturia for detailed differentiation and treatment of this condition.

15. Pain that improves with heat is not necessarily always a sign that cold is the initiating factor in the pain, because warmth will promote the movement of qi and lessen obstruction from any pathogenic factor, and thus reduce pain to some extent. One can only consider this a significant factor in differentiation if the pain is reduced to a great extent by the warmth. Pain which worsens with heat, likewise, is not inevitably caused by pathogenic heat: this can occur in severe stagnation, where the heat is insufficient to eliminate the obstruction but nonetheless attempts to move the blocked qi, and thus by increasing the local 'pressure' conversely causes more pain.

16. Once again, students may ask: 'If cold is contracting, why does it not contract and obstruct the urination?' The answer is that it can (for an example, the Shang Han Tai Yang fu-organ syndrome, treated with Wu Ling San 'Five-Ingredient Powder with Poria'), but this action will not be the same as the physiological consolidation of the Kidneys. The grasp of the concept of 'physiological' versus 'pathological' activity will clear up many problems and misconceptions in TCM.

17. For a detailed discussion of the mechanisms and the treatments involved in reduction of urinary output, see the chapter on edema. This may provide a more dexterous approach to the treatment of this symptom.

18. During the preparation of this chapter, a patient nearing the end of her treatment for another condition returned earlier than planned, because of a strange occurrence: over the previous four days she had suddenly developed lower abdominal distension from fluid retention, with dark scanty urine. The sudden onset of the problem immediately led me to ask whether she had noticed any swelling in the upper body, but she had not, and so the questioning continued along other lines until she mentioned that at the same time as the fluid retention she had developed pimples on the upper back and the face. When I described the reasoning behind my previous line of questioning she said 'Oh, like a virus?' and then it came out: five days previously she had developed a mild sore throat with cough and malaise, because she had been 'surrounded by kids with viruses'. I expressed surprise that such a mild exogenous wind invasion could obstruct the Lungs'

fluid metabolism functioning (as it was by then obvious that it had), and she then reported that 'she had never mentioned' that she had always reacted badly to wind, which caused migraines, and that she had another strange symptom: whenever she was exposed to cold, she would develop hives. This could be the result of something as innocuous as taking food from the freezer—hives would cause her hands to swell. I remarked that it sounded very much like damp lodged in the surface tissues, obstructing the circulation of protective qi and reacting to the presence of cold by congealing, and she replied that these symptoms had started after a trip to India during an intensely damp season, which had been immediately followed by a stay in England, where she had been thoroughly and continually chilled. This, then, was the reason for the ease with which a mild exogenous pathogen could interfere with the Lungs' regulation of the fluid metabolism: Lung qi was already obstructed by the pathogenic damp lodged in the skin, so that even a mild wind-heat pathogen could prevent its spread and descent. The heat, caught by the lodged damp, brought out the upper body pimples. Her pulse was floating, the tongue pale red with a thin slippery coat. My treatment principle was to restore the spread and descent of Lung qi and promote urination, which would deal with the immediate fluid retention, and would also begin to remove that lodged damp. I based the formula on Ma Huang Lian Qiao Chi Xiao Dou Tang ('Ephedra, Forsythia, and Phaseolus Calcaratus Decoction') with additions:

Ma Huang	3 g	Ephedrae, Herba
Chi Xiao Dou	24 g	Phaseoli Calcarati, Semen
Lian Qiao	15 g	Forsythiae Suspensae, Fructus
Sang Ye	12 g	Mori Albae, Folium
Xing Ren	9 g	Pruni Armeniacae, Semen
Gui Zhi	12 g	Cinnamomi Cassiae, Ramulus
Sang Bai Pi	12 g	Mori Albae Radicis, Cortex
Yi Yi Ren	18 g	Coicis Lachryma-jobi, Semen
Che Qian Cao	15 g	Plantaginis, Herba
Ze Xie	12 g	Alismatis Plantago-aquaticae, Rhizoma
Gan Cao	3 g	Glycyrrhizae Uralensis, Radix

Three packets. Decoct and take for four days.

With follow-up, the patient reported that the urine increased markedly, and the abdominal fluid retention disappeared after the second day on the herbs.

19. These symptoms associated with Kidney yang deficiency edema are well-documented in texts as early as the *Jin Gui Yao Lue* ('Essentials from the Golden Cabinet', *c*. 210 AD). Again, see the chapter on edema for more detailed information regarding mechanisms and treatment.

20. *Zhu Bing Yuan Hou Lun* ('General Treatise on the Etiology and Symptomatology of Disease', 610 AD) by Chao Yuan-Fang; People's Health Publishing, Beijing, 1983, p. 471.

21. For more information on this mechanism, see the chapters on damp-heat and edema.

22. There are at least twenty-five different conditions that can be treated with this ancient method (which was described in texts as early as the *Jin Gui Yao Lue* 'Essentials from the Golden Cabinet', *c*. 210 AD). The simplest is to tickle the nose. An only slightly more refined method is to ask the patient to hold water or oil in the mouth (this is not absolutely necessary), and then forcefully inhale herbal powder into the nose. Some of the herbs suitable for this condition which could be combined and finely powdered to accomplish this include:

Bo He	Menthae, Herba
Chuan Xiong	Ligustici Wallichii, Radix
Cang Zhu	Atractylodis, Rhizoma
Bai Zhi	Angelicae, Radix
Xi Xin	Asari cum Radice, Herba
Huang Qin	Scutellariae Baicalensis, Radix
Chi Xiao Dou	Phaseoli Calcarati, Semen
Zao Jiao	Gleditsiae Sinensis, Fructus
Peng Sha	Borax

Similarly, such herbs can be formed into a cone and inserted into the nose.

23. During my preparation of this section, I was thinking to myself that the distinction, in both this and the preceding section, between damp-heat and Liver channel qi blockage leading to both heat and damp, seemed somewhat pedantic. A patient presented serendipitously the very next day, however, who made the necessity for the distinction most clear. As the case also illustrates the interaction between a Western diagnosis, a Chinese diagnosis, and a Chinese differentiation, it seemed that it might be useful to include it here.

The case history is of a male, 30 years of age. The Western diagnosis was benign enlargement of the prostate. Cystoscopy revealed hyperplasia of the right lateral lobe, which biopsy confirmed was benign. Prolonged antibiotic treatment had little effect on the symptoms, after which Minipress (a vasodilator) was tried, again unfortunately without success.

For the last nine months, the patient had been experiencing hesitancy, frequency, urinary tenesmus (painful straining), scantiness, and a sensation of incompleteness following urination. The amount of urine ranged between 100–150 ml, with occasional cloudiness. The patient reported that all of the symptoms were worse in the morning, and exacerbated with stress, for which he was currently undergoing counselling. When he was relaxed, the color of the urine would be a strong yellow; when he was very anxious however, the color would become clear. Before these symptoms began, he had undergone a long course of treatment with L-tryptophan, which had been prescribed by his local GP for his symptoms of anxiety. Sleep, however, remained difficult throughout, and continued so.

Appetite and bowel movements were normal, and besides a life-long history of excessive nasal mucus and sinus headaches, there were few other symptoms. The pulse was thready, slippery and somewhat wiry and languid, the tongue was reddish with a moist, egg-white-like coat spread evenly over the surface.

This patient's condition is particularly apropos of the need to distinguish between damp-heat and Liver channel qi obstruction leading to heat and also to damp, for two reasons. The first is that the etiological mechanism is so clearly that of Liver qi blockage: chronic anxiety rules this patient's life, the symptoms worsen when he is anxious, and the pulse is wiry. The second is that while heat and damp symptoms both appear, they are not linked together as the dual pathogen damp-heat would be, but rather manifest in distinct areas: the heat shows in the redness of the tongue body and the occasional yellowness of the urine, the damp in the chronic sinus problems, the occasional cloudiness of the urine, the languid slipperiness of the pulse, and the moist egg-white-like tongue coat. The last sign is most significant: in damp-heat the tongue coat would most likely be yellow and greasy, showing that the heat was firmly enveloped within the damp. Here, though, the damp-phlegm appears on its own in the coat, while the heat manifests in the tongue body.

One interesting symptom is the tendency of the urine to become clear when anxious, and yellow when relaxed. This demonstrates the interference of the Liver qi blockage in the San Jiao fluid movement and the ability of the Urinary Bladder to separate clear and murky fluids: when the patient is relaxed and the qi movement throughout the body—and particularly the Shao Yang San Jiao—is less obstructed, then the pent-up heat can find its way down and out through the urine; when he is tense and anxious this openness is restricted, and the fluids available for excretion show only the pathogenic damp, clear in color but occasionally cloudy in consistency.

Chinese diagnosis is urinary obstruction, and Chinese differentiation is obstruction of the qi in the Liver channel leading to damp and mild heat.

Treatment principle is calm the Liver, open Liver channel qi flow, reduce swelling, and promote urination.

Prescription

Chai Hu	6 g	Bupleuri, Radix
He Huan Pi	18 g	Albizziae Julibrissin, Cortex
Bai Shao	9 g	Paeoniae Lactiflora, Radix
Chuan Shan Jia	9 g	Manitis Pentadactylae, Squama
Mu Tong	6 g	Mutong, Caulis
Wang Bu Liu Xing	9 g	Vaccariae Segetalis, Semen
Hua Shi	18 g	Talc
Che Qian Zi	12 g	Plantaginis, Semen
Ze Xie	12 g	Alismatis Plantago-aquaticae, Rhizoma
Xiang Fu	12 g	Cyperi Rotundi, Rhizoma
Chuan Xiong	9 g	Ligustici Wallichii, Radix
Zhi Shi	12 g	Citri seu Ponciri Immaturis, Fructus
Qing Pi	9 g	Citri Reticulatae Viride, Pericarpium
Zhe Bei Mu	9 g	Fritillariae Thunbergii, Bulbus
Gan Cao	3 g	Glycyrrhizae Uralensis, Radix

One week of herbal decoction, to be followed by one week of Qian Li Xian Wan ('Prostate Gland Pills', from the Peace Medicine Company, Guangdong, PROC), six pills TID.

This prescription is based upon the formula Chai Hu Shu Gan San ('Bupleurum Powder to Spread the Liver', *Formulas and Strategies*, p. 146). Below is a description of the added herbs:

He Huan Pi is a very effective calming herb which acts by moving Liver qi, nourishing Heart and Spleen, while also removing blood stagnation, reducing swelling, and stopping pain. Hence its rather large amount of 18 g.

Chuan Shan Jia and *Wang Bu Liu Xing* are both strongly moving and dispersing, and both enter the blood level of the Liver and Stomach channels to remove stagnation and reduce swelling.

Hua Shi and *Che Qian Zi* are both slippery in nature and thus help promote urination; while *Mu Tong* and *Ze Xie* both take heat out through the urine, and are also diuretic.

Qing Pi is a strong qi mover which enters the Liver and Gall Bladder channels to disperse accumulation and break up phlegm, and thus is often prescribed for hernial disorders; while *Zhi Shi* replaces *Zhi Ke* in the parent formula because the site of action is in the lower body rather than the chest.

Zhe Bei Mu is bitter, cold, pungent and dispersing, acting to cut phlegm and reduce nodular swelling, and is chosen here as the sole remaining representative of the formula Xiao Luo Wan ('Reduce Scrofula Pill', *Formulas and Strategies*, p. 441), which I follow my teachers in using for softening and dispersing swellings and nodes throughout the body. The other two constituents of Xiao Luo Wan are inappropriate, however: the *Mu Li* (Ostreae, Concha) because of its astringent tendency and the *Xuan Shen* (Scrophulariae Ningpoensis, Radix) because of its somewhat greasy nature.

As should be clear from the above discussion, this case demonstrates the need of a separate symptom pattern for Liver qi obstruction in the categories of 'difficult urination' and 'obstructed urination'.

It also illustrates, as mentioned previously, the interaction between the three levels of clinical analysis in a Western TCM setting: the Western diagnosis, the Chinese diagnosis and the Chinese differentiation. The Western diagnosis is clearly a distinct entity, as the two systems of medicine approach a patient in such different ways; it cannot, however, be disregarded, and its use in the treatment of this case is obvious in the choice of herbs that 'reduce swelling'. The difference between a Chinese diagnosis and a Chinese differentiation, though, is one which is often confusing for many students, but it is nonetheless crucial for focussed selection of treatment. The Chinese diagnosis is the identification of the major presenting problem. For example in gynecology it must be determined whether a patient with heavy bleeding is a case of a) heavy periods, b) extended periods, c) intermenstrual bleeding or d) irregular bleeding. Each is associated with distinct symptom patterns and will require a different approach in treatment. Differentiation identifies the symptom pattern and determines the mechanism by which the major problem arises, and also suggests the basic treatment strategy. As one will be continually reminded in China, if one's selection of diagnosis is incorrect the focus of treatment will be skewed, and then even proper identification of the symptom pattern differentiation will only serve to help the patient in a general way. The situation can be summed up in the story of Mulla Nasrudin, who was supposed to be taking his new and powerful but somewhat unruly horse to market. Someone called out that he was going in the wrong direction. 'I know', replied the Mulla proudly, 'But just look at the speed!'

24. *Zhong Xi Yi Jie He Zhi Liao Chang Jian Wai Ke Ji Fu Zheng* ('Combined Chinese-Western Treatment of Common Surgical Acute Abdominal Conditions'), Tianjin Science and Technology Press, 1982, p.391.
25. *ibid.*, pp. 391-392.
26. Quoted in *Zhong Yi Zheng Zhuang Jian Bie Zhen Duan Xue* ('Diagnostic Studies of Symptom Differentiation in Chinese Medicine'), People's Health Publishing, 1985, pp. 301-302.
27. From *Hunan Sheng Lao Zhong Yi Yi An Xuan* ('Selected Case Histories of Old Chinese Doctors in Hunan Province'), quoted in *Zhong Yi Zhen Duan Xue* ('TCM Diagnostics'), edited by Deng Tie–Tao, People's Health Publishing, 1987, p. 448.
28. The *Ling Shu* Chapter 10 says: 'The Luo-connecting channel separating from the Hand Tai Yin Lung channel [begins at the point] called Lie Que ... if there is deficiency, then yawning, urinary frequency and urinary incontinence [will result].' In the view of one of my acupuncture teachers in China, Lie Que (LU-7) was an essential point in Lung-related urinary disorders, not only because of the classical quote above but also due to its relationship with the Ren Mai. Thus its tonification in the present case can help to secure both the Lungs and the Ren Mai. On the other hand its action in the treatment of urinary obstruction, she said, 'is like lifting the lid on a pot of tea when it is too full: the air rushes in, the tea rushes out.'
29. This formula, a common choice for qi lin (painful urinary obstruction from qi blockage) is often attributed to the *Jin Gui Yi* ('Supplement to the Golden Cabinet') written by You Yi in 1768. But it actually appears much earlier, in the Song Dynasty work *San Yin Ji Yi Bing Zheng Fang Lun* ('Discussion of Illnesses, Patterns, and Formulas Related to the Unification of the Three Etiologies') written by Chen Yan in 1174. It can be found in chapter 12 of this book, on page 167 of the edition published in 1983 by the People's Health Publishing in Beijing.
30. *Jing Yue Quan Shu* ('Complete Works of Jing Yue'), 1624, by Zhang Jing-Yue; Shanghai Science and Technology Press, 1959, p. 506.
31. The 'Three Powers' are Heaven, Earth, and Man but here refer to the three Jiao which are regulated by the use of this formula: the *Tian Men Dong* tonifies the yin of the Lungs, the mother of Kidneys, as well as the Kidneys directly; the *Sha Ren* and *Gan Cao* ensure the normal functioning of the Spleen, both to protect it from the potentially greasy nature of the other herbs and also to ensure an on-going 'later Heaven' supplementation to the jing-essence; the *Ren Shen* tonifies the yuan qi of the whole body; and the *Shou Di, Rou Cong Rong* and *Huang Bo* act directly on the Kidneys in the lower Jiao.
32. *Bian Zheng Lu* ('Records of Syndrome Differentiation'), 1687, by Chen Shi-Duo; quoted in the *Zhong Yi Li Dai Yi Lun Xuan* ('Selected Medical Essays by Traditional Chinese Doctors of Past Generations'), 1983, edited by Wang Xin-Hua, published by the Jiangsu Science and Technology Press, 1983, pp. 70-71.
33. This statement appears in the *Jin Gui Yao Lue* ('Essentials from the Golden Cabinet', *c.* 210 AD), Chapter 12, section 18.

34. She 'to contract' 摄. It is the Metal-natured contracting energy of Lungs, gathering like autumn, that assists the storing Water-natured energy of Kidneys, like winter: no harvest, no storage. Without this beginning of contraction of the yin qi after yang has reached an extreme, the final stage of yin storage cannot be reached, and thus if Lung qi is weak the Kidneys lose power of consolidation.

35. *Jing Yue Quan Shu* ('Complete Works of Jing Yue'), 1624, by Zhang Jing-Yue; Shanghai Science and Technology Press, 1959, pp. 509-510.

Edema   5

In this chapter, the differentiation and treatment of edema will be described both from the modern TCM viewpoint (which in edema involves primarily Eight Principle and Zang Fu Internal Organ differentiation), and also from the Classical literature, starting from the *Nei Jing* and *Jin Gui Yao Lue*. Each approach has its value: the modern viewpoint for its simplicity and familiarity to Western students of TCM, the Classical for its precision and accumulated experience of some twenty centuries.

PATHOLOGY

Pathology is simply a disruption of normal physiological function. To obtain a good grasp of the pathological mechanisms leading to edema one must become familiar with TCM fluid metabolism, and the factors which can disturb it.

External factors most likely to interfere with fluid metabolism are the pathogens wind, damp and cold. Internal factors include either pathogenic excess or functional deficiency. The excess conditions most likely to cause internal interference with fluid metabolism are qi obstruction and disruption by the pathogens water, damp, heat and cold. The functional deficiencies most involved with fluid metabolism deterioration will be those of qi and yang, especially those of the Kidneys and Spleen, which will subsequently implicate the Lungs, the San Jiao and the Urinary Bladder. Abnormal interaction between the three substances qi, blood and fluids can also cause edema.

PATHOLOGICAL MECHANISMS

Exogenous (external) pathogens

Pathogens invading the skin and surface tissues can influence fluid metabolism in three ways: interference with Lung function through occupation of the skin, interference with the Urinary Bladder through invasion of the Tai Yang channel, and interference with the Spleen through exogenous damp accumulation in the flesh.

The Lungs are contiguous with the skin but also ensure the proper descent of fluids through the body by their descending action. A pathogen on the surface—

such as wind-cold—frequently affects this descent of Lung qi, which is why an early exogenous invasion is often signalled by a light cough and 'tickle' in the throat: Lung qi is prevented from descending normally. If Lungs cannot recover their descending ability, fluids will fail to be carried downward to the Urinary Bladder and will instead spread out through the skin.

The foot Tai Yang channel is one of the important pathways for the circulation of protective qi throughout the surface, and also runs over the most yang aspects of the body. These features predispose the Tai Yang channel to interference from exogenous pathogens, especially light rising yang pathogens such as wind. If wind-cold invades the Tai Yang channel, the most usual manifestations of this will be stiffening of the neck and shoulders due to pathogenic cold contracting and obstructing the flow of normal qi through the Tai Yang channel that supplies the area; however at the same time it is not uncommon for the pathogen to affect urination, either indirectly by hindering Urinary Bladder channel qi movement or directly by following the course of the channel and entering the Urinary Bladder itself. This is described in TCM Shang Han theory as 'Tai Yang Fu-organ Syndrome', and Wu Ling San ('Five-Ingredient Powder with Poria', *Formulas and Strategies*, p. 174) is the formula designed to deal with it.

Damp can enter the body either with pathogenic wind, which—because it is a yang dispersing pathogen—opens the pores, or by taking advantage of pores which have opened naturally, as, for example, with sweating. Once inside, damp (which is by nature Earth-related) gravitates to the flesh (again related to Earth) and remains there, where it continually obstructs the flow of Spleen's nourishing yang qi. This can eventually result in a weakening of Spleen yang, and a further build-up of internal damp. Even just locally, however, in the surface tissues, the pathogenic damp can interrupt normal fluid movement and cause edema. Damp can also produce heat, either through clogging the surface and preventing the dispersal of normal body heat or through conflicting with the flow of yang qi: the struggle generates heat, which then combines with the damp.

All of these three forms of exogenous pathogenic influence are able to affect the normal circulation of the protective qi throughout the surface, which will interfere with fluid metabolism in yet another way by preventing the orderly opening and closing of the pores, and thus causing chaos in another possible mechanism for dealing with a surplus of cutaneous fluids: perspiration.

Endogenous (internal) pathogens

Pathogenic excess

Water. In edema, excessive accumulation of pathogenic water is the immediate cause of the edematous swelling, and will therefore be involved in every case, regardless of etiology. Treatment, in some cases, will address only the 'root' of the problem, when it is felt that rectification of the root mechanisms will be sufficient to eliminate the water. In most cases, however, both the 'root' mechanisms and the 'branch' manifestations—the pathogenic water—will be considered. Elimination of the pathogenic water as the branch will usually involve either promotion of sweating, if the pathogenic water is on the surface or promotion of urination, if the water is in the interior.

Damp. Internal damp can lead to excessive accumulation of pathogenic water by overwhelming the Spleen's ability to transform and transport. If this happens water and damp are not carried downward to be excreted but instead spread out through the flesh and cause edema, as well as the other complications of surface damp noted in the discussion of exogenous damp above. Damp's pathogenic influence can also affect the movement in the San Jiao, both of the fluids themselves and also of the yuan qi necessary for the qi transformation processes in the body. Damp will cause edema in the middle and lower Jiao, mainly, due to the sinking nature of damp; the most direct effect being obstruction of the Urinary Bladder functioning by excessive damp.

Heat. Heat will be a factor in edema chiefly when it has combined with damp, which indeed may have produced it in the first place. Often, though, diet is the source of the damp-heat, through consumption of alcohol, hot spicy or rich foods or greasy hard-to-digest foods. Damp-heat can affect the Spleen and Stomach, the San Jiao or the Urinary Bladder, obstructing their normal functioning and thus causing edema. One peculiar identifying sign of damp-heat in this disease may be the appearance of boils, pimples and ulcerations in conjunction with the edema. (See the section on yellow sweat, p. 133.)

Cold. Internal cold will usually be the result of yang deficiency, either of the Spleen or the Kidneys, allowing cold to accumulate and eventually act as a pathogenic agent in its own right.[1] The cold can slow fluid movement through interference with the yang qi, and cause thickening by its contracting nature, congealing the fluids into damp, with which it then combines, forming cold-damp.

Functional deficiencies

Qi. Qi is both a function and a substance. In edema, it will be the functional aspect of qi which has the most influence: in its most general manifestation, weakness of the ability of the qi to carry fluids around the body can allow them to accumulate and flood (see 'qi edema' in the Classical differentiation section). Weakness of the yuan qi supporting qi transformation, especially in the Spleen and the Urinary Bladder, will result in retention of untransformed fluids, which can then spread into the surface tissues and cause edema. Specific weakness of the functioning of a particular organ such as, again, the Spleen or the Lungs or the Kidneys, can lead to edema: in Classical terms, Kidneys rule Water, Spleen and Stomach both rule Earth. The nature of Earth is to hold Water in check but if Stomach and Spleen are weak, the normal transformative capacity to maintain this check on water is reduced, pathogenic water qi builds up internally and attacks that which would normally restrain it: Earth. The Spleen, which hates damp, is especially oppressed and so fluids rush into the flesh of the limbs. The Kidneys, too, gradually become inundated with pathogenic water and so are unable to support the Urinary Bladder separation of fluids into murky and clear, and urine is reduced, thus cutting off a lower route of escape, and pathogenic fluids accumulate in the lower body and cause both edema and abdominal distention.

Yang. Yang deficiency is often the next stage after qi becomes weak, and this is especially true where such yin pathogens as water and damp are concerned, as their nature directly opposes yang and drains the yang warmth which is so crucial for the movement and transformation required by normal fluid metabolism. In the Spleen, weakness of the

yang (like the qi) will hamper both transformation of fluids and their transportation, allowing excess fluids to spread out to the flesh and then to the surface tissues and cause edema. A portion of these excess untransformed fluids can also be carried up to the Lungs, where they will commonly coalesce into phlegm or thin mucus; however, this process itself can interfere with the ability of the Lung qi to descend, thereby disrupting the Lung function of regulating the fluid pathways.

It is in the lower Jiao, however, that the most immediate and striking effects of yang qi deficiency will be found: Urinary Bladder qi transformation is directly supported by Kidney yang, which enables it to separate clear fluids from murky fluids, recovering the former to be recycled back into the body and expelling the latter through the urine. Weakness of Kidney yang quickly becomes apparent as scanty urine,[2] gradually followed by lower body edema.

San Jiao, as the organ responsible for the differentiation of yuan qi into its various functions, and the movement of yuan qi around the body, and again as the pathway for fluids, is the next to suffer from a lack of Kidney yang: Zhou Xue-Hai points out (in the essay concluding this chapter) that Kidney yang (as 'yuan qi') first must pass the Urinary Bladder, and then circulate in the San Jiao, ensuring both the movement of fluids and the warming ability to transform them. If the San Jiao is obstructed, normal ascent and descent of qi becomes chaotic, and fluids can flood and produce edema. As the *Zhong Zang Jing* ('Treasury Classic') says: 'If San Jiao is obstructed, nutritive and protective qi become blocked, qi and blood do not flow properly together, excess and deficiency intermix, water follows the flow of qi, and thus results in a water disease.'[3]

Interaction of qi, blood and fluids

These three substances support each other, often making up for a deficiency in one substance by transformation of another (see the section on relationship of qi, blood, and fluids in Chapter One). Obstruction of one substance can also affect the other two: qi blockage leading to blood stagnation is a well known example. Qi blockage can slow fluid movement, just as accumulated water will impede the circulation of qi. Blood stagnation can interfere with fluid metabolism, as in the syndrome known as 'xue fen' (blood separation); and accumulated fluids can also interrupt normal blood flow, as in the 'shui fen' (water separation) syndrome.

DIFFERENTIATION AND TREATMENT

Common symptom patterns

Wind-cold binding the Lungs. Rapid onset of edema beginning at the eyelids, face or head, continuing to the rest of the body and the limbs, accompanied by aversion to wind and cold, possible fever, dyspnea, aching joints, scanty urine, thin white tongue coat and a floating tight pulse.

Wind-heat disturbing the Lungs. Rapid onset of swelling of the eyelids and face, fever, aversion to wind, cough, sore red and swollen throat, scanty dark urine, tongue tip and edges slightly red, tongue coat thin yellow and a floating rapid pulse.

Damp combining with heat. Generalized edema, with moist glistening skin, abdominal distention, sensation of fullness in the chest and abdomen, feelings of restlessness and heat, thirst, scanty darkish urine, possible constipation, thick yellow tongue coat and, deep rapid pulse.

Water and damp oppressing the Spleen. Gradual onset of generalized edema of the limbs and trunk, starting usually at the limbs, and most obvious in the lower limbs and the abdomen, severe enough to hide a pressing finger. Accompanying symptoms will be a heavy sensation of the body, sleepiness and lethargy, stuffy chest and nausea, loss of taste and appetite for food, urine scanty but clear, white greasy tongue coat and a deep languid or deep slow pulse.

Spleen yang deficiency. Stubborn, recurring, edematous swelling most pronounced below the waist, which pits when pressed leaving a depression which is slow to resolve. Accompanying symptoms will be tiredness, cold limbs, sensations of epigastric fullness and abdominal distension, poor appetite, loose stool, scanty clear urine, pale tongue with a thin white slippery moist coat and a deep and languid pulse.

Kidney yang deficiency. Generalized edema which like the above is also pitting and slow to resolve, usually starting around the waist and in the feet, and most pronounced in the lower body,

especially around the medial ankles. Accompanying symptoms will be pale complexion possibly with dark areas under the eyes, cold aching of the lower back, sore weak knees that feel heavy, clammy cold moist feeling in the scrotum, chills and lethargy, cold limbs, scanty clear urine, pale flabby tongue, thin white tongue coat and a deep and thready weak pulse.

Qi and blood deficiency. Gradual onset of edematous swelling in the face and limbs, pale or sallow complexion, pale white lips, light-headedness, palpitations, shortness of breath, poor appetite, lethargy and tiredness, tongue body pale with little coat and a weak and thready pulse.

Differentiation

Wind-cold binding the Lungs versus wind-heat disturbing the Lungs causing edema. Both of these conditions result from an exogenous pathogenic wind invasion affecting the Lungs' fluid metabolism functioning. Lungs are known as 'the upper source of water' (shui zhi shang yuan), and also control the skin. If a pathogen prevents Lung qi from clearing, spreading, contracting and descending, then on the one hand the pores will fail to open and close properly so that excess fluids cannot be eliminated through the skin, while on the other, fluid movement downward will lose its pulsing regularity derived from Lung qi descent and be unable to flow smoothly to the Urinary Bladder. As a result, fluid distribution and excretion will suffer, leading to accumulation of water and damp, and finally scanty urine and edema.

Because the pathogen is exogenous wind, a yang pathogen with a quick upward-moving nature, the onset of the edematous swelling is sudden; and because of the location of the Lungs in the upper Jiao, the first location of the swelling will occur closest to the source of the disruption: the upper body. This is exacerbated by the rising tendency of the pathogenic wind, which will tend to carry the otherwise aimless fluids upward to the eyes, face and head.

However, although both conditions involve wind, they must be treated differently because the wind has allied itself with completely different types of pathogens: yin cold in the first case and yang heat in the second.

Differentiation of the two will be through the accompanying symptoms. For wind-cold binding the Lungs, the key symptoms to look for will be the more severe chills with milder fever, aching joints, no sweating and other typical symptoms of wind-cold invading the Tai Yang channel (as in the *Shang Han Lun*).

For wind-heat disturbing the Lungs causing edema, the fever will be more severe than the chills, the urine will be darker and there will also be sore red swollen throat.

The pulse in each instance will be very useful, as in wind-cold the pulse will be floating tight and languid (or slow), while for wind-heat it will be floating and rapid.

The tongue, too, will help differentiation: the coat in wind-cold binding the Lungs will be thin white, whereas in wind-heat it will be thin yellow, and the tip and edges in this case will also be slightly red if the heat has become a bit more entrenched.

Treatment requires dispersal of wind in both instances but with appropriate modifications. Wind-cold binding the Lungs causing edema should be treated with pungent warm wind-cold expellers, while also promoting Lung qi flow and the flow of water. Ma Huang Jia Zhu Tang ('Ephedra Decoction plus Atractylodes') was designed for this condition.

Wind-heat disturbing the Lungs causing edema should be treated with pungent cooling and Lung qi promoting herbs, plus cooling diuretics, with formulas such as Ma Huang Lian Qiao Chi Xiao Dou Tang ('Ephedra, Forsythia, and Phaseolus Calcaratus Decoction') or Yue Bi Jia Zhu Tang ('Maidservant from Yue Decoction plus Atractylodes').

If either of the above two conditions has sweating and aversion to wind, lethargy and stubborn edema which does not respond to these treatments, this indicates that the protective yang qi is already weak, and so the treatment should aim at promoting protective qi flow in order to move the pathogenic water and damp with Fang Ji Huang Qi Tang ('Stephania and Astragalus Decoction').

Formulas

Ma Huang Jia Zhu Tang ('Ephedra Decoction plus Atractylodes')

Ma Huang	Ephedrae, Herba
Xing Ren	Pruni Armeniacae, Semen
Gui Zhi	Cinnamomi Cassiae, Ramulus
Bai Zhu	Atractylodis Macrocephalae, Rhizoma
Gan Cao	Glycyrrhizae Uralensis, Radix

Source text: *Shang Han Lun* ('Discussion of Cold-induced Disorders', *c*.210AD) [*Formulas and Strategies*, p. 34]

Ma Huang Lian Qiao Chi Xiao Dou Tang ('Ephedra, Forsythia, and Phaseolus Calcaratus Decoction')

Ma Huang	6 g	Ephedrae, Herba
Lian Qiao	9 g	Forsythiae Suspensae, Fructus
Xing Ren	6 g	Pruni Armeniacae, Semen
Chi Xiao Dou	10 g	Phaseoli Calcarati, Semen
Sang Bai Pi	10 g	Mori Albae Radicis, Cortex
Zhi Gan Cao	6 g	Honey-fried Glycyrrhizae Uralensis, Radix
Da Zao	12 g	Zizyphi Jujubae, Fructus
Sheng Jiang	6 g	Zingiberis Officinalis Recens, Rhizoma

Take as decoction.

Source text: *Shang Han Lun* ('Discussion of Cold-Induced Disorders', 210AD)

Yue Bi Jia Zhu Tang ('Maidservant from Yue Decoction plus Atractylodes')

Ma Huang	Ephedrae, Herba
Shi Gao	Gypsum
Sheng Jiang	Zingiberis Officinalis Recens, Rhizoma
Bai Zhu	Atractylodis Macrocephalae, Rhizoma
Gan Cao	Glycyrrhizae Uralensis, Radix
Da Zao	Zizyphi Jujubae, Fructus

Source text: *Jin Gui Yao Lue* ('Essentials from the Golden Cabinet', *c*. 210 AD) [*Formulas and Strategies*, p. 89]

Fang Ji Huang Qi Tang ('Stephania and Astragalus Decoction')

Huang Qi	Astragali, Radix
Han Fang Ji	Stephaniae Tetrandrae, Radix
Bai Zhu	Atractylodis Macrocephalae, Rhizoma
Gan Cao	Glycyrrhizae Uralensis, Radix

Sheng Jiang	Zingiberis Officinalis Recens, Rhizoma
Da Zao	Zizyphi Jujubae, Fructus

Source text: *Jin Gui Yao Lue* ('Essentials from the Golden Cabinet', c. 210 AD) [*Formulas and Strategies*, p. 179]

Damp-heat. When pathogenic damp and heat combine to produce damp-heat, the flow of qi through the San Jiao is easily obstructed, the Urinary Bladder fluid separation function interrupted and fluids can accumulate to produce edema. While it can result from long-term accumulation of internal damp gradually producing heat, more usually the origins are in the diet. Zhang Jing-Yue, in the chapter on distension in his *Jing Yue Quan Shu* ('Complete Works of Jing Yue', 1624) says: 'Often youths who drink alcohol can develop damp-heat which they carry around despite the continuing vitality of their yuan qi; the pulse will be full and strong.'[4] Alcohol is not the only culprit, however: greasy rich foods, a taste for spice or sweets, or simply overeating habitually will provide fertile ground for the development of damp-heat. In damp-heat edema, the symptoms will be sensations of fullness in the chest, poor appetite, dry mouth but little thirst, dark scanty urine with a possible burning sensation or murkiness, red tongue with a yellow greasy coat and a slippery rapid or rapid floating and weak pulse.

The treatment of damp-heat edema requires separation of the two pathogens damp and heat, with expulsion of the damp, after which the heat will disperse by itself. The main formula is Shu Zao Yin Zi ('The Dispersing Chisel Decoction').

Formula

Shu Zao Yin Zi ('The Dispersing Chisel Decoction')

Shang Lu	Phytolaccae, Radix
Qiang Huo	Notopterygii, Rhizoma et Radix
Qin Jiao	Gentianae Macrophyllae, Radix
Bing Lang	Arecae Catechu, Semen
Da Fu Pi	Arecae Catechu, Pericarpium
Fu Ling Pi	Poriae Cocos, Cortex
Chuan Jiao	Zanthoxyli Bungeani, Fructus
Mu Tong	Mutong, Caulis
Ze Xie	Alismatis Plantago-aquaticae, Rhizoma
Chi Xiao Dou	Phaseoli Calcarati, Semen
Sheng Jiang Pi	Zingiberis Officinalis Recens, Cortex

Source text: *Ji Sheng Fang* ('Formulas to Aid the Living', 1253)

Note: This is a purging formula, and as such **must only be used with strong patients**. If the patient is somewhat weak, refer to the chapter on damp-heat for an appropriate strategy. *Shang Lu* (Phytolaccae, Radix) is poisonous and potentially dangerous in inexperienced hands, and so it would be best avoided (especially while TCM is seeking to establish a reputation in the West as a safe yet efficacious system of medicine). *Qian Niu Zi* (Pharbitidis, Semen) is a possible alternative, as the actions are quite similar, but if this is not available *Ting Li Zi* (Tinglizi, Semen) can be considered. If no herbs are used that strongly drive out excess water, the 'dispersing chisel' effect in the formula's name is lost, as there will be nothing to separate damp and heat.

Water and damp oppressing the Spleen versus Spleen yang deficiency causing edema. Water and damp oppressing the Spleen is an excess (shi) condition, formed by long-term residence in damp living conditions or damp working conditions, so that cold and damp permeate the body, invading the interior and accumulating in the location to which they have the most affinity: Earth, the middle Jiao. As this accumulation progresses, the normal transforming ability of the Spleen becomes overwhelmed, and a vicious cycle commences whereby ever more damp builds up and obstructs Spleen transformation and then transportation, so that water and damp are not carried downward to be excreted but instead spread out from the flesh (i.e. Earth) into the skin and surface tissues, causing edema. Because the limbs are mostly composed of muscle and flesh, it is in the limbs that the edematous swelling begins and so the body feels heavy and lethargic. The strength of the pathogenic damp qi is indicated by the thickness of the swelling, which is enough to partially obscure the investigating finger (especially on the abdomen) but the as-yet-unimpaired yang qi movement prevents pitting. Clear yang is prevented from rising normally because of the damp in the middle Jiao, leading to the heavy headache which feels as if the head has been wrapped up, and to the loss of taste discrimination. The damp in the middle Jiao not only affects the rise of clear yang but also affects the normal descent of Stomach qi, so that nausea and stuffy chest occur.

Damp being a sinking turbid yin pathogen, an excess amount seeping down into the Urinary Bladder can prevent transformation by the yang qi even here, and urine becomes scanty but still clear because there is, as yet, no build-up of heat.

The important point to grasp is the heaviness of pathogenic damp, which accounts for all the symptoms in this shi-type condition.

By contrast, Spleen yang weakness causing edema is based on deficiency. This is often a long-term consequence of failure to treat the excess type of edema from water and damp build-up, or it can be a result of constitutional Spleen qi deficiency, so that it is too weak to transform food and fluids completely, allowing them to build up into residual damp. Transport will be weak as well, and the damp and water will not be carried away to be eliminated but instead accumulate, spread and cause swelling. The important points in differentiating this from the excess damp condition will be the stubbornness of the problem, its constant recurrence and the inability of the weak yang qi to move within the surface tissues, so that when the edematous swelling is pressed upon it remains depressed like a pit. The other yang deficiency symptoms like cold limbs, exhaustion, poor appetite and loose stool should help differentiation.

So although there are many symptoms in common, the approach in differentiation is to focus on whether the condition is one of deficiency or one of excess. Upon this differentiation will rest the emphasis in treatment: whether to simply use warmth and diuretics to remove the excess damp, or to warm and tonify Spleen yang to transform damp. The correct choice of emphasis, and the proper degree of emphasis placed upon each aspect of the problem in treatment, will determine the degree of success.

Water and damp oppressing the Spleen should be treated by using warmth to open fluid metabolism and transform damp, while using diuretics, with a combination of Wei Ling Tang ('Calm the Stomach and Poria Decoction') and Wu Pi Yin ('Five-Peel Decoction').

Treatment of Spleen yang deficiency causing edema requires strengthening of Spleen yang transport, and the use of both damp transformation and diuretics simultaneously. A formula designed with this in mind is Shi Pi Yin ('Bolster the Spleen Decoction').

Formulas

Wei Ling Tang ('Calm the Stomach and Poria Decoction')

Cang Zhu	Atractylodis, Rhizoma
Chen Pi	Citri Reticulatae, Pericarpium
Hou Po	Magnoliae Officinalis, Cortex
Gan Cao	Glycyrrhizae Uralensis, Radix
Zhu Ling	Polypori Umbellati, Sclerotium
Fu Ling	Poriae Cocos, Sclerotium
Bai Zhu	Atractylodis Macrocephalae, Rhizoma
Gui Zhi	Cinnamomi Cassiae, Ramulus
Ze Xie	Alismatis Plantago-aquaticae, Rhizoma

Source text: *Dan Xi Xin Fa* ('Teachings of Dan Xi', 1481) [*Formulas and Strategies*, p. 176]

Wu Pi Yin ('Five-Peel Decoction')

Fu Ling Pi	Poriae Cocos, Cortex
Sang Bai Pi	Mori Albae Radicis, Cortex
Da Fu Pi	Arecae Catechu, Pericarpium
Sheng Jiang Pi	Zingiberis Officinalis Recens, Cortex
Chen Pi	Citri Reticulatae, Pericarpium

Source text: *Tai Ping Hui Min He Ji Ju Fang* ('Imperial Grace Formulary of the Tai Ping Era', 1078-85) [*Formulas and Strategies*, p. 179]

If more warmth is required to move the pathogenic water, add *Fu Zi* (Aconiti Carmichaeli Praeparata, Radix) and *Gan Jiang* (Zingiberis Officianalis, Rhizoma).

Shi Pi Yin ('Bolster the Spleen Decoction')

Fu Zi	Aconiti Carmichaeli Praeparata, Radix
Gan Jiang	Zingiberis Officianalis, Rhizoma
Fu Ling	Poriae Cocos, Sclerotium

Bai Zhu	Atractylodis Macrocephalae, Rhizoma
Mu Gua	Chaenomelis Lagenariae, Fructus
Hou Po	Magnoliae Officinalis, Cortex
Mu Xiang	Saussureae seu Vladimiriae, Radix
Da Fu Pi	Arecae Catechu, Pericarpium
Cao Guo	Amomi Tsao-ko, Fructus
Gan Cao	Glycyrrhizae Uralensis, Radix

Source text: *Shi Yi De Xiao Fang* ('Effective Formulas from Generations of Physicians', 1345) [*Formulas and Strategies*, p. 199]

If the damp has accumulated enough to become an excess pathogen in its own right, making this a combined excess-deficiency condition, then direct diuresis may be necessary to remove the pressure upon the Spleen. Add *Zhu Ling* (Polypori Umbellati, Sclerotium) and *Ze Xie* (Alismatis Plantago-aquaticae, Rhizoma). If the qi deficiency is extreme, add *Ren Shen* (Ginseng, Radix).

Spleen yang deficiency versus Kidney yang deficiency causing edema. Both are from yang deficiency and so are long-term problems, with pitting edematous swelling more pronounced below the waist, and pulse and tongue which are very similar in presentation. Furthermore, the two often occur together in clinic. Yet there are differences.

Kidneys are in the lower Jiao and provide the yang energy powering qi transformation throughout the body. But because this yang qi must pass through the Urinary Bladder, if Kidney yang is insufficient the Urinary Bladder function of separating the clear reusable fluids from the murky excretable fluids is impaired, urine becomes scanty and fluids accumulate, unable to exit. Thus lower Jiao fluid metabolism lacks support, and the edematous swelling begins in the lower body, around the waist and especially around the course of the Kidney channel on the feet. Accompanying symptoms will be darkening of the complexion, weak sore heavy knees, clammy cold scrotum, deep thready pulse— especially at the proximal (chi) position—and other typical Kidney yang deficiency signs.

Spleen yang deficiency edema, while it is most severe below the waist, tends to also involve the limbs and thus be more generalized. It will also have

digestive Spleen symptoms such as sensations of epigastric fullness, poor appetite and loose stool, and qi deficiency signs like tiredness.

With attention to details such as these, it should be possible to differentiate the relative degrees of Spleen or Kidney yang deficiency even if they occur together.

Treatment of Kidney yang deficiency should be to warm Kidney yang to enable it to support lower Jiao qi transformation of fluids in the Urinary Bladder, while encouraging diuresis; example formulas would be Ji Sheng Shen Qi Wan ('Kidney Qi Pill from *Formulas to Aid the Living*') or Zhen Wu Tang ('True Warrior Decoction') as a basis for additions.

Formulas

Ji Sheng Shen Qi Wan ('Kidney Qi Pill from *Formulas to Aid the Living*')

Shou Di	Rehmanniae Glutinosae Conquitae, Radix
Shan Zhu Yu	Corni Officinalis, Fructus
Shan Yao	Dioscoreae Oppositae, Radix
Fu Ling	Poriae Cocos, Sclerotium
Ze Xie	Alismatis Plantago-aquaticae, Rhizoma
Mu Dan Pi	Moutan Radicis, Cortex
Fu Zi	Aconiti Carmichaeli Praeparata, Radix
Rou Gui	Cinnamomi Cassiae, Cortex
Niu Xi	Achyranthis Bidentatae, Radix
Che Qian Zi	Plantaginis, Semen

Source text: *Ji Sheng Fang* ('Formulas to Aid the Living', Yan Yong–He, 1253) [*Formulas and Strategies*, p. 278]

Zhen Wu Tang ('True Warrior Decoction')

Fu Zi	Aconiti Carmichaeli Praeparata, Radix
Bai Zhu	Atractylodis Macrocephalae, Rhizoma
Fu Ling	Poriae Cocos, Sclerotium
Bai Shao	Paeoniae Lactiflora, Radix
Sheng Jiang	Zingiberis Officinalis Recens, Rhizoma

Source text: *Shang Han Lun* ('Discussion of Cold-induced Disorders', *c.*210AD) [*Formulas and Strategies*, p. 197]

If yang is extremely weak, add *Hu Lu Ba* (Trigonellae Foeni-graeci, Semen) and *Ba Ji Tian* (Morindae Officianalis, Radix).

If the qi itself is threatening collapse, with spontaneous perspiration, dyspnea and inability to lie flat, add *Ren Shen* (Ginseng, Radix), *Wu Wei Zi* (Schisandrae Chinensis, Fructus), *Duan Mu Li* (Ostreae, Concha, prepared) and *Zhi Gan Cao* (Glycyrrhizae Uralensis, Radix, honey-fried.)

Qi and blood deficiency causing edema. This again is internal deficiency but not involving yang. It is usually a result of reduced Spleen and Stomach function, so that transformation and transportation suffer, and the source of blood production is insufficient. Alternatively, damage to qi and blood over the course of a long illness will have the same effect: lack of support for zang-organ functioning so that fluid metabolism is disrupted and edema results. The *Wan Bing Hui Chun* ('Restoration of Health from the Myriad Diseases', Gong Ting-Xian, 1587) says: 'Relief in the morning, acute in the evening is blood deficiency; acute in the morning, relief in the evening is qi deficiency; acute both morning and evening is deficiency of both blood and qi.' The prime differentiating points between this condition and Spleen yang deficiency, which it most resembles, will be lack of Spleen cold symptoms, obvious blood deficiency symptoms (such as facial pallor, pale lips, scanty menstrual blood, dizziness and palpitations) and more pronounced qi deficiency symptoms (such as shortness of breath). The edema itself will also not be as severe as that of Spleen yang deficiency.

Treatment will focus on restoring qi (both functional qi and substantial qi) and tonifying blood. An example formula is Gui Pi Tang ('Restore the Spleen Decoction').

Formula

Gui Pi Tang ('Restore the Spleen Decoction')

Ren Shen	Ginseng, Radix
Huang Qi	Astragali, Radix
Bai Zhu	Atractylodis Macrocephalae, Rhizoma
Fu Ling	Poriae Cocos, Sclerotium
Suan Zao Ren	Ziziphi Spinosae, Semen
Long Yan Rou	Euphoriae Longanae, Arillus
Mu Xiang	Saussureae seu Vladimiriae, Radix
Dang Gui	Angelica Polymorpha, Radix
Yuan Zhi	Polygalae Tenuifoliae, Radix
Gan Cao	Glycyrrhizae Uralensis, Radix
Sheng Jiang	Zingiberis Officinalis Recens, Rhizoma
Da Zao	Zizyphi Jujubae, Fructus

Source text: *Ji Sheng Fang* ('Formulas to Aid the Living', Yan Yong-He, 1253) [*Formulas and Strategies*, p. 255]

Differentiations of edema in classical literature

Despite the complexity of the early classical theories of edema, the primary differentiations will be basically those of yin and yang, excess or deficient, surface or interior. The mechanisms are closely involved with the functioning of the three organs Lungs, Spleen and Kidneys, as well as the San Jiao which links them and forms the pathway for both the fluid movement around the body and the yuan qi which is required for fluid transformation.

The essential points to differentiate are:

1. whether the edema is yin edema or yang edema
2. whether the edema is the result of internal factors or external factors
3. whether the patient is deficient, or a pathogen is excessive
4. whether the location of the pathology is in the Lungs, the Spleen or the Kidneys.

It must also be borne in mind that the interaction between the qi, blood and fluids is extremely close: a disruption in one substance will sooner or later affect the other two. The gynecological conditions of 'xue fen' and 'shui fen' (introduced above and discussed more fully later in this chapter) are cogent examples.

Differentiating yin edema and yang edema

The yang syndrome is usually hot, acute and high in the body, being most often found in the early or middle stages of an edematous condition; while the yin syndrome is usually cold, gradual, deficient and low in the body, with pitting edema.

Yang edema. A yang pathogen acts rapidly, and so the condition is acute, usually becoming full-blown within several days. The edema proceeds from above to below, first affecting the face, head, shoulders, back and arms: i.e. involving the three yang channels of the hand. The accompanying symptoms will all be yang: red tongue with a white or yellow coat, floating and possibly tight or rapid pulse, heat in the chest, insatiable thirst, darkish difficult scanty urine and constipation. The patient will usually be young and strong, with a reddish complexion, rough breathing and usually a slippery strong pulse. The condition can begin with a sore throat, or perhaps boils or pimples, and then be followed by edema. Of the five edemas described in the *Jin Gui Yao Lue* (discussed below), wind edema, skin edema and yellow sweat fall into this category; of the five zang edemas, Lung water is considered yang.

Yin edema. Yin edema is the result of internal deficiency, and so has a gradual onset, only reaching its full extent after several months. The edema may begin on the surface but will gradually involve the interior; the swelling will often first become obvious in the lower body and then spread upwards, starting in the ankle, feet, shins and then the abdomen and waist: i.e. involving the three yin channels of the feet. The accompanying symptoms will all be yin: pale flabby tongue with a white moist coat, deep and possibly weak and slow pulse, lack of warmth, no thirst, possibly scanty or difficult but not dark urine, normal or loose stool, and the edema will be pitting because of the heavy turbidity of the pathogenic yin and the inability of the weak yang qi to circulate in the area. The patient will usually be thin and pallid, with a weak tired voice, and will often be middle-aged or old, weak, overworked or

overstressed. Yin edema can also occur following an illness, or after giving birth. Of the five edemas, righteous-edema and stone-edema are yin edema; also, most of the five zang edemas are yin edema.

Differentiation of the 'five edemas'

Wind-edema (feng shui). Wind-edema will have a floating pulse, aching joints and aversion to wind, in addition to fluid retention in the face and head. As the name suggests, it is the result of exogenous wind invading the Lungs. The Lungs are responsible for the skin and for regulating the downward movement of fluids; a wind pathogen on the surface will obstruct the flow of protective qi, leading to aversion to wind and also lessen nourishment to the joints, causing an ache. Wind is a yang pathogen with a rising nature and so will tend to lift the gathering fluids upwards, thereby bringing on facial edema. As usual in exogenous wind conditions, there will also be mild sweating, no thirst and only mild fever.

Skin-edema (pi shui). This will also have a floating pulse but no aversion to wind; the abdomen will be obviously swollen and distended, the edema will be in the lower legs, the swelling when prodded will leave a depression and there will be no thirst. This is a combined pathology of the Spleen and the Lungs, as the Spleen rules the flesh and the Lungs rule the skin. The focus of the pathology is on the surface, which accounts for the floating pulse but there is no exogenous pathogenic wind involvement and thus no aversion to wind, and nothing to carry the fluids upward so the fluids sink to the abdomen and legs. They will build up until unable to move, and the edema, when prodded, will leave a depression. As there is no pathogenic yang involvement or heat to dry the fluids, there is no thirst.

Because wind-edema and skin-edema are both situated in the surface tissues, they fall into the (historically) later theoretical category of 'yang edema', and so should be treated by promotion of sweating.

Righteous-edema (zheng shui). In righteous-edema[5] as described in the *Jin Gui Yao Lue*, the pulse is deep and slow, and its special characteristic is dyspnea. The pathological mechanism is weak-

Table 5.1 Differentiation of yang edema and yin edema

	Yang Edema	Yin Edema
Location	begins in the head	begins in the legs
Onset	rapid	gradual
Duration	recent	chronic
Skin color	glossy	sallow, lusterless
Urine	scanty dark and difficult	scanty and difficult
Stool	dry constipation	loose
Tongue color	pale red or red	pale, flabby
Tongue coat	white or yellow & perhaps greasy	white moist & perhaps greasy
Pulse	floating or deep, and perhaps rapid	deep, & perhaps slow

ness of Kidney yang allowing water to accumulate internally. It then follows the pathway of the Kidney channel upward into the Lungs, preventing the Lung qi from descending normally and thus causing dyspnea. Kidney deficiency edema will have more symptoms than those described in the original text of the *Jin Gui's* righteous-edema category, however: even the earlier *Su Wen* Chapter 61 describes a more complete picture: 'Edema: below, there is swelling of the shins and upper abdomen; above, there is dyspnea and rough breathing, with inability to recline; the branch and root are both diseased, therefore the Lungs cause dyspnea, the Kidneys cause edema'. Thus in righteous-edema there will certainly be edema in the legs and upper abdomen, as well as a deep slow pulse and dyspnea.

Stone-edema (shi shui). Stone-edema's pulse is also deep but there is no dyspnea, and the lower abdominal swelling and fullness is particularly severe, even hard to the touch, hence the name. The pathology is again the result of Kidney yang deficiency allowing water to accumulate in the lower body but in this condition there is no Lung involvement.

Both righteous-edema and stone-edema are located internally, have deep pulses and abdominal distension, and therefore both belong to the later theoretical category of 'yin edema'. However, in righteous-edema the location is somewhat higher than that of stone-edema, as the abdominal distension is in the upper rather than the lower abdomen, and the limbs are also swollen. In stone-edema the lower abdomen is swollen and hard as a stone, and only subsequently will there be edema of the limbs.

Yellow sweat (huang han). Yellow sweat has a deep and slow pulse, with fever, sensation of fullness in the chest, swelling of the arms, legs, face and head. Once the disease has become chronic, ulcers and boils may appear. Yellow sweat is classically caused by immersion in cold water while sweating, so that pathogenic cold-damp can invade the pores which are open and vulnerable. The cold then tightly contracts them, obstructing the flow of nutritive and protective qi, causing heat, which both steams a yellowish sweaty fluid out of the body and leads to fever. Both cold and damp easily obstruct the flow of yang qi, resulting in the stuffy full chest and the deep slow pulse. After the pathogen has remained in the surface tissues for

an extended period of time, the lack of nourishment from the nutritive and protective qi, and the continual action of the pathogenic cold, damp and subsequent heat, make the normal structure of the tissues break down so that they putrefy and become ulcerated.

Special categories of edema differentiation in Classical literature

Qi edema. This condition is also known as 'qi fen' ('qi separation') and involves initial disruption of the qi movement, which causes the flow of fluids to be 'separated' into normal and abnormal courses, so that some fluids seep out of their normal pathways and into the skin and surface tissues, resulting in edema. This disruption can be of two types, according to the *Jin Gui Yao Lue*: excess or deficiency.

In qi excess, the mechanism is one of obstruction to the flow of qi, so that fluids also slow and become obstructed, leading to edema. The symptoms mentioned in the *Jin Gui Yao Lue* are numbness of the limbs, cold hands and feet, borborygmus, belching and flatulence; but there will often be signs of emotional disturbance.[6] Here, moving the qi will eliminate the edema.

In qi deficiency, the possible ramifications in the fluid metabolism are extensive; however the most basic will be that resulting from weakness of the yuan qi, which is responsible for each qi transformation process occurring throughout the body. If the yuan qi is sufficient, then qi transformation can proceed normally; if it is insufficient, the qi transformation process will at some point fail, and fluids will not be transformed but rather become pathogenic water. This can cause edema and other signs of qi transformation dysfunction. Thus the symptom mentioned in the *Jin Gui Yao Lue* is 'if deficient, then urinary incontinence'. The treatment, naturally, is to tonify the yuan qi, which will involve strengthening the Kidneys, its basis.

Xue fen (blood separation) and shui fen (water separation). The 'xue fen' and 'shui fen' syndromes are a common feature in TCM gynecology, although rather less well known in other departments of Chinese medicine. But they provide another illustration of the close relationship between fluids and blood.

Xue fen is 'amenorrhea followed by edema', shui fen is 'edema followed by amenorrhea'. The names of these syndromes first appeared in the *Jin Gui Yao Lue*, Chapter 14 but a more complete explanation occurs in Chapter 153 of the *Sheng Ji Zong Lu* ('Comprehensive Recording of the Sages' Benefits', *c*. 1117):

> The meaning of 'xue fen' in the discourses is that as the menses begin to flow, cold-damp damages the Chong and Ren and causes menstruation to cease; qi accumulates and cannot move, and spreads into the skin [becoming pathological qi]; the [pathological] qi and the [still normal] qi struggle, the menstrual blood separates and becomes water, which disperses and causes cutaneous edema; hence the name 'xue fen' (blood separation).

Shui fen (water separation) results from Spleen weakness unable to control water, which accumulates internally and overwhelms the ability of the qi transformation function of the Urinary Bladder to deal with the problem by transforming the excess water into reusable qi. The water spreads out through the surface tissues and disperses, so that edema appears first; however the excess water also has a dispersing effect on the locally gathered menstrual blood, separating it pathologically into water and qi so that the blood cannot flow into the uterine vessels, thus causing amenorrhea.

CLASSICAL TREATMENTS

Any treatment of edema must be based firmly upon precise differentiation of the strength or weakness of both the patient and the pathogen, as well as its location and stage of development, as described above. Simply promoting urination to deal with every case of edema that presents is a sign of immaturity in practice. Using a purge to expel water without careful consideration beforehand, however, is worse.

Zhang Zhong–Jing: diaphoresis and diuresis

In the *Jin Gui Yao Lue*, Zhang Zhong–Jing established the principle of promoting sweating for edema in the upper body, using formulas such as Ma Xing Yi Gan Tang ('Ephedra, Apricot Kernel,

Coicis, and Licorice Decoction', *Formulas and Strategies*, p. 35), Yue Bi Tang ('Maidservant from Yue Decoction', *Formulas and Strategies*, p. 89) and Yue Bi Jia Zhu Tang ('Maidservant from Yue Decoction plus Atractylodes', *Formulas and Strategies*, p. 89). For edema in the lower body, he proposed diuresis, using such formulas as Wu Ling San ('Five-Ingredient Powder with Poria', *Formulas and Strategies*, p. 174) and Fang Ji Fu Ling Tang ('Stephania and Poria Decoction', *Formulas and Strategies*, p. 180).

Zhu Dan-Xi: tonify Spleen and Lung, harmonize Liver

If the pathogen is strong, promotion of sweating or urination will usually be appropriate but if the patient is weak, they must be tonified. Zhu Dan-Xi therefore emphasized the tonification of Spleen to strengthen its ability to transform and transport, and the support of Lung function so that Lungs can ensure open fluid pathways and the subsequent descent of fluids carried upwards to the Lungs from the Spleen. If these two aspects are normal, he pointed out, then fluids will not be able to build up in the Spleen and oppress its activity. He also recommended that if qi is weak and cannot rise, that *Sheng Ma* (Cimicifugae, Rhizoma) be added to help lift the clear yang of the middle Jiao and *Chai Hu* (Bupleuri, Radix) be added to encourage Liver qi to rise, so that it can assist Spleen transport. If Liver qi flow is disrupted, however, and adversely affects the Spleen, then *Huang Qin* (Scutellariae Baicalensis, Radix), *Mai Men Dong* (Ophiopogonis Japonici, Tuber) and *Shan Zhi Zi* (Gardeniae Jasminoidis, Fructus) can be added to control the Liver Wood: Earth qi achieves stability, and will then control Water.

Zhang Jing-Yue: Kidney yang is the basis

As mentioned previously, the basis for all of the qi transformation processes in the body is the yuan qi, which in turn has its root in the Kidneys. Zhang Jing-Yue stressed that although edema must be approached by 'first treating water, [nonetheless] treating water [requires] first treating the qi'. He emphasized that the activity of the yuan qi from the lower Jiao is essential, and recommended Jin

Gui Shen Qi Wan ('Kidney Qi Pill from the Golden Cabinet', *Formulas and Strategies*, p. 275) to restore its normal function.

Specific treatments and formulas

The treatment methods and formulas that follow are those which have been suggested by the medical authors of the last eighteen centuries.

Yang edema. In general, the initial approach in yang edema will be to use Wu Pi Yin ('Five-Peel Decoction', *Formulas and Strategies*, p. 179) to eliminate cutaneous edema, plus Si Mo Tang ('Four Milled-Herb Decoction', *Formulas and Strategies*, p. 301) to promote the descent of Lung qi.

If the condition is still in the early stages, and is the result of exogenous invasion of pathogenic wind, with obvious surface symptoms, then one can select the most appropriate formula from the following:

   Xiao Qing Long Tang ('Minor Bluegreen Dragon Decoction', *Formulas and Strategies*, p. 38)

   Yue Bi Tang ('Maidservant from Yue Decoction', *Formulas and Strategies*, p. 89)

   Fang Ji Huang Qi Tang ('Stephania and Astragalus Decoction' *Formulas and Strategies*, p. 179).

If only the face is swollen with fluid, then one should use Su Zi Jiang Qi Tang ('Perilla Fruit Decoction for Directing the Qi Downward', *Formulas and Strategies*, p. 299).

If exogenous damp is the predominant pathogen, Fang Ji Huang Qi Tang should be combined with Wu Ling San ('Five-Ingredient Powder with Poria', *Formulas and Strategies*, p. 174).

If the edema in the upper body is extreme, one can add several of the following herbs:

Qiang Huo	Notopterygii, Rhizoma et Radix
Zi Su Ye	Perillae Fructescentis, Folium
Fang Feng	Ledebouriellae Sesloidis, Radix
Sheng Ma	Cimicifugae, Rhizoma
Bai Zhi	Angelicae, Radix

Yin edema. The basic approach is to support Spleen transformation and transportation, assist Lung qi descent and warm the Kidney yang. Shi Pi Yin ('Bolster the Spleen Decoction', *Formulas and Strategies*, p. 199) can do all of these things, while re-establishing the pivotal function of the middle Jiao in the ascent and descent of qi through the San Jiao.

If Lung and Spleen qi is deficient, Liu Jun Zi Tang ('Six-Gentlemen Decoction', *Formulas and Strategies*, p. 238) or Bu Zhong Yi Qi Tang ('Tonify the Middle and Augment the Qi Decoction', *Formulas and Strategies*, p. 241) can be used.

If the Spleen qi is oppressed by damp, so that the stool is loose, Shen Ling Bai Zhu San ('Ginseng, Poria and Atractylodes Macrocephala Powder', *Formulas and Strategies*, p. 239) is appropriate.

If bowel movements are difficult (but not dry), with abdominal fullness, one can assist the downward movement of qi with Si Mo Tang ('Four Milled-Herb Decoction', *Formulas and Strategies*, p. 301).

If both the Spleen qi and the Kidney qi are deficient, then Shen Qi Si Jun Zi Tang ('Four Gentlemen Decoction', *Formulas and Strategies*, p. 236), with added *Huang Qi* (Astragali) can be combined with Jin Gui Shen Qi Wan ('Kidney Qi Pill from the Golden Cabinet', *Formulas and Strategies*, p. 275).

If Kidney yang weakness is the primary focus, Zhen Wu Tang ('True Warrior Decoction', *Formulas and Strategies*, p. 197) should be used.

If Kidney yin is too weak to control yang, so that fire surges upward, Liu Wei Di Huang Wan ('Six-Ingredient Pill with Rehmannia', *Formulas and Strategies*, p. 263) plus the following herbs can be used:

Niu Xi	Achyranthis Bidentatae, Radix
Che Qian Zi	Plantaginis, Semen
Mai Men Dong	Ophiopogonis Japonici, Tuber

If the heat is severe, Zi Shen Tong Guan Wan ('Enrich the Kidneys and Open the Gates Pill', *Formulas and Strategies*, p. 268) can be added.

If the edema of the lower body is severe, Wu Ling San ('Five-Ingredient Powder with Poria', *Formulas and Strategies*, p. 174) plus *Cang Zhu* (Atractylodis, Rhizoma) and *Mu Tong* (Mutong, Caulis) should be used.

ACUPUNCTURE TREATMENT OF YIN AND YANG EDEMA

The following point selection is not from ancient texts but still uses the yin edema and yang edema categories—as many modern TCM texts continue to do.

Yang edema

San Jiao Shu	BL-22
Fei Shu	BL-13
Yin Ling Quan	SP-9
Shui Fen	CV-9
He Gu	LI-4
Shang Ju Xu	ST-37

All of the above points should be reduced, both because the disease is acute and because the pathogen is excess (shi). Moxa can be used at Shui Fen (CV-9).

Explanation

San Jiao Shu (BL-22) has the functions of regulating qi flow in the San Jiao channel, and promoting urination. As the Tang Dynasty *Qian Jin Yao Fang* ('Thousand Ducat Formulas', 652AD) records in Chapter 30, it is indicated for 'lower abdominal hardness [and distension] as big as a bowl, fullness and distension of the chest and abdomen, failure of food and fluids to be dispersed, and gynecological masses: moxa together with Qi Hai (CV-6), each 100 cones.'

Fei Shu (BL-13) regulates Lung qi flow, and so can restore descent to Lungs which have been disrupted by pathogenic wind. This point is particularly indicated in edema resulting from exogenous edema, since both the Lungs—which rule the skin—and the Tai Yang channel—which rules the surface—will be the primary focus of pathogenic influence. This point is able to rectify the functioning of both, since it is the back Shu-point for the Lungs and is located on the foot Tai Yang Urinary Bladder channel.

Yin Ling Quan (SP-9) is a major point for fluid problems, as it is the He-sea point on the Spleen channel, and also related to Kidneys through its attribute as a Water point. The *Nei Jing* says: 'Any damp, swelling and fullness, all belong to Spleen'. The *Bai Zheng Fu* ('Song of the Hundred Symptoms') says: 'Yin Ling [Quan] and Shui Fen treat umbilical fullness from edema'; and the *Tong Xuan Zhi Yao Fu* ('Ode of the Essentials for Penetrating the Dark Mystery') says: 'Yin Ling [Quan] can open the water pathways'.

Shui Fen (CV-9), according to the *Zhen Jiu Ju Ying* ('Collection of the Essentials of Acupuncture and Moxibustion', by Gao Wu, 1529) is 'the point at the lower opening of the Small Intestine, at which the murky and turbid are dispersed, fluids enter the Urinary Bladder, and substantial dross enters the Large Intestine, therefore its name is Shui Fen ('Water Separating').[7] Hence its importance in edema treatment can be appreciated.

The function of He Gu (LI-4) in this point prescription is primarily to strengthen the surface clearing effects of Fei Shu (BL-13) but its status as a Yuan-source point gives it further significance: through its connection with the yuan qi of the San Jiao, it can influence the qi transformation processes throughout the body. This, indeed, is the origin of its general tonic abilities, which are enhanced by the Yang Ming channel attributes of having 'ample qi and ample blood'. Furthermore, because of its actions on the head and face, He Gu (LI-4) is an excellent point to reduce the edema of the face and head characteristic of yang edema.

Shang Ju Xu (ST-37) as the lower He-sea point for the Large Intestine, can promote expulsion of excess fluids by this route, thus encouraging Lung qi descent and preventing it from rebelling upward, and also support the action of Shui Fen (CV-9) mentioned above.

Yin edema

Pi Shu	BL-20
Shen Shu	Bl-23
Zu San Li	ST-36
Qi Hai	CV-6
San Yin Jiao	SP-6
Wei Yang	Bl-39
Shui Fen	CV-9

The first three points should be tonified with both needles and moxa; the next two points should be first tonified and then reduced, with moxa permitted at Qi Hai (CV-6); the last two points should be reduced, with reducing moxa at Shui Fen (CV-9) but none at Wei Yang (Bl-39).

Explanation

Pi Shu (BL-20) and Shen Shu (Bl-23) are both located on the Urinary Bladder channel, and so have the ability not only to regulate the functioning of their respective organs, so important for fluid metabolism, but also to promote the functioning of the Urinary Bladder itself. They should be tonified, to improve the 'functional qi' of these organs.

Zu San Li (ST-36) assists Pi Shu (BL-20) to improve Spleen and Stomach function. Also, as it is the Earth point on the yang Earth channel of the feet, its ability to strengthen Earth's control of Water is significant and thus it should be tonified. It is also an essential point for the treatment of abdominal distension but for this it must be reduced (as the pathogenic water and qi obstruction is excess) and then tonified.

Qi Hai (CV-6) can both restore the flow of yuan qi from the Kidneys, and also regulate the lower Jiao qi transformation process to enable Urinary Bladder to separate the clear and murky fluids. It should be first tonified, to restore the flow of Kidney yuan qi necessary for Urinary Bladder qi transformation, and then reduced to expel the murky fluids remaining in the Urinary Bladder after recovery of the clear fluid qi.

San Yin Jiao (SP-6) links the Spleen, Kidney and Liver channels and, through promoting the functioning of the Spleen and the Kidneys, is itself able to promote urination and thus support the action of Pi Shu (BL-20) and Shen Shu (Bl-23). It should be first tonified to restore the qi flow in the Spleen and Kidney channels, and then reduced to ensure that the Liver channel (which intersects itself directly over the Urinary Bladder) has no obstruction which might interfere with lower Jiao fluid metabolism.

Wei Yang (Bl-39), itself a Urinary Bladder channel point, is also the lower He-sea point for the San Jiao, and thus of double importance in the treatment of edema. Its major actions are promoting San Jiao functioning, opening the fluid pathways and assisting Urinary Bladder activity. It should be reduced because both the Urinary Bladder and the San Jiao have become inundated with pathogenic water, which must be drained away. While moxa is not absolutely contraindicated, its proximity to Wei Zhong (UB-40)—which is so contraindicated—suggests caution.

Shui Fen (CV-9)—see above under yang edema.

Treatment of the 'Five Edemas' (wu shui)

Wind-edema (feng shui)

The symptoms of floating pulse, heavy aching body, mild sweating and aversion to wind show that the location of the problem is the surface, and thus promotion of mild sweating can be used to expel the excess pathogen. Formulas such as Fang Ji Huang Qi Tang ('Stephania and Astragalus Decoction', *Formulas and Strategies*, p. 179), Yue Bi Tang ('Maidservant from Yue Decoction', *Formulas and Strategies*, p. 89) and Yue Bi Jia Zhu Tang ('Maidservant from Yue Decoction plus Atractylodes', *Formulas and Strategies*, p. 89) can be selected according to the accompanying symptoms.

Skin-edema (pi shui)

Subcutaneous edema of the limbs, while not due here to an exogenous invasion, is still a surface location; again diaphoresis is indicated, using formulas such as Fang Ji Fu Ling Tang ('Stephania and Poria Decoction', *Formulas and Strategies*, p. 180) or Wu Pi Yin ('Five-Peel Decoction', *Formulas and Strategies*, p. 179).

Righteous-edema (zheng shui)

A deep slow pulse accompanied by dyspnea requires warming of the yang qi in order to restore its normal descent and the ability to transform fluids. Shi Pi Yin ('Bolster the Spleen Decoction', *Formulas and Strategies*, p. 199) can be used to accomplish this.

Stone-edema (shi shui)

Characterized by lower abdominal hardness and distension, stone edema, like righteous edema, is also the result of Kidney yang deficiency allowing water to accumulate in the lower body. It can be treated with either Jin Gui Shen Qi Wan ('Kidney Qi Pill from the Golden Cabinet', *Formulas and Strategies*, p. 275) or Zhen Wu Tang ('True Warrior Decoction', *Formulas and Strategies*, p. 197).

Yellow sweat (huang han)

This can also be categorized as a type of jaundice, and treated with Huang Qi Shao Yao Gui Zhi Ku Jiu Tang ('Astragalus, Peony, Cinnamon and Vinegar Decoction')

Huang Qi	15 g	Astragali, Radix
Bai Shao	9 g	Paeoniae Lactiflora, Radix

Gui Zhi 9 g Cinnamomi Cassiae, Ramulus

Cook in two cups of water and one cup of vinegar, until only one cup remains, and drink.

Qi edema

For qi obstruction from emotional disturbance leading to edema, Liu Jun Zi Tang ('Six-Gentlemen Decoction', *Formulas and Strategies*, p. 238) plus *Mu Xiang* (Saussureae seu Vladimiriae, Radix) and *Mu Tong* (Mutong, Caulis) can be combined with Xiao Yao San ('Rambling Powder', *Formulas and Strategies*, p. 147). If there is abdominal distension and constipation, Liu Mo Tang ('Six Milled-Herb Decoction', *Formulas and Strategies*, p. 302) or Mu Xiang Bing Lang Wan ('Aucklandia and Betel Nut Pill', *Formulas and Strategies*, p. 457) can be used (the latter with caution in weak patients).

Treatment of xue fen (blood separation)

Because, in xue fen, the period stops first and is then followed by edema, the treatment is primarily aimed at regulating menstruation, after which the edema will disperse by itself. Tao Hong Si Wu Tang ('Four-Substance Decoction with Safflower and Peach Pit', *Formulas and Strategies*, p. 250) or Xue Fu Zhu Yu Tang ('Drive Out Stasis in the Mansion of the Blood Decoction', *Formulas and Strategies*, p. 314) can be used if blood stagnation has halted the flow of blood; if cold is the culprit, use Shao Fu Zhu Yu Tang ('Drive Out Blood Stasis in the Lower Abdomen Decoction', *Formulas and Strategies*, p. 316).

Treatment of shui fen (water separation)

Shui fen is just the opposite of the above: the edema appears first and then the menstruation ceases.

Treatment in this case is, therefore, opposite to that of xue fen: the Spleen must be strengthened and the qi transformation of the Urinary Bladder encouraged, so that the pathogenic water is transformed or eliminated, and then the menstruation will revert to its normal flow. The formula of choice in this case is Dao Shui Fu Ling Tang ('Lead the Water Poria Decoction'), a formula introduced to me very early on by my teacher as eliminating fluid retention 'and regulating the endocrine system'. On

that basis I have used it successfully in many gynecological cases, ranging from menopause to PMS: but always involving edema.

Dao Shui Fu Ling Tang ('Lead the Water Poria Decoction')

Fu Ling	12 g	Poriae Cocos, Cortex
Bai Zhu	12 g	Atractylodes Macrocephalae, Rhizoma
Che Qian Zi	12 g	Plantaginis, Semen
Mai Men Dong	12 g	Ophiopogonis Japonici, Tuber
Sang Bai Pi	9 g	Mori Albae Radicis, Cortex
Zi Su Ye	9 g	Perilla Frutescentis, Folium
Mu Gua	9 g	Chaenomelis Lagenariae, Fructus
Sha Ren	3 g	Amomi, Fructus seu Semen
Bing Lang	9 g	Areca Catechu, Semen
Da Fu Pi	12 g	Areca Catechu, Pericarpium
Chen Pi	6 g	Citri Reticulatae, Pericarpium

Source text: *Pu Ji Ben Shi Fang* ('Formulas of Universal Benefit from My Practice') by Xu Shu-Wei, 1132) Chapter 191.

HISTORICAL OVERVIEW OF THE DEVELOPMENT OF EDEMA PATHOLOGY

The Su Wen Chapter 7 says: 'When the [single channel system of the] third yin [i.e. Hand and Foot Tai Yin, Lungs and Spleen] knots [and becomes blocked, the result is] called 'Water' [retention].'

The seventy-fourth Chapter says: 'All damp, swelling, and fullness are related to the Spleen'.

The sixty-first Chapter says: 'The Kidneys are the floodgate of the Stomach; if the floodgate cannot move smoothly, the water will accumulate and gather with its kind'.[8] The first part of Chapter 61 in the *Su Wen* says:

Huang Di asked: Why does Shao Yin control the Kidneys? And why do the Kidneys control Water?

Qi Bo answered: Kidneys are the most yin of the zang organs, and the most yin-natured thing is an abundance of water. Lungs are Tai Yin; [but] Shao Yin is the channel most influenced by Winter [with its quiet, stored, yin nature]. Thus the root [of edema] is in the Kidneys, its branch is in the Lungs; [if these two organs do not function normally], both can cause accumulated water.

The Emperor said: How can the Kidneys accumulate water to cause disease?

Qi Bo answered: The Kidneys are the floodgate of the Stomach; if the floodgate cannot move smoothly, the water will accumulate and gather with its kind. Above and below, flooding out to the skin, and there producing edema (fu zhong). The meaning of edema is accumulation of water to cause disease.[9]

All of the above statements identify the source of fluid retention as difficulties in the functioning of the Lungs, Spleen and Kidneys.

The *Su Wen* also discusses the etiology, pathology, certain symptoms and treatment of edema in Chapter 14:

Huang Di said: There are also [edematous] illnesses which do not originate from [exogenous invasions of] the skin but instead result from the obstruction of the yang qi of the Five Zang organs. Yang qi is unable to transform jin and ye fluids, which then [become pathological and] suffuse the surface tissues, the chest and the abdomen. With the yin predominant internally, the yang is unable to spread and thus is externally insufficient. Pathogenic water then floods, causing edematous swelling around the body and the clothing no longer fits. When edema becomes severe in the limbs, the movement of qi is disrupted inside the body [and pathogenic water rebels upward], causing dyspnea. This is the result of the impediment to the flow of qi inside, which is shown by the swelling outside. How can this be treated?

Qi Bo said: This must be determined by judging the severity and pace of the disease [but the basic goal is to] eliminate the obstructed stagnant water. If the disease is mild, exercise the limbs and wear warmer clothing [to assist the flow of yang qi, then] use the 'cross-needling' method[10] to reduce the swelling and restore the body to its original shape. [In more severe cases] one can also use laxative or diuretic methods to eliminate the pathogenic water, which will free the essential qi to circulate normally around the body, and thus restore the ability of the yang qi of the Five Zang organs to scour away the remaining

pathogenic water internally. Thereafter jing-essence will again be produced, the body will become stronger, the tendons and bones will be maintained in a healthy state and the zheng qi will flourish.

There are several implications of this section which should be mentioned. One is the implied acknowledgment of exogenous factors in the etiology of edema: the section begins with the words: 'There are also [edematous] illnesses which do not originate from [exogenous invasions] of the skin but instead result from the obstruction of the yang qi of the Five Zang organs.' Although there is, in this section, no elaboration of which illnesses do originate 'from the skin', Chapter 61 of the *Su Wen* says: 'Kidney sweat emerges and encounters wind, the pores become obstructed and the fluids cannot return internally to the zang fu organs, nor can they be expelled outward through the surface. Instead the fluids are arrested around the pores, and flood the surface tissues, causing edema. The root of the problem is in the Kidneys, and it is called wind edema (feng shui 风水).' 'Kidney sweat' is the sweat resulting from overexertion or sexual activity injuring the Kidneys. This is a clear indication that although 'wind water' type edema is brought on by exogenous invasion, the root cause of edema remains in the Kidneys.

The other implication requiring mention is that of yang qi obstruction, so that it cannot warm, transform or transport fluids properly around the body, leading to accumulation of these fluids and finally edema. This section, again, does not mention directly how yang qi becomes obstructed. But the context of Chapter 14, which discusses (among other things) how unrestricted eating and drinking, and continual worry, can damage the spirit, suggests that emotional factors are likely to play a large part in this obstruction. If we look at the second section of Chapter 14, which appears before the section quoted above, it says:

In high antiquity the sages prepared decoctions and wines to treat diseases. But at that time people were strong, and such measures were not used very much. In middle antiquity, the virtues in society became somewhat eroded, and people's physiques likewise became weaker; pathogens were then able to occasionally become predominant. At those times [decoctions and wines] could be used to good effect.

Huang Di said: But why are decoctions and wines not always effective nowadays?

Qi Bo answered: The people of the present time require potent medicines to attack internal illnesses, and needles and moxa to treat external illnesses [before they will respond].

Huang Di said: But some are treated for a long time, even until the body, the qi and the blood become exhausted, and yet still do not respond. Why is this?

Qi Bo replied: The shen does not work.[11]

Huang Di said: Why does the shen not work?

Qi Bo said: This is the Dao of needling: to promote the patient's essence and spirit. If the essence and spirit (jing shen) are not enhanced, and the will and intent (zhi yi 志意 yuan zhi de zhi, yisi de yi) not controlled, then illness cannot be cured. In the present era, people's essence is ruined and their spirit is gone, the nutritive and protective qi cannot circulate fully. And why is this? [Because] there is no limit to eating and drinking, and [people] worry ceaselessly. [Thus] essential qi is ruined, nutritive qi leaks out and protective qi is lost, [and the gradual end] result is loss of spirit and failure of the disease to be cured.

A brief section follows describing how an illness proceeds from the surface, and how to deal with such a mild affliction, and then the section quoted above in relation to edema begins: 'There are also [edematous] illnesses which do not originate from [exogenous invasions] of the skin but instead result from the obstruction of the yang qi of the Five Zang organs.' Therefore the role of emotional factors in obstructing the flow of qi around the body and interfering with fluid metabolism, and thus possibly resulting in edema, should be recalled in clinic, as well as the advice that without a settled and balanced consciousness any disease—and not just edema—will be difficult to cure.

So it is apparent, even from these partial selections, that quite an extensive amount of information about edema was available in the *Nei Jing*, ranging from causative factors, pathological mechanisms, symptomatology and treatments, to prognosis and

even psychological considerations in therapy. Most later writings base their discussions of edema pathology on the *Nei Jing*, which is the reason for the relatively detailed review above.

The *Zhong Zang Jing* ('Treasury Classic', attributed to Hua Tuo, probably Six Dynasties Period, 317-618AD) records ten different types of edema but, like the *Nei Jing*, emphasizes the crucial role of the Kidneys in fluid metabolism. In Chapter 43, which is entitled 'Discussion of Edema (shui zhong), Symptoms and Prognosis', it says:

> Of the Hundred Diseases suffered by people, nothing is harder to treat than [pathogenic] water. Water is controlled by the Kidneys; Kidneys are a person's foundation (ben). When the Kidney qi is strong, the water will return to the sea;[12] when the Kidney qi is deficient, the water will spread to the skin. Again, if San Jiao is obstructed, nutritive and protective qi become blocked, qi and blood do not flow properly together, excess and deficiency intermix, water follows the flow of qi and thus results in a water disease.[13]

In the *Jin Gui Yao Lue*, Zhang Zhong-Jing devotes a full chapter to the discussion of edema, listing two sets of edema differentiation, the first being 'feng shui' (wind water), 'shi shui' (stone water), 'pi shui' (skin water), 'zheng shui' (righteous water) and 'huang han' (yellow sweat); the second set being attributed to the Five Zang organs, for example 'Xin shui' (Heart-edema), 'Gan shui' (Liver-edema), 'Pi shui' (Spleen-edema) and so on. Most later authors adopted the first set of differentiations and largely ignored the second.[14]

Zhang described several principles of edema treatment, such as promotion of urination for edema below the waist, and promotion of sweating for edema above the waist, which have also been adopted in later medical writings.

The *Zhu Bing Yuan Hou Lun* ('General Treatise on the Etiology and Symptomatology of Disease', 610AD) by Chao Yuan-Fang describes edema as predominantly a result of combined deficiency of both the Spleen and Kidneys. In the twenty-second Discussion 'Symptoms of Edema' (shui zhong bing) it says:

> Kidneys control Water, Spleen and Stomach both control Earth; the nature of Earth is to conquer

Water. Spleen and Stomach are united, being in exterior-interior relationship with each other. The Stomach is the Sea of Food and Fluids, [but] in this situation Stomach is deficient and unable to transform the qi of water, causing water qi to seep into the channels and collaterals and suffuse the zang fu organs. The Spleen [which hates damp] becomes diseased through the addition of excess water, and a diseased Spleen [Earth] then cannot control Water; thereafter the water qi all descends upon the Kidneys. The San Jiao is unable to drain [itself of the excess water], the channels and vessels (jing mai) become obstructed and thus water qi floods the skin, bringing about swelling. ...

Edema has five [signs which indicate that it is] incurable: the first is blackening of the lips, [which show that] Liver is injured; the second is [swelling of] the supraclavicular region [until it becomes] level, [which shows that] Heart is injured; the third is protrusion of the umbilicus, [which shows that] Spleen is injured; the fourth is swelling of the sole until it is flat, [which shows that] the Kidneys are injured; the fifth is swelling until [the normal curvature of the] back is flat, [which shows that] the Lungs are injured.

A deep pulse indicates water. If the pulse is tidal (hong) and big (da), it can be treated; thready and indistinct is a bad sign (literally 'means death').[15]

The *Qian Jin Yao Fang* ('Thousand Ducat Formulas', Sun Si-Miao, 652AD) describes ten types of edema, five of which are incurable. Sun Si-Miao also describes other factors affecting edema treatment (as well as medical ethics) in Chapter 21, Section 4:

In general water diseases are hard to treat. Once they are cured, one must be especially careful about diet. Those which relapse into edema are usually the people who cannot restrict their taste for food. That is why this disease is difficult to cure. Now, there are doctors who go along with [the patient's] whims of the moment, with their mind on riches, and not based on [maintaining] life. The patient wants to eat meat—[usually those in] rich and beautiful surroundings—[and the doctor] encourages them to eat meat from lamb's head or pig's trotters—I have never seen [even] one cure in this type of situation!

The *Ji Sheng Fang* ('Formulas to Aid the Living', Yan Yong-He, 1253) was the first to make the differentiation into yin edema and yang edema, later to be elaborated by Zhu Dan-Xi, who says in the *Dan Xi Xin Fa* ('Teachings of Dan Xi', Zhu Dan-Xi, 1481): '[In] yang disease, [there is] edema with yang symptoms; [in] yin disease, [there is] edema with yin symptoms. Water pathology is not all the same.' This differentiation into yin and yang edema is followed in the *Qi Xiao Liang Fang* ('Remarkably Effective Fine Formulas', 1470, by Dong Su and Fang Xian), the *Yi Xue Ru Men* ('Introduction to Medicine', 1575, by Li Chan) and the *Yi Bian* ('Fundamentals of Medicine', 1751, by He Meng-Yao). In the *Yi Xue Ru Men*, which is composed of a series of seven character rhyming verses to assist memorization by students, Li Chan says in the elucidation of the first two lines under 'Edema':

'Edema Above and Below: the Subtlety of Yin and Yang'

Yang edema is usually brought on by external factors, [either] wading or getting soaked by rain; or in conjunction with wind-cold or summerheat qi; and yang symptoms will be seen. Yin edema is usually the result of internal factors, [such as] excessive consumption of water, tea or wine; or fasting and overeating, overwork or sexual desire; yin symptoms will be seen.

Yang edema first swells the upper body, the shoulders, back, hands and arms, [i.e.] the three hand yang channels. Yin edema first swells the lower body, the waist, abdomen, shins and ankles, [i.e.] the three foot yin channels. If males begin to swell from the feet up, or females have edema first on the head, this is abnormal [and thus unfavourable]: such is the subtlety of yin and yang.

'Damp-heat Alterations Always Belong to Spleen'

The True Water and True Fire in a person's body transform the ten thousand things in order to nourish life. If the Spleen is diseased, water flows and becomes damp, fire flares and produces heat; over an extended period of time damp and heat obstruct, and the channels and collaterals are completely filled with turbid rotten qi: jin-ye fluids and the blood also transform into [pathogenic] water. ... [17]

The *Yi Zong Bi Du* ('Required Readings from the Masters of Medicine', Li Zhong-Zi, 1637) and the *Jing Yue Quan Shu* ('Complete Works of Jing Yue', 1624) both emphasize the role of deficiency in the development of the illness. In the *Jing Yue Quan Shu*, Zhang Jing-Yue observes:

> In all of the diseases related to edema, the three zang organs Lungs, Spleen and Kidneys are involved. This is because water is the most yin, thus its root is in the Kidneys; water is transformed from qi, thus its branch is in the Lungs; Water only fears Earth, thus its control is in the Spleen. In this situation, if the Lungs are deficient, then qi cannot be transformed into jing-essence and instead transforms into water; if Spleen is deficient, then Earth cannot control Water, which instead rebels upon it; if Kidneys are deficient, then water has no master and moves unrestrainedly. Water not returning into its [normal] channels will then rebel upwards and spread: thus if the fluids exclusively enter the Spleen [i.e. 'rebelling upon it'], the muscles and tissues become swollen; if the fluids exclusively enter the Lungs then rough breathing and dyspnea [result].
>
> When we discuss them separately, the three organs each have [an aspect] of which they are in charge but when we discuss [the problem] as a whole, the damage is wholly from preponderance of yin, and the root of the disease is in the Kidneys.[18]

Classical Essays

The following translation of the section 'Edema' (shui zhong) in the *Yi Xue Xin Wu* ('Medical Revelations', 1732, by Cheng Guo–Peng) is a fine example of the coverage given to edema in medical texts during the early Qing dynasty, and also a source of practical clinical advice.[19]

> The symptom of edema can be differentiated into internal, external, cold, heat, Kidneys, and Stomach. In general, if the four limbs are swollen but the abdomen is not, this is external (biao). If the four limbs are swollen and the abdomen is also swollen, this is internal. [Edema] with insatiable thirst with parched mouth, darkish urine, constipation and a desire for cold food and drink belongs to Yang Ming, and is heat. [Edema] without insatiable thirst, [but] with regular bowel motions and a desire for warm food and drinks, belongs to [the category of] yin edema, and is cold. Dyspnea followed by swelling is accumulated water in the Kidney channel; swelling followed by dyspnea—or only swelling without dyspnea—is water held in the Stomach channel. The Classics say: Kidneys are the floodgate of the Stomach. If the floodgate is closed then water will amass; in the same way, if the Stomach is diseased the floodgate will close by itself. To treat the Stomach, the main formula should be Wu Pi Yin with suitable alterations; to treat the Kidneys, the main formula should be Shen Qi Wan with suitable alterations.
>
> It may be asked: 'The books say, first dyspnea and then swelling, the disease is in the Lungs—how is this?'
>
> The answer: 'Dyspnea, although a Lung disease, has its root in the Kidneys; the saying in the Classics that 'All atrophy, dyspnea and nausea are from below' is both true and to the point here. If an exogenous invasion causes dyspnea, some [cases may] belong exclusively to a pathogen affecting the Lung channel; [but] internal injury bringing on dyspnea will not have one that is not from the Kidneys: therapists be cautious!'

Wu Pi Yin

Wu Pi Yin ('Five-Peel Decoction', *Formulas and Strategies*, p. 179) treats accumulated water in the Stomach channel and is commonly used as a prescription. It is a formula from Hua Tuo's *Zhong Zang Jing* ('Treasury Classic'), used again and again with good results.

Wu Pi Yin ('Five-Peel Decoction')

Da Fu Pi	5 g	Arecae Catechu, Pericarpium (wash in the juice of black soybeans)
Fu Ling Pi	5 g	Poriae Cocos, Cortex
Chen Pi	5 g	Citri Reticulatae, Pericarpium
Sang Bai Pi	5 g	Mori Albae Radicis, Cortex
Sheng Jiang Pi	2.6 g	Zingiberis Officinalis Recens, Cortex

Decoct in water and drink.

[Zhang] Zhong-Jing says: 'Edema above the waist should [be treated by] promotion of sweating'; [thus one should] add *Zi Su Ye* (Perillae Fructescentis, Folium), *Qin Jiao* (Gentianae Macrophyllae, Radix), *Jing Jie* (Schizonepetae Tenuifoliae, Herba et Flos) [and] *Fang Feng* (Ledebouriellae Sesloidis, Radix).

'Edema below the waist should [be treated by] promotion of urination'; [thus one should] add *Chi Xiao Dou* (Phaseoli Calcarati, Semen), *Chi Fu Ling* (Poriae, Cocos Rubrae, Sclerotium), *Ze Xie* (Alismatis Plantago-aquaticae, Rhizoma), *Che Qian Zi* (Plantaginis, Semen), *Bei Xie* (Dioscoreae, Rhizoma) [and] *Fang Ji* (Stephaniae Tetrandrae, Radix).

If there is constipation, one should purge, adding *Da Huang* (Rhei, Rhizoma) [and] *Ting Li Zi* (Tinglizi, Semen).

If there is fullness and distension of the abdomen, add *Lai Fu Zi* (Raphani Sativi, Semen), *Hou Po* (Magnoliae Officinalis, Cortex), *Chen Pi* (Citri Reticulatae, Pericarpium), *Mai Ya* (Hordei Vulgaris Germinantus, Fructus) [and] *Shan Zha* (Crataegi, Fructus).

For deficient patients, add *Bai Zhu* (Atractylodis Macrocephalae, Rhizoma), *Ren Shen* (Ginseng, Radix) [and] *Fu Ling* (Poriae Cocos, Sclerotium).

If examination finds that it is yin edema, add *Fu Zi* (Aconiti Carmichaeli Praeparata, Radix), *Gan Jiang* (Zingiberis Officianalis, Rhizoma) [and] *Rou Gui* (Cinnamomi Cassiae, Cortex).

If examination finds that it is yang shui, add *Lian Qiao* (Forsythiae Suspensae, Fructus), *Huang Bo* (Phellodendri, Cortex) [and] *Huang Qin* (Scutellariae Baicalensis, Radix).

If there is also phlegm, add *Ban Xia* (Pinelliae Ternata, Rhizoma) [and] *Sheng Jiang* (Zingiberis Officinalis Recens, Rhizoma).

Once the edema has receded, then Li Zhong Wan ('Settle the Middle Pill', *Formulas and Strategies*, p. 219) should be used to strengthen the Spleen and Stomach, or use Jin Gui Shen Qi Wan ('Kidney Qi Pill from the Golden Cabinet', *Formulas and Strategies*, p. 275) to warm Mingmen, or Liu Wei Di Huang Wan ('Six-Ingredient Pill with Rehmannia', *Formulas and Strategies*, p. 263) adding *Niu Xi* (Achyranthis Bidentatae, Radix), and *Che Qian Zi* (Plantaginis, Semen) can be used to moisten Kidney Water and cool remaining heat. [In this way one can] expect to achieve a complete effect.

Jin Gui Shen Qi Wan

Jin Gui Shen Qi Wan ('Kidney Qi Pill from the Golden Cabinet', *Formulas and Strategies*, p. 275) treats accumulated water in the Kidney channel, with difficult urination, abdominal distension, swelling of the limbs, and possibly phlegm dyspnea and rough breathing gradually developing into ascites: its effect is almost miraculous.

Now accumulated water in the Kidney channel has a yin category and a yang category, which must be differentiated. The Classics say: 'Yin without yang has nothing to [provide the power] for growth (sheng), yang without yin has nothing to transform.' The Classics also say: 'Urinary Bladder is the official in charge of irrigation, the place where jin and ye fluids are stored, through qi transformation [these fluids] are able to come out.' If the Kidney channel yang is deficient, then yin has nothing for growth, [therefore] in those cases where the True Fire cannot control water, this pill (i.e. Shen Qi Wan) should be used.

If Kidney channel yin is deficient, then yang has nothing to transform, [therefore] in those cases where True Yin cannot be transformed into qi this formula should be used, removing the *Fu Zi* (Aconiti Carmichaeli Praeparata, Radix) and *Rou Gui* (Cinnamomi Cassiae, Cortex).

[Li] Dong-Yuan says: 'Earth in the midst of rain transforms into mud: this is the image of yin edema.'

He–Jian [i.e. Liu Wan-Su] says: 'In the extreme summer heat, all the earth steams and swelters: this is the image of yang edema. Those who know the meaning of this have the ability to treat edema.'

Shou Di	240 g	Rehmanniae Glutinosae Conquitae, Radix
Shan Yao	120 g	Dioscoreae Oppositae, Radix
Shan Zhu Yu	60 g	Corni Officinalis, Fructus
Mu Dan Pi	60 g	Moutan Radicis, Cortex
Ze Xie	60 g	Alismatis Plantago-aquaticae, Rhizoma
Che Qian Zi	60 g	Plantaginis, Semen
Niu Xi	60 g	Achyranthis Bidentatae, Radix
Fu Ling	180 g	Poriae Cocos, Sclerotium
Rou Gui	30 g	Cinnamomi Cassiae, Cortex
Fu Zi	10 g	Aconiti Carmichaeli Praeparata, Radix

Use Wu Jia Pi 240 g (Acanthopanacis Radicis, Cortex) boiled in a large bowl of water and then strained, combine [with all of the above] herbs; add honey and make into small pills. Each morning 12 g [of pills] should be taken with boiled water.

If the previous condition belongs to the category of yin edema, remove the *Rou Gui* (Cinnamomi Cassiae, Cortex) and *Fu Zi* (Aconiti Carmichaeli Praeparata, Radix) from this formula, and add 60 g each of *Ge Ke* (Cyclinae Sinensis, Concha) and *Mu Li* (Ostreae, Concha).

If damp-heat is severe, add 15 g of *Huang Bo* (Phellodendri, Cortex), and substitute 240 g of *Bei Xie* (Dioscoreae, Rhizoma) cooked into syrup instead of using *Wu Jia Pi* (Acanthopanacis Radicis, Cortex).'

Discussion of xue fen and shui fen

When a woman's menses stops first, and then edema appears, this is called xue fen, and the main formula is Tong Jing Wan ('Promote Menses Pill', designed by Cheng Guo Peng himself). If the edema appears first, followed by amenorrhea, this is called shui fen, and should be treated by using Wu Pi Yin ('Five-Peel Decoction', *Formulas and Strategies*, p. 179) to wash down Tong Jing Wan ('Promote Menses Pill').

Tong Jing Wan ('Promote Menses Pill')

Dang Gui Wei	30 g	Angelica Polymorpha, Radix
Chi Shao	30 g	Paeoniae Rubra, Radix
Sheng Di	30 g	Rehmannia Glutinosae, Radix
Chuan Xiong	30 g	Ligustici Wallichii, Radix
Niu Xi	30 g	Achyranthis Bidentatae, Radix
Wu Ling Zhi	30 g	Trogopterori seu pteromi, Excrementum
Hong Hua	15 g	Carthami Tinctorii, Flos
Tao Ren	15 g	Persicae, Semen
Xiang Fu	60 g	Cyperi Rotundi, Rhizoma
Hu Po	22.5 g	Succinum

Use 60 g of *Su Mu* (Sappan, Lignum) shavings, and cook with the above herbs in wine, add granulated sugar, then gradually decoct [until thick and suitable to] make small pills. The dose is 9g [of pills], taken with wine. If the patient is weak, use Li Zhong Tang ('Regulate the Middle Decoction', *Formulas and Strategies*, p. 219) to wash the pills down. If the blood is cold, add 15 g of *Rou Gui* (Cinnamomi Cassiae, Cortex) to the formula.[20]

Du Yi Sui Bi ('Random Notes while Reading Medicine' 1898) 'On Promotion of Urination'

Everyone knows the damage to the qi from diarrhea (da bian hua li) but they do not realize that the damage that excessive urination can cause is even worse. They know that frequent urination can injure yin but do not know that using herbs like *Zhu Ling* (Polypori Umbellati, Sclerotium), *Fu Ling* (Poriae Cocos, Sclerotium), *Ze Xie* (Alismatis Plantago-aquaticae, Rhizoma) and *Mu Tong* (Mutong, Caulis) to force urination with patients whose urination, even with these herbs, refuses to pass, will be even more injurious to the yang than it is to the yin. These days, doctors misled by talk about how the ancients used diuresis as a shortcut in the treatment of disease [21]—never mind what type of disease—they blithely use *Zhu Ling* (Polypori Umbellati, Sclerotium), *Fu Ling* (Poriae Cocos, Sclerotium) and *Ze Xie* (Alismatis Plantago-aquaticae, Rhizoma), and more often than not the True Qi (zhen qi) collapses downward, the pathogenic qi sinks into the interior and [the disease] becomes a tangled knot they cannot unravel. They really do not understand what the ancients meant when they said that 'the free and open qi transformation of the San Jiao is from free passage of the urine, which is called 'internal harmony'.' [What they meant was that] the clear passage of the urine was the indication of internal harmony. Later generations should look for the methods of bringing about internal harmony, not just promote the passage of urine.

Now the Urinary Bladder is joined with Ming Men, and is the first portal for the emission of Ming Men's yuan qi. The *Nei Jing* says that San Jiao and Urinary Bladder correspond to the hairs of the skin (hao mao) and the surface tissues (cou li), [which means that] the yuan qi travels through the Urinary Bladder to suffuse the San Jiao and reach the skin and surface tissues. Thus my contemporaries' draining of the Urinary Bladder is directly draining the root of the yuan qi emission! This is why, if promotion of urination would not be used with yin deficient patients, even more should it not be used with yang deficient patients.

Qian Zhong-Yang[22] said: 'For mild fevers relieve toxins, for high fevers promote urination'. Li Dong-Yuan said: 'When the Lungs suffer from pathogenic heat, the source of the jin and ye fluid's qi transformation is cut off. Then the flow of cold water is interrupted, the Urinary Bladder suffers damp-heat and becomes bound with urinary obstruction so that the urine does not flow freely: one should use *Mu Tong* (Mutong, Caulis) to treat this.' Zhu Er-Yun[23] said: 'When the urine passes freely, then the pathogenic fire in any of the channels will all pass downward through the urine'. [But] this fire which is pent up internally [has two types]: there are those for whom promoting the passage of stool is appropriate, when the heat has combined with the dross in the Intestines and Stomach, and is in the murky passageway (i.e. the bowels), not the clear passageway (i.e. the urinary tract); there are those for whom the promotion of urination is appropriate, when the pathogenic heat has infiltrated the blood vessels (xue mai) of the San Jiao, and the clear passageway is arrested by the murky heat. [In this case one] should use yin nourishing herbs, such as *Sheng Di* (Rehmannia Glutinosae, Radix) and *Tian Hua Fen* (Trichosanthis, Radix), to restore the jin and ye fluids, making the pathogenic heat float and drift out of the blood vessels within the fluids, and then use diuretic herbs so that both the fluids and the heat are taken downwards together. Thus the urine passes freely, yin is produced, and the fire recedes.

There is also [the situation in which] pathogenic heat and murky turbidity knot up both [the stool and the urine], for which Zhang Zi-He designed Yu Zhu San ('Jade Candle Powder', *Formulas and Strategies*, p. 250), and Tao Jie-An[24] had Qing Long Tang ('Bluegreen Dragon Decoction'), both of which formulas combined Si Wu [Tang] ('Four-Substances Decoction', *Formulas and Strategies*, p. 248) and the Cheng Qi [Tang]s ('Order the Qi Decoctions', *Formulas and Strategies*, pp. 115-117). Hu Zong-Xian (c. 1780), again, said to first nourish the yin and move the blood, to make the toxin not adhere in the Liver, after which a Cheng Qi [Tang] ('Order the Qi Decoction') can be used to purge: this also uses first one treatment method and then another. Thus for internal accumulation of water, one should promote urination; but when fire is pent up inside, one can also consider promoting urination.

[Zhang] Zhong-Jing's method of treating shang han [syndrome with] accumulated water, using Wu Ling San ('Five-Ingredient Powder with Poria', *Formulas and Strategies*, p. 174) with increased intake of warm water: [with this approach] how could the accumulated water be too scanty to use diuresis? In fact this syndrome has not only accumulated water, but also accumulated heat; the water and heat each occupy the area. *Ze Xie* (Alismatis Plantago-aquaticae, Rhizoma), *Fu Ling* (Poriae Cocos, Sclerotium) and the warm water being taken in together will cause both of the pathogens to be expelled simultaneously, not causing [an imbalance whereby] the water is expelled [but] the heat increased. Furthermore, if at this time the surface pathogen [which gave rise to the syndrome in the first place] has not been completely cleared, the *Gui Zhi* (Cinnamomi Cassiae, Ramulus) in the formula will both free up the Urinary Bladder ability to transform qi, and will also clear the surface pathogen and regulate [the flow of nutritive and protective qi through the surface tissues]. Pathogenic water cannot produce sweat; the essence of the [imbibed] warm water must be borrowed to generate sweat: where could there be a technique as subtle as this? Using one formula and one method to resolve two internal pathogens and one external pathogen, where could there be a technique as rapid as this?

The methods of the ancients in promoting urination cannot all be listed but in general either nourishing yin or regulating qi movement will be used before diuretic herbs are tried: the sudden free flow of urine, just when the situation is crucial, truly verifies [the efficacy of] this approach!

Nowadays people do not seek the reason for encouraging a free flow of urine but vaguely use it for any type of illness; nor do they look for the [appropriate] method of promoting urination but simply select *Ze Xie* (Alismatis Plantago-aquaticae, Rhizoma) or *Fu Ling* (Poriae Cocos, Sclerotium) and just use these all the time. [If they do this] with an exogenous pathogen present, then the pathogenic qi sinks into the interior; with internal injury, then the True Yang drains away below; there is also the saying that [inappropriate diuresis] will destroy the Heart[25]. Promotion of urination causes the qi on the surface to suddenly sink and the rising qi to be concealed: because of this, the manifestations of the illness will temporarily recede: [these doctors] point to this as an improvement in the condition, thus misleading the patient, and then immediately deny any further responsibility, dumping the disaster onto the next doctor.

Everyone knows that incorrect use of *Ma Huang* (Ephedrae, Herba) and *Gui Zhi* (Cinnamomi Cassiae, Ramulus) will cause collapse through sweating, and that incorrect use of *Mang Xiao* (Mirabilitum) and *Da Huang* (Rhei, Rhizoma) will cause collapse through purging, but no one knows that mistaken use of *Ze Xie* (Alismatis Plantago-aquaticae, Rhizoma) and *Fu Ling* (Poriae Cocos, Sclerotium) will cause collapse through diuresis. Even when diuretic herbs do not cause a perceptible increase in urination, the yuan qi—which is insubstantial—can still be lost.'[26]

NOTES

1. New students of TCM in the West may need to be reminded that, in Chinese medicine, 'cold' is not simply 'the absence of heat' but actively asserts its cooling, contracting nature. This is why there is a separate category of herbs and formulas that warm internal cold, rather than just formulas and herbs that tonify yang.

2. New students, again, may also have difficulty here, thinking 'Wait a minute, I thought frequent urination was a sign of Kidney yang deficiency. How could the same thing now suddenly cause scanty urine?' The answer is that when Kidney yang deficiency leads to frequent urination, the Kidney-Urinary Bladder functions both of transforming fluids, and of storing

('gu' to consolidate) fluids are impaired. In the present situation, Kidney consolidation is normal but Urinary Bladder is unable to transform, and then expel, fluids, which accumulate internally (see also Chapter 4).

3. *Zhong Zang Jing Wu Yi*, 'Vernacular Translation of the Treasury Classic', 1990, Beijing, People's Health Publishing, p. 83.

4. Zhang Jing-Yue continues: 'But these cases would not respond well to warm tonification: here one should [use purging to] expel the damp-heat, and the effect will be quick. One can use formulas like Yu Gong San ('Legendary Yu's Effective Powder') and Jun Chuan San ('Dredge the River Powder').

Yu Gong San ('Legendary Yu's Effective Powder')

Hei Qian Niu Zi	Pharbitidis, Semen: black morning glory seeds
Xiao Hui Xiang	Foeniculi Vulgaris, Fructus

Xia Yu was the legendary hero who first controlled flood waters and established irrigation, and thus promoted the development of agriculture in China.

Jun Chuan San ('Dredge the River Powder')

Da Huang	Rhei, Rhizoma
Qian Niu Zi	Pharbitidis, Semen
Yu Li Ren	Pruni, Semen
Mang Xiao	Mirabilitum
Gan Sui	Euphorbiae Kansui, Radix
Mu Xiang	Saussureae seu Vladimiriae, Radix.

Jing Yue Quan Shu ('Complete Works of Jing Yue', 1624), Shanghai Science and Technology Press, 1959, p. 398).

5. The name 'zheng shui' is difficult to translate: even the New World Press English translation of the *Jin Gui Yao Lue* prefers to leave it as 'zheng-edema', while translating all of the other Five Edema names. Most of the modern and relatively shallow introductions to the *Jin Gui* in Chinese say that 'The symptoms of zheng edema are the principal (zheng) signs of edematous disease', which is clearly off the mark. My own opinion—unsubstantiated (so far as I can find) by Classical reference—is that zheng edema refers to zheng qi weakness allowing pathogenic water to accumulate. My reasoning is as follows: zheng edema involves all of the organs most related to the production and proper functioning of the zheng qi: the Kidneys, Spleen and Lungs; the depth of the pathology is neither as shallow as the surface, nor as deep as stone edema, as zheng edema is centered in the middle Jiao; and the description of 'zheng shui' comes immediately after the descriptions of the yang edemas, and is the first of the yin edemas, preceding stone edema, which is deep in the lower Jiao and involves only the Kidneys. Therefore my translation as 'righteous' as in 'righteous qi'.

6. See the discussion on shen and edema in the Su Wen, in the history section later in this chapter.

7. *Zhen Jiu Ju Ying* ('Collection of the Essentials of Acupuncture and Moxibustion', Gao Wu, 1529), Shanghai Science and Technology Press, 1961, p. 128. (See also note 30 in Chapter 1).

8. 'Shen zhe, Wei zhi guan ye, guan men bu li, gu ju shui er cong qi lei ye.' 肾者，胃之关也，关门不利，故聚水而从其类也. When fluids are taken into the body, they first pass the Stomach. After passing through the various organs and transformations in the metabolism of fluids, they are finally processed in the Urinary Bladder, under the control of the Kidney yang. Thus the Stomach can be likened to the upper gate of a lock in a waterway and the Kidneys to the lower gate. If the upper gate continues to take in water when the lower gate is not opening in concert with it, the level of water in the lock will rise and flood. At a slightly deeper level of meaning, the passage should remind us that all of the qi transformations in the process of fluid metabolism have their basic motive power in the Kidney yang. As far as the meaning of 'gather with its kind' is concerned, Wang Bing explains: 'If the floodgate is closed, water will accumulate; accumulation of water will stop the [flow of] qi; stopped qi will cause [further] production of [pathogenic] water, which will cause increased qi [obstruction, and so on]. Qi and water are similar in kind, thus the statement: if the floodgate cannot move smoothly, water will accumulate and gather with its kind'.

In my own naive opinion, 'gather with its kind' (or 'conform' with its 'type'): er cong qi lei 而从其类 more likely means that water, which is yin, tends to reduce its movement, which is yang, thus becoming quiet and static and thus 'conform with yin-nature'. The end result is the same: stagnant water.

9. This too has several layers of meaning. Zhang Yin-An, in his *Huang Di Nei Jing Su Wen Ji Zhu* ('Collected Annotations to the *Huang Di Nei Jing Su Wen*'), has an interesting gloss to the first part of this passage, after 'both can cause accumulated water':

This refers to water being produced from the midst of earth, and then [some] rising to the heavens above, while [the rest] returns to its spring. The qi of heaven and the qi of water are in communication above and below. Therefore, on the earth is water, while in the heavens is cold. Now the heavens are yang, and the earth is yin. A spring is under the earth, and thus it is the most yin, with an abundance of water. Abundance means a plenitude of content.

The Lungs control the Heavens [because of their place as the uppermost yin organ, and through their direct contact during breathing with the qi of heaven], and the qi of Tai Yin controls damp earth [because Tai Yin is also Spleen]. Earthly qi rises to the heavens and produces clouds.

Heavenly qi falls and becomes water. Thus water falls from heaven, and clouds are produced from earth, and so it says: Lungs are Tai Yin, referring to the mutual connection between the qi of heaven and earth.

Shao Yin controls water, and is the agent of Winter; its channel [i.e. the Kidney channel] passes through the diaphragm and enters into the midst of the Lungs. Thus its root is in the Kidneys, while its branch is in the Lungs: above and below, all accumulate water.

Zhao Huang [a previous commentator on the *Su Wen*] says: 'The Lungs rule the qi but their generative source is in the Kidneys. Thus qi is produced from below, and water also rises from below. [In the normal course of things] if it descends, it becomes urine; if it rises, it becomes sweat; [but pathologically] if it halts and gathers then floods outward to the skin, it becomes edema.' Zhang Yin-An, *Huang Di Nei Jing Su Wen Ji Zhu* ('Collected Annotations to the *Huang Di Nei Jing Su Wen*') Chapter 61, Shanghai Science and Technology Press, 1959, p. 220.

One of the interesting things about this gloss is the clear picture it gives of the TCM concept of the interior of the body as 'a small cosmos'. The Lungs cover the other organs like the heavens, within which (although not mentioned here) moves the Heart like the sun; in the middle is the Spleen earth, moist and damp; within which again is water springing up from the water organ: the Kidneys. Just as water falls, evaporates and rises in a meteorological cycle, within the body a similar process is described, the qi of water rising from a damp earth to form clouds in the heavens of the upper Jiao or falling from heaven as rain, just as the Lungs move fluids downward in the body, to return beneath the earth, where they will either well up again as a clear spring or be carried away by the murky river of the urine.

Many Western commentators seem unable to control their tendency to view this scenario as quaint proof of the simple-mindedness of the ancient Chinese (a tendency scathingly described at length in Edward Said's *Orientalism* in relation to the European view of Arab culture). But such superciliousness has a price: it prevents them from realising that this view of the body's process is useful as an effective *shorthand analogy* of the physiological functioning of the fluid metabolism within the body.

Western physiology is undeniably accurate, aiming at precise descriptions down to the microscopic and sub-microscopic levels of how each cell and its components function in the body, but this very precision results in a complexity which is often overwhelming in a clinical situation: the effect which one drug will have on an *individual* patient—as opposed to a statistical generality—is difficult to predict; the combined effect of two or more drugs becomes almost impossible.

Chinese medicine, though, without denying the accuracy and place of Western physiology in medical science, is based squarely in clinic. The theoretical structure of Chinese medicine, such as the scenario described above, is a simplified description of the body's processes, a shorthand which can be kept in the mind of the practitioner, and which helps not only to explain how the fluids (in this case) move but also both to predict the likely outcome of a fluid pathology and to chose an effective treatment. The underlying practicality of the approach is evident from the fact that the ancient Chinese medical authors carry this description just as far as it is useful as an analogy and stop there, without elaborating into an ever more fantastic internal cosmology.

On the other hand, I have found that it is Western students of Chinese medicine who tend to get carried away with 'fantastic' elaborations of Chinese medical theory, and must be repeatedly reminded that such descriptions are not 'true' but rather intended as a clinical tool, with practical applications and limitations. Chinese medicine has many such tools, each designed for a particular use, and unwieldy or inappropriate for other uses. For example, the yin-organ theory (zang xiang) is useful for describing disruptions of internal functioning but less effective for predicting the progress of an exogenous invasion. Again, in the exogenous invasion sphere, there are two tools: the Shang Han six-channel theory and the combined wei-qi-ying-xue and San Jiao theories of the febrile disease school: both are extremely detailed accounts of the processes and treatments of exogenous diseases but one is designed for pathogenic cold, the other for pathogenic heat. 'Scholars' who delight in pointing out the 'inconsistencies' of the various theories of traditional Chinese medicine show about as much understanding as the man who accused the carpenter of being 'inconsistent' when he used a screwdriver for one job, then suddenly picked up a hammer for another!

10. 'miu ci' 繆刺, a technique to which the whole of Chapter 63 in the *Su Wen* is devoted, involves needling the left for disease on the right, and vice versa.

11. Zhang Jing-Yue, in the *Lei Jing* ('Systematic Categorization of the *Nei Jing*', 1624), explains:

The Dao of treatment is thus: attacking the pathogen is accomplished through needles and herbs, [but] the herbs [and needles] act through the shen qi (spirit). Therefore if a treatment is to act on the root, then the shen must move within it, causing that which should ascend to ascend, and that which should descend to fall: these are the workings of the spirit. If herbal prescriptions are used to treat the inside, but the qi of the zang-organs does not respond, or needles are used to treat the outside, but the qi in the channels does not respond, this shows that the shen qi has departed, and cannot perform its work. One can exhaust all of one's strength—and that of the patient—in treatment, but the end result will be only exhaustion. This is what is meant by 'the shen does not work'.

12. See the scenario discussed in note 9 above.
13. *Zhong Zang Jing Wu Yi*, 'Vernacular Translation of the Treasury Classic', 1990, Beijing, People's Health Publishing, p. 83.
14. Although the theory did not play a major historical role in later TCM, I offer a brief outline. 'Xin shui' (Heart water) results from insufficiency of Heart yang, so that cold constricts fluid movement, causing it to gather and disturb the Heart, leading to symptoms of swelling and sensations of heaviness; shortness of breath as water accumulates in the chest; inability to lie down because pathogenic water will rise and further limit the breathing; irritability and restlessness as the predominant yin prevents the free flow of yang, which, becoming pent-up, intensifies into pathogenic heat which disturbs the shen; and swelling of the genitals due to Heart Yang failing to warm the Kidneys, and thus yang is unable to transform the water that sinks into the lower Jiao.

'Gan shui' (Liver water) results from obstruction to the movement of Liver qi, so that qi and blood become blocked, the Liver collaterals become full and blood transforms into pathogenic water, leading to symptoms of abdominal distension with inability to turn freely side-to-side due to the obstruction of the Liver—and therefore Gall Bladder—channels; pain in the subcostal and abdominal regions from the same blockage; variation in the amount of salivary fluid produced because, when Liver qi is blocked, fluid metabolism is unable to carry fluids upward to the mouth, but when the blockage becomes extreme, qi rebels upward and carries pathogenic fluid with it so that saliva becomes temporarily excessive; and urination will be affected in the same way for the same reason: obstruction to the qi flow will occasionally prevent fluids from entering the Urinary Bladder (which is directly below the intersection of the bilateral branches of the Liver channel), while at other times the supply will be unaffected and so urine will be normal. (See the case history in note 23 of Chapter 4 for an interesting variation of this.)

'Fei shui' (Lung water) results from Lung qi failure to spread, contract and descend, and thus inability to ensure the normal downward movement of the fluid pathways, so that the body swells (especially the upper body); the urine becomes difficult because fluids do not enter the Urinary Bladder but instead pour into the counterpart of the Lungs, the Large Intestine, and the stool becomes frequent and loose 'like that of a duck'. Many commentators mention that this last symptom is a distinctive sign of edema from Lung pathology.

'Pi shui' (Spleen water) occurs when Spleen transport fails and pathogenic damp gathers internally, affects the Spleen, and pours out to flood the tissues, so that the limbs ache from lack of nourishment and excessive edema; the abdomen swells; there is lack of energy and the mouth becomes dry because most food and fluids are not transformed by the oppressed Spleen yang, and the already transformed fluid that is available cannot be carried upward to the mouth due to this oppression; and the urine becomes difficult as water simply gathers internally.

'Shen shui' (Kidney water) results from failure of Kidney yang qi transformation in the lower Jiao, so that urine ceases and the abdomen and the umbilicus swell; the local excess fluid seeps out in the groin causing continual wetness 'like the sweat on the nose of cattle'; the lower back hurts due to lack of nourishment from the weak Kidneys; the feet become cold as the sinking water obstructs the flow of already weak Kidney yang through its channels; and because jing-essence and blood cannot be carried upward due to the weakness of yang, 'the face alone becomes thin' ('alone' because the rest of the body is swollen).

When this section of the *Jin Gui Yao Lue* ('Essentials from the Golden Cabinet') is analyzed, it can be seen that although each of the Five Zang organs has its characteristic symptom patterns, the Liver, Spleen and Kidneys form one group and the Lungs and Heart form another. The Liver, Spleen and Kidneys are yin zang organs, located in the abdomen, with their pathology centered in the lower and interior parts of the body, and all share symptoms of abdominal swelling, distension and fullness. Heart and Lungs, on the other hand, are yang zang organs, located in the chest, with their center of pathological activity in the upper body and surface. Thus Heart and Lungs water will have swelling and heaviness of the body, irritability and inability to lie down, but the original text does not mention abdominal enlargement.

Thus later medical authors—such as Xu Zhong-Ke in the *Jin Gui Yao Lue Lun Zhu* ('Annotated Discussion of the Golden Cabinet', 1671)—felt that the edema described under the Liver, Spleen and Kidneys was merely an elaboration of the two categories 'zheng shui' (righteous water) and 'shi shui' (stone water); while that of the Heart and the Lungs could be subsumed under the category of 'pi shui' (skin water). This argument is supported by the fact that no specific treatment is provided for any zang water category. This conclusion by the commentators on the *Jin Gui Yao Lue* is the reason why the theory of the Five Zang edema played a lesser role in later TCM development of edema pathology.

15. *Zhu Bing Yuan Hou Lun Jiao Shi* ('Annotated Explanation of the General Treatise on the Etiology and Symptomatology of Disease', 610AD) by Chao Yuan-Fang, annotated by the Nanjing TCM College, published by People's Health Publishing, 1982, pp. 635-636.

16. *Qian Jin Yao Fang* ('Thousand Ducat Formulas', Sun Si-Miao, 652), Beijing, 1982, People's Health Publishing, p. 382.
17. *Yi Xue Ru Men* ('Introduction to Medicine', 1575, Li Chan), Jiangxi Science and Technology Press, 1988, pp. 799-800.
18. *Jing Yue Quan Shu* ('Collected Treatises of Zhang Jing-Yue'), 1624, Shanghai Science and Technology Press, 1959, pp. 397-398.
19. My teacher in internal medicine at the Zhejiang TCM College, Prof. Wu Song-Kang, highly recommended the *Yi Xue Xin Wu* for TCM interns. Cheng Guo-Peng's outstanding contribution to TCM development was his clarification of the eight treatment methods used in the *Shang Han Lun*: diaphoresis, emesis purging, harmonization, warming, cooling, tonifying and dispersal; a scheme of treatment categorization which is still used in modern TCM education. He was also very active in promoting medical education in his time, emphasizing the importance of practical experience as well as theoretical study.
20. *Yi Xue Xin Wu* ('Medical Revelations'), 1732, Cheng Guo-Peng'; People's Health Publishing, Beijing, 1982, pp. 143-144.
21. Zhou Xue-Hai is probably referring to the passage in the *Jing Yue Quan Shu* where Zhang Jing–Yue says:

   The ancient methods of treating fluid retention almost never employed tonification, but instead usually used water expelling herbs: in mild cases [herbs would be used to promote Urinary Bladder] separation and diuresis, while in severe cases [herbs that would] drive out [excessive water through the intestines]. For example, formulas such as Wu Ling San ('Five-Ingredient Powder with Poria', *Formulas and Strategies*, p. 174), Wu Lin San ('Five-Ingredient Powder for Painful Urinary Dysfunction', *Formulas and Strategies*, p. 194), Wu Pi San ('Five-Peel Powder', *Formulas and Strategies*, p. 179) or Dao Shui Fu Ling Tang ('Lead Water Decoction with Poria') would be used for diuresis; while formulas like Zhou Che Wan ('Vessel and Vehicle Pill', *Formulas and Strategies*, p. 129), Jun Chuan San ('Dredge the River Powder'), Yu Gong San ('Legendary Yu's Effective Powder') (see note 4 in this chapter for constituents of the last two formulas) and Shi Zao Tang ('Ten-Jujube Decoction', *Formulas and Strategies*, p. 128) are all [examples of] water expelling.'(*Jing Yue Quan Shu*, Shanghai Science and Technology Press, 1959, pp. 398-399.)

   Zhang Jing-Yue quickly follows this up, though, by noting that these methods can only be contemplated in conditions of excess:

   otherwise one must be very cautious. Nowadays these 'witch doctors' only know this type of treatment, and thus [their patients] take a dose in the evening and by morning [the flow of urine is] opened, or they use [the herbs] in the morning and by evening they evacuate a cupful of fluid; the edema is immediately reduced, the effect is indeed rapid. But they do not consider the deficiency or excess of people, nor care about their life or death: as soon as they see an effect, they ask for thanks and go. They do not know that following the relief, the edema returns, and that after a few days it will be worse than ever (*ibid.*, p. 399).

22. Proper name Qian Yi, 1035-1117, a very famous pediatrician, author of *Xiao Er Yao Zheng Zhi Jue* ('Craft of Medicinal Treatment for Childhood Disease Patterns'), 1119.
23. Although extensive checking failed to confirm this, Zhou Xue-Hai is probably referring to Zhu Gong, the Song dynasty author of the *Nan Yang Huo Ren Shu* ('The Nan Yang Book to Safeguard Life', 1108). This book was so named because Zhu Gong was a widely read commentator on the *Shang Han Lun*, which Hua Tuo referred to as 'The Book to Safeguard Life' (Huo Ren Shu), and because the author of the *Shang Han Lun*, Zhang Zhong-Jing, was from the area of Nan Yang).
24. A prolific medical author in the Shang Han tradition, *c.* 1445.
25. See the section on the relationship between fluids and the shen in Chapter 1.
26 *Du Yi Sui Bi* ('Random Notes while Reading Medicine'), 1898, by Zhou Xue-Hai, Jiangsu Science and Technology Press, 1983, pp.185-187.

Thin mucus syndromes

6

INTRODUCTION

Thin mucus conditions are the earliest recorded instances of thickened fluid pathology in traditional Chinese medicine. While they are mentioned in the *Nei Jing*, for example in Chapter 74 and again in Chapter 69, their first complete description appears in the *Jin Gui Yao Lue* ('Essentials of the Golden Cabinet'), Chapter 12, by Zhang Zhong-Jing, written about 210AD.[1]

Despite their antiquity, the Classical descriptions of thin mucus syndromes remain highly useful frameworks for the diagnosis and treatment of certain symptom patterns in conditions such as asthma, cough, palpitations, epigastric discomfort, edema, borborygmus and diarrhea.

PATHOLOGY

There are two common features in all thin mucus pathology. The first is that all etiological mechanisms in thin mucus involve the slowing of fluid transformation and transportation. The second feature is that the focus of pathology in thin mucus syndromes centers on three zang organs: the Lungs, the Spleen and the Kidneys. Thus thin mucus can result from Lung inability to regulate the descent of body fluids, from Spleen failure to distribute and transform or from Kidney incapacity to support the Urinary Bladder's assimilation of fluids. The primary mechanisms are weakness of Spleen and Kidney yang qi: Spleen yang must be able to both transform fluids taken into the body and also distribute the resulting essential fluid qi; if it cannot, thin mucus can accumulate in the middle Jiao and even be carried up to the Lungs. This is summed up in the *Su Wen*, Chapter 21, where it says:

> When fluids enter the Stomach, its warming steaming action lifts the essential qi of these fluids up to the Spleen. The Spleen then transports this qi up to the Lungs, where regulation of the fluid pathways is initiated [through the Lung's clearing and rhythmic descent]: fluids are transported downward to the Urinary Bladder, and the essential qi [of the fluids] is spread outward in the four directions, reaching the skin and pouring into the channels of the Five Zang organs. This is in accord with [the nature of] the four seasons and the yin yang of the five organs, and is part of the normal activity of the channels and vessels (jing mai).

Kidney yang must be able to support the Spleen in the middle Jiao and also sustain lower Jiao qi transformation of fluids in the Urinary Bladder. If it is unable to do so the Spleen yang will become further weakened in the middle, while in the lower body edema can result from fluids which are untransformed and unable to be either reclaimed or excreted. Because of the crucial role of the yang qi in both fluid metabolism and in thin mucus pathology, the general treatment method outlined in the *Jin Gui Yao Lue* for these conditions is 'Those with phlegm and thin mucus should be harmonized with warming herbs'.

The San Jiao is another important component in thin mucus pathology. In the *Sheng Ji Zong Lu* ('Comprehensive Recording of the Sages' Benefits', compiled *circa* 1117AD by the Song Emperor's new Tai Yi Medical College) the functioning of the San Jiao is well described:

The San Jiao is the pathway of the fluids and food, and the location for all qi transformation. If the San Jiao is regulated in its course, then the vessels of the qi (qi mai) will be calm and even, and able to smoothly move the water and fluids into the channels so that they can be transformed into blood and irrigate the whole body. If the San Jiao qi is obstructed, the pathways of the vessels will be blocked, and then the water and fluids will stop, gather and be unable to move. [They will then] accumulate into phlegm and thin mucus.

If we look at the functioning of the zang organs in the context of the San Jiao, then the organization of the fluid metabolism, and thus the formation of thin mucus, becomes clearer. The Lungs reside in the upper Jiao and through the inspiration of qi can move and ensure the openness and regularity of the fluid propulsion, and so are called 'the uppermost source of water'. The Spleen rules the middle Jiao, transforming and then transporting the qi essence of fluids, and acting as the axis, with the Stomach, for the ascent and descent of yin and yang. The Kidneys occupy the lower Jiao, steaming and transforming fluids which have arrived in the lower body in order to separate the clear re-useable fluids from the murky unredeemable fluids which then are excreted. The interconnection of these organs lies in the San Jiao: the lifting of fluid essence from the Spleen, the descending activity of the Lungs, the re-deployment of recovered fluids from the Kidneys, all occur along the fluid pathway of the San Jiao. Likewise, obstruction at any point can lead to thin mucus.

Categories of thin mucus syndromes

History

In the *Jin Gui Yao Lue* ('Essentials of the Golden Cabinet', 210AD) four types of thin mucus syndrome are described: tan yin (痰饮 'phlegm and thin mucus', which Maciocia calls 'Phlegm-fluids in the Stomach and Intestines').[2], xuan yin (悬饮 'suspended thin mucus', which Maciocia calls 'Phlegm-fluids in the hypochondrium'), yi yin (溢饮 'flooding thin mucus', which Maciocia calls 'Phlegm-fluids in the limbs') and zhi yin (支饮 'prodding thin mucus', which Maciocia calls 'Phlegm-fluids above the diaphragm').

This categorization is based upon the locations of the focus of the pathology within the body, each causing different symptoms.

There are also two other types of thin mucus, included in the *Jin Gui Yao Lue* section discussing thin mucus. These are really descriptions of the above four types which have become chronic and aggravated, sinking deep within the body. These are liu yin (留饮 'lingering thin mucus') and fu yin (伏饮 'lurking thin mucus'). These are not separate categories but rather examples of thin mucus pathologies which have progressed to a later stage.

In the Tang dynasty *Qian Jin Yi Fang* ('Supplement to the Thousand Ducat Formulas', 682AD) Sun Si-Miao has five classes of thin mucus: liu yin (留饮 'lingering thin mucus'), pi yin (澼饮 'gurgling thin mucus'), dan yin (淡饮 'bland thin mucus'), liu yin (流饮 'flowing thin mucus') and yi yin (溢饮 'flooding thin mucus'). He does not include zhi yin ('prodding thin mucus') and xuan yin ('suspended thin mucus'). In Sun Si–Miao's scheme, the locations are: tan (or dan) yin is pathogenic thin mucus in the Stomach, liu yin ('flowing thin mucus') is located in the Intestines and pi yin ('gurgling thin mucus') is the pathogen in the subcostal area, which is the same as the *Jin Gui Yao Lue*'s xuan yin ('suspended thin mucus').

The *Zhu Bing Yuan Hou Lun* ('General Treatise on the Symptomatology and Etiology of Disease', 610 AD, written by Chao Yuan-Fang) contains the original four types of thin mucus listed in the *Jin Gui Yao Lue*, plus three more: liu yin ('lingering thin mucus') which is pathogenic thin mucus lodged in the chest and diaphragm, liu yin ('flowing thin mucus') which is pathogenic thin mucus in the Stomach and Intestines (Chao puts tan yin's location in the chest) and pi yin (癖饮 'occluded thin mucus') which is thin mucus accumulated bilaterally in the ribs and forming nodes.

From the Tang dynasty to the present, almost all medical authors have categorized thin mucus syndromes according to the original descriptions in the *Jin Gui Yao Lue*. In modern textbooks of TCM, the descriptions are slightly different: thin mucus syndromes are described according to their locations rather than by name, as set out in Maciocia's *Foundations of Chinese Medicine*, for example, 'Phlegm-fluids in the Stomach and Intestines' (equivalent to tan yin); 'Phlegm-fluids in the hypochondrium' (equivalent to xuan yin); 'Phlegm-fluids in the limbs' (equivalent to yi yin); and 'Phlegm-fluids above the diaphragm' (equivalent to zhi yin). This is clear and easy to understand and is still based on Zhang Zhong-Jing's original layout, so this will be the method used in the discussion below.

Types of thin mucus syndrome and treatment[3]

Thin mucus in the Stomach and Intestines

This is called tan-yin (痰饮 'phlegm and thin mucus'). The cause is weakness of Spleen and Kidney yang unable to transform fluids, so that they remain in the Stomach and Intestines. However, treatments will differ according to the relative degree of weakness of the physiological functioning and the strength of the pathogen.

The *Jin Gui Yao Lue* gives this definition: 'The patient was hefty but is now thin, with the sound of water sloshing in the Intestines; this is called tan yin'. Beyond these few symptoms however, one will often find sensations of fullness in the chest and flanks, palpitations and shortness of breath, nausea and vomiting of frothy fluid, light-headedness and

vertigo, dry mouth without desire to drink, scanty urine, white tongue coat and a wiry pulse.

The patient becomes thin due to the lack of normal nourishment from the essence of food and fluids, which have not been properly transformed and transported throughout the body. The borborygmus results from untransformed fluids moving in the Intestines. Water and fluids rushing upwards in an uncontrolled manner lead to palpitations and shortness of breath, and the white tongue coat and wiry pulse are signs of internal cold, resulting from the yang deficiency.

The treatment of tan yin will be either warming of transportation or the purging of Intestinal water. The *Jin Gui Yao Lue* says: 'When the epigastric region has tan yin, with a sensation of fullness in the chest and flanks, and vertigo, the main formula will be Ling Gui Zhu Gan Tang'. This formula stimulates the middle Jiao yang qi to transform and transport water and fluids, promote urination, and give the now transformed thin mucus a route out of the body. If the Kidney qi is weak and unable to steam and transform fluids, the treatment should be Ji Sheng Shen Qi Wan, to warm the Kidneys and promote fluid movement.

Formulas

Ling Gui Zhu Gan Tang ('Poria, Cinnamon Twig, Atractylodes Macrocephalae and Licorice Decoction')

Fu Ling	Poriae Cocos, Sclerotium
Gui Zhi	Cinnamomi Cassiae, Ramulus
Bai Zhu	Atractylodis Macrocephalae, Rhizoma
Gan Cao	Glycyrrhizae Uralensis, Radix

Source text: *Shang Han Lun* ('Discussion of Cold-induced Disorders') [*Formulas and Strategies*, p. 443]

Ji Sheng Shen Qi Wan ('Kidney Qi Pill from *Formulas that Aid the Living*')

Shou Di	Rehmanniae Glutinosae Conquitae, Radix
Shan Yao	Dioscoreae Oppositae, Radix
Shan Zhu Yu	Corni Officinalis, Fructus
Mu Dan Pi	Moutan Radicis, Cortex
Fu Ling	Poriae Cocos, Sclerotium

Ze Xie	Alismatis Plantago-aquaticae, Rhizoma
Fu Zi	Aconiti Carmichaeli Praeparata, Radix)
Rou Gui	Cinnamomi Cassiae, Cortex)
Che Qian Zi	Plantaginis, Semen
Chuan Niu Xi	Cyathulae, Radix

Source text: *Ji Sheng Fang* ('Formulas that Aid the Living', 1253) [*Formulas and Strategies*, p. 278]

In excess conditions, where the strength of the pathogenic water exceeds the degree of weakness of the zang organ functioning, the treatment will be expulsion of pathogenic water. The *Jin Gui Yao Lue* says: 'If the patient's pulse is hidden (extremely deep), with an urge to move the bowels, after which movement they feel better but still have a feeling of hard fullness in the epigastric region, this is liu yin ('lingering thin mucus') wanting expulsion. The main formula should be Gan Sui Ban Xia Tang ('Euphorbia and Pinellia Decoction').'

Formula

Gan Sui Ban Xia Tang ('Euphorbia and Pinellia Decoction')

Gan Sui	Euphorbiae Kansui, Radix
Ban Xia	Pinelliae Ternata, Rhizoma
Bai Shao	Paeoniae Lactiflora, Radix
Zhi Gan Cao	Glycyrrhizae Uralensis, Radix.'

Source text: *Jin Gui Yao Lue* ('Essentials from the Golden Cabinet', *c*. 210 AD)

These lines are an example of the use of fluid expulsion in thin mucus syndrome. The 'hidden pulse' shows that the thin mucus has accumulated deep within the body so that the yang qi is unable to circulate. The 'hard fullness in the epigastric region' results from the gathering of the pathogen into an excess (shi) knot. In this type of situation, the usual warming and promoting movement approach will not be sufficient and so the pathogenic water must be expelled. Gan Sui Ban Xia Tang can both expel the water and also nourish normal fluids, to eliminate the pathogen while protecting the body.

If the thin mucus has obstructed the Intestines and caused constipation, Ji Jiao Li Huang Wan ('Stephania, Zanthoxylum, Descurainia, and Rhubarb Pill') plus *Mang Xiao* (Mirabilitum) can be used to soften the accumulated hardness in the

Intestines and flush out the pathogenic water. This is another example of a purging expulsion.

Formula

Ji Jiao Li Huang Wan ('Stephania, Zanthoxylum, Descurainia, and Rhubarb Pill')

Han Fang Ji	Stephaniae Tetrandrae, Radix
Chuan Jiao	Zanthoxyli Bungeani, Fructus
Ting Li Zi	Tinglizi, Semen
Da Huang	Rhei, Rhizoma

Source text: *Jin Gui Yao Lue* ('Essentials from the Golden Cabinet', *c*. 210 AD) [*Formulas and Strategies*, p. 130]

Treatment for associated symptoms of thin mucus in the Stomach and Intestines. When tan yin leads to vertigo, palpitations, nausea and vomiting, this indicates water and thin mucus rushing upwards affecting the Heart, with turbid yin obstructing the normal ascent of clear yang. The treatment should be Xiao Ban Xia Jia Fu Ling Tang ('Minor Pinellia Decoction with Poria').

Xiao Ban Xia Jia Fu Ling Tang ('Minor Pinellia Decoction with Poria')

Ban Xia	Pinelliae Ternata, Rhizoma
Sheng Jiang	Zingiberis Officinalis Recens, Rhizoma
Fu Ling	Poriae Cocos, Sclerotium

Source text: *Jin Gui Yao Lue* ('Essentials from the Golden Cabinet', *c*. 210 AD)

This will harmonize the Stomach and settle rebelling qi.

If there is thin mucus in the Stomach and Intestines causing abdominal fullness, with blockage of the qi of these two fu organs and consequent constipation, Hou Po Da Huang Tang ('Magnolia and Rhubarb Decoction') should be used to open the fu organ blockage and expel the thin mucus.

Hou Po Da Huang Tang ('Magnolia and Rhubarb Decoction')

Hou Po	15 g	Magnoliae Officinalis, Cortex
Da Huang	18 g	Rhei, Rhizoma
Zhi Shi	9 g	Citri seu Ponciri Immaturis, Fructus

Source text: *Jin Gui Yao Lue* ('Essentials from the Golden Cabinet', *c*. 210 AD)

Professor Wu (upon whose lectures this discussion is based) described one of his cases which had thin mucus in the Stomach and Intestines, saying:

I once treated a patient with tan yin that was exacerbated by emotions. The patient was completely normal until stressed, after which the abdomen would become distended, followed by borborygmus, scanty urine, stuffy chest, poor appetite, white tongue coat and wiry pulse. I tried Wu Ling San ('Five-Ingredient Powder with Poria', *Formulas and Strategies*, p. 174), then Wu Pi Yin ('Five-Peel Decoction', *Formulas and Strategies*, p. 179), but without success. However, with deeper thought as to the cause of the problem, I realized that the emotional stress was damaging the Liver and blocking Liver qi assistance to normal Spleen transport and digestion, thus leading to the build up of pathogenic fluids. So I used Dao Shui Fu Ling Tang ('Lead the Water Poria Decoction') and Si Ni San ('Frigid Extremities Powder', *Formulas and Strategies*, p. 145) to open the Liver qi flow so that vigorous Spleen transport could be restored. After several doses, the urine increased and the abdominal distention disappeared. I ordered the patient to take Xiang Sha Liu Jun Zi Wan ('Six-Gentlemen Pill with Aucklandia and Amomum', *Formulas and Strategies*, p. 238) for an extended period of time, in order to strengthen the Spleen and regulate the qi. Follow-up showed no recurrence.

Dao Shui Fu Ling Tang ('Lead the Water Poria Decoction')

Fu Ling	12 g	Poriae Cocos, Sclerotium
Bai Zhu	12 g	Atractylodis Macrocephalae, Rhizoma
Sha Ren	6 g	Amomi, Fructus et Semen
Chen Pi	9 g	Citri Reticulatae, Pericarpium
Zi Su Ye	9 g	Perillae Fructescentis, Folium
Sang Bai Pi	9 g	Mori Albae Radicis, Cortex
Che Qian Zi	12 g	Plantaginis, Semen
Mai Men Dong	9 g	Ophiopogonis Japonici, Tuber
Bing Lang	9 g	Arecae Catechu, Semen
Da Fu Pi	12 g	Arecae Catechu, Pericarpium
Mu Gua	9 g	Chaenomelis Lagenariae, Fructus

Source text: *Pu Ji Ben Shi Fang* ('Formulas of Universal Benefit from My Practice', by Xu Shu-Wei, 1132), Chapter 191.

(Note: In the original text, equal weights were used of each herb, *Ze Xie* (Alismatis Plantago-aquaticae, Rhizoma) and *Zhu Ling* (Polypori Umbellati, Sclerotium) were added, and the *Mai Men Dong* (Ophiopogonis Japonici, Tuber) was not included. The above formula contains the constituents and weights which Professor Wu commonly used.

Si Ni San ('Frigid Extremities Powder')

Chai Hu	Bupleuri, Radix
Zhi Shi	Citri seu Ponciri Immaturis, Fructus
Bai Shao	Paeoniae Lactiflora, Radix
Zhi Gan Cao	Honey-fried Glycyrrhizae Uralensis, Radix

Source text: *Shang Han Lun* ('Discussion of Cold-induced Disorders') [*Formulas and Strategies*, p. 145]

Thin mucus in the hypochondrium

This is called xuan yin ('suspended thin mucus') because the thin mucus is not distributed around the body but instead gathers in the chest and costal regions as if suspended. The *Jin Gui Yao Lue* says: 'After drinking, the fluids flow under the ribs, coughing and expectoration bring on pain: this is called xuan yin'. The main symptoms are pulling pain in the chest and flanks worsened by coughing or turning the trunk, so that sometimes the patient will only be able to recline on one side; shortness of breath and rough breathing, white tongue coat and deep wiry pulse. When thin mucus accumulates in the chest and flanks, the flow of qi is obstructed, and this leads to pain, limits the ability to turn the body, and also causes the wiry pulse. Fluids rushing up to the Lungs cause cough and shortness of breath, and thin mucus in the interior causes the pulse to be deep.[4]

The treatment of thin mucus in the hypochondrium has remained the same from Zhang Zhong-Jing's time up to the present: all physicians have used expulsion of water and thin mucus with Shi Zao Tang ('Ten-Jujube Decoction', *Formulas and Strategies*, p. 128). Because it contains *Gan Sui* (Euphorbiae Kansui, Radix), *Yuan Hua* (Daphnes Genkwa, Flos) and *Da Ji* (Euphorbiae seu Knoxiae, Radix) together, it has a very strong and rapid action. It should be taken, initially in small doses, in the morning on an empty stomach. Professor Wu emphasized that when this is used in clinic there are several factors to note: the first is that there should be no pathogen remaining on the surface, because a purge such as this can drag the pathogen into the interior of the body. The *Shang Han Lun* points out: 'A purge can only be used if the surface has already been released [from the pathogen] ... a hard fullness in the epigastric area, a pulling pain in the lower ribs, dry retching, shortness of breath, sweating but no aversion to cold: this means that the surface has been released but the interior is not harmonized. The main formula is Shi Zao Tang.' This is essential to remember when contemplating the use of this approach.

The second factor to note is the constitution of the patient. If the patient is still strong and the pathogen has not yet sunk too deeply within the body, the use of Shi Zao Tang will often be quickly effective. If there is not an obvious effect with the first dose, the patient should not continue to take it but rather wait several days and then try again. This waiting will not only improve the effect but will also prevent damage to the zheng qi. If the patient is rather weak but definitely requires this purging expulsion of the pathogen, then tonification should be employed together with the purge in order to both eliminate the pathogen and also harmonize the normal qi within the body.

The third factor is careful observation of the patient after using this type of purge. Clinically, 2.4-3 g of Shi Zao Wan ('Ten-Jujube Pill')—which is actually stronger than the decoction from the same herbs—will achieve a purging effect; in some patients, though, it can lead to severe and continual diarrhea. So the patient's relatives must be told that if this occurs, cold rice porridge will be effective in stopping it.

Formula

Shi Zao Tang ('Ten-Jujube Decoction')

Gan Sui	Euphorbiae Kansui, Radix
Yuan Hua	Daphnes Genkwa, Flos
Da Ji	Euphorbiae seu Knoxiae, Radix

Source text: *Shang Han Lun* ('Discussion of Cold-induced Disorders') [*Formulas and Strategies*, p. 128]

Professor Wu outlined three types of thin mucus in the hypochondrium (xuan yin) which

he encountered in clinic, often with the Western bio-medical diagnosis of pleurisy with pleural effusion:

Pent-up-heat in the Lungs. This is treated with Sang Bai Pi Tang ('Morus Root Decoction')

Sang Bai Pi	Mori Albae Radicis, Cortex
Huang Qin	Scutellariae Baicalensis, Radix
Huang Lian	Coptidis, Rhizoma
Xing Ren	Pruni Armeniacae, Semen
Chuan Bei Mu	Fritillariae Cirrhosae, Bulbus
Shan Zhi Zi	Gardeniae Jasminoidis, Fructus
Zi Su Zi	Perillae Fructescentis, Fructus
Ban Xia	Pinelliae Ternata, Rhizoma
Sheng Jiang	Zingiberis Officinalis Recens, Rhizoma

Each herb 2.4 g.

Source text: *Gu Jin Yi Tong* ('Unification of Medicine Past and Present', 1556)

to which he would add

| Bai Bu | Stemonae, Radix and |
| Bai Guo | Ginkgo Bilobae, Semen |

The patient would also take 1.5 g of Shi Zao Wan ('Ten-Jujube Pill') in order to cool heat, clear the Lungs and expel pathogenic water.

Qi obstruction and excess phlegm. This is treated with Dao Tan Tang ('Guide Out the Phlegm Decoction') to promote qi flow and transform phlegm, while also using 3g of Kong Xian Dan ('Control Mucus Special Pill', *Formulas and Strategies*, p. 129). He noted that while his standard treatment for xuan yin is based upon the formula Shi Zao Wan ('Ten-Jujube Pill'), if phlegm is found with the thin mucus he will switch to Kong Xian Dan, which instead of *Yuan Hua* (Daphnes Genkwa, Flos) has *Bai Jie Zi* (Sinapsis Albae, Semen), and thus will not only expel pathogenic thin mucus but also break up cold-phlegm.

Formulas

Dao Tan Tang ('Guide Out Phlegm Decoction')

Ju Hong	Citri Erythrocarpae, Pericarpium
Ban Xia	Pinelliae Ternata, Rhizoma
Fu Ling	Poriae Cocos, Sclerotium
Gan Cao	Glycyrrhizae Uralensis, Radix

| Zhi Shi | Citri seu Ponciri Immaturis, Fructus |
| Dan Nan Xing | Arisaemae cum Felle Bovis, Pulvis |

Source text: *Ji Sheng Fang* ('Formulas to Aid the Living', 1253) [*Formulas and Strategies*, p. 448]

Kong Xian Dan ('Control Mucus Special Pill')

Gan Sui	Euphorbiae Kansui, Radix
Da Ji	Euphorbiae seu Knoxiae, Radix
Bai Jie Zi	Sinapsis Albae, Semen

Source text: *San Yin Ji Yi Bing Zheng Fang Lun* ('Discussion of Illnesses, Patterns, and Formulas Related to the Unification of the Three Etiologies', 1174), [*Formulas and Strategies*, p. 129]

Chest pain from knotted qi is treated with Xuan Fu Hua Tang ('Inula Flower Decoction')

Xuan Fu Hua	9 g	Inulae, Flos
Cong Bai	14 stalks	Allii Fistulosi, Herba
Qian Cao Gen	9 g	Rubiae Cordifoliae, Radix (as a substitute for Xin Jiang)

Source text: *Jin Gui Yao Lue* ('Essentials from the Golden Cabinet' *c.* 210 AD)

to which he would add *Xiang Fu* (Cyperi Rotundi, Rhizoma) and *Wa Leng Zi* (Arcae, Concha) to promote qi flow and stop pain, while using this decoction to wash down Shi Zao Wan ('Ten-Jujube Pill').

Thin mucus in the limbs

This is called yi yin ('flooding thin mucus') because the fluids spill over into the four limbs and cause edema. The *Jin Gui Yao Lue* says: 'Those with yi yin should be treated by bringing on a sweat, with the main formulas being Da Qing Long Tang ('Major Bluegreen Dragon Decoction', *Formulas and Strategies*, p.34) and Xiao Qing Long Tang ('Minor Bluegreen Dragon Decoction', *Formulas and Strategies*, p. 38).' But no symptoms are mentioned in the *Jin Gui*, only the treatment methods. According to later authors, the main symptoms of thin mucus in the limbs (yi yin) are chills, no sweating, edema in the limbs, generalized aching, lethargy, lack of thirst, profuse white frothy phlegm and possible dyspnea, white tongue coat and a floating wiry or tight pulse. The condition originates from disorder of the Lungs and Spleen

distributive functioning, so that fluids are retained in the superficial tissues (i.e. between the skin and flesh) of the limbs and cause edema. Obstruction of the flow of qi through these tissues leads to generalized aching and chills with lack of sweating from the interruption of protective qi flow. Because of the location of the pathogenic fluids in the superficial tissues of the limbs, warm transformation or purging will not touch them at all, because these methods act on the interior of the body. The only approach which will work is to use warm diaphoretics to bring on sweating, which will expel the pathogen by the shortest route: through the skin.

In some cases, particularly in strong patients, heat will build up internally either from normal exertion or from the struggle of the protective qi and the pathogen. But with the pathogenic fluids obstructing the surface tissues this heat will be unable to escape through the surface, so that restless irritability and fever will result. In these cases Da Qing Long Tang ('Major Bluegreen Dragon Decoction') is the formula of choice, to open the surface while cooling internal heat.

In other cases, especially in weak or cold patients, the surface obstruction by pathogenic fluids will be complicated by the presence of internal xu-cold, and thus treatment requires not only surface opening but also internal warming to remove the cold, using Xiao Qing Long Tang ('Minor Bluegreen Dragon Decoction'), which will accomplish this goal while also regulating Lung function.[5]

Both of the above formulas are diaphoretic but each has a different emphasis; both use *Ma Huang* (Ephedrae, Herba) and *Gui Zhi* (Cinnamomi Cassiae, Ramulus) together to bring on sweating but the herbs to treat the interior are completely different. Da Qing Long Tang ('Major Bluegreen Dragon Decoction') uses *Shi Gao* (Gypsum)'s pungent nature to assist the opening of the surface but employs its coldness to cool the heat beneath the surface. Xiao Qing Long Tang ('Minor Bluegreen Dragon Decoction') uses the pungent heat of *Xi Xin* (Asari cum Radice, Herba) and *Gan Jiang* (Zingiberis Officinalis, Rhizoma) to warm the interior and disperse pathogenic cold.

Thin mucus in the limbs is similar to the condition known as 'wind-water' (feng shui 风水), in that both are pathogenic fluids in the surface tissues. The difference is that yi yin is localized to the limbs, while in wind-water the edema is generalized, including not only the limbs but also the trunk and the face.

Formulas

Da Qing Long Tang ('Major Bluegreen Dragon Decoction')

Ma Huang	Ephedrae, Herba
Xing Ren	Pruni Armeniacae, Semen
Gui Zhi	Cinnamomi Cassiae, Ramulus
Zhi Gan Cao	Glycyrrhizae Uralensis, Radix
Shi Gao	Gypsum
Sheng Jiang	Zingiberis Officinalis Recens, Rhizoma
Da Zao	Zizyphi Jujubae, Fructus

Source text: *Shang Han Lun* ('Discussion of Cold-induced Disorders') [*Formulas and Strategies*, p. 34]

Xiao Qing Long Tang ('Minor Bluegreen Dragon Decoction')

Ma Huang	Ephedrae, Herba
Gui Zhi	Cinnamomi Cassiae, Ramulus
Gan Jiang	Zingiberis Officianalis, Rhizoma
Xi Xin	Asari cum Radice, Herba
Wu Wei Zi	Schisandrae Chinensis, Fructus
Bai Shao	Paeoniae Lactiflora, Radix
Ban Xia	Pinelliae Ternata, Rhizoma
Zhi Gan Cao	Honey-fried Glycyrrhizae Uralensis, Radix

Source text: *Shang Han Lun* ('Discussion of Cold-induced Disorders'), [*Formulas and Strategies*, p. 38]

Thin mucus above the diaphragm

This is called zhi yin ('prodding thin mucus') because the pathogen is propped, as it were, like a stanchion above the diaphragm, pushing up into the chest against the Lungs. In the *Jin Gui Yao Lue*, the main symptoms of zhi yin are described: 'Cough and rebelling qi, with the patient leaning upon something to breath, dyspnea upon reclining so that the patient cannot continue to lie flat. The face appears swollen. This is called zhi yin.' This is a remarkably accurate description of some of the manifestations of severe asthma, even to the observation of the patient's need to use the accessory muscles of the chest to help the breathing: 'leaning upon something to breath'.

Professor Wu was the student of Dr. Ye Xi-Chun, a 'famous old Chinese doctor' (ming lao zhong yi) in the region of central China. Dr. Ye explained that the symptoms mentioned in the above passage would not necessarily all appear in the early phase of thin mucus above the diaphragm but covered the range of symptoms to be found at all stages of the disease. In the early phase, the strength of the pathogen is the primary characteristic of the condition. At this time the symptoms will be cough, Lung qi rebelling upward, chills, profuse white thick phlegm, white tongue coat and a wiry pulse. All of these symptoms result from the pathogenic thin mucus thrusting upward and interfering with the Lungs' contraction and descent.

If however the thin mucus above the diaphragm is not eliminated and the illness continues for an extended period of time, the condition will change, progressively weakening the yang of the Lungs, Spleen and Kidneys. The symptoms will also worsen: cough, dyspnea to the extent that the patient cannot lie flat, chills, profuse white thick phlegm, aching of both the upper and lower back, and eventually edema of the face, eyes or limbs. The tongue coat will be white, the pulse will be wiry and thready, or wiry and tight. Once this stage is reached, the situation is that of a weak constitution fighting a strong pathogen, and the emphasis in treatment will have to be on the weak constitution. Thus the approach is different from that in the first phase of the illness.

Dr. Ye's treatment of thin mucus above the diaphragm was based on the general principle of 'harmonizing with warm herbs'. He would determine the strength or weakness of the patient's yang qi and the depth of the pathogen, before deciding on treatment. In the early stages of zhi yin, the strength of the pathogen is the main concern and so treatment must focus on opening the surface, warming the interior and transforming the thin mucus. The basic formula is Xiao Qing Long Tang ('Minor Bluegreen Dragon Decoction', see above), with changes in the use of the three constituents *Gan Jiang* (Zingiberis, dried ginger), *Xi Xin* (Asari cum Radice, Herba) and *Wu Wei Zi* (Schisandrae Chinensis, Fructus) depending upon the nature of the illness.

Dr. Ye felt that if the cough and dyspnea were severe, *Wu Wei Zi* (Schisandrae) could be increased to assist Lungs' contraction, while the *Gan Jiang* (Zingiberis) and *Xi Xin* (Asari) should be reduced to lessen the dispersing effect of their pungency, which would exacerbate Lung qi's difficulty to constrict and descend.

If the phlegm was difficult to cough out, Dr. Ye would remove the *Bai Shao* (Paeoniae Lactiflora, Radix) in the formula and decrease the amount of *Wu Wei Zi* (Schisandrae), so that phlegm would not be improperly held in by the sour-contraction of these two herbs.

He also insisted that at any stage of the zhi yin syndrome, the treatment could not do without the three herbs *Gui Zhi* (Cinnamomi Cassiae, Ramulus), *Ban Xia* (Pinelliae Ternata, Rhizoma) and *Fu Ling* (Poriae Cocos, Sclerotium), and so he would always add the latter herb to Xiao Qing Long Tang ('Minor Bluegreen Dragon Decoction') in order to strengthen the Spleen and increase urination to provide a route out of the body for the thin mucus dispersed through the warm transformation of *Gui Zhi* (Cinnamomi) and *Ban Xia* (Pinelliae). *Ban Xia* also brings down rebelling qi and thus stops the cough resulting from Lung qi descent unable to resist the upward push of the pathogenic fluids. For these reasons, all three are also important herbs in the treatment of thin mucus.

If the thin mucus has accumulated in the body for a long time and produced heat, the symptoms will be cough, Lung qi rebelling upward, phlegm beginning to turn yellow and a wiry rapid pulse. In this situation, Xiao Qing Long Tang ('Minor Bluegreen Dragon Decoction') should have *Shi Gao* (Gypsum) added, both to cool the internal heat and to control the still necessary pungent-warmth of *Ma Huang* (Ephedrae) and *Gui Zhi* (Cinnamomi Cassiae, Ramulus).

If the zhi yin problem is complicated by an exogenous wind attack, the symptoms will be chills, cough, dyspnea, audible wheeze in the throat and floating pulse. Here the treatment requires She Gan Ma Huang Tang ('Belamcanda and Ephedra Decoction') to disperse cold and ventilate the Lungs while bringing down rebelling qi and transforming phlegm.

Formulas

Da Qing Long Tang ('Major Bluegreen Dragon Decoction') [*Formulas and Strategies*, p. 34] *(See above)*

Xiao Qing Long Tang ('Minor Bluegreen Dragon Decoction') [*Formulas and Strategies*, p. 38] *(See above)*

She Gan Ma Huang Tang ('Belamcanda and Ephedra Decoction')

She Gan	Belamcandae Chinensis, Rhizoma
Ma Huang	Ephedrae, Herba
Zi Wan	Asteris Tatarici, Radix
Kuan Dong Hua	Tussilagi Farfarae, Flos
Ban Xia	Pinelliae Ternata, Rhizoma
Xi Xin	Asari cum Radice, Herba
Wu Wei Zi	Schisandrae Chinensis, Fructus
Sheng Jiang	Zingiberis Officinalis Recens, Rhizoma
Da Zao	Zizyphi Jujubae, Fructus

Source text: *Jin Gui Yao Lue* ('Essentials from the Golden Cabinet', *c.* 210 AD) [*Formulas and Strategies*, p. 39]

Xiao Qing Long Tang ('Minor Bluegreen Dragon Decoction') is the standard formula for thin mucus above the diaphragm. But that does not mean that it can be used in every case. If the zhi yin has continued for years without relief, the yang of the Lungs, Spleen and Kidneys will become weak. The symptoms of this will then be cough, dyspnea to the extent that the patient cannot lie flat, white thick phlegm, chills, aching of the lower and upper back, and edema most noticeable in the face and lower limbs. The tongue coat will be white and the pulse thready and wiry or tight. These symptoms show that cold thin mucus is internally predominant, with a weak yang qi. If *Ma Huang* (Ephedrae) were to be used at this time, it could well prove too pungent and dispersing, and result in severe damage to the already weakened yang qi by allowing it to leak away through surface tissues opened by the diaphoretic action of the *Ma Huang*. Therefore the appropriate formula is Gui Ling Wu Wei Gan Cao Tang ('Cinnamon Twig, Poria, Schizandra, and Licorice Decoction').

Formula

Gui Ling Wu Wei Gan Cao Tang ('Cinnamon Twig, Poria, Schizandra, and Licorice Decoction')

Gui Zhi	Cinnamomi Cassiae, Ramulus
Fu Ling	Poriae Cocos, Sclerotium
Wu Wei Zi	Schisandrae Chinensis, Fructus
Gan Cao	Glycyrrhizae Uralensis, Radix

Source text: *Jin Gui Yao Lue* ('Essentials from the Golden Cabinet', *c.* 210 AD) [*Formulas and Strategies*, p. 445]

In the *Jin Gui Yao Lue*, this formula was originally used as the main remedy for qi rushing upward excessively after using Xiao Qing Long Tang ('Minor Bluegreen Dragon Decoction') in treatment. Gui Ling Wu Wei Gan Cao Tang can warm yang, transform thin mucus, constrict the qi and settle dyspnea. With the addition of *Ban Xia* (Pinelliae) and *Xi Xin* (Asari), the formula's effect of transforming thin mucus is somewhat improved.

Having to lean on something or sit up in order to breath is caused by the water and thin mucus prodding upward into the Lungs. When one sits up the water and thin mucus sink down and so the dyspnea and cough are lessened. The *Jin Gui Yao Lue* says: 'Thin mucus above the diaphragm, unable to breath; the main formula is Ting Li Da Zao Xie Fei Tang ('Descurainia and Jujube Decoction to Drain the Lungs').

Formula

Ting Li Da Zao Xie Fei Tang ('Descurainia and Jujube Decoction to Drain the Lungs')

| Ting Li Zi | Tinglizi, Semen |
| Da Zao | Zizyphi Jujubae, Fructus |

Source text: *Jin Gui Yao Lue* ('Essentials from the Golden Cabinet', c. 210 AD) [*Formulas and Strategies*, p. 91]

Ting Li Zi is bitter, cold and descending, acting to drain a pathogen in the Lungs and promoting movement of pathogenic water. If *Zi Su Zi* (Perillae Fructescentis, Fructus) is added to the formula, the effect is improved.

The edema that appears with zhi yin is most often seen in the face and the lower limbs. This results from Spleen and Kidney yang deficiency, so that fluid transformation suffers, pathogenic fluids accumulate and fail to be expeditiously removed from the body, and thus urine is always reduced. The treatment principle must be to open the flow of yang and promote urination. This is accomplished, while still using Xiao Qing Long Tang ('Minor Bluegreen Dragon Decoction') or Gui Ling Wu Wei Gan Cao Tang ('Cinnamon Twig, Poria, Schizandra, and Licorice Decoction'), by increasing the amount of *Gui Zhi* (Cinnamomi Cassiae, Ramulus) to the formula, and also adding herbs such as *Zhu Ling* (Polypori Umbellati, Sclerotium), *Ze Xie* (Alismatis Plantago-aquaticae, Rhizoma), and *Che Qian Zi* (Plantaginis, Semen).

If the Kidney yang has become extremely weak through protracted struggle with the zhi yin pathogen, the symptoms will be cough and dyspnea with inability to lie flat, chills, greyish black tinge to the face, spontaneous lacrimation with cold tears, edema and scanty urine. The tongue coat will be white and the pulse deep, thready and wiry, with noticeable weakness at the chi (proximal) position. The treatment should be to warm the Kidneys to grasp qi, open the flow of yang and transform the thin mucus, using Ji Sheng Shen Qi Wan ('Kidney Qi Pill form Formulas that Aid the Living') but removing the *Mu Dan Pi* (Moutan Radicis, Cortex) and adding *Hu Lu Ba* (Trigonellae Foeni-graeci, Semen), *Ba Ji Tian* (Morindae Officinalis, Radix), *Rou Cong Rong* (Cistanches, Herba) and *Tong Ji Li* (Astragali, Semen). In the most severe cases, *Ge Jie* (Gecko) or even .5 g of powdered human umbilical cord (*Qi Dai*) can be taken to increase the warming of Kidney yang and assisting it to grasp qi, and thus settle the dyspnea.

Formula

Ji Sheng Shen Qi Wan ('Kidney Qi Pill from *Formulas that Aid the Living*')

Shou Di	Rehmanniae Glutinosae Conquitae, Radix
Shan Yao	Dioscoreae Oppositae, Radix
Shan Zhu Yu	Corni Officinalis, Fructus
Mu Dan Pi	Moutan Radicis, Cortex
Fu Ling	Poriae Cocos, Sclerotium
Ze Xie	Alismatis Plantago-aquaticae, Rhizoma
Fu Zi	Aconiti Carmichaeli Praeparata, Radix)
Rou Gui	Cinnamomi Cassiae, Cortex
Che Qian Zi	Plantaginis, Semen
Chuan Niu Xi	Cyathulae, Radix

Source text: *Ji Sheng Fang* ('Formulas to Aid the Living', 1253) [*Formulas and Strategies*, p. 278]

To summarize the discussion of thin mucus syndromes, one of the case histories of Xu Shu-Wei (1079),[6] in which he himself figured as the patient, is most illustrative.

Case history from Xu Shu-Wei: pocketed thin mucus syndrome

I suffered from pi yin (癖饮 'occluded thin mucus' which is thin mucus accumulated bilaterally in the ribs and forming nodes) for thirty years. It started because as a youth I would sit up at night writing, and always leant against the table with my left side, and thus the food and drink would predominantly amass on the left. In the middle of the night it was my custom to have several cups of wine and again lie down on my left. With the strength of my youthful years, I did not notice, until about five years later I started to feel the wine under the left ribs and hear it making a noise. My ribs ached, my appetite lessened—to be replaced with an indefinable gnawing hunger-like feeling. After half a cup of wine, I would have to stop, and every ten days or so would vomit several bowls-full of sour watery fluid. In the summer, only my right side would sweat, with absolutely no moisture on the left! I visited famous doctors and tried every formula and secret prescription known to man: some of them would work for a while, the illness would stop for a month or so and then recur ... My own conjecture was that the pathogen must be gathered into a knot and contained in a pocket (pi nang 癖囊), as it were: like water in a measuring cup, it will not overflow until the measure is full (this last line is a quote from the philosopher Meng Zi; by 'pocket' Xu Shu-Wei is referring to the Spleen). But only the clear portion could flow, while the turbid portion remained occluded with no course of escape, and thus it would accumulate until every week or so, through vomiting, it could be released. Now Spleen Earth abhors damp, but this pathogenic fluid movement brings on damp; thus by my reckoning the best approach was to parch the Spleen to eliminate damp: upholding the Earth to fill the measuring cup (i.e. with normal, as opposed to pathological, fluids). Thus, after systematic evaluation and elimination of all the potential herbs, I took one jin (approximately 500 g) of *Cang Zhu* (Atractylodis, Rhizoma), removed the outer layer and sliced it, added sesame oil and a bit of water, ground it, and filtered out the fluid. Then I steamed fifty *Da Zao* (Zizyphi Jujubae, Fructus), removed the skin and stones, and pounded this [together with the *Cang Zhu*] and made small pills. I would take fifty pills with warm water, every day, on an empty stomach and gradually increased this to one or two hundred pills. I avoided eating peaches, pears and sparrow meat; and within three months, the phlegm had been expelled. Since then I have taken this often: there is no nausea or pain, the chest and diaphragm feel open and spacious, I eat and drink as before, in the summer months sweat appears over the whole body, and now even in lamp-light I can write tiny characters. This is all due to the potency of the *Cang Zhu*. In the early stages of taking it, there will necessarily be some slight feeling of dryness; this can be relieved by briefly decocting *Shan Zhi Zi* (Gardeniae Jasminoidis, Fructus) powder and using this to take the pills. After a period of time, this sensation of dryness will disappear.

A later commentator notes:

> Using *Cang Zhu* to treat pocketed thin mucus is the idea that 'those with phlegm and thin mucus should be harmonized with warming herbs', but this is not completely the same as the idea behind Ling Gui Zhu Gan Tang ('Poria, Cinnamon Twig, Atractylodis Macrocephala, and Licorice Decoction', *Formulas and Strategies*, p. 443), because only the single parching *Cang Zhu* is used, without all the other herbs. He also tells us about the side effects and how to relieve them with *Shan Zhi Zi* powder. This is an example of the medical ethics of the ancients!

This short essay by Xu Shu-Wei is well-known and often commented upon in the medical literature. See for example 'The Pathological Mechanisms and Treatment of Phlegm and Thin Mucus' (from the *Lei Zheng Zhi Cai* by Lin Pei-Qin, d. 1839), at the end of the Appendix on the history of phlegm theory development.

NOTES

1. Maciocia refers to thin mucus (yin 饮) as 'Phlegm-fluids', Bensky refers to them as 'congested fluids'.
2. Before the Tang dynasty, in Classical literature such as the *Mai Jing* ('Pulse Classic') and the *Qian Jin Yao Fang* ('Thousand Ducat Formulas')—but not the *Jin Gui Yao Lue*—the character 'tan' was often written 'dan' 淡 which means 'bland', so that the meaning would be 'a clear bland thin type of pathological fluid which has accumulated within the body to cause disease'. After the Tang dynasty, the character was always written with the illness radical, as 'tan'.
3. This discussion of thin mucus types and their treatment is based upon lectures and articles by my internal medicine teacher at the Zhejiang College of TCM, associate professor Wu Song-Kang.
4. Xuan yin syndrome can be found in such bio-medically defined conditions as pleurisy.
5. The use of Xiao Qing Long Tang ('Minor Bluegreen Dragon Decoction') in the treatment of thin mucus in the limbs, as described in the *Jin Gui Yao Lue*, is slightly different from the usage described for it in the *Shang Han Lun*. In the latter text, a wind-cold pathogen is responsible for stirring up internally retained thin mucus (which is already in place below the diaphragm), and the formula is used to expel the wind-cold from the surface while breaking up the internal retention of pathogenic fluids. In yi yin, the formula uses the same herbs to expel thin mucus on the surface, while warming internal cold from constitutional deficiency. It is this kind of methodological elegance, demonstrated again and again throughout each of Zhang Zhong-Jing's two works *Shang Han Lun* and *Jin Gui Yao Lue*, which has stimulated the almost universal admiration for Zhang Zhong-Jing amongst Chinese physicians of later ages. The real clincher is that, far from being 'mere theoretical speculation', these methods work astoundingly well.
6. Xu Shu-Wei was a well-known physician and author of numerous works in the *Shang Han Lun* tradition, among which are the *Lei Zheng Pu Ji Ben Shi Fang* ('Classified Formulas of Universal Benefit from My Practice'), the *Shang Han Jiu Shi Lun* ('Ninety Discussions on the *Shang Han Lun*') and the *Zhu Jie Shang Han Bai Zheng Ge* ('Annotated Songs of One Hundred Shang Han Conditions'). Xu Shu-Wei was also known as Xu Xue-Shi—'Xu the Scholar'.

Phlegm: etiology and symptomatology

7

The concept of phlegm as both a product and a cause of disease is not unique to Chinese medicine, being a component of medical systems as widely dispersed as Tibet and Greece. But no other medical system has developed a theory as comprehensive in regard to its pathogenesis and development, its symptomatology and its relationship with each organ in the body. It is primarily these aspects of the phlegm theory in Chinese medicine which will be discussed in this chapter, while reviewing briefly the physiology of normal fluid metabolism in order to provide a context in which this theory may be viewed.

CONCEPT OF PHLEGM IN TRADITIONAL CHINESE MEDICINE

Traditional Chinese medicine has two general categories of phlegm, a 'broadly defined' phlegm and a 'narrowly defined' phlegm.

The narrowly defined phlegm is generally regarded as the visible substance secreted by the Lungs and upper respiratory tract which can be either coughed or spat out, or vomited up. This is also often known as 'external phlegm' (wai tan 外痰) or 'substantial phlegm'.

Broadly defined phlegm is often the consequence of internal disruption of the body's fluid metabolism, either through qi stasis, yang qi deficiency or similar reasons. Because this type of phlegm is not visually obvious to an observer, and because the etiology is internal, it is also known as 'internal phlegm'. It should not be referred to as 'insubstantial phlegm', although the term has been used both in Chinese and in English, because this type of phlegm is quite capable of producing very substantial nodules indeed.

However, the two categories of phlegm are not totally independent, indeed external phlegm may be a concrete indication of the existence of internal phlegm. Nonetheless, it is internal phlegm which is responsible for the incredibly varied symptoms and conditions of phlegm diseases, and thus TCM phlegm theory is especially rich in the area of internal phlegm differentiation and treatment.

Scope of phlegm influence

Normal fluid metabolism depends on Spleen's transport, Lung's rhythmic descent and Kidney's normal qi transformation function. The least malfunction in any one of these organs can allow fluids to slow in circulation, accumulate and thicken into phlegm. Similarly, the influence of Shao Yang's San Jiao (Triple Warmer) is extraordinarily broad, as San Jiao is the pathway for the ascent and descent of qi and is also the pathway for fluids, reaching outward to the surface tissues, inward to the zang fu, up to the vertex and down to the feet. Therefore, any phlegm which accumulates due to a Spleen, Lung or Kidney imbalance can be carried through the qi or fluid system of the San Jiao to lodge anywhere in the body. In the same way, fluid at any point in the San Jiao network can accumulate into phlegm, given the right conditions.

For these reasons, diseases involving phlegm are among the most complicated of any in TCM. For example, if phlegm lodges in the chest and ribs causing local obstruction, it can variously lead to uncomfortable fullness in the epigastric area, pain in the ribs or flanks or a feeling of coldness running between the heart and the back. If the phlegm obstructs the ascent and descent of yin and yang, then Heart and Kidneys can become unbalanced, the Heart shen disturbed, and symptoms such as insomnia, palpitations and lower backache result. If phlegm obstructs the Stomach, Stomach qi can rebel upward causing nausea and vomiting. Phlegm descending into the Intestine can cause diarrhea or, following the San Jiao up to the vertex of the head, can cause dizziness and headaches. If phlegm accumulates in the Lungs, cough and dyspnea result; in the Heart, palpitations and anxiety. Phlegm misting the Pericardium, Heart or the vessels can even cause stroke or epilepsy. Gynecologically, it can cause leukorrhea, irregular periods, abdominal mass and infertility. If phlegm remains in the tissues of the limbs, numbness and pain can result, or nodes and swelling.

There is a famous quote in TCM which says: 'Phlegm does not move upward in the body by itself, just as water cannot flow uphill. So to treat phlegm, forget the phlegm and treat the qi. When the qi moves smoothly, all the fluids of the body will follow it and move smoothly'.

Because phlegm follows the flow of qi around the body, and can potentially reach any place where the qi can flow—every organ, every tissue, inside or out, high or low—phlegm theory therefore influences every department of traditional Chinese medicine. The combined clinical experiences of several millennia, recorded in TCM medical literature, show that phlegm should be considered as a possible etiological factor in almost any disease. Traditional Chinese medical texts record long lists of phlegm-related conditions, such as phlegm constipation, phlegm vertigo, phlegm misting the Heart, phlegm paralysis, phlegm infertility, phlegm skin ulceration, sublingual phlegm swelling the tongue, and so on.

Shen Jin-Ao, in his *Za Bing Yuan Liu Xi Zhu* ('Wondrous Lantern for Peering into the Origin and Development of Miscellaneous Diseases', 1773), says: 'The nature of phlegm is to flow unpredictably, thus the damage from phlegm can stretch from the vertex of the head to Yong Quan (K.1) on the soles as it is carried by the qi through its ascent and descent, arriving everywhere in the body, interior or exterior, so that each of the Five Zang and Six Fu has it.'[1]

It does not take long in actual practice before the TCM statement 'the Hundred Afflictions [all] coexist with phlegm' begins to look like less of an exaggeration.

Summary

Phlegm (tan 痰), thin mucus (yin 饮) and water (shui 水) are all products of disruption to normal food and fluid transformation, a phenomenon which has been termed 'one root and three branches'. But the sheer variety of locations and symptoms for phlegm cannot be matched by either thin mucus or water, and so clinical differentiation of these three pathogens is essential, because a treatment designed for one will not necessarily be effective for another.

However, broadly defined phlegm presents such complex symptomatology in clinic that it can be difficult for beginners to recognize, differentiate and treat. The ancients often noted that 'strange afflictions are usually phlegm', even to the extent that Zhu Dan-Xi remarked: '[These phlegm] illnesses appear [the result of] an evil spirit, only when obstructed phlegm is expelled will the illness be allayed.'[2]

This very complexity of symptoms is in itself one of the most characteristic signs of broadly defined phlegm. If one is able to become familiar with the special points of TCM phlegm theory, though, one will be able to recognize and flexibly deal with phlegm in all of its manifestations, and thus achieve results where other methods may have failed.

ROLE OF THE ZANG ORGANS IN THE PRODUCTION OF PHLEGM

Brief review of fluid metabolism

The food we consume is composed of solids and fluids. After ingestion, the solids are digested, absorbed and transported by the combined functions of the Stomach, Spleen, Small Intestine and Large Intestine, and essential qi from these solids forms the nourishing qi and blood distributed throughout the body to meet the needs of the tissues. The non-essential portion is carried downward to the Large Intestine, formed into feces and excreted. This is the function of the digestive system.

Fluids, after entering the Stomach, rely on the transport function of the Spleen for absorption and transport to the Lungs. The Lungs reside in the upper Jiao and are functionally linked with all the channels through the flow of channel qi, which is itself composed of the combination of the zong qi of the chest and the essential qi derived from food and fluids. In terms of fluid processes, the Lungs have the function of regulating and keeping clear the fluid passageways by their rhythmic descending qi; and again, the clearing qi transformation of the Lungs separates out excess fluids from those carried upward from the Spleen and the Kidneys and sends them directly to the Urinary Bladder, where they will pass through another qi transformation process, supported by the Kidney yang, before excretion. By virtue of the linkage with all the channels and the descending regularity of Lung qi, the Lungs are able to maintain a smooth and continuous circulation of the proper amount of fluids, blood and qi through the channels, each interacting with the other, under normal circumstances, in supportive harmony.

While the jin and ye fluids fulfil their nutrient function, the remaining murky portion of the fluids absorbed by the Spleen is sent through the San Jiao to the Urinary Bladder in the lower Jiao. From the solid waste passed downward by the Stomach, other fluids are further extracted by the Intestines, and the murky portion of these fluids are also sent directly to the Urinary Bladder.

Here, the yang qi of the Kidneys performs a vital function: 'separating the Clear [to be reused by the body] and expelling the Murky'. The 'clear' or pure portions of the fluids, which nourish and moisten, are reabsorbed and lifted through the Kidney channel and the San Jiao to the Lungs to be distributed again throughout the whole body. The 'murky' portion, left over after the steaming Kidney qi transformation in the Urinary Bladder, is excreted as urine.

Another excretory route is available for waste fluids, which likewise helps maintain a condition of metabolic harmony in the body fluids. A small portion of the jin and ye fluids circulating through the muscles and skin is 'vaporized' by the yang protective qi into sweat, a process which both assists fluid harmony and also aids the organism's adjustment to changing environmental conditions.

Liver too, has a hand in clear fluid passage through its involvement in the channel qi flow mechanism and its close relationship through the Shao Yang San Jiao.

INTRODUCTION TO PHLEGM PATHOLOGY

Chinese medicine has two categories of fluid metabolism disruption: one, in which for whatever reason the body's fluids are depleted, leading to a state of 'damage to fluids' or, if severe, to 'insufficiency of yin'; the other being retention of pathogenic fluids due to problems of transformation, distribution or excretion.

It must be re-emphasized here that 'jin-ye' and 'water' (shui) are strictly differentiated in traditional Chinese medicine. The designation 'jin and ye fluids' does not constitute a general term for all the liquids in the body but refers to nourishing fluid substance; the term covers all physiologically normal fluids within the organism. Water, conversely, is pathological. It may result from the mutation of jin and ye fluids after contact with pathogens, or it may be made up of unexcreted waste material formed during normal metabolism. In either case, the retention of water is deleterious to the health of the body.

Water retention may be categorized according to cause, location and quality: if its nature is thin, light and clear, and the location fixed (e.g. Stomach-Intestines, flanks, epigastric area, or in the limbs), this is thin mucus (yin).[3]

If its nature is fine, like clear water, accumulating and spreading subcutaneously, leading to generalized edema, this is called edema (shui zhong, 'water-swelling').

If there is water retention which begins to congeal, becoming thick and viscous and carried to every part of the body, this is called phlegm (痰 'tan').

As described previously, normal fluid metabolism relies upon the harmonious functioning of Spleen qi, Lung qi, Kidney yang, San Jiao and the qi of the channels. But disharmony in the qi transformation of these three organs or disruption of the normal yuan qi flow in the San Jiao may be precipitated by a number of factors. These include invasion by exogenous pathogens, stress from emotional excitement, inappropriate intake of food, with accumulation and eventual coagulation of the food into phlegm.

Pathogenic fire is a factor in phlegm formation which does not affect the qi transformation process described above but acts directly on the fluid metabolism to produce phlegm. In fact, pathogenic fire leads to phlegm as often as it does to wind, insufficient yin and extravasated blood. Recognition of this close relationship is reflected in the ancient saying 'phlegm is merely fire with form; fire is merely formless phlegm'.

'Pathogenic fire' does not mean just an invasion of exogenous heat into the body; other pathogens often have a tendency to become fire under the proper conditions. Emotional overactivity in the form of fury, joy, worry, grief and fear can also cause fire to be produced. Constitutional deficiency of yin leads to xu-fire (i.e. fire resulting from this deficiency). In short, fire is such a common clinical phenomenon that it must always be taken into account when dealing with diseases resulting from or complicated by phlegm.

Based on the above points, we can summarize the most influential factors in the production of phlegm from the zang and fu organs as follows: the functional irregularity of Lung qi, Spleen qi, Kidney (yang) qi, San Jiao yuan qi and the overactivity of pathogenic fire. This is the origin of the Chinese saying that phlegm is formed through 'the Four Qi and the One Pathogen'.

Individual zang organ activity

Lungs

Physiology. Lungs rule the qi of the whole body as well as maintaining regular water passage. Under normal conditions, the essence of food and fluids absorbed by the Spleen and Stomach are purified, carried to the upper Jiao, and murky fluids are separated out and directed downward by the Lungs. This, in conjunction with the qi transformation of the San Jiao, insures thorough and even distribution of nourishing body fluids—jin-ye—around the body, at the same time allowing for the excretion of waste fluids through the medium of urine, tears, nasal mucus and so on.

Lungs and phlegm. Lungs, as 'the tender organ' (Fei wei jiao zang), are very susceptible to attack by exogenous pathogens, and such attacks are frequently the cause of Lung phlegm, as will be described in later sections. This section, however, will concern itself mainly with the effects of internal disruption of Lung functioning.

If the physiological functions described above are upset, the fluids can collect and form phlegm, hence the saying: 'Lungs are the storehouse of phlegm'. This obviously points to the role of the Lungs in phlegm syndromes and diseases such as phlegm-dyspnea and other phlegm-related respiratory diseases; but less obviously, in a broader sense, refers to the unequal distribution and accumulation of body fluids in different areas of the body as a result of an abnormal or interrupted descent of Lung qi.

These examples do not completely define the relationship of the Lungs to phlegm pathology, though. For instance, fire resulting from an insufficiency of Lung yin, or from exogenous pathogenic attack, could lead to a depletion of fluids and so to phlegm. Conversely, a weakness of Kidney qi might lead to an inundation of the Lungs with excess fluids, a situation described by the saying 'excess water leads to phlegm'. So we see that the statement 'Lungs are the storehouse of phlegm' not only refers to phlegm produced by the Lungs themselves but also to disruption of fluid distribution due to Lung dysfunction; desiccation of fluids by fire from yin deficiency; and storage in the Lungs of phlegm formed by the Spleen and Kidneys.

Spleen

Physiology and phlegm production. The function of Spleen qi is to distribute the extracted jing-essence of food and fluids to every part of the body. If this function is disrupted due to weak Spleen qi or an abnormal ascending tendency of Stomach qi, then distribution will be hampered, the essential jing-qi will tend to stagnate, gather and become phlegm.

Spleen and Stomach in the middle Jiao are pivotal in the ascent and descent of qi from the upper and lower Jiao: if Spleen qi is too weak to lift or Stomach qi obstructed from descending, then the qi movement throughout the body suffers and phlegm can be produced anywhere.

The Ming dynasty text *Yi Zong Bi Du* ('Required Readings from the Masters of Medicine', 1637) contains the comment: 'When throughout the body there is an even distribution of the qi of foods and fluids, and smooth harmonious movement in the channels of the Five Zang, where could there be phlegm?' It also points out 'when Spleen Earth is weak, the clear finds it hard to rise, the turbid has difficulty descending, and both lodge in the center, obstructing the diaphragm and accumulating to form phlegm'.

The *Zhu Bing Yuan Hou Lun* ('Comprehensive Treatise on Origins and Signs of Disease') records: 'Phlegm [means] congealed fluid' and occurs in 'people who suffer from overexertion, which weakens their Stomach and Spleen so that these organs no longer control water and fluids. Undispersed fluids become tan-yin'.

It was the *Zhu Bing Yuan Hou Lun* which first contained the statement 'phlegm is formed by weakness of the Spleen and Stomach' which became the basis for the later doctrine 'Spleen is the source of phlegm.'[4]

The Yuan dynasty physician Zhu Dan-Xi explains: 'Spleen qi is the [type of] yang qi responsible for transportation in the body. It can be likened to the sun in the sky. When yin congeals so that all the Four [Directions] are obstructed, the sun is shut out of its rightful place. Regulating the Spleen, then, resembles [the reappearance of] a fierce sun in a cloudless sky, naturally dispersing the congealed yin and the turbid phlegm.'[5]

Zhang Jing-Yue agrees: 'Excess phlegm is a condition invariably caused by Central deficiency'.

His 'Central deficiency' mainly refers to a weakened Stomach and Spleen in the central Jiao, where the ascending and descending functions have become disordered. So he says:

> The fact is, the transformation of phlegm is based on fluids and food, and if the Spleen is strong and the Stomach healthy like that of a young person's, then whatever is eaten will be transformed, and it all becomes qi and blood; where could retention occur to become phlegm?
>
> It is only when there is incomplete transformation, where one or two parts out of ten are retained, that those one or two parts become phlegm. If three or four parts are retained, then those three or four parts become phlegm.[6]

Wang Ang points out that it is not only Spleen deficiency that can lead to phlegm: 'Spleen patients' phlegm can be a result either of excess or of deficiency. For example, if pathogenic damp is too obstructive, this is Spleen excess; if Earth is debilitated and unable to control Water, this is Spleen deficiency'.[7]

This reminder that the originating mechanism of phlegm may be different even though the originating location is the same is essential for the proper selection of treatment principle: if the origin is excess, reduction of the pathogen is required; if the origin is in deficiency, then only tonification can treat the root. Nonetheless, even reduction of the pathogen will require some attention to Spleen functioning. Thus Wang Ang notes: 'To treat phlegm, first tonify the Spleen; if the Spleen's normal healthy transport is restored, the phlegm will disperse by itself.'[8]

The Spleen may also be influenced by the dysfunction of other zang-organs, especially the Lungs, the Liver and the Kidneys. If the Lung qi cannot clear and descend normally so that phlegm accumulates in the Lungs, this can back up onto the Spleen. If the Liver qi does not assist Spleen transport but instead Wood becomes obstructed and overcomes Spleen Earth, first damp and then phlegm will result. It is the Kidneys, though, which perhaps have the greatest influence upon the Spleen, because of the Spleen requirement of the support of Kidney yang for both transformation and transportation. Kidney yang deficiency will not only fail to support the Spleen but will also deprive the San Jiao of the warming yuan qi necessary for fluid movement and for qi transformation of fluids. Less directly, failure of the Kidney yang to steam the fluids held by the Urinary Bladder can result in pathogenic water flooding upwards, which can both overcome the Spleen and also result in phlegm.

Improper treatment is a further causative factor in the production of Spleen damp and phlegm. If excessively cold herbs are used, Spleen yang may be damaged. If diuresis or purging is employed in too heavy-handed a way, Spleen yang may be dragged downward instead of rising. Overly greasy herbs can also dampen Spleen functioning. Awareness of the dangers can help to reduce the unfortunately frequent incidence of such iatrogenic injury.

Physiology of Kidneys

Kidneys are entrusted with the primal yin (yuan yin), storing this inherited constitutional essence within which moves primal yang (yuan yang), the motive life force. At the same time, the Kidneys are continually receiving and storing the jing-essence transformed from food and fluids, which is re-supplied to the other organs as required. Consequently the amount of these essential substances present within the Kidney at any given time depends on the strength or weakness of the other organs. If the Kidneys are depleted, this can have far-reaching effects on every organ in the body. Chen Shi-Duo stresses this in his *Shi Shi Mi Lu* ('Secret Records of the Stone Chamber', 1687):

> Only when the Heart has access to Mingmen ('gate of vitality') fire can it rule consciousness, only when the Liver has access to Mingmen fire can it control reflection, only when the Gall-bladder has access to Mingmen fire can it exercise decision. With Mingmen fire, the Stomach is able to accept food, the Spleen can transport and distribute jin-ye, and the Lungs may provide rhythmic regulation [over the qi of the whole body]. If the Large Intestine obtains Mingmen fire it can provide passage [to the solid waste], if the Small Intestine obtains Mingmen fire it can distribute and transform [fluids], if the Kidneys obtain Mingmen fire they can act strongly, if the San Jiao obtains Mingmen fire it can rule fluid passage, if the Urinary Bladder obtains Mingmen fire it can receive and

hold [fluids]. None of these but borrows the nourishing warmth of Mingmen fire.[9]

The qi transformation in the Urinary Bladder supported by the warmth of Kidney yang is the last stage in the metabolism of fluids before excretion. The fluids separated out as useless by the other organs in the body are sent downward to the Urinary Bladder to undergo transformation by Kidney yang, after which the still useable portion is 'vaporized' and carried upward to the Lungs, and the rest are excreted. The intimately supportive role which the Kidneys play in relationship with both the San Jiao and the Spleen is also of crucial importance in the maintenance of healthy fluid mechanisms.

Kidneys and phlegm. In the context of phlegm or phlegm diseases, the relationship with the Kidneys is almost always one of deficiency. The phlegm may be a direct result of Kidney deficiency, such as a breakdown in water transport, or the connection may be less obvious. There may be a gradual lack of support in the functioning of the San Jiao or the Spleen, or impaired Kidney vitality may cause a steady worsening in an already existing phlegm condition. Kidney involvement is always to be suspected in long-standing phlegm diseases, where weak Kidney yang or imbalance of Kidney yin-yang is so often the cause that traditional Chinese medicine calls the Kidneys 'the Root of Phlegm'.

This quote from the Chapter 239 of the *Gu Jin Tu Shu Ji Cheng: Yi Bu Hui Lu* ('Collection of Books and Illustrations Past and Present: Records of the Medical Section' 1725) outlines some of the pathological processes involved and indicates the relationship of the Kidneys to phlegm production in long term diseases:

> Kidneys produce phlegm—mostly xu (deficient) phlegm. Long term illnesses often involve a great deal of phlegm. However this cannot be explained by the 'Spleen damp leads to phlegm' theory. Those diseases which drag on without improvement inevitably involve deficiency of Kidney yin. So if it is not Kidney water welling upward, then Kidney fire has boiled into phlegm (i.e. referring to fire from Kidney yin deficiency desiccating the fluids which then become phlegm). This is the phlegm of long-term disease.[10]

Phlegm produced from Kidney deficiency may then go on to invade the Heart or the Lungs by the avenue of the Kidney channel which communicates directly with these organs. Spleen yang may be weakened by such a build-up of phlegm, in which case the disease often becomes very protracted and hard to cure. Zhang Jing-Yue says: 'This phlegm is really pathogenic water: its root (ben) is the Kidney, its branch (biao) is the Spleen. Phlegm is produced in the Kidneys as water returns to its source, overflows and becomes phlegm. It is produced in the Spleen when [lacking the support of Kidney yang] foods and fluids are not transformed properly, and thus Earth does not control Water'. He goes on to remark 'Shi (excess) phlegm is nothing to worry about' and 'the thing most to be feared is xu (deficient) phlegm'. This is because, in the case of shi phlegm, 'its onset is rapid and recovery quick', because the root of the disease is shallow. Deficient (xu) phlegm, however, 'comes on gradually and is slow to depart', consequently it is very difficult to eradicate completely. This xu phlegm is the result of failed transformation of foods and fluids by the Spleen due to a lack of Kidney yang. Therefore he feels that xu phlegm must never be 'attacked' as a method of treatment; since this phlegm is a product of the mis-transformation of foods and fluids, it can be produced as fast as it is expelled. Furthermore, attacking treatments can damage the constitutional (yuan) qi, and the use of preparations such as Gun Tan Wan ('Vaporize Phlegm Pill', *Formulas and Strategies*, p. 424) is 'looking only at the present with no thought for what follows.'

Zhang Jing-Yue taught that the best principle of treatment in phlegm disease is to 'cause it not to be produced', which is to say, in certain long-term cases of stubborn phlegm, one needs to warm and tonify Kidney yang, 'tonifying fire to support Earth' in order to disperse the knot of phlegm. In the same context he goes on to say: 'Phlegm may be produced in any disorder of the five zang-organs ... therefore the transformation of phlegm must occur from the Spleen but the Root of Phlegm is none other than the Kidneys'. Obviously the key point in the development of xu (deficient) phlegm is a weakness of Kidney yang, especially in so far as this is related to 'fire not supporting Earth' and an overflow of pathogenic water building up into phlegm.[11]

Similar theoretical descriptions from the Ming and Qing dynasties are numerous, from such authors as Lin Pei-Qin and Chen Xiu-Yuan who also spoke of the Kidneys as the source of phlegm, the Spleen as its transport and the Lungs as the storehouse; all showing clearly that the development of phlegm is closely related to Kidney yang or Kidney yin deficiency, or a disruption of the yin-yang balance in the Kidneys.

Physiology of San Jiao

The yuan qi of the Kidneys is the source of warming energy for the San Jiao. This heat enables the San Jiao to control qi transformation, the products of which, according to Chapter 36 of the *Ling Shu*, go to warm and nourish the muscles and flesh, and to make firm the skin. The first chapter of the *Jin Gui Yao Lue* ('Essentials from the Golden Cabinet', c. 210 AD) states: 'The crevices in the surface tissues on the exterior of the body and the organs are the place where the San Jiao moves and gathers the Original True [qi], the area suffused with qi and blood.' Thus the transformation and then transportation of qi, blood and fluids by the Five Zang and Six Fu require the qi transformation and movement of the San Jiao. This is its first function.

The San Jiao and the Urinary Bladder are connected, and the action of the San Jiao is to maintain clear fluid passage, transporting fluids throughout the body and supplying the Urinary Bladder with cast-off fluids. Because of this, the *Nei Jing* names the Urinary Bladder 'the Ditch Official', which ensures that no backlog of water or disruption of flow occur. The San Jiao must act closely with the Lungs and the Kidneys, however, if this function is to be performed properly. The Lungs are responsible for transporting the essential part of the fluids (received from the Spleen) to the rest of the body, and separately sending the remainder to the Urinary Bladder. This function is mirrored in the Kidneys, which 'distil' the still useful portion of the fluids sent for disposal, and that portion is returned upward for redistribution. The pathway for all this movement is the San Jiao. This is its second function.

San Jiao and phlegm. Again it was the *Zhu Bing Yuan Hou Lun* that first suggested the mechanisms of the relationship between the San Jiao and phlegm, saying such things as 'phlegm and thin mucus disease is a result of weak yang qi failing to maintain open pathways for qi, so that the body fluids are unable to transit smoothly', and 'the qi of yin and yang cannot circulate smoothly [so that] the upper Jiao blockage produces heat [and thereafter phlegm]'. Because of this book's influence on traditional Chinese medicine, later works such as *Sheng Ji Zong Lu* ('Comprehensive Recording of the Sages' Benefits', c. 1117 AD) and *Ji Sheng Fang* ('Formulas to Aid the Living', 1253) all contain passages like this: 'If the San Jiao qi is blocked, channel flow will be obstructed causing water and fluids to stop and gather without proper circulation, collecting to form phlegm and leading to diseases innumerable.' In the *Zheng Zhi Zhun Sheng* ('Standards of Patterns and Treatments', 1602) Wang Ken-Tang observes: 'A long-term accumulation of phlegm resembles a ditch which has been backed-up for a long time, the water running contrary to its normal direction of flow so that everywhere is clogged with stagnating filth. If one seeks to avoid opening the ditch, and tries to purify the standing water, this simply shows lack of sense.'[12]

When Wang says 'open the ditch', he is referring to the normalization of the San Jiao qi transformation process, clearing the water passages and so dispelling phlegm.

There are two related conditions which should be clarified here. Although San Jiao functioning depends on the heat of Kidney yang, a breakdown of San Jiao qi transformation is different from weak Kidney yang unable to 'vaporize' the qi of water. The latter is a Kidney deficiency leading to a state known as 'excess water producing phlegm', the Primal Yang (yuan yang) is exhausted, and symptoms will be serious. A blockage of the qi transformation function of the San Jiao means interruption in the flow of fluids, which then gather and congeal to form phlegm. In this case the symptoms will be less severe and deep rooted.

Zhang Jing-Yue observes: 'Qi can transform water and distribute fluids', and also says: 'Qi is the Mother of Water, and those who know that the Way of regulating water lies in the principle "The transformation of qi leads to the excretion of water [from the Urinary Bladder]", they are the ones who have grasped a large part of the process.'[13] This again refers to the qi transformation process of the San Jiao, functioning to clear and harmonize the passage of fluids, water and damp. Thus when phlegm-damp or stagnation of water is found in a clinical situation, warming San Jiao and promoting its qi transformation process is an essential part of treatment.

Physiology of Liver

Both physiologically and pathologically, the Liver is the most complex of the five organs. Actively yang while structurally yin, the Liver not only exercises functions of dispersion but also of storage, at once hard and at the same time yielding. It has earned the title 'the Bandit of the 10 000 Illnesses' because of the many different types of disease to which it gives rise: emotional problems, respiratory, digestive, circulatory and reproductive disorders among them. The section on Liver qi in the *Lei Zheng Zhi Cai* ('Tailored Treatments Arranged According to Pattern') by Lin Pei-Qin, (d. 1839), lists twenty-five different symptoms attributed to Liver qi disharmony, including cough, distention, nausea, fainting, subcostal pain, and so on. Beyond all these, Liver also has a hand in the development of certain types of phlegm.

Liver and phlegm. The 'shu-xie' function of the Liver—which is the rising and spreading of Liver qi—not only maintains the yin, yang, qi and blood equilibrium of the Liver organ itself, ensuring against the tendencies of Liver qi to stagnate or rebel upward, but also exercises a tremendous influence on the Spleen and Stomach. If the Liver qi movement is obstructed, the digestion and distribution abilities of the Spleen and Stomach are directly affected, causing a reduction in transportation and the gradual production of phlegm. This is a pathological mechanism with which the ancient physicians were well familiar, often discussing in the same breath the theories 'Spleen is the source of phlegm' and 'Phlegm is produced from stagnation of qi'. Li Shi-Zhen states: 'Excessive Wind and Wood come to oppress Spleen Earth, so that the transportation of qi is interrupted, obstruction occurs and phlegm is formed'.[14] Note that despite the involvement of the Spleen, the root cause of the phlegm here is the problem in the Liver.

But it is not only by affecting the functioning of the Spleen that obstruction of the Liver qi can lead to phlegm. Because qi must carry the fluids around the body, any slow-down in this movement can allow fluids to coalesce and become phlegm. It was

Zhu Dan-Xi who said: 'Those who treat phlegm effectively do not treat the phlegm, but first treat the qi. When the circulation of the qi is smooth and ordered, this will lead the body fluids in a smooth and ordered circulation as well'. He explains: 'the substance of phlegm follows the qi in its rise or fall, so that every place in the body may be reached'.

The Song dynasty physician Chen Wu-Ze in the *San Yin Ji Yi Bing Zheng Fang Lun* ('Discussion of Illnesses, Patterns, and Formulas Related to the Unification of the Three Etiologies', 1174) says:

> The reasons that people have phlegm and thin mucus disease are: lack of clearness in the nutritive and protective qi (ying wei bu qing) so that qi and blood fail (bai) and become turbid, then form knots and produce [phlegm]. Internally, the seven emotions cause havoc, the zang-organ qi cannot move, it stops and produces thickened fluid, which in its turn produces thin mucus.[15]

Zhao Xian-Ke says: 'The seven emotions cause internal damage, occlusion, and finally, phlegm'; Yan Yong-He also discusses the relationship between emotional disturbance leading to a blockage of qi and the consequent development of phlegm disease, and finally Li Yong-Cui records: 'Shock, fury, sadness, and worry: phlegm stems therefrom'. In many ancient medical works, again, mention is made of qi-tan (qi-phlegm), feng-tan (wind-phlegm), jing-tan (shock-phlegm), and tan-jue (phlegm-coma) and so on, all of which can be linked with Liver qi disharmony.

Besides directly slowing the flow of fluids by failing to move qi, there are several other mechanisms by which Liver dysfunction can indirectly cause the production of phlegm. One is through heat or fire resulting from Liver qi obstruction or even Liver yin deficiency. This can dry the fluids into phlegm. Another is through the Liver channel influence on the San Jiao, which like Gall Bladder is Shao Yang, and thus linked to the state of the qi flow in the Jue Yin Liver channel. Yet another, even more indirect, is qi blockage leading to blood stagnation, so that the fluids within the stagnated blood also coagulate into phlegm.

Thus the state of the Liver is an extremely crucial factor in the healthy transport of fluids, since any abnormality of Liver can so easily result in the production of phlegm.

Physiology of the Heart

Although every functional activity in the body influences the whole, this does not mean that each activity is influentially equal. In the production of phlegm, for example, the Lungs, Spleen and Kidneys are primarily significant, the San Jiao and Liver secondarily so, and the Heart and the six fu organs of the least consequence. This is not, of course, to say irrelevant. The Heart controls consciousness (shen ming) and rules emotion. In the *Lei Jing* ('Systematic Categorization of the *Nei Jing*', 1624), it says:

> In terms of the injury from emotions, although each of the Five Zang has its own attribution, if one is looking for the source, it is nowhere but the Heart. ... The *Ling Shu*, Chapter 28, says: 'Sorrow, sadness and worry all move the Heart, when the Heart is moved, then the Five Zang and Six Fu are agitated'. Thus it can be seen that the Heart is the Supreme Master (da zhu) of the Five Zang and Six Fu, and presides over the hun (ethereal soul) and the po (corporeal soul), while encompassing thought (yi) and will (zhi) as well. Therefore when sadness moves in the Heart, the Lungs respond; when thought moves in the Heart, the Spleen responds; when anger moves in the Heart, the Liver responds; [and] when fear moves in the Heart, the Kidneys respond. This is why only the Heart controls the Five Emotions. If one can cultivate this Heart well, living in a safe and quiet place, without fear, without rapture, agreeably going along with things without strife, and accepting without Self the changes of Time, then the will and the thought harmonize, the spirit (jing shen) settles, regret and anger do not arise, the hun and po do not scatter, and the Five Zang and Six Fu are totally peaceful. What, then, can a pathogen do to one?[16]

The Heart also controls blood, a major component of which is fluid, and which requires the warming action of Heart yang for continuous circulation. (The relationship of the blood and the fluids, and also with the sweat, was discussed in an earlier chapter.)

Heart and phlegm. It is interesting to note that while the Heart is the zang organ least involved in phlegm production, it suffers some of the most grievous consequences, such as coma and epilepsy from 'phlegm misting the Heart', palpitations, insomnia and other disturbed Heart shen disorders, and even pain in the cardiac region resulting from the combination of stagnant blood and phlegm. In contradistinction to this suffering by the Heart, the Kidneys—which are deeply involved in phlegm development—are subject to little direct harm from phlegm, so that it is even said 'phlegm is never found in the Kidneys'.[17]

The mechanisms by which the Heart does contribute to phlegm production are primarily through the activities of Heart fire and the deficiencies of Heart yin or yang.

Heart fire, like any fire, can dry the fluids, in this case particularly the fluids of the blood, leading to the condition known as 'phlegm-fire disturbing the Heart'. This will require bitter-cold herbs to drain the excess fire, with salty-cold herbs to cut hot phlegm, and some pungent cooling blood-movers to ensure Heart blood circulation.

Deficiency of Heart yin can also produce fire but of a different nature, and requiring a different approach in treatment, even though it too can be called 'phlegm-fire disturbing the Heart'. Here the treatment method must be to moisten yin fluids to settle deficient-fire, while lightly using cooling bitter and pungent herbs to break up that phlegm which has already formed. Unless the Spleen is also deficient, one need not worry overmuch that the use of yin-moistening herbs will increase the phlegm: this phlegm is the consequence of xu-fire drying already weakened fluids, not the result of weak Spleen transformation. Moistening the yin fluids will in fact help to 'float' the pathogenic phlegm and allow it to be eliminated even more easily.

Heart yang deficiency is well-documented as a contributor to phlegm production. Six of the ten formulas introduced to treat thoracic-bi syndrome and heart pain in the *Jin Gui Yao Lue* ('Essentials from the Golden Cabinet') contain herbs to transform phlegm and open the flow of yang qi. In the Qing dynasty, Li Yong-Cui in the section discussing palpitations in the *Zheng Zhi Hui Bu* ('A Supplement to Diagnosis and Treatment'), says: 'The master of the body is the Heart, the nourishment of the Heart is the blood. If the Heart blood is deficient, the shen departs and its residence is left empty. The empty residence [without the direction of shen] becomes stuffy and phlegm builds up. Phlegm collecting in the position of the Heart: this is the origin of fright (jing) and palpitations.'[18]

This describes the actions of both the Heart yin (blood) and the Heart yang (shen), saying that if the Heart yang activity is not supported by the yin blood, it will fail to move, and fluids will collect into phlegm. It also implies that as this phlegm is the result of deficiency, its treatment will require tonification rather than attack.

Summary

The role of each of the five zang organs in the production of phlegm is closely determined by the part each plays in normal fluid metabolism, and by its susceptibility to the influence of other pathogenic factors. Each of these aspects will have a bearing upon the manifestations of phlegm in the individual patient. Awareness of the possible range of involvement each zang may have with phlegm production, and the mechanisms by which such involvement occurs, will allow accurate interpretation of those symptoms with which a patient may present. Some further considerations in symptom interpretation are presented below.

CONSTITUTIONAL INDICATIONS OF PHLEGM

1. Extended illness without weakening; repeated attacks and remissions; typically middle age and above
2. Eye movements are lackadaisical; eye sockets are dark; there may be exudate in the corners of the eyes. Complexion is dull and wan; the face appears puffy
3. Obviously greasy skin; moist, often odorous, secretions from the armpits, genitals, palms and soles. Shiny face as if oiled
4. Heavy-set, with thick fingers and hands, especially if the flesh is not muscular but soft and flabby

5. Aching distended feeling in the hands and feet
6. Tongue coat usually white and greasy
7. Tongue body is more slack and flabby than normal
8. Pulse usually deep and rolling; but could also be wiry; soft, floating and rolling; or just deep
9. Dislike for oily greasy food and diary products, prefers bland foods and drinks. Odors like petrol or perfume can cause headaches, dizziness and nausea
10. Lack of concentration and poor memory; or when severe, even depression, paranoia or hyperactivity
11. Excessive salivation, or even uncontrolled dribbling. Constant expectoration of phlegm or saliva
12. Lethargy or excessive sleep
13. Sluggish incomplete bowel movements, but not dry stool. Stool may contain mucus
14. Symptoms may worsen with weather or seasonal changes

Explanation of the constitutional indications of phlegm

Extended illness without weakening; repeated attacks and remissions; typically middle-age and above

'Without weakening' means that the patient's strength, appetite, musculature and even voice show no signs of illness.

In those patients who do become somewhat emaciated, their energy and voice seem normal. At the time when phlegm accumulates and obstructs there may be temporary lethargy—and this is when it is easiest to mis-diagnose as deficiency—but as soon as the phlegm breaks up slightly, the patient's energy returns. This is because although the zheng qi is obstructed by the phlegm, it is not deficient. In fact, some patients look stronger than before the illness, due to a gain in weight.

'Repeated remissions and attacks' occur because of the tendency of phlegm to disperse, so that symptoms disappear, and then accumulate again, so that symptoms reappear.

Case history: Alternating dispersal and collection of phlegm and damp

My patient was an Australian male, 30 years of age, who had been noticing over the last few years an unusual cycle of symptoms: for several weeks he would be happy and energetic, with good urine flow and a clear tongue coat, but after a period of time he would start to feel heavy and tired, the urine would become frequent but scanty, the bowels irregular—either loose or constipated—and he would notice a 'line of tenderness' which traced exactly the right side Gall Bladder channel, from Feng Chi (GB-20) to the foot. The most telling sign was perhaps the tongue coat, which would change from relatively clear to thick greasy yellow at the root.

It was plain that the condition stemmed from the alternating dispersal and collection of phlegm and damp, combined with obstruction of the qi in the Liver and Gall Bladder channels, with each blockage able to provoke the other. Liver qi stasis failing to move fluids and failing to support the Spleen could begin the process of phlegm and damp gathering, which itself could further obstruct qi flow, initiating a vicious cycle that would culminate in the above constellation of symptoms. Alternatively, overeating or the wrong type of foods could begin the process with Spleen damp and phlegm assembling and then hampering Liver and Gall Bladder qi flow, with the same result.

The scantiness of the urine was the result of damp and phlegm preventing normal Urinary Bladder function, while the irregular bowel functions demonstrated the twin processes of the condition: when the qi flow was obstructed, the peristaltic action of the bowels was arrhythmic and led to constipation; the build-up of heavy sinking damp and phlegm, on the other hand, finally resulted in loose stool.

Treatment combined removal of phlegm and damp with support for both the Spleen and the Liver function, using a combination of Xiang Sha Liu Jun Zi Tang ('Six Gentlemen Decoction with Aucklandia and Amomum', *Formulas and Strategies*, p. 238) and Xiao Yao San ('Rambling Powder', *Formulas and Strategies*, p. 147).

Phlegm diseases are most likely to begin in middle age, as the yang qi starts to decline, years of stress and tension continually slowing the flow of qi allow fluids to gradually thicken and accumulate into phlegm, and over-rich foods have wrought their wrack on the Spleen's digestive and distributive functions.

If, of course, the phlegm is itself the result of deficiency—e.g. Spleen and Kidney yang deficiency eventually allowing untransformed food and fluids to accumulate and become phlegm—then of course the patient will show the deficiency and not have 'extended illness without weakening'.

Eye movements are lackadaisical; eye sockets are dark; there may be exudate in the corners of the eyes.
Complexion is dull and unfresh; the face appears puffy

In TCM theory, the essential jing-qi of the Five Zang and Six Fu pours upwards into the eyes, allowing them to move freely, in a lively manner, and providing sharp vision.

But as damp and phlegm can follow the qi anywhere, the eyes too can be affected. Patients occasionally report an unusual sticky yet stretchy substance secreted from the corners of the eyes, which is often a sign of Liver phlegm-fire. If the jing-qi is prevented from rising to the eyes, the eye movement slows and becomes lethargic.

In China, dark or black areas around, and especially under, the eyes are (in certain levels of society) called 'leukorrhea circles' in women, as leukorrhea is itself due to an accumulation of damp and phlegm. Puffy face and dark complexion result from the superficial accumulation of phlegm and damp obstructing the normal circulation of nutritive and protective qi in the face.

Obviously greasy skin; moist, often odorous, secretions from the armpits, genitals, palms and soles. Shiny face as if oiled

This is a reflection of phlegm-heat. Heat is a yang pathogen and so by nature is active and spreads outward. When heat and phlegm combine, phlegm is pushed outward toward the surface. A shiny oily face, therefore, is an important diagnostic sign of phlegm-heat, while a dull black complexion signals phlegm-damp or turbid phlegm obstructing physiological yang qi.

Both are phlegm signs but they need to be differentiated for proper treatment.

Heavy-set, with thick fingers and hands, especially if the flesh is not muscular but soft and flabby

Phlegm is heavy and murky and by nature tends to obstruct Spleen, which hates damp. Digestion and distribution suffer, leaving residue which adds to the already excessive phlegm, and the person 'gains weight'. Traditional axioms such as 'fat people usually have excessive phlegm' and 'skinny people usually have excessive fire' are quite dependable as clinical reminders, although not sufficient for a diagnosis on their own. An initial impression of 'overweight' or 'underweight' signals the experienced Chinese doctor to specifically look for phlegm and damp, say, in the former case, and fire symptoms in the latter. There must be other confirming symptoms for a reliable diagnosis.

Aching distended feeling in the hands and feet

Fullness or distended feeling in the hands, feet, neck and upper back can often be traced to phlegm obstructing the flow of qi and preventing the required nourishment from reaching the tissues, thus causing aching; distention will be the result of accumulation of both qi and phlegm. The limbs are ruled by the Spleen, because of the identity of both with Earth; phlegm being of the same nature as damp, is also related to Earth: like calls to like.

Tongue coat usually white and greasy

The tongue coat will usually be white and greasy, and may stay this way for years, or may disappear and reappear repeatedly. It may appear only on the sides, or may just be permanently greasy at the root.

The coat will vary depending upon the nature of the phlegm: whether it is mixed with hot or cold, or the result of a deficiency or another shi-pathogen, or has caused qi blockage or blood stagnation, and so on. The location of the phlegm accumulation or the stage of the illness will also affect the tongue coat, making it thick in the middle, say, for middle Jiao phlegm damp, or pooled just behind the tip for phlegm gathered in the Lungs, and so on.

One important fact to recognize is that a peeled coat (or a coat peeled only in the center) can point to phlegm as well as to yin deficiency. The differentiating factor is whether or not the patient has a yin deficient body type, or any yin deficiency symptoms. If not, it is probably phlegm.

However, it is also said 'stubborn phlegm [brings out] strange symptoms', and sometimes the tongue may, surprisingly, have little coat at all. In these cases one must balance the rest of the symptoms against the solitary contradiction of the tongue, and make a reasoned judgement. In some cases this will be a signal that the phlegm is simply not involved with the digestive system, and so is less likely to manifest on the tongue coat. In other situations, such as the case history described above, the phlegm is lodged deep within the body, and only appears when stirred up by a precipitating factor.

Tongue body is more slack and flabby than normal

A slack tongue is a cardinal sign of qi deficiency with phlegm retention. But the slack tongue of phlegm disease is not as severe as that of a stroke victim, where the tongue body is often lolling, drooling and difficult to retract. Slack tongue in phlegm disease is very slight and extremely easy to miss unless watched for carefully. When the illness is at a peak, it may be more obvious.

Qi deficient patients with retained phlegm usually have a pale white tongue. Phlegm and blood stagnation occurring together show up as a dull purplish tongue.

Pulse usually deep and rolling; but could also be wiry; soft, floating and rolling; or just deep

The pulse typically manifests as deep and slippery, or soft floating and slippery (ru 濡), but it could be wiry, or just deep.

Dislike for oily greasy food and dairy products, preference for bland foods and drinks. Odors like petrol or perfume can cause headaches, dizziness and nausea

If the person is not addicted to junk food and is somewhat in touch with what makes them feel physically better, they will prefer simple bland food, and report that greasy foods, even the icing on cakes, will make them nauseous. Greasy foods have what the Chinese call a 'heavy' flavor and odor, like phlegm itself, and so tend to increase damp and phlegm.

Bland, as a flavor, is classed as yang and encourages diuresis, thus reducing damp. Heat, too, is yang, while phlegm is yin, and so heated foods and drinks can temporarily reduce excessive internal yin. Certain fragrant foods such as coriander or basil can disperse and dry damp and also provide some relief to the patient.

But piercingly strong fragrant odors like petrol or perfume will break up phlegm because of the yang-expanding nature of fragrance. This is even used in herbal treatment as a principle of damp treatment: fragrance to disperse damp and phlegm. Here, though, the effect is from the environment and therefore uncontrolled. Once the phlegm is broken up by these odors, the yang nature of the fragrance starts it on its rise upward, and then the phlegm is lifted with the normal flow of clear yang to the head, obstructing the orifice of the mind, and bringing on dizziness and headaches. Nausea is caused because of the rising phlegm's interference with the normal descent of Stomach qi.[19]

Lack of concentration and poor memory; or when severe, even depression, paranoia or hyperactivity

Lack of concentration and poor memory are extremely common symptoms of phlegm and damp obstructing the flow of clear yang to the head. As such it will usually be most noticeable in the early morning, before the excessive yin which has settled over the night-time has had a chance to be dispersed by the activity of yang. It will also be poor after eating, when Spleen yang is fully engaged in digestion and unable to break through the already-formed phlegm-damp to lift clear yang to the head. The depression, paranoia and hyperactivity are symptoms of phlegm disturbing the Heart shen and may be obvious and severe, as in mental illness or stroke.[20]

Excessive salivation, or even uncontrolled dribbling. Constant expectoration of phlegm or saliva

Stool examination to eliminate intestinal parasites as a possible causative factor is necessary with this symptom. While frequently a result of Spleen or Kidney deficiency, excess phlegm obstructing the normal descent of Stomach qi is another possible origin. If Stomach qi cannot descend it will rebel upward, carrying the accumulated untransformed fluids with it, producing excessive saliva. A characteristic sign of phlegm, though, is that this symptom is worse when the patient is depressed, or has nothing to distract them. This is because the excess saliva is often related to an impairment of Liver assistance in the proper ascent and descent of Spleen and Stomach qi. 'Spleen and Stomach are the pathway for ascent and descent, while Liver is the pivot', observed the Qing dynasty physician Zhou Xue-Hai.

For proper treatment when this symptom is the main presenting complaint—as it may well be, due to the distress it can cause to the patient and their family—it is important to distinguish deficiency and excess, as suggested above. Excess conditions result from functional disharmony of the Liver, Spleen, Stomach and Lungs; whereas the deficiency conditions (which involve primarily the Spleen and Kidneys) result from yang qi not transforming fluids.[21]

Lethargy or excessive sleep

This can be the outcome of either excessive phlegm-damp (i.e. an excess condition), or deficient Spleen producing phlegm (which is a mixed xu-shi state). In both cases Spleen yang is fatigued and the urge to sleep increased.

But there is a difference: in the case of excessive phlegm, the urge to sleep and then the sleep itself is heavy, while the lethargy is less marked.

On the other hand, when qi is deficient, blood too is affected and fails to nourish the Heart. The patient is constantly sitting, lying or leaning against something to rest, but when it comes to actually sleeping, this is difficult. Often they cannot get to sleep due to recurring thoughts. If they do manage to sleep, they awaken easily. The whole clinical picture is strikingly different to the log-like sleep of excess-type phlegm suppressing the yang qi, and was in fact noted centuries ago. The *Zhu Bing Yuan*

Hou Lun ('General Treatise on the Etiology and Symptomatology of Disease', 610 AD) by Chao Yuan-Fang recorded: 'Shortness of breath and desire to sleep is a sign of phlegm.'[22]

This hypersomnolence can itself be a presenting symptom, or of course can be admixed with other symptoms. If it is the presenting symptom, usually it will be found to be excess-type phlegm suppressing yang qi. If admixed, all the other factors must be considered before determining treatment.

Sluggish incomplete bowel movements, but not dry stool. The stool may contain mucus

If the sluggishness is minor, it may only be accompanied by abdominal distention, or epigastric fullness and discomfort. If the constipation is more serious, there may be symptoms such as restless feelings of agitation in the chest, fullness and distention in the head and disorientation, disturbing normal thinking, eating and sleeping. Symptoms like these are not life-threatening but are very annoying. A tell-tale indication of the root cause of the whole syndrome is that on those occasions when the bowels move well, the patient suddenly feels light and clear, 'on top of the world'.[23]

The underlying mechanism in this type of constipation is deep internal phlegm obstructing the descent of fu-organ qi. A common associated factor is Liver qi stasis, which by overcoming the Spleen can cause damp and eventually phlegm. It can also directly influence the descent of qi through the Stomach and Intestines.

It should be noted that this is not parched phlegm (zao tan 燥痰) or phlegm-fire causing the constipation by drying out the stool but rather turbid phlegm: the stool is not dry, and may even contain mucus. 'Phlegm-constipation', however, is a diagnosis often overlooked by even experienced Chinese doctors amongst the myriad of other causes: fire, heat, parching dryness, cold, qi obstruction, qi deficiency, yin deficiency, and so on. But it has to be considered, if only to understand why certain treatments fail.[24]

Symptoms may worsen with weather or seasonal changes

Many illnesses are affected by the weather but phlegm diseases are the most obvious. This is due to the nature of phlegm, which follows the flow of qi anywhere in the body and therefore reacts as much to meteorological conditions as the qi does itself.

For example, if cold phlegm has accumulated internally and the weather changes to an overcast or damp state, this increase in yin influence can cause worsening of the heaviness in the head, stuffy chest, nausea, excess salivation, insomnia and heavy limbs, to the extent that the patient may have to stop whatever they are doing and rest.

But in summer, or a very dry autumn, these symptoms will lessen or even disappear altogether.

On the other hand, hot phlegm that has accumulated inside the body will react to weather that is hot or warm and muggy, or a work environment that is at a high temperature, or a noisy disturbing or dirty environment. Symptoms such as distension in the head, palpitations, anxiety, distension of the hands, feet and neck, greasy skin and bitter taste or sticky feeling in the mouth will all worsen. When the temperature is cool, the symptoms can lessen or be relieved, or even in some cases disappear.

TYPICAL PHLEGM SYMPTOMS

1. Vertigo, headache and heavy head
2. Nausea, vomiting, borborygmus; sticky greasy feeling in the mouth; or dry mouth with no desire to drink
3. Intermittent plum-stone throat
4. Difficulty swallowing; vomiting of thin phlegm
5. Chronic chest tightness and stuffiness (this may be described as 'shortness of breath' by the patient); possible sudden heart pain like pressure, heaviness, or compression
6. Palpitations, anxiety, easily startled; insomnia; even fainting and convulsions, or mental disturbance. But neurological signs and symptoms are normal; also no signs of yin xu with yang rising
7. Heavy body, low grade fever; or subjective fever only
8. Local heat sensations (e.g. in the limbs or trunk); or local chills (e.g. a hand-sized cold feeling on the back); or numbness without pain or itching; or a local swelling on the limbs that feels different from the surrounding areas. Western diagnosis is inconclusive
9. Sores and ulcers, or tissue necrosis with weeping or exudation of a sticky phlegm-like material. Long-term failure of such sores to heal-over. Also local thickening of the skin with flaking but no weeping
10. Stuffy chest, distended or cool feeling in the back, that improves with massage or beating; and frequent sighing. These symptoms become more obvious in muggy, overcast or rainy days, or in rapid weather changes
11. Masses or nodes (for example, subcutaneous nodules or abdominal masses), with little change to the overlying skin except perhaps a slight feeling of coolness or darkening of the skin
12. Raw pain in the mouth
13. Subcostal swelling and fullness, possibly with slight pain
14. Variable pulse manifestations.

Explanation of the special characteristics of typical phlegm symptoms

Vertigo, headache and heavy head

In Chinese medicine, the head is considered 'the mansion of clear expanse' (qing xu zhi fu 清虚之府), the residence of original shen (yuan shen 元神)[25] which requires the nourishment of qi, blood, essence and marrow, and which cannot endure interference from unclean murky pathogens.

For example, if phlegm or damp rise up and disturb the 'clear expanse', then the result can be vertigo, headache and a stuffy full feeling in the head. The pathogens phlegm and damp are heavy, turbid and substantial, and as the TCM dictum states: 'It is the nature of phlegm, when causing disease, to follow qi in its ascent and descent, reaching every place without exception.' Thus phlegm-damp can rise, impede clear yang and also enter and choke the circulation both inside and outside of the blood vessels. In bio-medical terms, the resulting condition is similar to that of hypertension with loss of vascular elasticity and eventually sclerosis. It is noteworthy, too, that hypertensive patients with symptoms of phlegm rising and clouding the clear yang usually respond well to treatment based upon transforming and clearing phlegm-damp.

There is a fundamental difference between the mechanisms involved in phlegm-induced vertigo, headache and heavy head, and the similar condition resulting from deficiency of qi and blood. They both may be constant and chronic, or intermittent, but in the case of phlegm the use of qi lifting and tonifying will worsen the condition.

Nausea, vomiting, borborygmus; sticky greasy feeling in the mouth; or dry mouth with no desire to drink

Phlegm and damp hindering the normal descent of Stomach and Intestinal qi will lead to nausea, vomiting and the sound of fluids sloshing about the abdomen.

Phlegm and mucus being carried upward will lead to a sticky feeling in the mouth and a greasy taste.

Phlegm and mucus are originally derived from physiological fluids (jin-ye): when normal fluid transformation fails, the jin-ye condense, and the end result is a pathological production of phlegm. As this pathogen begins to build up, however, its very accumulation further retards the normal fluid transformation and transportation. The inability of the Spleen to transport fluids upward, because of phlegm-damp oppression, leads to dryness of the mouth. Moreover, the ever-growing impediment to Spleen transport means that less and less normal fluids are being produced, which further exacerbates the situation. The most effective treatment approach is to warm and assist Spleen transformation of phlegm and damp, with a formula such as Ping Wei San (Calm the Stomach Powder, *Formulas and Strategies*, p. 181), or moxa on Zhong Wan (CV-12) with reduction of Feng Long (ST-40). In some cases it may be necessary to open the Liver qi flow to assist Spleen transport.

The differentiating point in this symptom is the lack of desire to drink. If questioned closely, the patient will often report that, even though they have a dry mouth, drinking water will not help, and that they even feel epigastric discomfort or nausea. This is because adding water to an excess of damp will additionally hamper Spleen and Stomach function.

Intermittent plum-stone throat

Usually this is a consequence of Liver qi knotting up due to emotional imbalance. As it gets worse, Spleen is affected, normal transport and digestion is diminished and body fluids coalesce into phlegm. This phlegm follows the qi up to the throat and jams there, bringing on a feeling of something physically stuck in the throat, which cannot be swallowed or brought up.

One of the characteristics of phlegm, as noted previously, is its cyclical accumulation and dispersal. In this case the cycle depends on the emotional state and the effect of that emotional state on the qi. When the qi flows openly without restraint, the throat is clear; but with stress or pressure, the feeling in the throat returns. If this process continues for an extended period of time deficiency of yin may occur, because Spleen production of normal yin fluids is reduced, while pathological fluids such as phlegm and damp increase. As yin decreases, xu-fire builds up which further damages the yin. This results in a combined yin-deficiency and phlegm-excess condition. At this stage, simply attempting to remove phlegm would be disastrous. Normal fluids would be severely injured and the dry obstructed throat symptoms would become worse. Yin-moistening herbs must be added to support fluids, and dispersal becomes secondary.

Difficulty swallowing; vomiting of thin phlegm

Here again emotions precipitate the symptoms. The qi flow is impaired, jin-ye dries, phlegm forms and it may even reach the stage where blood stagnates and fuses with the phlegm.

This is the difference between the former symptom of plum-stone throat and the present dysphagia: in the previous condition, despite a feeling of obstruction, there was no actual difficulty swallowing. In the present state, the barrier is substantial.

If, however, the mass is not located in the throat but in or around the stomach, the result can be a inhibition of downward movement from the Stomach, with a consequent vomiting upward of thin phlegm.

Chronic chest tightness and stuffiness (this may be described as 'shortness of breath' by the patient); possible sudden heart pain like pressure, heaviness or compression

In this case phlegm is impeding the Heart yang, yang qi is failing to circulate properly, and the patient will feel, first, a tightness in the chest and then, as the yang qi becomes more obstructed, pain.

Alternatively, it may initially be the Heart yang itself which is deficient, so that a yin 'mist' arises and clouds the Heart yang, finally ending in phlegm oppressing the chest.

These symptoms are similar to the bio-medical disorder of coronary heart disease. But for patients whose TCM etiology involves phlegm, the use of blood stagnation removers[26] of any description will not be enough. They must be accompanied by herbs that warm yang and transform phlegm in order to achieve effect.

Palpitations, anxiety, easily startled; insomnia; even fainting and convulsions, or mental disturbance. But neurological signs and symptoms are normal; also no signs of yin xu with yang rising

Zhu Dan-Xi says in regard to severe palpitations: 'This is generally blood deficiency. If it is worse with worry or anxiety, it is from deficiency, and usually lack of blood. If it comes and goes, this is phlegm being moved by fire. In thin people, lack of blood will usually be the cause; in fat people it is almost always from phlegm.'[27] The other symptoms too can result from phlegm misting the Heart, and occluding the shen.

Heavy body, low grade fever; or subjective fever only

Phlegm is a yin pathogen, with a sticky nature that easily lies latent deep inside the body. This latent deep-lying phlegm can hinder the yang qi from expanding properly, so that yang increases internally and heat builds up.

This is different from exogenous fever and also from yin, blood, or qi deficient fever. The special differentiating point is the *heavy body* and low fever.

Clinically, idiopathic low-grade fever is quite common. As a rule, if it is not in the category of yin deficiency or qi deficiency, it is probably phlegm. Careless use of yin or qi tonifying herbs in this case will add to the phlegm and turn the condition into a long drawn-out affair. To avoid this, symptoms such as pulse and tongue should be painstakingly checked to determine the real underlying cause.

Local heat sensations (e.g. in limbs or trunk); or local chills (e.g. palm-sized cold feeling on the back); or numbness without pain or itching; or a local swelling on the limbs that feels different from the surrounding areas. Western diagnosis is inconclusive

These symptoms result from local phlegm build up obstructing the flow of protective and nutritive qi through the surface tissues. Numbness from patho-genic wind tends to be fleeting and not fixed in position, whereas numbness from phlegm will not move as quickly. Over a period of time, if not dispersed, the phlegm can collect and form nodes and lumps. As the saying has it: '[Phlegm's] accompanying symptoms may all be different, and there may be hundreds of possible pathological permutations'.

Sores and ulcers, or tissue necrosis with weeping or exudation of a sticky phlegm-like material. Long-term failure of sores to heal-over. Also local thickening of the skin with flaking but no weeping

Phlegm and damp, or hot phlegm accumulation, affect the local flow of qi and blood, and can cause exudation of the substantial phlegm. When this becomes severe, it can lead to ulceration.

Long term cases will have weak zheng qi, plus an open wound allowing exogenous invasion of wind, cold or heat. Under these conditions, normal nutritive and protective qi cannot reach the area to heal it in the usual way.

This can start as turbid phlegm accumulation but end as qi and yin deficiency plus stubborn-phlegm (wan tan 頑痰). Once at this stage, the skin often thickens and scales, the lack of exudate showing that normal fluids are exhausted.

Stuffy chest, distended or cool feeling in the back, that improves with massage or beating; and frequent sighing. These symptoms become more obvious in muggy, overcast, or rainy days, or in rapid weather changes

Phlegm frustrates yang qi flow, including the spread and dispersal of Lung qi. Massage, beating and even sighing helps qi move, thus providing relief, although only temporarily.

If phlegm stalls in the back, the hindering of yang qi flow generates a feeling of distension or cold.

As noted previously, the symptoms' responsiveness to weather changes is an indication of phlegm (or damp) involvement.

Masses or nodes (for example, subcutaneous nodules or abdominal masses), with little change to the overlying skin except perhaps a slight feeling of coolness or darkening of the skin

Yang qi deficiency or emotions leading to qi obstruction can weaken Spleen's ability to transport, so that damp and finally phlegm gather and begin to interfere with the flow of qi. Once turbid phlegm collects, the flow of qi becomes even more clogged and the phlegm can coalesce into knots or swellings. The patient often worries about this and a vicious cycle of increasing qi stasis and phlegm build-up occurs, with the nodes becoming ever more firm and difficult to break up.

If the skin or complexion is obviously darkened, this means the accumulation is formed of stubborn phlegm and 'dead' blood (si xue 死血). This can only be treated by both transforming stubborn phlegm and breaking up dead blood. If the condition is chronic, attacking and tonifying will have to be used in combination by adding yang warming and yin nourishing herbs, plus fragrant piercing substances such as musk or insect drugs to enter the lump and disperse. This will help prevent a further development of the mass.

Raw pain in the mouth

This is intermittent raw pain in the mouth, with a tender red tongue that is sensitive to pungent, spicy, salty, hot, sour or astringent foods; or even acid foods such as oranges. The symptom can be very debilitating, influencing eating, work and finally overall health.

Usually mouth pain is considered a fire or heat symptom. While this is not exactly wrong, most often the symptom is a result of combined yin deficiency and phlegm, occurring most frequently in women patients with damaged blood and fluids.

There are three facets to treatment: nourishing yin, moistening dryness and transforming hot phlegm. If the phlegm transformation is ignored, the results will not be satisfactory. Raw pain in the mouth should always alert one to look for yin deficiency with parched phlegm. (See the case history 'Stubborn phlegm lodged in the San Jiao' later in this chapter.)

Subcostal swelling and fullness, possibly with slight pain

Subcostal swelling, stuffiness and pain is related, usually, to the stresses of work and living, through the chronic inhibition of Liver qi. But such a chronic condition rarely leaves the Spleen unscathed, and

phlegm is then the almost inevitable result. This is especially so because impairment of the flow of qi will slow fluid circulation in general around the body, so that even a tiny local obstruction of fluids can, under these conditions, grow into phlegm. Thus subcostal fullness should be a reminder to look for symptoms of phlegm.

Variable pulse manifestations

The most usual types of pulse in phlegm cases are slippery, wiry, deep and slow.

Strong hot phlegm internally is shown by a slippery and wiry pulse.

Knotted stubborn phlegm internally produces deep or slow pulses.

Li Shi-Zhen, in his *Bin Hu Mai Xue* ('The Pulse Studies of Bin Hu', 1564), says:

1. Rapid means heat, slow is cold, slippery is phlegm.[28]
2. Deep cun (distal) position means phlegm obstruction or stagnant pathological water in the chest.[29]
3. Slow shows a zang illness or abundant phlegm.[30]
4. Cun (distal) slippery means phlegm around the diaphragm causing nausea and vomiting.[31]

Clinically, however, it is difficult to predict exactly what type of pulse a patient with phlegm may present, due to the numerous variables involved in phlegm pathology. Therefore a diagnosis of phlegm—or no phlegm—should not be based solely on the pulse but should include all symptoms, equally weighed.

Summary

The symptoms described in the two sections above are typical clinical manifestations of phlegm, in regard to both symptoms and body types.

But it must be remembered that not every patient will have every manifestation. Factors such as climate (hot or cold, wet or dry), work (mental or physical), age, sex, standard of living, life-style habits, and so on, will all make a big difference in the presenting symptoms of individual patients. For example, a sedentary office worker who fancies himself a gourmet will tend to grow fat, become dizzy and have palpitations: all highly likely symptoms. Or, a late-middle-aged woman with Liver qi stasis failing to assist Spleen transport will likely have phlegm obstructing the chest, back, flanks or epigastric area, or obstructing the throat. Because of the feelings of obstruction, she will probably often sigh a lot to disperse the phlegm, and feel temporary relief after massage. Thus the special characteristics of phlegm symptoms and the constitutional indications of phlegm must be considered in the light of the patient's actual living situation to appreciate their diagnostic significance.

COMBINATION OF PHLEGM AND OTHER PATHOGENS

Phlegm has a tendency to combine with other pathogens, often those which led to the phlegm formation in the first place. These are therefore often described in the TCM literature, both Classical and modern, in terms of a combined nomenclature. For example, accumulation of damp into phlegm, with some pathogenic damp still remaining in con-

junction with the phlegm is usually termed 'phlegm-damp' (tan shi 痰湿) or 'damp-phlegm' (shi tan 湿痰). Wind and phlegm existing together is called 'wind-phlegm' (feng tan 风痰), although the problem then remains as to whether the wind referred to is exogenous or endogenous—this is solved by calling it 'wai feng feng tan' ('exogenous-wind wind-phlegm' 外风风痰) or 'nei feng feng tan' ('endogenous-wind wind-phlegm 內风风痰); phlegm resulting from the invasion of a zao-drying pathogen which desiccates the fluids is called 'dry-phlegm' (or 'parched-phlegm'—zao tan 燥痰); phlegm building up as the consequence of stagnating food in the middle Jiao is called 'food-phlegm' (shi tan 食痰); phlegm resulting from deficiency of either yin or yang is called 'deficient-phlegm' (xu tan 虚痰); while all other types of phlegm are known as 'excess-phlegm' (shi tan 实痰); and so on. The seeming complexity of the terminology reflects the extent to which Chinese medicine has investigated phlegm pathology but there is little actual difficulty when the terms are found in context.

Figures 7.1-7.8 are examples of how and where these pathogenic combinations interact and the symptoms engendered by this interaction.[32]

Fig. 7.1 Production of exogenous wind-phlegm (wai feng feng tan)

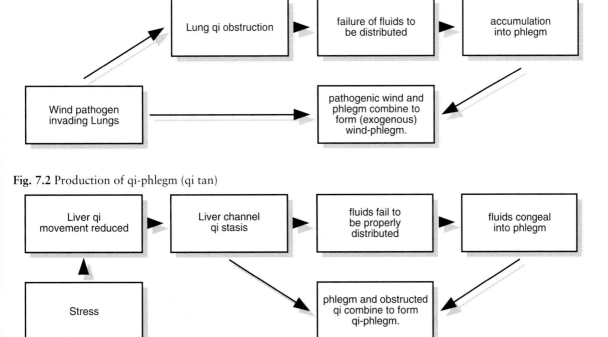

Fig. 7.2 Production of qi-phlegm (qi tan)

Fig. 7.3 Production of hot-phlegm or phlegm-fire (re tan, tan huo)

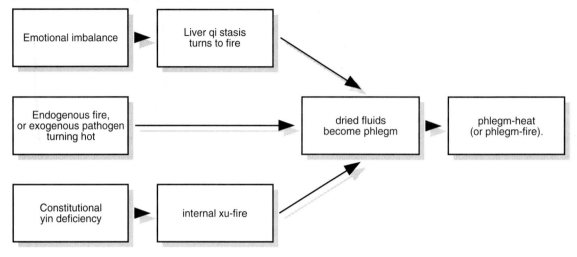

Fig. 7.4 Production of endogenous wind-phlegm (nei feng feng tan)

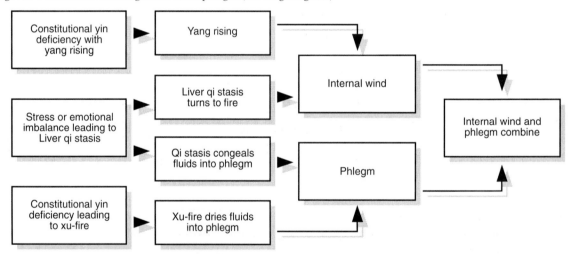

Fig. 7.5 Production of damp-phlegm (shi tan)

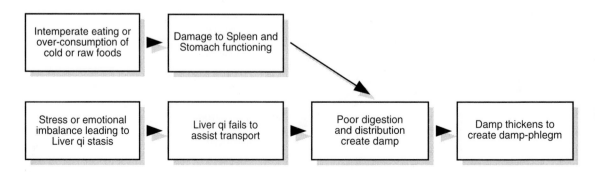

Fig. 7.6 Production of stagnation-phlegm (tan yu)

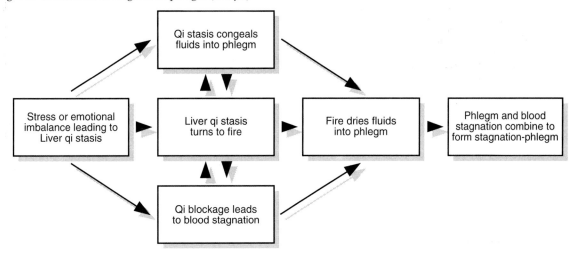

Fig. 7.7 Production of parched-phlegm (zao tan)

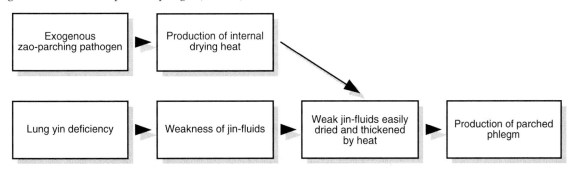

Fig. 7.8 Production of cold-phlegm (han tan)

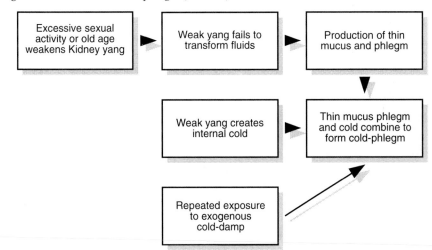

Notes. See also Appendix 3

1. Wind phlegm will be located in the Lungs and have a white, thin, frothy appearance. It may be accompanied by surface symptoms such as chills, fever and recently developed cough; and the tongue coat will be thin white.
2. Qi-phlegm will be located either in the channels and collaterals, the Liver or the Heart. The telling symptoms may be soft painless nodes in the neck, breast, or inguinal region that do not have any changes in skin color; 'plum-stone throat'; sensation of fullness in the chest; mood swings; apathy; or the loss of concentration and mental 'presence'. The tongue coat will usually be thin and greasy.
3. Hot-phlegm will be located in the Lungs and have sticky thick yellow phlegm, possibly with pus or even blood in it. The face may be red, there may be thirst and possibly fever. The tongue body will be red, the tongue coat yellow and greasy.
    Phlegm-fire will be located in the Heart or the Liver and because these organs are not open to the surface, may not have visible phlegm unless phlegm is also affecting another area. The symptoms may be an anxious feeling of restlessness in the chest (xin fan), nightmares, bitter taste and dry mouth, fury or other loss of mental equilibrium, red eyes, sound of phlegm in the throat, stroke, or even coma. The tongue and coat will be as in phlegm-heat.
4. Endogenous wind-phlegm will be located in the Liver and have symptoms of hemiplegia, facial paralysis, cramps, epilepsy and difficulty swallowing, plus bringing up phlegm and the sound of phlegm in the throat. The tongue coat may be thin white or thin greasy.
5. Damp-phlegm will be located either in the Lungs, or in the Liver, Heart, or Spleen and Stomach. If in the Lungs, the phlegm will be visible: appearing white, sticky, profuse and easy to cough out, with a thick phlegmy sound to the cough, and there may be a feeling of tightness in the chest, loss of appetite and possibly loose stool.
    If the damp-phlegm is in the Liver, Heart, or Spleen and Stomach, the phlegm may not be visible (e.g. coughed out), but these locations can share the following symptoms: the patient will be heavy-set, there may be dizziness and a heavy head as if wrapped up in something, there may be excessive saliva, sensation of fullness in the chest, variable concentration, reduced appetite and a possible vomiting of thin phlegm.
    The tongue coat in damp-phlegm will usually be white greasy.
6. Stagnant blood phlegm can be located in the Heart, Liver, channels and collaterals, or the Spleen and Stomach. In the Heart, the symptoms may be a feeling of tightness in the chest with occasional bouts of chest pain. In the Liver, the symptoms may be sequela of stroke, numbness of the limbs and stiffness of the tongue with difficult speech. In the channels and collaterals, there may be joint pain and swelling with restricted movement and deformity of the joint. In the Spleen and Stomach, there may be pain in the epigastric region or the chest, difficulty swallowing and vomiting of phlegm and/or dark blood.
7. Exogenous parching (zao) pathogen combining with phlegm will be located in the Lungs, where it will manifest a dry cough, possibly producing a slight amount of sticky stretchy phlegm which will be difficult to cough out. Accompanying symptoms will show obvious damage to body fluids: dry nose and throat, dry mouth, dry stool, scanty urine, dry skin and possibly fever. The tongue coat will be thin white and dry. The tongue itself may have a red tip.
8. Cold phlegm can be located either in the Lungs, or in the channels and collaterals.
    If in the Lungs, the phlegm will be white, thin, profuse and easy to cough out. The patient will have a sound of thick phlegm in the throat. There may also be wheeze, dyspnea, chills and pallor with perhaps a slightly bluish tinge. The tongue coat will be white and slippery, the tongue pale, the pulse deep wiry, deep tight, or deep and slow, unless the phlegm is welling upwards—as in an attack of asthma—during which time it may be floating-tight or floating-slippery.
    If the cold-phlegm is in the channels and collaterals, there may be sore aching joints with local swelling but no change in skin color and no local heat. Again the tongue coat will be white and slippery and the tongue itself pale.

Other common phlegm combinations

Some other examples of phlegm combinations which are commonly seen are food-phlegm (shi tan 食痰), stubborn-phlegm (wan tan 頑痰), and turbid-phlegm (tan zhuo 痰濁).

Food phlegm is the result of frequent consumption of alcohol and rich foods which damage the Spleen and Stomach and prevent complete digestion, so that undigested food builds up in the middle Jiao and eventually creates phlegm. This is related to phlegm-damp.

Stubborn phlegm is phlegm that is difficult to eliminate despite protracted therapy, and that may have caused stubborn, hard-to-dissolve nodes and accumulations.

Turbid-phlegm is a very frequently mentioned phlegm combination in traditional Chinese medicine. The term 'turbid' (zhuo 濁) is often used in contradistinction to 'clear' (qing 清), and thus turbid phlegm is often used for situations in which upper body symptoms manifest, especially in the head and the chest, such as vertigo, coma and chest pain (i.e. where phlegm is obstructing the 'ascent of clear yang' or misting the Heart shen—the 'clear spirit': shen ming 神明). However, it can also be used for visible phlegm, if it is particularly sticky thick and murky, or when damp-phlegm produces an especially thick greasy tongue coat.

The following case history from Zhu Ceng–Bo illustrates the importance of understanding the mechanisms involved in phlegm formation.

Case history: Chronic phlegm–heat

The patient, a female aged 48 years presented on 6 October 1977. For five years she had experienced extensive and frequent ulcerations of the oral cavity, including the upper and lower gums and tongue, with burning pain.

Seven years previously, the patient began to experience occasional mild ulcerations of the mouth, with minor pain and heat sensations which responded to symptomatic treatment but would recur. These would appear every several weeks, with rare remissions of one or two months. Over the last three years the condition has worsened, so that the areas of ulceration began to merge, and began to appear more and more frequently, until five or six days pain free days per month seemed like a godsend.

During the ulcerations, the mouth would be burning, there would be a sensation of restless anxiety in the chest, the urine would be dark, and the palms and soles would feel heat as if she had been scalded. The mouth was dry but without desire to drink much water.

The continuous ulcerations affected eating and the patient reported that she had lost 20 kg over the last three years, going from stout to quite thin.

The complexion was red and moist, the voice strong and the patient's energy relatively good. The pulse was deep, slippery and strong; the tongue body red, completely covered with a thin yellow coat.

Besides reporting that she preferred bland foods (mainly because the least taste of salt or spice would set off her mouth ulcers), there were no other notable food preferences, and there was no other remarkable medical history.

Over the last several years the patient had consulted many doctors, all without success, and she was at her wits' end.

Comment

This condition is chronic phlegm-heat lying deep within the body, alternatively affecting the Heart, Lungs, Liver, Gall Bladder, Spleen, Stomach and Kidneys. Because it influences such a wide area, it can be called a 'stubborn phlegm deep in the San Jiao' syndrome.

According to the TCM theory of the internal organs, the various areas of the mouth—left and right, above and below, upper and lower gums, the top and bottom of the tongue—each belong to different organs within the body. These different areas of influence each being affected at different times by burning and ulceration, accompanied by agitation in the chest, darkish urine, burning heat in the palms and soles, and so on, plus the signs of the pulse and tongue coating, indicate without doubt that the condition is one of hot phlegm lodged within the San Jiao.

Once the body's fluids have coalesced into phlegm, this phlegm can become arrested within any of the body's tissues or organs, as it is said: 'Phlegm follows the qi to accumulate, and there is no place it cannot reach'.

Since the phlegm is deep-lying, it requires a stimulus before it becomes stirred up, which in this case is Liver and Kidney fire. When Liver and Kidney fire has subsided, the fire is dormant, the phlegm at rest, and the condition goes into remission. When the Liver and Kidney fire becomes aroused, all of the channels are affected, phlegm is stirred and rises with the qi, setting off an attack.

The burning of the oral cavity and the agitation in the chest are signs of the blazing upward of the lower Jiao fire, while the dry mouth without desire to drink is the peculiar characteristic of phlegm and body fluid obstruction.

The patient's preference for bland food is due to the diuretic effect of the bland flavor, which reduces the dominance of damp and phlegm, and is an important clue to the differentiation of phlegm disease which should never be overlooked.

The tenacity of the condition is the result of its etiology: the patient became worried about her illness and this impediment to the flow of qi led both to accumulation of fluids and to heat, and then fire which dried the fluids into phlegm. This type of vicious cycle is not amenable to the usual forms of treatment for mouth ulcers but instead requires cooling of the fire in each of the organs comprising the 'San Jiao', as well as transformation of the stubborn phlegm.

Prescription

Xuan Shen	30 g	Scrophulariae Ningpoensis, Radix
Quan Gua Lou	30 g	Trichosanthis, Fructus et Pericarpium
Zhe Bei Mu	9 g	Fritillariae Thunbergii, Bulbus
Xing Ren	15 g	Pruni Armeniacae, Semen
Long Gu	30 g	Draconis, Os
Mu Li	30 g	Ostreae, Concha
Shi Gao	30 g	Gypsum
Huang Qin	15 g	Scutellariae Baicalensis, Radix
Huang Lian	6 g	Coptidis, Rhizoma
Qing Dai	9 g	Indigo Pulverata Levis
Mu Dan Pi	15 g	Moutan Radicis, Cortex
Ge Ke	30 g	Cyclinae Sinensis, Concha
Ze Xie	24 g	Alismatis Plantago-aquaticae, Rhizoma

5 bags total, 1 bag per day, each bag decocted twice to provide a morning and night dose.

Explanation

Xuan Shen (Scrophulariae), *Zhe Bei Mu* (Fritillariae), *Quan Gua Lou* (Trichosanthis) and *Xing Ren* (Pruni Armeniacae) combined into the same formula will clear and transform hot-phlegm, and when combined with *Mu Li* (Ostreae, Concha), *Qing Dai* (Indigo) and *Ge Ke* (Cyclinae) will strengthen the ability to disperse phlegm-heat's cohesiveness. Raw *Shi Gao* (Gypsum) and raw *Long Gu* (Draconis, Os), used together, will not only clear the fire and heat from the Lungs and Stomach but also will suppress the ascending tendency of the lower Jiao fire. It is only when the lower Jiao Liver and Kidney fire is quiet and collected that the instigating factor in this condition can be removed, thus reducing the opportunity for attacks.

Huang Qin (Scutellariae) and *Huang Lian* (Coptidis) combined can cool the heat of the Heart, Lungs, Liver, Gall Bladder, Spleen and Stomach and their associated channels, for when this heat is removed, the cohesiveness of the phlegm—which is the consequence of heat drying fluids—is reduced as well.

Although this patient has suffered from her problem for many years, her energy and constitution remain strong, which is a characteristic sign of phlegm excess (shi tan 实痰). Because of the acutely excess nature of the condition, the bitter coldness of the prescription will not be harmful.

The *Mu Dan Pi* (Moutan) cools the blood and drains heat, and the large dosage of *Ze Xie* (Alisma) functions to drain away the dispersed phlegm through diuresis, providing another route for the removal of phlegm from the body.

After these five days of herbs, the ulcerations in the oral cavity were 80-90% cleared. The patient reported that as she drank the herbs, the restless anxious feeling in the chest would disappear, which is the result to be expected if the pent-up heat and phlegm are being dispersed by the herbs.

On the second consultation, *Xuan Fu Hua* (Inulae, Flos) 15 g was added to further transform and disperse stubborn phlegm.

After ten days of taking herbs (one bag per day), the lesions had cleared. Follow-up two years after this revealed no recurrence, and a further communication five years later confirmed that the condition was completely cured.[33]

DIFFERENT TREATMENT METHODS IN PHLEGM CONDITIONS

The principles of treatment in phlegm disease are based upon the differentiation of the origin, nature and location of the phlegm. If this differentiation is incorrect, the principle of treatment will be inappropriate, and thus the herbs or points selected will not match the condition of the patient. Under these circumstances, a successful treatment will be simply a fluke.

To illustrate the importance of proper differentiation, a list of some of the possible treatment principles in phlegm disease is presented below. For a full discussion of these and other treatments see both the following chapter and the Appendix on the history and development of phlegm disease theory in traditional Chinese medicine.

1. Weak Spleen transport, allowing phlegm to accumulate from damp, is treated by restoring normal transformation and transportation, while parching damp and transforming phlegm

2. Kidney yang deficiency failing to support Spleen transformation of food and fluids is treated by warm transformation of damp and thin-mucus, followed by tonification of both Spleen and Kidney yang

3. Kidney yang deficiency failing to support Urinary Bladder qi transformation, allowing lower Jiao fluids to flood and become phlegm, is treated by restoration of Urinary Bladder qi transformation through tonification of Kidney yang

4. Yin deficiency with fire drying fluids into phlegm is treated by moistening and transforming phlegm

5. Pent-up heat in San Jiao drying fluids into phlegm is treated by cooling heat, moving qi and transforming phlegm[34]

6. Severe accumulation of thin mucus resulting from Spleen and/or Kidney yang deficiency is treated by first eliminating the thin mucus, then tonifying Spleen and Kidney yang

7. Exogenous pathogenic factors invading the Lungs can bring about phlegm accumulation by disturbing the clearing and descending function of the Lungs. This must be treated by restoring Lung function and transforming phlegm

8. Phlegm collecting into nodules must be softened with salty-cold herbs and then dispersed

9. Food stagnation in the Stomach requires dispersal of the accumulated food and leading it downward into the Intestines for expulsion from the body

10. Liver wind can be (and often is) complicated by phlegm, so that when Liver wind rises phlegm follows, and the mind is disturbed. Wind must be extinguished while phlegm is dispersed

11. Phlegm obstructing the movement of Heart yang can cause chest pain, palpitations, epilepsy and depression. Phlegm must be scoured away to free Heart yang circulation.

12. Phlegm blocking the orifices is treated by opening the orifices and transforming phlegm

13. Phlegm in the channels, collaterals and surface tissues is treated by opening collaterals and removing phlegm.

NOTES

1. Quoted in *Zhong Yi Tan Bing Xue* ('TCM Phlegm Disease Studies'), by Zhu Ceng-Bo, Hubei Science and Technology Press, 1984, p. 3. Most of this chapter is based on selections from this book.

2. Bing si xie gui, dao qu zhi tan, bing nai ke an 病似邪鬼，导去滞痰，病乃可安. Quoted in *Zhong Yi Tan Bing Xue* ('TCM Phlegm Disease Studies'), by Zhu Ceng-Bo, Hubei Science and Technology Press, 1984, p. 3.

3. See Chapter 6 for a detailed discussion of these types of pathologies.

4. *Zhu Bing Yuan Hou Lun Jiao Shi* (Annotated Explanation of the 'Generalized Treatise on the Etiology and Symptomatolgy of Diseases'), annotated by the Nanjing College of TCM, People's Health Publishing, 1983, pp. 607-611. See the Appendix on the development of phlegm theory in traditional Chinese medicine where this essay is translated in full. Ever since the Tang dynasty, this book, which discusses etiology and symptomatology exclusively, has had a huge developmental influence on traditional medicine in China.

5. Quoted in *Zhong Yi Tan Bing Xue* ('TCM Phlegm Disease Studies'), by Zhu Ceng-Bo, Hubei Science and Technology Press, 1984, p. 25.

6. *Jing Yue Quan Shu* ('Complete Works of Jing Yue', 1624) Shanghai Science and Technology Press, 1959, p. 531. See the Appendix on the development of phlegm theory in traditional Chinese medicine for a full translation of this essay.

7. Quoted in *Zhong Yi Tan Bing Xue* ('TCM Phlegm Disease Studies'), by Zhu Ceng-Bo, Hubei Science and Technology Press, 1984, p. 25.

8. *Yi Fang Ji Jie Bei Yao* ('Essentials from the Analytic Collection of Medical Formulas'), Chao Ren Publishing, Taichong, Taiwan, 1981, p. 290.

9. It probably need not be said that Chen Shi–Duo was a strong proponent of the Mingmen school, along the same lines as Zhao Xian-Ke in his *Yi Guan* ('Key Link of Medicine', 1683), which contains an almost identical passage as that just quoted. Chen Shi-Duo went a bit farther to provide support for his ideas, however, claiming that the *Shi Shi Mi Lu* ('Secret Records of the Stone Chamber') was a record of conversations between Huang Di and his ministers, passed down by Qi Bo, and further annotated by Zhang Ji, Hua Tuo and later Lei Gong. The above quote is taken from the *Zhong Yi Ji Chu Li Lun Xiang Jie* ('Detailed Explanation of TCM Basic Theory'), Fujian Science and Technology Press, 1981, p. 63.

10. Quoted in *Zhong Yi Tan Bing Xue* ('TCM Phlegm Disease Studies'), by Zhu Ceng-Bo, Hubei Science and Technology Press, 1984, p.27.

11. See the Appendix on the development of phlegm theory in traditional Chinese medicine for a full translation of this essay.

12. Quoted in *Zhong Yi Tan Bing Xue* ('TCM Phlegm Disease Studies'), by Zhu Ceng-Bo, Hubei Science and Technology Press, 1984, p. 33.

13. For those who wish to know the 'Way' mentioned by Jing–Yue, see the essay by Zhou Xue-Hai in his *Du Yi Sui Bi* ('Random Notes while Reading Medicine', 1898) at the end of the Appendix on the development of phlegm theory in traditional Chinese medicine, where he discusses this quote from the *Su Wen*, Chapter 8.

14. Quoted in *Zhong Yi Tan Bing Xue* ('TCM Phlegm Disease Studies'), by Zhu Ceng-Bo, Hubei Science and Technology Press, 1984, p. 29.

15. *San Yin Ji Yi Bing Zheng Fang Lun* ('Discussion of Illnesses, Patterns, and Formulas Related to the Unification of the Three Etiologies'), 1174, by Chen Yan (zi-name Wu–Ze); People's Health Publishing, Beijing, 1957, p. 174.

16. *Lei Jing* ('Systematic Categorization of the *Nei Jing*'), 1624, by Zhang Jing-Yue; People's Health Publishing, Beijing, 1982, p. 465.

17. 'Shen wu tan zheng'. This refers to the locus of activity of the pathogenic phlegm, not to its pathogenesis, with which (as noted) Kidneys play an extremely important role. The above sentiments are in line with the general observation that 'Kidneys have no shi (excess) conditions'.

18. Quoted in *Zhong Yi Tan Bing Xue* ('TCM Phlegm Disease Studies'), by Zhu Ceng–Bo, Hubei Science and Technology Press, 1984, p. 32.

19. These symptoms must be differentiated from qi or blood deficient headaches and dizziness, which can be done by determining precipitating factors, such as whether the symptoms are brought on by odors or instead, for example, by over-exertion if the cause is lack of qi. Patients may, of course, have both qi and blood deficiency and phlegm accumulation. In Western cultures, dairy products such as milk and cheese have long been considered to increase phlegm and patients will often consciously avoid them for that reason.

It must be recognized, though, that the yang-lifting effect of pungent fragrance will also trigger an up-rush of yang where this tendency already exists, such as in Liver-yang-rising patients.

20. Here, too, the cause may be deficiency of qi or blood but the sensitive patient can tell the difference: phlegm vagueness seems to 'cloud' the mind, they can almost grasp the elusive idea, which they know is there behind a veil of fog or smoke. With qi or blood deficiency, however, the mind feels 'empty'. Treatment in the first case will necessitate the use of herbs such as *Yuan Zhi* (Polygalae Tenuifoliae, Radix) and *Shi Chang Pu* (Acori Graminei, Rhizoma); while in the second case, a formula such as Bu Zhong Yi Qi Tang ('Tonify the Middle and Augment the Qi Decoction', *Formulas and Strategies*, p. 241) is more appropriate, to lift the clear yang to the head.

21 See Chapter Two, under 'Salivation'.

22. *Zhu Bing Yuan Hou Lun* ('General Treatise on the Etiology and Symptomatology of Disease'), 610 AD, by Chao Yuan-Fang, in 2 volumes, annotated by the Nanjing TCM College, People's Publishing, Beijing, 1983, p. 608.

23. This is so to such an extent that it led one (past) U.S. President to exclaim 'I have long been convinced that a good reliable set of bowels is worth any amount of brains!'

24. For example, Ma Zi Ren Wan ('Hemp Seed Pill', *Formulas and Strategies*, p. 123) is the most common formula in the treatment of constipation. But in this case it would not only not cure the problem, it would even make the constipation worse and the abdomen more distended. The reason is that Hemp Seed Pill is designed for a dry type constipation and so consists of intestinal moistening herbs. But as we have seen, the stool is not dry. The moistening herbs only exacerbate the problem, like adding oil to grease.

What is needed are herbs to restore qi flow and cut phlegm. Zhu Ceng-Bo, a modern author who has written extensively on TCM phlegm theory, advocates the use of the following herbs:

Bai Zhu	Atractylodis Macrocephalae, Rhizoma
Zhi Shi	Citri seu Ponciri Immaturis, Fructus
Qiang Huo	Notopterygii, Rhizoma et Radix
Fang Feng	Ledebouriellae Sesloidis, Radix
Chai Hu	Bupleuri, Radix
Bai Jie Zi	Sinapsis Albae, Semen

He comments 'When Spleen qi rises, and phlegm is dispersed, the results exceed all expectation'. The lifting of Spleen qi is necessary as an initial step in the restoration of the normal flow of qi, because it will have been dragged downward by the heavy damp and phlegm.

25. This term originated in the *Ben Cao Gang Mu*. Yuan originally meant the head. The head is also called jing ming zhi fu 精明之府, 'mansion of the clear essence', because the jing-essence of the zang and fu organs rise and collect in the head and especially in the eyes, where the shen is manifest.

26. A very effective single herb for angina, of the blood stagnation removing variety, is *San Qi* (Pseudoginseng, Radix).

27. *Dan Xi Zhi Fa Xin Yao* ('Essentials from the Treatments of [Zhu] Dan-Xi'), Shandong Science and Technology Press, 1985, p. 136.

28. *Bin Hu Mai Xue Xin Shi* ('New Explanation of The Pulse Studies of Bin Hu'), Henan Science and Technology Press, 1983, p. 11.

29. *Ibid.*, p 11.

30. *Ibid.*, p. 17.

31. *Ibid.*, p. 29.

32. The charts and diagrams in this section were based on those in the book *Tan He Tan Zheng* ('Phlegm and Phlegm Symptoms') by He Xi–Yan, Jiangsu Science and Technology Press, 1978, pp. 6-7 and pp. 12-13.

33. This case history was taken from *Zhong Yi Tan Bing Xue* ('TCM Phlegm Disease Studies') by Zhu Ceng-Bo, Hubei Science and Technology Press, 1984, pp. 78-80.

34. It may be asked: 'What is the difference between this and number four: yin deficiency with fire drying fluids into phlegm?' The answer is that the situation in number four is xu-fire, from yin deficiency, while that in number five is shi-fire, from pent-up heat.
Q: Is this difference important?
A: It is crucial. The methods of treatment and herbs used are all different. Yin-xu fire is treated with moistening yin-tonics, while shi-fire is treated with bitter cold herbs.
Q: So what if you make a mistake?
A: Think of it: pent-up San Jiao further blocked by greasy yin-tonics, or weak yin further drained by bitter herbs. Can you afford to be careless?

Phlegm treatment: principles and methods

8

This chapter will introduce both the general principles involved in the treatment of phlegm, and specific methods with suggested formulas for common classes of phlegm disease. Because of the variability of phlegm conditions, it is not possible to cover every possible circumstance in which phlegm is a factor. If the principles and methods are mastered, however, and the diagnosis is correct, then it will be possible to make an appropriate choice of method for the condition, with adjustments for the individual patient.

INTRODUCTION

As mentioned in the previous chapter, phlegm is both the product of pathological processes and a disease-causing agent in its own right. Thus the overall guiding principle for dealing with phlegm disease can be contained in the Chinese phrase 'fu zheng qu xie'—restore the Correct and eliminate the Deviant (or 'strengthen the zheng qi and eliminate the pathogen').[1]

One very common principle of phlegm treatment is restoration of qi flow with herbs to transform phlegm, followed by harmonization of the middle Jiao to eliminate the thin mucus which often precipitates it. Once the qi moves, the fluids which have hitherto accumulated begin to be properly distributed, and so the phlegm disperses.

Another common principle is warming transformation. Because phlegm is a yin pathogen, it will tend to move with warmth and coalesce with cold, and thus warmth is applied to reduce the congealing effects of cold, and transformation (hua) used to break up the phlegm. This was established as early as the *Jin Gui Yao Lue* in its chapter on thin mucus, where it says: 'Cases of phlegm and mucus should be harmonized with warming herbs.' In order to keep this statement in perspective, however, we should remember that Zhang Zhong-Jing in both the *Shang Han Lun* ('Discussion of Cold-induced Disorders') and the *Jing Gui Yao Lue* ('Essentials from the Golden Cabinet') emphasized warming treatments in almost *all* diseases. This may not be appropriate for other situations, though, as for example in phlegm-fire accumulations.

As a general rule, phlegm treatments should first act to restore harmony to the body by eliminating the phlegm, and then proceed to correct the processes that created it. Thus for cold phlegm, one should warm yang to transform phlegm; for hot phlegm, one should clear heat to eliminate phlegm; in exogenous invasions, the aim is to restore normal Lung qi spread and descent in order to transform phlegm; if Spleen is weak, the goal is to support the Spleen transport and transformation of phlegm. Fluids being dried into phlegm must be moistened and the drying factor eliminated; if food stagnation is producing phlegm, the stagnant food must be removed before the digestion can be strengthened: the phlegm will naturally be eliminated if the food stagnation does not exist. Qi blockage leading to phlegm, which is very common in the West, will have as its primary principle the restoration of normal qi flow, which itself will carry away the phlegm.

Most of the above principles may seem obvious but it is remarkable how easily the 'simple principles' are forgotten in clinic! The following are not so straightforward: phlegm which has entered the channels and collaterals requires attention to opening the collaterals before the phlegm can be expelled; phlegm which has formed knots and nodes needs to be softened before it can be dissolved; if the phlegm proves to be stubborn, it must be aggressively flushed away. Phlegm misting the Heart requires not only the removal of phlegm (and whatever caused it), but also opening the Heart orifice and restoration of healthy blood to nourish the Heart and its shen.

APPROACHES TO PHLEGM TREATMENT

Phlegm treatments can be divided into two categories: those which treat the mechanism which produces the phlegm, which is called 'treating the root', and those which treat the phlegm itself to alleviate the condition, which is called 'treating the branch (or manifestation)'.

The first section below contains examples of treatments which aim at rectifying the underlying mechanism producing the phlegm, treating the root of the problem so that the source of the phlegm is eliminated. This is the ideal approach, as Zhang Jing-Yue says: 'for phlegm to become pathological, there must be a cause, for example, wind or fire producing phlegm. If one treats the wind or fire, though, and the wind or fire is extinguished, then

the phlegm will be cleared in and of itself. ... One will never hear of wind or fire extinguishing themselves simply by treating the phlegm which results from it! ... The reason for this is that phlegm is necessarily a product of disease, not disease a product of phlegm.'[2] Therefore, for a phlegm treatment to be permanently successful, the source of the phlegm must be found and restored to a normally functioning condition. Phlegm, lacking a source, will then cease to exist.

Under certain conditions, however, the symptoms resulting from the phlegm are so severe that treatment of the root would simply take too much time: the symptoms must first be pacified by reducing the ravages of the phlegm, which is called 'treating the branch'. Once this has been accomplished, as a follow-up approach the root source of the phlegm is addressed in order to prevent the return of the condition. Examples of these kind of treatments are given in the second section below.

Many standard phlegm formulas are designed with some constituents which treat the root and others which treat the branch manifestations. Recognizing the difference between the two approaches will allow one to adjust the emphasis of an individual prescription to take into account the patient's requirements.

For example, a patient with underlying Spleen deficiency leading to build-up of phlegm which is then carried up to the Lungs, resulting in a severe asthma attack, will first require an alleviation of the Lung condition, with minimum emphasis on the Spleen. Once the asthma has settled, primary emphasis can then be shifted back to the Spleen to eliminate the source of the phlegm.

If the asthma is usually mild, the prescription can contain both herbs which expel the phlegm accumulated in the Lungs—treating the branch—and also herbs which regulate Spleen transformation and transport—treating the root. Here the emphasis is equal.

If the patient is little bothered by the asthma, a treatment aimed solely at the root will be most efficient: strengthening Spleen transformation and transportation will itself eliminate the source of the phlegm; with no more phlegm coming in, and with better qi lifted from the Spleen, the Lungs will themselves eliminate any vestiges of phlegm which may remain within them. This is a pure root treatment.

Root treatments

The following are examples of treatments addressed to the mechanisms producing phlegm: treating the root.

Restoring normal transformation and transportation

Weak Spleen transport allowing phlegm to accumulate from damp is treated by restoring normal transformation and transportation, while parching damp and transforming phlegm. Symptoms will include relatively long-term digestive problems such as poor appetite, cravings for sweets, nausea and fullness after a small amount of food; possibly accompanied by lethargy, poor concentration, flabby tongue with a white tongue coat and a languid slippery pulse. The standard formula for this is Liu Jun Zi Tang ('Six-Gentlemen Decoction'); if the phlegm and damp have thoroughly oppressed the Spleen, slightly more emphasis can be addressed to the 'branch' by adding herbs which use the yang-dispersing quality of fragrance to break up the damp and phlegm, and allow Spleen transport to take effect. A good formula to do this is Xiang Sha Liu Jun Zi Tang ('Six Gentlemen Decoction with Aucklandia and Amomum').

Formulas

Liu Jun Zi Tang ('Six Gentlemen Decoction')

Ren Shen	Ginseng, Radix
Bai Zhu	Atractylodis Macrocephalae, Rhizoma
Fu Ling	Poriae Cocos, Sclerotium
Ban Xia	Pinelliae Ternata, Rhizoma
Chen Pi	Citri Reticulatae, Pericarpium
Gan Cao	Glycyrrhizae Uralensis, Radix

Source text: *Yi Xue Zheng Chuan* ('True Lineage of Medicine', 1515) [*Formulas and Strategies*, p. 238]

Xiang Sha Liu Jun Zi Tang ('Six Gentlemen Decoction with Aucklandia and Amomum')

Ren Shen	Ginseng, Radix
Bai Zhu	Atractylodis Macrocephalae, Rhizoma
Fu Ling	Poriae Cocos, Sclerotium
Zhi Gan Cao	Honey-fried Glycyrrhizae Uralensis, Radix
Chen Pi	Citri Reticulatae, Pericarpium
Sha Ren	Amomi, Fructus et Semen
Mu Xiang	Saussureae seu Vladimiriae, Radix

Source text: *Zhang Shi Yi Tong* ('Comprehensive Medicine According to Master Zhang', 1695) [*Formulas and Strategies*, p. 238]

Tonifying Spleen and Kidney yang

Spleen and Kidney yang deficiency allowing cold thin mucus to accumulate internally is treated by warm transformation of damp and thin mucus, assisted by tonification of Spleen and Kidney yang. Symptoms will include generalized edematous fluid retention which is more pronounced in the lower body, lethargy and heaviness which is worse in the morning, cold aching in the lower back and knees, poor appetite, thin clear phlegm in the throat and chest, loose stool which is worse in the morning containing sticky mucus and perhaps undigested food, abdominal distension and possibly cold abdominal pain, scanty difficult urination, general chills and cold limbs, pale face, pale flabby tongue with a white slippery or greasy tongue coat, and a deep thready slow or languid pulse. The initial formula should be Shi Pi Yin ('Bolster the Spleen Decoction') to warm Kidneys and Spleen, move qi, and eliminate pathogenic water. Once the edema and thin phlegm have been substantially reduced, follow up formulas can be used, perhaps in pill or powder form. If the Spleen yang is more deficient than Kidney yang, Shen Ling Bai Zhu San ('Ginseng, Poria, and Atractylodes Macrocephala Powder') should be used. If Kidney yang is weakest, Ji Sheng Shen Qi Wan ('Kidney Qi Pill from *Formulas to Aid the Living*') is best.

Formulas

Shi Pi Yin ('Bolster the Spleen Decoction')

Fu Zi	Aconiti Carmichaeli Praeparata, Radix
Gan Jiang	Zingiberis Officianalis, Rhizoma
Fu Ling	Poriae Cocos, Sclerotium
Bai Zhu	Atractylodis Macrocephalae, Rhizoma
Mu Gua	Chaenomelis Lagenariae, Fructus
Hou Po	Magnoliae Officinalis, Cortex

Mu Xiang	Saussureae seu Vladimiriae, Radix
Da Fu Pi	Arecae Catechu, Pericarpium
Cao Guo	Amomi Tsao-ko, Fructus
Gan Cao	Glycyrrhizae Uralensis, Radix

Source text: *Shi Yi De Xiao Fang* ('Effective Formulas from Generations of Physicians', 1345) [*Formulas and Strategies*, p. 199]

Shen Ling Bai Zhu San ('Ginseng, Poria and Atractylodes Macrocephala Powder')

Dang Shen	Codonopsis Pilosulae, Radix
Bai Zhu	Atractylodis Macrocephalae, Rhizoma
Fu Ling	Poriae Cocos, Sclerotium
Gan Cao	Glycyrrhizae Uralensis, Radix
Shan Yao	Dioscoreae Oppositae, Radix
Bai Bian Dou	Dolichos Lablab, Semen
Lian Zi	Nelumbinis Nuciferae, Semen
Yi Yi Ren	Coicis Lachryma-jobi, Semen
Sha Ren	Amomi, Fructus et Semen
Jie Geng	Platycodi Grandiflori, Radix

Source text: *Tai Ping Hui Min He Ji Ju Fang* ('Imperial Grace Formulary of the Tai Ping Era', 1078-85) [*Formulas and Strategies*, p. 239]

Ji Sheng Shen Qi Wan ('Kidney Qi Pill from *Formulas to Aid the Living*')

Shou Di	Rehmanniae Glutinosae Conquitae, Radix
Shan Zhu Yu	Corni Officinalis, Fructus
Shan Yao	Dioscoreae Oppositae, Radix
Fu Ling	Poriae Cocos, Sclerotium
Ze Xie	Alismatis Plantago-aquaticae, Rhizoma
Mu Dan Pi	Moutan Radicis, Cortex
Fu Zi	Aconiti Carmichaeli Praeparata, Radix
Rou Gui	Cinnamomi Cassiae, Cortex
Niu Xi	Achyranthis Bidentatae, Radix
Che Qian Zi	Plantaginis, Semen

Source text: *Ji Sheng Fang* ('Formulas to Aid the Living', 1253) [*Formulas and Strategies*, p. 278]

Warming Kidney yang to support Urinary Bladder

Kidney yang deficiency allowing pathogenic water to flood and become thin mucus and phlegm is treated by warming Kidney yang to restore Urinary Bladder qi transformation, so that reusable 'clear' fluids are recovered, and 'murky' waste fluids are converted to urine and expelled from the body.

This condition is quite different from the one above, in both mechanism and location: in the former, the focus of the problem is in the middle Jiao where Spleen transformation is unsupported by Kidney yang, and damp (and then phlegm) accumulates from the untransformed food and fluids. In the present case, the problem is not in the Spleen, but the Urinary Bladder; not in the middle Jiao, but the lower; and the fluids which accumulate are those which have already undergone several qi transformation processes before they arrive at the Urinary Bladder, for the final separation into either 'clear' fluids which will be recycled back into the body, or 'murky' fluids to be eliminated. Kidney yang weakness is the origin in both cases but from then on the mechanism—and therefore the treatment—is different. Symptoms will be scanty but clear urination, edema worse in the lower body, chills and cold aching of the lower back, knees and legs, darkness under the eyes, tinnitus, and cold lower abdominal pain and distension. In females, there may be watery vaginal discharge and infertility; in males, sexual dysfunction such as impotence or spermatorrhea. The tongue will be flabby and pale, with a white slippery tongue coat more pronounced at the root of the tongue, and a deep thready weak pulse, especially at the chi (proximal) position. The initial formula should be Zhen Wu Tang ('True Warrior Decoction'); when this has achieved stable results, Ji Sheng Shen Qi Wan ('Kidney Qi Pill from *Formulas to Aid the Living*') will consolidate the effects so that the root—the Kidney yang—is stable.

Formulas

Zhen Wu Tang ('True Warrior Decoction')

Fu Zi	Aconiti Carmichaeli Praeparata, Radix
Bai Zhu	Atractylodis Macrocephalae, Rhizoma
Fu Ling	Poriae Cocos, Sclerotium
Bai Shao	Paeoniae Lactiflora, Radix
Sheng Jiang	Zingiberis Officinalis Recens, Rhizoma

Source text: *Shang Han Lun* ('Discussion of Cold-induced Disorders', c. 210AD) [*Formulas and Strategies*, p. 197]

Ji Sheng Shen Qi Wan ('Kidney Qi Pill from Formulas to Aid the Living') [*Formulas and Strategies*, p. 278]
(See above)

Tonifying yin fluids

Yin deficiency with fire drying fluids into phlegm is treated by moistening yin fluids to reduce fire, cooling heat, and transforming phlegm. This can occur anywhere in the body, and so specific treatments will need to be designed for each individual but, because all of the yin in the body is based upon Kidney yin and jing-essence, the follow-up consolidation will usually involve tonification of Kidney yin. The general presentation will include typical yin deficiency symptoms such as malar flush, heat at night with nightsweats, thirst but only for small amounts of water, dry skin and hair, heat in the palms and soles, scanty dark urine and so on; plus symptoms of dried hot phlegm: a sticky sensation in the mouth, yellow sticky phlegm, feelings of heaviness worse in the morning and absent at night, urine dark and scanty as above but also murky, constipation perhaps with dried yellow mucus in the stool, and increased body odor.[3] The tongue body will be red, the tongue coat will be peeled, but the coat that remains will be thick and greasy. In cases where the phlegm is not involved with the digestive system at all (i.e. in 'broadly defined' phlegm situations where it does not manifest visually), there may be little sign of it on the tongue coat. The pulse will be thready and rapid, as is usual for yin deficiency, but will also be slippery or wiry. The location of the most noticeable threadiness on the pulse positions will indicate the focus of the yin deficiency, while the location of the phlegm accumulation in the body can be indicated by the pulse position with the most pronounced slippery feeling.

The pathological mechanism is somewhat complicated: yin weakness fails to balance yang activity and warmth, so that a portion of the body's own heat (which in a balanced state can perform physiological functions) builds up and becomes pathological (which means that this portion can no longer function as normal beneficially warming energy but instead creates disorder). This heat dries the body fluids, which thicken and become phlegm. The phlegm—a yin pathogen—and the pathogenic heat—a yang pathogen—then can combine into phlegm-heat, each acting on the other in a vicious cycle which exacerbates the problem: the heat continues to dry and jell the phlegm, the phlegm holds and concentrates the heat, resulting in an extremely stubborn and difficult to treat condition. Zhang Jing-Yue quotes Pang An-Shi in regard to treatment:

> Pang An-Shi says if yin water is deficient, yin fire will flare up to the Lungs, where the pathogenic fire will prevent Lungs' clearing, contracting and descending action. Because of this [obstruction to the Lungs influence on the fluid metabolism], jin and ye fluids thicken, become murky, and produce phlegm instead of [moving into the Heart and] producing blood. This should be treated with a moistening prescription which includes such herbs as *Mai Men Dong* (Ophiopogonis Japonici, Tuber), *Di Huang* (Rehmannia Glutinosae, Radix) and *Gou Qi Zi* (Lycii Chinensis, Fructus). Moistening the yin will lead the rebelling fire downward into its proper place, and the phlegm will clear of itself.[4]

Zhang Jing-Yue also quotes Xue Ji, who says 'If Kidneys are deficient, with yin fire flaring up, Liu Wei Di Huang Wan ('Six-Ingredient Pill with Rehmannia', *Formulas and Strategies*, p.263) is indicated'.[5] Thus the treatment for the root of the problem should be based on the formulas Liu Wei Di Huang Wan ('Six-Ingredient Pill with Rehmannia'), Zhi Bai Di Huang Wan ('Anemarrhena, Phellodendron, and Rehmannia'), or a formula similarly aimed at nourishing the yin but perhaps more suitable for the unique condition of the individual patient.[6]

Formulas

Liu Wei Di Huang Wan ('Six-Ingredient Pill with Rehmannia')

Shou Di	Rehmanniae Glutinosae Conquitae, Radix
Shan Zhu Yu	Corni Officinalis, Fructus
Shan Yao	Dioscoreae Oppositae, Radix
Fu Ling	Poriae Cocos, Sclerotium
Mu Dan Pi	Moutan Radicis, Cortex
Ze Xie	Alismatis Plantago-aquaticae, Rhizoma

Source text: *Xiao Er Yao Zheng Zhi Jue* ('Craft of Medicinal Treatment for Childhood Disease Patterns', 1119). [*Formulas and Strategies*, p. 263]

Zhi Bai Di Huang Wan ('Anemarrhena, Phellodendron, and Rehmannia')

Shou Di	Rehmanniae Glutinosae Conquitae, Radix
Shan Zhu Yu	Corni Officinalis, Fructus
Shan Yao	Dioscoreae Oppositae, Radix
Fu Ling	Poriae Cocos, Sclerotium
Mu Dan Pi	Moutan Radicis, Cortex
Ze Xie	Alismatis Plantago-aquaticae, Rhizoma
Zhi Mu	Anemarrhenae Asphodeloidis, Radix
Huang Bo	Phellodendri, Cortex

Source text: *Zheng Yin Mai Zhi* ('Pattern, Cause, Pulse, and Treatment', 1702) [*Formulas and Strategies*, p. 265]

Cooling heat, restoring qi flow and transforming phlegm

Pent-up heat in San Jiao drying fluids into phlegm is treated by cooling heat, restoring normal qi flow and transforming phlegm. 'In the San Jiao' means anywhere in the upper, middle or lower body; the heat is from pathogenic excess and therefore is 'excess' (shi) heat. The most common mechanisms leading to heat combining with phlegm include:

1. Exogenous invasion of wind-heat (or zao-drying pathogen) becoming pent up in the Lungs and affecting Lung fluid metabolism so that fluids dry into phlegm instead of descending thoughout the body
2. Liver qi blockage turning hot and either combining with Spleen damp or affecting Hand Shao Yang San Jiao channel fluid pathway function, so that the qi blockage slows the movement of the fluids, and the heat then jells the fluids into phlegm
3. Heart fire parching the fluids of the blood into phlegm.

The treatment, then, requires the use of bitter-cold herbs to cool the excess heat, combined with herbs to restore San Jiao qi flow and expel excess phlegm, and also herbs directed at restoring the malfunctioning of the affected zang organ or channel. Symptoms will vary depending upon the location of the heat and the phlegm but will share some common features: the phlegm itself will be yellow and thick, and may even contain blood; there will often be emotional imbalance; the pulse will be slippery and/or wiry, rapid and strong; the tongue body will be red, especially where the heat predominates; and the tongue coat will be yellow and greasy. Treatment of the root in this case is the elimination of fire: once the fire has ceased drying fluids into phlegm, the problem will disappear. Simply eliminating hot phlegm, which is the product of the disease process, will not succeed. Typical formulas of use in this condition are:

Exogenous heat in the Lungs: Ma Xing Shi Gan Tang ('Ephedra, Apricot Seed, Gypsum and Licorice Decoction') will eliminate the exogenous heat.

Formula

Ma Xing Shi Gan Tang ('Ephedra, Apricot Seed, Gypsum and Licorice Decoction')

Ma Huang	Ephedrae, Herba
Xing Ren	Pruni Armeniacae, Semen
Shi Gao	Gypsum
Gan Cao	Glycyrrhizae Uralensis, Radix

Source text: *Shang Han Lun* ('Discussion of Cold-Induced Disorders', *c.* 210AD) [*Formulas and Strategies*, p. 88]

Liver qi turning to fire: Wen Dan Tang ('Warm the Gallbladder Decoction') plus *Shan Zhi Zi* (Gardeniae) to cool heat; *Yu Jin* (Curcumae) and *He Huan Hua* (Albizziae Julibrissin, Flos) to move qi; *Long Gu* (Draconis, Os) and *Ye Jiao Teng* (Polygoni Multiflori, Caulis) to settle the spirit.

Formula

Wen Dan Tang ('Warm the Gall Bladder Decoction')

Zhu Ru	Bambusae in Taeniis, Caulis
Zhi Shi	Citri seu Ponciri Immaturis, Fructus
Ban Xia	Pinelliae Ternata, Rhizoma
Chen Pi	Citri Reticulatae, Pericarpium
Fu Ling	Poriae Cocos, Sclerotium
Gan Cao	Glycyrrhizae Uralensis, Radix
Sheng Jiang	Zingiberis Officinalis Recens, Rhizoma

Source text: *Yi Zong Jin Jian* ('Golden Mirror of the Medical Tradition', 1742) [*Formulas and Strategies*, p. 435]

Heart fire: Sheng Tie Luo Yin ('Iron Filings Decoction') or An Gong Niu Huang Wan ('Calm the Palace Pill with Cattle Gallstone') plus Gun Tan Wan ('Vaporize Phlegm Pill'). Follow up treatment will require blood replenishing herbs.

Formulas

Sheng Tie Luo Yin ('Iron Filings Decoction')

Sheng Tie Luo	Frusta Ferri
Dan Nan Xing	Arisaemae cum Felle Bovis, Pulvis
Zhe Bei Mu	Fritillariae Thunbergii, Bulbus
Xuan Shen	Scrophulariae Ningpoensis, Radix
Tian Men Dong	Asparagi Cochinchinensis, Tuber
Mai Men Dong	Ophiopogonis Japonici, Tuber
Lian Qiao	Forsythiae Suspensae, Fructus
Gou Teng	Uncariae Cum Uncis, Ramulus
Dan Shen	Salviae Miltiorrhizae, Radix
Fu Ling	Poriae Cocos, Sclerotium
Fu Shen	Poriae Cocos Paradicis, Sclerotium
Chen Pi	Citri Reticulatae, Pericarpium
Yuan Zhi	Polygalae Tenuifoliae, Radix
Zhu Sha	Cinnabaris

Source text: *Yi Xue Xin Wu* ('Medical Revelations', 1732) [*Formulas and Strategies*, p. 386]

An Gong Niu Huang Wan ('Calm the Palace Pill with Cattle Gallstone')

Niu Huang	Bovis, Calculus
Xi Jiao	Rhinoceri, Cornu
She Xiang	Moschus Moschiferi, Secretio
Huang Lian	Coptidis, Rhizoma
Huang Qin	Scutellariae Baicalensis, Radix
Shan Zhi Zi	Gardeniae Jasminoidis, Fructus
Xiong Huang	Realgar
Bing Pian	Borneol
Yu Jin	Curcumae, Tuber
Zhu Sha	Cinnabaris
Zhen Zhu	Margarita

Source text: *Wen Bing Tiao Bian* ('Systematic Differentiation of Warm Diseases', 1798) [*Formulas and Strategies*, p. 416]

Gun Tan Wan ('Vaporize Phlegm Pill')

Duan Meng Shi	Calcined Lapis Micae seu Chloriti
Da Huang	Rhei, Rhizoma
Huang Qin	Scutellariae Baicalensis, Radix
Chen Xiang	Aquilariae, Lignum

Source text: *Tai Ding Yang Sheng Zhu Lun* ('Treatises on the Calm and Settled Nourishment of the Director of Life'), 1338[7]

Branch treatments

The following are examples of treatments addressed primarily at the branch manifestations, in order to alleviate severe symptoms. These are usually followed by treatment of the root to prevent recurrence of the problem.

Warm transformation of thin mucus

If Spleen yang is deficient then water and thin mucus will accumulate. If the thin mucus is severe enough to require a 'branch' treatment first, the basic approach is to use either Ling Gui Zhu Gan Tang ('Poria, Cinnamon Twig, Atractylodes Macrocephala and Licorice Decoction') or Shi Pi Yin ('Bolster the Spleen Decoction').

When Kidney yang is weak, water can flood and become thin mucus, leading to symptoms such as chills and cold limbs, difficult urination, severe fluid retention, pale flabby tongue with a white slippery or greasy tongue coat, and deep weak slow pulse. The standard treatment approach is to use Zhen Wu Tang ('True Warrior Decoction') first, followed by Ji Sheng Shen Qi Wan ('Kidney Qi Pill from *Formulas to Aid the Living*') to consolidate the treatment after the excess fluids have been reduced.

If both the Kidneys and the Spleen are weak, then these treatments should be used together.

Formulas

Ling Gui Zhu Gan Tang ('Poria, Cinnamon Twig, Atractylodes Macrocephalae and Licorice Decoction')

Fu Ling	Poriae Cocos, Sclerotium
Gui Zhi	Cinnamomi Cassiae, Ramulus
Bai Zhu	Atractylodis Macrocephalae, Rhizoma
Gan Cao	Glycyrrhizae Uralensis, Radix

Source text: *Shang Han Lun* ('Discussion of Cold-induced Disorders', c. 210AD) [*Formulas and Strategies*, p. 443]

Shi Pi Yin ('Bolster the Spleen Decoction') [*Formulas and Strategies*, p. 199]
(*See above*)

Zhen Wu Tang ('True Warrior Decoction') [*Formulas and Strategies*, p. 197)
(*See above*)

Ji Sheng Shen Qi Wan ('Kidney Qi Pill from *Formulas to Aid the Living*') [*Formulas and Strategies*, p. 278)
(*See above*)

Attack to expel thin mucus

This is used in 'thin mucus conditions' (yin zheng)[8] where these fluids have halted in the area around the chest and ribs. Common symptoms include a pulling pain in the lower costal region, worse with breathing, coughing and turning the body; with the possible result of shortness of breath and rough breathing; plus a white tongue coat, and deep wiry pulse. Classically, Shi Zao Tang ('Ten Jujube Decoction') is used as a purging treatment for severe conditions; in other cases, and perhaps especially in the West, Xiang Fu Xuan Fu Hua Tang ('Cyperus and Inula Decoction') is more suitable.

Formulas

Shi Zao Tang ('Ten-Jujube Decoction')

Gan Sui	Euphorbiae Kansui, Radix
Yuan Hua	Daphnes Genkwa, Flos
Da Ji	Euphorbiae seu Knoxiae, Radix
Da Zao	Zizyphi Jujubae

Source text: *Shang Han Lun* ('Discussion of Cold-induced Disorders', *c.* 210AD) [*Formulas and Strategies*, p. 128]

Xiang Fu Xuan Fu Hua Tang ('Cyperus and Inula Decoction')

Xiang Fu	Cyperi Rotundi, Rhizoma
Xuan Fu Hua	Inulae, Flos
Zi Su Zi	Perillae Fructescentis, Fructus
Chen Pi	Citri Reticulatae, Pericarpium
Fu Ling	Poriae Cocos, Sclerotium

Yi Yi Ren	Coicis Lachryma-jobi, Semen
Ban Xia	Pinelliae Ternata, Rhizoma

Source text: *Wen Bing Tiao Bian* ('Systematic Differentiation of Warm Diseases', 1798) [*Formulas and Strategies*, p. 434]

Unblocking the surface to transform thin mucus

This is employed for thin mucus seeping into the surface tissues (yi yin 溢饮 'flooding thin mucus')[9] causing heaviness and aching of the muscles and joints, lack of appropriate sweating, the appearance of swelling in the body, white tongue coat, and tight and wiry pulse. The best formula is Xiao Qing Long Tang ('Minor Blue-Green Dragon Decoction').

If the thin mucus obstruction has existed for a long time it can produce heat, which will manifest as restlessness and irritability. Da Qing Long Tang ('Major Blue-Green Dragon Decoction') will both transform the thin mucus and cool the heat.

If pathogenic thin mucus affects the Lungs, leading to cough with profuse clear white phlegm and dyspnea worsened with lying flat, then Xiao Qing Long Tang ('Minor Blue-Green Dragon Decoction') is again the formula of choice.

Formulas

Xiao Qing Long Tang ('Minor Bluegreen Dragon Decoction')

Ma Huang	Ephedrae, Herba
Gui Zhi	Cinnamomi Cassiae, Ramulus
Gan Jiang	Zingiberis Officinalis, Rhizoma
Xi Xin	Asari cum Radice, Herba
Wu Wei Zi	Schisandrae Chinensis, Fructus
Bai Shao	Paeoniae Lactiflora, Radix
Ban Xia	Pinelliae Ternata, Rhizoma
Zhi Gan Cao	Honey-fried Glycyrrhizae Uralensis, Radix

Source text: *Shang Han Lun* ('Discussion of Cold-induced Disorders', *c.* 210AD) [*Formulas and Strategies*, p. 38]

Da Qing Long Tang ('Major Bluegreen Dragon Decoction')

Ma Huang	Ephedrae, Herba
Xing Ren	Pruni Armeniacae, Semen
Gui Zhi	Cinnamomi Cassiae, Ramulus
Zhi Gan Cao	Honey-fried Glycyrrhizae Uralensis, Radix
Shi Gao	Gypsum
Sheng Jiang	Zingiberis Officinalis Recens, Rhizoma
Da Zao	Zizyphi Jujubae, Fructus

Source text: *Shang Han Lun* ('Discussion of Cold-induced Disorders', c. 210AD) [*Formulas and Strategies*, p. 34]

Transform phlegm to settle dyspnea

This is used for dyspnea from phlegm and pathogenic fluids clogging the Lungs, with rough difficult breathing. Because this condition can result from a number of different causes, and also can be influenced by so many different factors, the scenarios provided below are only examples.

In one situation, the phlegm is thick and profuse, with a sensation of tightness and fullness in the chest, nausea and thick white greasy tongue coat. This is phlegm-damp, and two suggested formulas are San Zi Yang Qin Tang ('Three Seed Decoction to Nourish One's Parents') and Su Zi Jiang Qi Tang ('Perilla Fruit Decoction for Directing Qi Downward').

Formulas

San Zi Yang Qin Tang ('Three Seed Decoction to Nourish One's Parents')

Bai Jie Zi	Sinapsis Albae, Semen
Zi Su Zi	Perillae Fructescentis, Fructus
Lai Fu Zi	Raphani Sativi, Semen

Source text: *Han Shi Yi Tong* ('Comprehensive Medicine According to Master Han', 1522) [*Formulas and Strategies*, p. 445]

Su Zi Jiang Qi Tang ('Perilla Fruit Decoction for Directing Qi Downward')

Zi Su Zi	Perillae Fructescentis, Fructus
Ban Xia	Pinelliae Ternata, Rhizoma
Dang Gui	Angelica Polymorpha, Radix
Zhi Gan Cao	Honey-fried Glycyrrhizae Uralensis, Radix
Hou Po	Magnoliae Officinalis, Cortex
Qian Hu	Peucedani, Radix
Rou Gui	Cinnamomi Cassiae, Cortex
Sheng Jiang	Zingiberis Officinalis Recens, Rhizoma
Da Zao	Zizyphi Jujubae, Fructus

Source text: *Tai Ping Hui Min He Ji Ju Fang* ('Imperial Grace Formulary of the Tai Ping Era', 1078-85) [*Formulas and Strategies*, p. 299]

In another situation the phlegm is hot, the chest feels both full and heated, the mouth is dry and the cough produces thick yellow phlegm, the tongue is red with a yellow greasy dry coat, and the pulse is slippery and rapid. Ma Xing Shi Gan Tang ('Ephedra, Apricot Seed, Gypsum and Licorice Decoction') is appropriate, with added *Huang Qin* (Scutellariae) and *Jin Yin Hua* (Lonicerae) to cool heat, and *Gua Lou Pi* (Trichosanthes, Pericarpium), *Dong Gua Ren* (Benincasae Hispidae, Semen), *Chuan Bei Mu* (Fritillariae Cirrhosae, Bulbus), and *Ban Xia* (Pinelliae) prepared with *Zhu Li* (Bambusae, Succus) to cut hot phlegm.

Formula

Ma Xing Shi Gan Tang ('Ephedra, Apricot Seed, Gypsum, and Licorice Decoction') [*Formulas and Strategies*, p. 88]
(See above)

In a third situation, that of exogenous cold with internal heat leading to dyspnea, there will also be chills and fever, little or no sweating, irritable heat obstructing the chest, yellow phlegm, thirst, thin whitish yellow tongue coat, and floating rapid pulse. The formula of choice in this case is Ding Chuan Tang ('Arrest Wheezing Decoction').

Formula

Ding Chuan Tang ('Arrest Wheezing Decoction')

Yin Xing	Ginkgo Bilobae, Semen
Ma Huang	Ephedrae, Herba
Zi Su Zi	Perillae Fructescentis, Fructus
Gan Cao	Glycyrrhizae Uralensis, Radix

Kuan Dong Hua	Tussilagi Farfarae, Flos
Xing Ren	Pruni Armeniacae, Semen
Sang Bai Pi	Mori Albae Radicis, Cortex
Huang Qin	Scutellariae Baicalensis, Radix
Ban Xia	Pinelliae Ternata, Rhizoma

Source text: *Fu Shou Jing Fang* ('Exquisite Formulas for Fostering Longevity', 1530) [*Formulas and Strategies*, p. 300]

Transforming phlegm to stop cough

In this condition phlegm fluids are again obstructing the Lungs ability to spread and descend but the most obvious result of this is cough rather than dyspnea.

If the cause is phlegm-damp, the symptoms will be profuse white sticky phlegm, tightness in the chest and epigastric area, lassitude, poor appetite, white greasy tongue coat, and floating thin forceless slippery pulse. Er Chen Tang ('Two-Cured Decoction') should be used with appropriate additions.

Formula

Er Chen Tang ('Two-Cured Decoction')

Ban Xia	Pinelliae Ternata, Rhizoma
Chen Pi	Citri Reticulatae, Pericarpium
Fu Ling	Poriae Cocos, Sclerotium
Gan Cao	Glycyrrhizae Uralensis, Radix

Source text: *Tai Ping Hui Min He Ji Ju Fang* ('Imperial Grace Formulary of the Tai Ping Era', 1078-85) [*Formulas and Strategies*, p. 432]

If the phlegm is hot, it will be sticky and hard to cough out, there will be a dry mouth and a bitter taste, sore throat, a rapid slippery pulse, and a tongue coat that is either yellow and greasy or, if the heat is less, both yellow and white. Qing Qi Hua Tan Wan ('Clear the Qi and Transform Phlegm Pill') should be used.

Formula

Qing Qi Hua Tan Wan ('Clear the Qi and Transform Phlegm Pill')

Dan Nan Xing	Arisaemae cum Felle Bovis, Pulvis
Ban Xia	Pinelliae Ternata, Rhizoma
Gua Lou Ren	Trichosanthes, Semen
Huang Qin	Scutellariae Baicalensis, Radix
Chen Pi	Citri Reticulatae, Pericarpium
Xing Ren	Pruni Armeniacae, Semen

Zhi Shi	Citri seu Ponciri Immaturis, Fructus
Fu Ling	Poriae Cocos, Sclerotium

Source text: *Yi Fang Kao* ('Investigations of Medical Formulas', 1584) [*Formulas and Strategies*, p. 437]

If the heat has hardened the phlegm, the cough will be worse at night, with little or no phlegm produced. That which can be coughed out will be sticky and hard. There will be a desire for sweet moistening liquids, after which the cough will be somewhat reduced; the chest will be tight and irritated, the mouth dry, the stool dry and constipated, the pulse wiry and rapid, and the tongue red with a yellow greasy coat. Salty cold herbs must be used to soften the phlegm, such as *Hai Fu Shi* (Pumice), *Ge Ke* (Cyclinae Sinensis, Concha), or *Kun Bu* (Algae, Thallus). These can be combined with the formula Bei Mu Gua Lou San ('Fritillaria and Trichosanthes Fruit Powder').

Formula

Bei Mu Gua Lou San ('Fritillaria and Trichosanthes Fruit Powder')

Chuan Bei Mu	Fritillariae Cirrhosae, Bulbus
Gua Lou Ren	Trichosanthes, Fructus
Tian Hua Fen	Trichosanthis, Radix
Fu Ling	Poriae Cocos, Sclerotium
Ju Hong	Citri Erythrocarpae, Pericarpium
Jie Geng	Platycodi Grandiflori, Radix

Source text: *Yi Xue Xin Wu* ('Medical Revelations', 1732) [*Formulas and Strategies*, p. 439]

If Liver heat is scorching the Lungs, there may be blood in the phlegm, with piercing pain in the chest and flanks, irritability and anger, bitter taste, dry irritation in the throat, red face and eyes, a thin yellow tongue coat, and a wiry rapid pulse. Sang Dan Xie Bai Tang ('Mulberry Leaf and Moutan Decoction to Drain the White') should be used.

Formula

Sang Dan Xie Bai Tang ('Mulberry Leaf and Moutan Decoction to Drain the White')

Sang Bai Pi	Mori Albae Radicis, Cortex
Sang Ye	Mori Albae, Folium
Di Gu Pi	Lycii Chinensis Radicis, Cortex

Mu Dan Pi	Moutan Radicis, Cortex
Zhu Ru	Bambusae in Taeniis, Caulis
Chuan Bei Mu	Fritillariae Cirrhosae, Bulbus
Jing Mi	Oryza Sativae, semen
Zhi Gan Cao	Honey-fried Glycyrrhizae Uralensis, Radix
Da Zao	Zizyphi Jujubae, Fructus

Source text: *Chong Ding Tong Su Shang Han Lun* ('Revised Popular Guide to the Discussion of Cold-induced Disorders', Ming) [*Formulas and Strategies*, p. 91]

Transforming phlegm to disperse nodular masses

This method is employed to treat goiter, scrofula, and other nodular masses around the body which have arisen through the coagulation of turbid-phlegm (zhuo tan) into knot-like nodes (tan he). This often occurs on the neck, either bilaterally or on one side only, but may just as frequently be seen in the breasts or lower abdomen along the Liver or Dai channels. Phlegm nodules will begin as relatively soft and painless masses with indistinct edges, no discoloration of the skin and a glossy appearance, and may coalesce and disperse depending upon the movement of the qi. As time passes, they can become hard and firm. If the nodule is recent, red, tender and inflamed, with general signs of fever, this is unlikely to be phlegm.

Phlegm nodules should be treated by softening the hardness and dispersing the knots, with salty-cold herbs such as are contained in formulas like Xiao Luo Wan ('Reduce Scrofula Pill') or Hai Zao Yu Hu Tang ('Sargassum Decoction for the Jade Flask'), although this treatment, once effective, must be followed with Liver qi regulating herbs for better long-term results.

Formulas

Xiao Luo Wan ('Reduce Scrofula Pill')

Xuan Shen	Scrophulariae Ningpoensis, Radix
Mu Li	Ostreae, Concha
Zhe Bei Mu	Fritillariae Thunbergii, Bulbus

Source text: *Yi Xue Xin Wu* ('Medical Revelations', 1732) [*Formulas and Strategies*, p. 441]

Hai Zao Yu Hu Tang ('Sargassum Decoction for the Jade Flask')

Hai Zao	Sargassi, Herba
Kun Bu	Algae, Thallus
Hai Dai	Laminariae Japonicae, Herba
Zhe Bei Mu	Fritillariae Thunbergii, Bulbus
Ban Xia	Pinelliae Ternata, Rhizoma
Du Huo	Duhuo, Radix
Chuan Xiong	Ligustici Wallichii, Radix
Dang Gui	Angelica Polymorpha, Radix
Qing Pi	Citri Reticulatae Viride, Pericarpium
Chen Pi	Citri Reticulatae, Pericarpium
Lian Qiao	Forsythiae Suspensae, Fructus
Gan Cao	Glycyrrhizae Uralensis, Radix

Source text: *Wai Ke Zheng Zong* ('True Lineage of External Medicine', 1617) [*Formulas and Strategies*, p. 442]

Removing food stagnation to eliminate phlegm

Phlegm can result from long-term over-consumption of rich foods which fail to be digested by the Spleen and Stomach, and thus accumulate in the middle Jiao. This leads to symptoms of fullness and distension in the epigastric area and abdomen, aversion to rich food with desire only for light bland foods, foul-smelling eructation, acid regurgitation, nausea and vomiting, greasy tongue coat, and a slippery pulse. The condition requires dispersal of the accumulated food, then leading it downward into the Intestines for expulsion from the body.

Appropriate formulas include Bao He Wan ('Preserve Harmony Pill') for relatively mild or early-stage cases; if the phlegm has accumulated to the stage where it is being carried up to the Lungs, Bao He Wan can be combined with San Zi Yang Qin Tang ('Three Seed Decoction to Nourish One's Parents'); if the Spleen has been weakened by the continual strain on its energy, then support for the Spleen takes precedence, and Jian Pi Wan ('Support the Spleen Pill') can be washed down with a decoction of Er Chen Tang ('Two-Cured Decoction') and raw ginger.

Formulas

Bao He Wan ('Preserve Harmony Pill')

| Shan Zha | Crataegi, Fructus |
| Shen Qu | Massa Fermentata |

Lai Fu Zi	Raphani Sativi, Semen
Chen Pi	Citri Reticulatae, Pericarpium
Ban Xia	Pinelliae Ternata, Rhizoma
Fu Ling	Poriae Cocos, Sclerotium
Lian Qiao	Forsythiae Suspensae, Fructus

Source text: *Dan Xi Xin Fa* ('Teachings of Dan Xi', 1481) [*Formulas and Strategies*, p. 455]

San Zi Yang Qin Tang ('Three Seed Decoction to Nourish One's Parents') [*Formulas and Strategies*, p. 445]
(See above)

Jian Pi Wan ('Support the Spleen Pill')

Chao Bai Zhu	Fried Atractylodis Macrocephalae, Rhizoma
Fu Ling	Poriae Cocos, Sclerotium
Ren Shen	Ginseng, Radix
Shan Yao	Dioscoreae Oppositae, Radix
Rou Dou Kou	Myristicae Fragranticis, Semen
Shan Zha	Crataegi, Fructus
Shen Qu	Massa Fermentata
Chao Mai Ya	Fried Hordei Vulgaris Germinantus, Fructus
Mu Xiang	Saussureae seu Vladimiriae, Radix
Chen Pi	Citri Reticulatae, Pericarpium
Sha Ren	Amomi, Fructus et Semen
Jiu Chao Huang Lian	Wine-fried Coptidis, Rhizoma
Gan Cao	Glycyrrhizae Uralensis, Radix

Source text: *Zheng Zhi Zhun Sheng* ('Standards of Patterns and Treatments', 1602) [*Formulas and Strategies*, p. 458]

Er Chen Tang ('Two-Cured Decoction') [*Formulas and Strategies*, p. 432]
(See above)

Transforming phlegm and extinguishing wind

The wind referred to here is internal wind, which carries phlegm upward causing headache and vertigo. The head will be heavy, with loss of concentration, the chest will feel stuffy and tight, the tongue flabby with a thick white moist coat, and the pulse will be wiry, slippery and rapid. Wind must be extinguished while phlegm is dispersed. The standard formula for this is Ban Xia Bai Zhu Tian Ma Tang ('Pinellia, Atractylodes Macrocephalae and Gastrodia Decoction').

Formula

Ban Xia Bai Zhu Tian Ma Tang ('Pinellia, Atractylodes Macrocephalae and Gastrodia Decoction')

Ban Xia	Pinelliae Ternata, Rhizoma
Tian Ma	Gastrodiae Elatae, Rhizoma
Bai Zhu	Atractylodis Macrocephalae, Rhizoma
Ju Hong	Citri Erythrocarpae, Pericarpium
Fu Ling	Poriae Cocos, Sclerotium
Gan Cao	Glycyrrhizae Uralensis, Radix
Sheng Jiang	Zingiberis Officinalis Recens, Rhizoma
Da Zao	Zizyphi Jujubae, Fructus

Source text: *Yi Xue Xin Wu* ('Medical Revelations', 1732) [*Formulas and Strategies*, p. 447]

If there is also anger, red face and eyes, and pain in the flanks, this signifies that phlegm, wind and fire have combined. Er Chen Tang ('Two-Cured Decoction') should be used to wash down Dang Gui Long Hui Wan ('Tangkuei, Gentiana Longdancao, and Aloe Pill').

Formulas

Er Chen Tang ('Two-Cured Decoction') [*Formulas and Strategies*, p. 432]
(See above)

Dang Gui Long Hui Wan ('Tangkuei, Gentiana Longdancao, and Aloe Pill')

Dang Gui	Angelica Polymorpha, Radix
Long Dan Cao	Gentianae Scabrae, Radix
Zhi Shi	Citri seu Ponciri Immaturis, Fructus
Huang Lian	Coptidis, Rhizoma
Huang Bo	Phellodendri, Cortex
Huang Qin	Scutellariae Baicalensis, Radix
Lu Hui	Aloes, Herba
Da Huang	Rhei, Rhizoma
Mu Xiang	Saussureae seu Vladimiriae, Radix
She Xiang	Moschus Moschiferi, Secretio
Sheng Jiang	Zingiberis Officinalis Recens, Rhizoma

Source text: *Dan Xi Xin Fa* ('Teachings of Dan Xi', 1481) [*Formulas and Strategies*, p. 98]

Transforming phlegm to calm the Heart

One cause of palpitations can be turbid-phlegm obstructing the flow of Heart qi, which leads to symptoms such as palpitations, shortness of breath, tightness in the chest or focal distension, profuse phlegm, loss of appetite, abdominal distension and possible nausea, white greasy and possibly slippery tongue coat, and a slippery wiry pulse. Dao Tan Tang ('Guide Out the Phlegm Decoction') can be used or, if there is heat involved, Huang Lian Wen Dan Tang ('Coptis Decoction to Warm the Gall Bladder').

Formulas

Dao Tan Tang ('Guide Out Phlegm Decoction')

Ju Hong	Citri Erythrocarpae, Pericarpium
Ban Xia	Pinelliae Ternata, Rhizoma
Fu Ling	Poriae Cocos, Sclerotium
Gan Cao	Glycyrrhizae Uralensis, Radix
Zhi Shi	Citri seu Ponciri Immaturis, Fructus
Dan Nan Xing	Arisaemae cum Felle Bovis, Pulvis

Source text: *Ji Sheng Fang* ('Formulas to Aid the Living', 1253) [*Formulas and Strategies*, p. 448]

Huang Lian Wen Dan Tang ('Coptis Decoction to Warm the Gall Bladder')

Huang Lian	Coptidis, Rhizoma
Zhu Ru	Bambusae in Taeniis, Caulis
Zhi Shi	Citri seu Ponciri Immaturis, Fructus
Ban Xia	Pinelliae Ternata, Rhizoma
Chen Pi	Citri Reticulatae, Pericarpium
Fu Ling	Poriae Cocos, Sclerotium
Gan Cao	Glycyrrhizae Uralensis, Radix
Sheng Jiang	Zingiberis Officinalis Recens, Rhizoma

Source text: *Wen Re Jing Wei* ('Warp and Woof of Warm-febrile Diseases', 1852) [*Formulas and Strategies*, p. 436]

Transforming phlegm to open painful chest obstruction

When turbid-phlegm blocks the flow of Heart yang, it can cause tightness and pain in the chest which radiates through to the back, or conversely pain in the back penetrating through to the heart area, especially noticeable in overcast or rainy weather. There may also be shortness of breath, cough with profuse thin phlegm, white greasy or slippery tongue coat, and a slippery or slippery-wiry pulse. Two ancient but still highly effective formulas can be used for this: Gua Lou Xie Bai Ban Xia Tang ('Trichosanthes Fruit, Chinese Chive and Pinellia Decoction') and Zhi Shi Gua Lou Gui Zhi Tang ('Immature Bitter Orange, Trichosanthes Fruit and Cinnamon Twig Decoction').

Formulas

Gua Lou Xie Bai Ban Xia Tang ('Trichosanthes Fruit, Chinese Chive, and Pinellia Decoction')

Gua Lou Pi	Trichosanthes, Pericarpium
Xie Bai	Alii, Bulbus
Bai Jiu	White wine
Ban Xia	Pinelliae Ternata, Rhizoma

Source text: *Shang Han Lun* ('Discussion of Cold-Induced Disorders', *c*. 210AD) [*Formulas and Strategies*, p. 293]

Zhi Shi Gua Lou Gui Zhi Tang ('Immature Bitter Orange, Trichosanthes Fruit, and Cinnamon Twig Decoction')

Gua Lou Ren	Trichosanthes, Fructus
Xie Bai	Alii, Bulbus
Zhi Shi	Citri seu Ponciri Immaturis, Fructus
Hou Po	Magnoliae Officinalis, Cortex
Gui Zhi	Cinnamomi Cassiae, Ramulus

Source text: *Jin Gui Yao Lue* ('Essentials from the Golden Cabinet', *c*. 210AD) [*Formulas and Strategies*, p. 293]

Expelling phlegm to settle epilepsy

This method can be used to treat epilepsy resulting from either wind phlegm rebelling upward or phlegm misting the Heart orifice. The symptoms will be sudden collapse and unconsciousness, or temporary 'absence' of consciousness, with mental confusion, incontinence of bowels and urine, and vomiting of white phlegm; there may be clenching of the jaws, and upturned eyes. The tongue coat will be greasy white or yellow, the pulse either deep thready and slow, or wiry slippery and rapid. The most commonly used formula is Ding Xian Wan ('Arrest Seizures Pill').

Formula

Ding Xian Wan ('Arrest Seizures Pill')

Tian Ma	Gastrodiae Elatae, Rhizoma
Chuan Bei Mu	Fritillariae Cirrhosae, Bulbus
Jiang Ban Xia	Ginger-fried Pinelliae Ternata, Rhizoma
Fu Ling	Poriae Cocos, Sclerotium
Fu Shen	Poriae Cocos Paradicis, Sclerotium
Dan Nan Xing	Arisaemae cum Felle Bovis, Pulvis
Shi Chang Pu	Acori Graminei, Rhizoma
Quan Xie	Buthus Martensi
Jiang Can	Bombyx Batryticatus
Hou Po	Magnoliae Officinalis, Cortex
Deng Xin Cao	Junci Effusi, Medulla
Chen Pi	Citri Reticulatae, Pericarpium
Yuan Zhi	Polygalae Tenuifoliae, Radix
Dan Shen	Salviae Miltiorrhizae, Radix
Mai Men Dong	Ophiopogonis Japonici, Tuber
Zhu Sha	Cinnabaris
Gan Cao	Glycyrrhizae Uralensis, Radix
Zhu Li	Bambusae, Succus

Source text: *Yi Xue Xin Wu* ('Medical Revelations', 1732) [*Formulas and Strategies*, p. 448]

Scouring phlegm to relieve depression

In epilepsy which results from phlegm and qi obstruction, there will be depression, lack of expression, impairment of mental functions and confusion, mood swings and speech impairment. When the condition is severe, there will be withdrawal and refusal of food and drink. The tongue coat will be white and greasy, the pulse wiry and slippery. Di Tan Tang ('Scour Phlegm Decoction') and Xiao Yao San ('Rambling Powder') should be combined.

Formulas

Di Tan Tang ('Scour Phlegm Decoction')

Ban Xia	Pinelliae Ternata, Rhizoma
Ju Hong	Citri Erythrocarpae, Pericarpium
Fu Ling	Poriae Cocos, Sclerotium
Zhi Shi	Citri seu Ponciri Immaturis, Fructus
Zhu Ru	Bambusae in Taeniis, Caulis
Dan Nan Xing	Arisaemae cum Felle Bovis, Pulvis
Shi Chang Pu	Acori Graminei, Rhizoma

Ren Shen	Ginseng, Radix
Gan Cao	Glycyrrhizae Uralensis, Radix
Sheng Jiang	Zingiberis Officinalis Recens, Rhizoma
Da Zao	Zizyphi Jujubae, Fructus

Source text: *Ji Sheng Fang* ('Formulas to Aid the Living', 1253) [*Formulas and Strategies*, p. 424]

Xiao Yao San ('Rambling Powder')

Chai Hu	Bupleuri, Radix
Dang Gui	Angelica Polymorpha, Radix
Bai Shao	Paeoniae Lactiflora, Radix
Bai Zhu	Atractylodis Macrocephalae, Rhizoma
Fu Ling	Poriae Cocos, Sclerotium
Gan Cao	Glycyrrhizae Uralensis, Radix
Sheng Jiang	Zingiberis Officinalis Recens, Rhizoma
Bo He	Menthae, Herba

Source text: *Tai Ping Hui Min He Ji Ju Fang* ('Imperial Grace Formulary of the Tai Ping Era', 1078-85) [*Formulas and Strategies*, p. 147]

Draining fire to eradicate phlegm

This is used in mania (kuang) from phlegm-fire disturbing the Heart, with symptoms of restlessness, irritability, headache, insomnia, furious expression in the eyes, red face and ears, possible sudden explosions of anger and violence with super-human strength, high emotions, irrational speech, singing and cursing and the stripping-off of clothing. There will also be desire for cold drinks, constipation, darkish urine, refusal to eat or sleep, scarlet red tongue usually with a greasy yellow coat, and a wiry slippery rapid pulse. Emesis can be used in this case, brought about with San Sheng San ('Three Sage Powder') followed by Gun Tan Wan ('Vaporize Phlegm Pill') swallowed with a decoction of Xie Xin Tang ('Drain The Epigastrium Decoction').

Formulas

San Sheng San ('Three Sage Powder')

Fang Feng	Ledebouriellae Sesloidis, Radix
Gua Di	Curcumae, Pedicellus
Li Lu	Veratri, Radix and Rhizoma

Source text: *Ru Men Shi Qin* ('Confucians' Duties to Their Parents', 1228) [*Formulas and Strategies*, p. 450]

Gun Tan Wan ('Vaporize Phlegm Pill')[*Formulas and Strategies*, p. 42]
(See above)

Xie Xin Tang ('Drain The Epigastrium Decoction')

Da Huang	Rhei, Rhizoma
Huang Lian	Coptidis, Rhizoma
Huang Qin	Scutellariae Baicalensis, Radix

Source text: *Jin Gui Yao Lue* ('Essentials from the Golden Cabinet', c. 210AD) [*Formulas and Strategies*, p. 79]

Transforming phlegm to open the orifice of the Spirit

When qi blockage leads to phlegm accumulation, the 'orifice of clear intelligence' becomes obstructed, leading to dementia and impairment of the intellect. Symptoms include dulled expression, refusal to talk, drink or eat, mood swings and, when severe, the patient is unable to look after himself. There will often be shortness of breath, lassitude, facial pallor with lack of gloss to the skin, flabby pale tongue body with a white greasy coat, and a thready slippery pulse. A suggested formula is Xi Xin Tang ('Wash the Heart Decoction').

Formula

Xi Xin Tang ('Wash the Heart Decoction')

Ren Shen	30 g	Ginseng, Radix
Fu Shen	30 g	Poriae Cocos Paradicis, Sclerotium
Ban Xia	15 g	Pinelliae Ternata, Rhizoma
Chen Pi	9 g	Citri Reticulatae, Pericarpium
Shen Qu	9 g	Massa Fermentata
Gan Cao	3 g	Glycyrrhizae Uralensis, Radix
Fu Zi	3 g	Aconiti Carmichaeli Praeparata, Radix
Shi Chang Pu	3 g	Acori Graminei, Rhizoma
Suan Zao Ren	30 g	Ziziphi Spinosae, Semen

Source text: *Bian Zheng Lu* ('Record of Differentiation of Syndromes', 1687).

The above herbs should be decocted, and 120 mls should be taken in one dose, after which the patient should sleep deeply. On no account should they be awakened.

The constituents of this formula are primarily phlegm cutting and shen calming, with *Shi Chang*

Pu (Acori) to open orifices, a small amount of *Fu Zi* (Aconiti) to warm and open the flow of yang qi, and *Shen Qu* (Massa Fermentata) to eliminate phlegm and strengthen the Stomach. Because the original source of the turbid-phlegm is related to weakness of the zheng qi, an especially heavy dose of ginseng is used, assisted by the *Gan Cao* (Glycyrrhizae). The source text says: 'If the phlegm is not expelled, the zheng qi is hard to restore, [but] once the zheng qi is restored the pathogen is much more easily eliminated'. It also says 'When the pathogen sees the vigor of the zheng qi, no wonder it disappears without a trace!'. This formula is a good example of the combined use of tonification and expulsion ('fu zheng qu xie', discussed above in the introduction to this chapter).

Scouring phlegm to calm the shen

Insomnia resulting from internal disturbance by phlegm-heat will be accompanied by symptoms of restless anxiety, bitter taste, vertigo, tight chest, yellow greasy tongue coat with a somewhat reddish tongue body, and a rapid slippery pulse. The formula of choice is Qing Xin Di Tan Tang ('Clear the Heart and Scour the Phlegm Decoction').

Formula

Qing Xin Di Tan Tang ('Clear the Heart and Scour the Phlegm Decoction')

Ban Xia	Pinelliae Ternata, Rhizoma
Ju Hong	Citri Erythrocarpae, Pericarpium
Fu Ling	Poriae Cocos, Sclerotium
Zhi Shi	Citri seu Ponciri Immaturis, Fructus
Zhu Ru	Bambusae in Taeniis, Caulis
Dan Nan Xing	Arisaemae cum Felle Bovis, Pulvis
Shi Chang Pu	Acori Graminei, Rhizoma
Ren Shen	Ginseng, Radix
Mai Men Dong	Ophiopogonis Japonici, Tuber
Huang Lian	Coptidis, Rhizoma
Suan Zao Ren	Ziziphi Spinosae, Semen
Gan Cao	Glycyrrhizae Uralensis, Radix
Sheng Jiang	Zingiberis Officinalis Recens, Rhizoma
Da Zao	Zizyphi Jujubae, Fructus

Source text: *Yi Zong Jin Jian* ('Golden Mirror of the Medical Tradition', 1742)

Breaking up phlegm to restore consciousness

This is used for phlegm obstructing the qi flow in the channels, leading to sudden collapse and loss of consciousness, with the sound of phlegm in the throat or vomiting of thin phlegm, rough breathing, white greasy tongue coat, and deep slippery pulse. Chen Shi-Duo's *Qi Mi Dan* ('Awaken the Enchanted Pill') is effective, or one can powder *Qian Niu Zi* (Pharbitidis, Semen) and *Gan Sui* (Euphorbiae Kansui, Radix), combine the powder with flour, and paste it to the soles of the feet. Absorbed through the skin, this will have a similar effect of restoring consciousness.

Formula

Qi Mi Dan ('Awaken the Enchanted Pill')

Ban Xia	15 g	Pinelliae Ternata, Rhizoma
Ren Shen	15 g	Ginseng, Radix
Shi Chang Pu	6 g	Acori Graminei, Rhizoma
Tu Si Zi	30 g	Cuscutae, Semen
Gan Cao	0.9 g	Glycyrrhizae Uralensis, Radix
Fu Shen	9 g	Poriae Cocos Paradicis, Sclerotium
Zao Jiao	3 g	Gleditsiae Sinensis, Fructus
Sheng Jiang	3 g	Zingiberis Officinalis Recens, Rhizoma

Source text: *Shi Shi Mi Lu* ('Secret Records of the Stone Chamber', 1687).

Taken as a decoction for sudden fainting, inability to talk, eyes closed and hands uncontrolled, gurgling in the throat and very profuse phlegm.

Cutting phlegm to open the collaterals

When phlegm and stagnant blood combine, the result can be as mild as numbness or as severe as paralysis. This pathogenic combination is often a component of long term bi-syndrome (painful obstruction syndrome) where wind, damp and cold have slowed both the blood and the fluids to the extent that they have congealed. If heat is engendered by the obstruction, this too can lead to phlegm and stagnant blood by drying the fluids. The most characteristic sign is the tongue, which will have both purplish areas and either a greasy or a slippery coat. Da Huo Luo Dan ('Major Invigorate the Collaterals Pill') and Xiao Huo Luo Dan ('Minor Invigorate the Collaterals Special Pill') can be used, the former if the patient is somewhat deficient, the latter for strong patients.

Formulas

Da Huo Luo Dan ('Major Invigorate the Collaterals Pill')

This formula is readily available in prepared form, and rarely used as a decoction, due to the number and expense of the constituents.

Source text: *Ji Sheng Fang* ('Formulas to Aid the Living', 1253)

Xiao Huo Luo Dan ('Minor Invigorate the Collaterals Special Pill')

Zhi Chuan Wu	Aconiti Carmicheali Praeparata, Radix
Zhi Cao Wu	Aconiti Kusnezoffii Praeparata, Radix
Dan Nan Xing	Arisaemae cum Felle Bovis, Pulvis
Ru Xiang	Olibanum, Gummi
Mo Yao	Myrrha
Di Long	Lumbricus

Source text: *Tai Ping Hui Min He Ji Ju Fang* ('Imperial Grace Formulary of the Tai Ping Era', 1078-85) [*Formulas and Strategies*, p. 398]

Summary of phlegm treatment methods

Knowledge of the mechanism is essential

A thorough grasp of the mechanisms producing the phlegm in the individual patient is an essential prerequisite to the competent design of an effective formula for that patient. For example, in his *Jing Yue Quan Shu* ('Complete Works of Jing Yue', 1624), Zhang Jing–Yue discusses the phenomenon, occurring in some blood stagnation cases, of the yin-fluid aspect of the blood and jing-essence congealing to become phlegm in the channels and collaterals: 'there will be a lack of qi amidst the water, jin-fluids will coalesce and blood fail [to move] and go bad, both of which can transform into phlegm!' Here the phlegm is the direct result of the blood stagnation, not phlegm invading the channels from some outside source, as Zhang notes: 'This yield of phlegm or [the converse, normal] production of jing-essence and blood, how could it be external to the jing and blood, from some unrelated pathogenic phlegm?'

So one cannot simply hope to eliminate phlegm with pungent-parching phlegm-cutting herbs, which would not only not reach the phlegm but would also damage the blood. Zhang continues: 'If it is said that phlegm in the channels must be attacked in order to be eliminated, then the jing-essence and the blood must also be completely eliminated, before that would be possible. He suggests, in this case, that if both qi and yin are weak, to use Jin Shui Liu Jun Jian ('Six Gentlemen of Metal and Water Decoction') and if yin alone is deficient, to use a formula like Li Yin Jian ('Regulate the Yin Decoction').

Formulas

Jin Shui Liu Jun Jian ('Six Gentlemen of Metal and Water Decoction')

Ban Xia	Pinelliae Ternata, Rhizoma
Chen Pi	Citri Reticulatae, Pericarpium
Fu Ling	Poriae Cocos, Sclerotium
Zhi Gan Cao	Honey-fried Glycyrrhizae Uralensis, Radix
Dang Gui	Angelica Polymorpha, Radix
Sheng Di	Rehmannia Glutinosae, Radix
Sheng Jiang	Zingiberis Officinalis Recens, Rhizoma

Source text: *Jing Yue Quan Shu* ('Complete Works of Jing Yue', 1624) [*Formulas and Strategies*, p. 433]

Li Yin Jian ('Regulate the Yin Decoction')

Shou Di	9-30 g	Rehmanniae Glutinosae Conquitae, Radix
Dang Gui	6-21 g	Angelica Polymorpha, Radix
Zhi Gan Cao	3-6 g	Glycyrrhizae Uralensis, Radix
Gan Jiang	6-9 g	Zingiberis Officianalis, Rhizoma, (fried until yellow)
with the possible addition of		
Rou Gui	3-6 g	(Cinnamomi Cassiae, Cortex)

Source text: *Jing Yue Quan Shu* ('Complete Works of Jing Yue', 1624)

Zhang Jing-Yue notes: 'With phlegm, *Fu Ling* (Poriae Cocos, Sclerotium) or *Bai Jie Zi* (Sinapsis Albae, Semen) can be added in small amounts to promote movement'.[10]

Note. In both of these formulas, *Dang Gui* (Angelica Polymorpha, Radix) and *Shou Di* (Rehmanniae) are the main herbs, to restore blood and jing-essence, supported by qi tonic herbs to ensure the flow of qi to lead the blood. The herbs to transform phlegm, while essential, are only used in small amounts to facilitate the restoration of normal blood and jing-essence circulation, by removing obstruction from already existing phlegm.

A principle like this can be adjusted to suit slightly different cases, however. In a stronger patient with phlegm at the blood level—that is, moving with it in the channels, or perhaps interfering with menstruation—one can use stronger phlegm removing herbs combined with smaller amounts of *Dang Gui* (Angelica) and *Shou Di* (Rehmanniae) to lead them into the blood. Without these guiding herbs, the formula would miss the mark.

Once the mechanism is known, the appropriate principle—or even combination of principles—can be applied. As might have been appreciated from the above example, one needs to know not only which processes are involved in a pathological mechanism, but also the relative strengths of those processes, so that the amounts of the individual herbs which deal with those processes can be adjusted accordingly.[11]

Herbs used in phlegm treatments

In the early days of Chinese treatments for phlegm and thin mucus, the watchword was 'harmonize with warming herbs', because 'phlegm is a yin pathogen, without warmth it will not transform'. However, this is only relevant to a partial range of phlegm conditions, such as yang deficiency or thin mucus accumulation; it cannot be taken as the single principle upon which to base all phlegm treatments. We now know that for an approach to be effective it must take into account differences between hot and cold, deficiency and excess, obstruction, dryness, fire and so on, as well as the length of the illness, the strength of the patient, and the thickness and turbidity of the phlegm itself. Thus, as we have seen, in clinic a variety of methods may be applied, e.g. moving qi to transform phlegm, softening hardness to break up phlegm, cooling heat to eliminate phlegm, and even using insect drugs to open the collaterals and expel stagnant blood and phlegm. Deep-seated phlegm, for example, will require a completely different strategy than recent phlegm-cold in the Lungs; while in another case the incorrect use of phlegm-parching herbs would have a disastrous effect if used incorrectly with a zao-dryness pathogen desiccating the fluids to produce phlegm.

The patient's age, sex, strength, medical history, working and living conditions are all factors that will influence the choice of therapy. For example, in a young strong athlete, emesis or purging is an option; whereas with an old, weak or sedentary intellectual, treatment would have to focus on the Spleen, Liver or Kidneys. This applies not only to the choice of formula but also to the selection of individual herbs with which to alter that formula. Little has been written in English on the precise use of Chinese herbs; even modern Chinese medicine textbooks never mention 'phlegm' for many herbs classically described as extremely useful in phlegm treatments. *Long Gu* (Draconis, Os), *Mu Li* (Ostreae, Concha), *Jiang Can* (Bombyx Batryticatus), *Quan Xie* (Buthus Martensi) and *Wu Gong* (Scolopendra Subspinipes) are good examples: these are usually described as wind-extinguishing or spirit-calming, and phlegm is not listed. In classic texts, however, *Long Gu* (Draconis, Os) and *Mu Li* (Ostreae, Concha) are described as 'marvellous articles' for the expulsion of phlegm, and the others are often utilized in phlegm formulas.

Thus to increase the armory of those engaged in treating phlegm with Chinese herbal medicine, and to encourage precision in the use of herbs, some of the most useful—and most ignored—herbs for eliminating phlegm will be described in detail; other herbs whose phlegm dispelling effects are better known will be covered mainly in the comparison sections of the herbs described below.[12]

Xuan Fu Hua (Inulae, Flos)

Classed under 'herbs that stop cough and wheezing' in some modern texts, and under 'warm herbs that transform cold-phlegm' in others, *Xuan Fu Hua* is bitter (so it drains downward), pungent (so it disperses), salty (so it softens hardened phlegm) and

is slightly warm. It enters the Lungs, Stomach and Large Intestine channels, settles nausea, and has the ability to 'disperse knotted phlegm above the diaphragm, phlegm which when expectorated has the appearance of glue or lacquer, and phlegm-water in the costal and cardiac region' (*Ming Yi Bie Lu*).[13] 'Xuan Fu Hua is the herb to disperse phlegm, expel water, and carry qi downward! Hot-phlegm, damp-phlegm, cold-phlegm, phlegm from food stagnation, thin mucus and phlegm, any of these conditions will respond well to *Xuan Fu Hua*; with excess or deficiency, heat or cold, if used in the appropriate combinations, it will never fail to get good results' (*Ben Cao Hui Yan*).[14]

Comparison with Ban Xia (Pinelliae). Both herbs can disperse knotted phlegm, settle the Stomach and stop nausea, and are often combined to do just this. But the main action of *Xuan Fu Hua* (Inulae) is to bring down qi, break up knotted accumulation, and move water, while *Ban Xia* (Pinelliae) primarily parches damp to transform phlegm. So the *Xuan Fu Hua* is more appropriate for thick sticky, hard-to-cough-out phlegm, or flank pain with distension and fullness of the chest and abdomen from accumulated pathogenic water and thin mucus, or middle Jiao qi deficiency allowing water and damp to build up in the Spleen and Stomach causing nausea. *Ban Xia* is best for profuse thin clear phlegm that is easy to cough out.

Comparison with Hai Fu Shi (Pumice). Both of these herbs are salty and so are able to soften hardened phlegm, and in fact they are often combined to treat clumped sticky phlegm difficult to cough out. But *Xuan Fu Hua* (Inulae) is warm, with both bitter and pungent flavors that enable it to bring qi downward in the treatment of cough, wheeze, and nausea. *Hai Fu Shi* (Pumice) is cold, and better for hot sticky phlegm, or Lung heat injuring the collaterals and leading to coughing of blood.

Hou Po (Magnoliae Officianalis, Cortex)

Bitter, pungent, warm and parching, *Hou Po* (Magnoliae) is best at dispelling 'insubstantial' cold and damp qi blockage, and at dispersing 'substantial' food and phlegm stagnation. Li Dong-Yuan says: '*Hou Po*: bitter can bring down qi, and so it can drain excess (shi) fullness; warmth can benefit qi, and so it can dispel damp fullness'. *The Tang Ye Ben Cao*[15] says: '*Hou Po* can disperse phlegm and bring down qi'. Therefore *Hou Po* can be used to warm the center, bring down qi, parch damp and disperse phlegm; but because of its warmth and bitterness, it is most often used in cases of damp phlegm, cold phlegm and phlegm from qi obstruction.

Comparison with Zhi Shi *(Citri seu Ponciri Immaturis, Fructus)*. *Zhi Shi* is best at busting qi blockage, and it is through this action that its phlegm dispersing effects are achieved. *Hou Po* is warm and parching, pungent and dispersing, and so the warmth and parching strengthen the Spleen, while the pungency dispels knotted qi and thus eliminates distension and fullness.

Zhi Shi *(Citri seu Ponciri Immaturis, Fructus)*

This is an important herb for removing qi obstruction through its bitter draining and descending actions. The *Ben Cao Yan Yi Bu Yi*[16] records: '*Zhi Shi* drains phlegm; it can attack barriers and break down walls, and is a herb which can make slippery the orifices and drain qi'. The *Yao Pin Hua Yi* says: '*Zhi Shi* specializes in draining excess in the Stomach (and Intestines), opening and leading away hard knots, dispersing phlegm accumulations and phlegm water, and expelling accumulated food'. The *Shi Yi De Xiao Fang*[17] records that *Zhi Shi* combined with *Zao Jiao* (Gleditsiae Sinensis, Fructus) and powdered, then formed into a pill with rice paste, can be used to treat constipation resulting from phlegm obstructing the qi flow through the fu organs (i.e. here meaning the Stomach and Intestines).

Comparison with Zhi Ke *(Citri seu Ponciri, Fructus)*. The reason that the above treatment is effective can be seen from the comments of Wu Ju–Tong in his *Yi Yi Bing Shu*:

> *Zhi Shi* is firm and sinking, and moves specifically to the pylorus (you men). The pylorus is the lower opening of the Stomach and the upper opening of the Small Intestine. Expelling sedimentary dross, phlegm and thin mucus, [it] makes it move from the Stomach into the Small Intestine, and from the Small Intestine into the Large Intestine. *Zhi Ke* (Citri seu Ponciri, Fructus) has empty pockets [while *Zhi Shi* is

solid inside], and thus *Zhi Ke* is light and rises, specifically moving to the upper mouth of the Stomach. The prescription books say that mistaken use of *Zhi Ke* will harm the highest qi (gao qi) in the chest. Nowadays people do not dare to use *Zhi Shi* because the recent *Ben Cao* (Materia Medica) texts say that it 'can attack barriers and break down walls', and instead use *Zhi Ke*. This only mistakenly damages places which have no problem, while the sedimentary dross around the pylorus, conversely, is not expelled!'[18]

Bing Lang *(Arecae Catechu, Semen)*

Classed as a 'herb that expels parasites', *Bing Lang* (Arecae Catechu, Semen) also breaks up qi obstruction through its pungency, leads qi downward because of its bitterness, and moves water with its warmth. The sum of these actions provides a good effect on phlegm accumulation, especially in the channels which it enters: the Stomach and Large Intestine. Thus Li Shi-Zhen states: *Bing Lang* 'treats wheeze and dyspnea from phlegm and qi [obstruction], and qi obstruction in the Large and Small Intestines leading to constipation and urinary blockage'. The *Ben Cao Yue Yan*[19] explains: '*Bing Lang* enters the chest and abdomen, breaking up blocked qi, and then continues into the Stomach and Intestines to expel phlegm occlusion and take it directly downward; it can lead other herbs downward, expelling water to deal with swelling pain and numbness of the foot … it is due to its descending action that it can expel intestinal parasites'.

Comparison with Da Fu Pi *(Arecae Catechu, Pericarpium)*. *Da Fu Pi* is the shell of Bing Lang (Arecae Catechu, Semen), and is classed as a qi mover, pungent and slightly warm. *Da Fu Pi* is better at dispersing 'insubstantial' qi blockage, eliminating distension and promoting urination to reduce fluid retention. *Bing Lang* (Arecae Catechu, Semen) is better at dispersing 'substantial' accumulations, including phlegm, and of course can expel parasites.

Da Huang *(Rhei, Rhizoma)*

Da Huang is not only a good purgative and blood mover (if prepared with alcohol) but can also be used with excellent effect to expel hot phlegm through the intestines. The *Ben Cao Jing Shu* (1809) says:

> *Da Huang* is very cold and very bitter, with a direct nature, best at opening the lower body, and is therefore an important herb in the treatment of heat knotted in the middle and lower Jiao as a result of injury by cold (shang han), febrile diseases, heat conditions, and damp-heat, leading to constipation and urinary difficulty. It is also good for damp and heat jelling into phlegm in the middle and lower Jiao. It expels the pathogen and stops the violence [of pathogenic interference], with the special ability to uproot chaos and restore normality.[20]

Zi Su Zi (Perillae Fructescentis, Fructus)

Zi Su Zi is pungent, warm and fragrant, with a moistening nature that descends, and is well-known as a herb to stop cough and wheeze. But its other effects are often ignored. According to the *Ri Hua Ben Cao*,[21] *Zi Su Zi* can also 'break up (movable) abdominal masses and knots'; and the *Yao Pin Hua Yi* says 'Because it both descends and disperses, it is specific for qi blockage leading to phlegm' especially in the Intestines, and so *Zi Su Zi* can be used for phlegm constipation.

Comparison with Zi Su Ye (Perillae Fructescentis, Folium) and Zi Su Geng (Perillae Fructescentis, Ramulus). All three can harmonize the qi but the leaves (ye) expel surface pathogens and harmonize the middle Jiao qi, the stalks (geng) open the middle Jiao qi and regulate the qi flow in the chest and diaphragm, and the seeds (zi) help Lung qi to descend and transform turbid-phlegm.

Comparison with Ma Huang (Ephedrae, Herba). Both herbs settle dyspnea, and are used together for cough and asthma from cold phlegm leading to Lung qi rebelling upward. But because of the stronger phlegm-transforming effect of *Zi Su Zi* (Perillae Fructescentis, Fructus), it is more appropriate for cough and asthma with profuse phlegm blocking the flow of Lung qi; while *Ma Huang* is a stronger surface opening herb, and more appropriate for exogenous wind cold pathogen blocking the Lung qi.

Lai Fu Zi (Raphani Sativi, Semen)

Often classed as a herb to relieve food stagnation, or a herb to cut phlegm and stop cough, *Lai Fu Zi* is actually best at moving qi, with the special ability to lift if used in its raw state, and descend if prepared (by frying it over a moderate flame). In its raw state it is pungent, sweet and neutral, and, because of its lifting function, liable to cause nausea if used in too great amounts; if prepared it is warm, and will not lead to nausea. So in many parts of China, if '*Lai Fu Zi*' is written, the herb shop will provide fried *Lai Fu Zi*, and will only supply raw if specified on the prescription. When fried, it can enter the Lung channel to help Lung qi to descend and transform phlegm, and also enters the Spleen and Stomach channels to move qi and disperse food stagnation. In its raw state many doctors, including Zhu Dan-Xi, have used its ascending nature to bring on vomiting in cases of profuse phlegm and food stagnation obstructing the middle Jiao, where emesis is the quickest and most effective treatment.

Comparison with Bai Jie Zi (Sinapsis Albae, Semen). Both are good at dispelling phlegm in the treatment of cough and dyspnea. But the nature of *Lai Fu Zi* is moderate and harmonious, and it tends to move into the zang fu organs, with its emphasis on regulating the functioning of the Lungs, Stomach, and Large Intestine to relieve fullness and distension. It can be used for either hot phlegm or cold phlegm.

Bai Jie Zi, on the other hand, is pungent, warm and strongly parching; it moves through the channels and collaterals, moving qi and eradicating knots of phlegm, with its specialty being phlegm 'beneath the skin but outside the membranes'. Because of its warmth, *Bai Jie Zi* is only appropriate for cold phlegm.

Zao Jiao (Gleditsiae Sinensis, Fructus)

With its pungent warmth, softening saltiness and sharp piercing nature, *Zao Jiao* is excellent for expelling stubborn phlegm and 'scouring thick grease', as the *Ben Cao Jing Shu* notes: 'Any thick greasy dirty turbid qi in the Intestines or the Stomach, *Zao Jiao* (Gleditsiae Sinensis, Fructus) can scour and flush it away, leaving the Stomach and Intestines clean and pure'. This 'qi' mentioned above is referring to phlegm, as we know from the *Ben*

Jing Feng Yuan:[22] '*Zao Jiao* expels stubborn thick greasy phlegm'. It is not only effective in the Stomach and Intestines but also works for thick jelled phlegm in the upper Jiao, as the *Jin Gui Yao Lue* ('Essentials from the Golden Cabinet') formula Zao Jiao Wan (made up of the single herb, peeled, and made into pills with honey) was designed to treat. In Chapter 7, section 6, it says: 'Cough with qi rebelling upward and frequent expectoration of turbid fluid, [the patient is] only able to sit up so that sleep is impossible: Zao Jiao Wan is the main formula'. *Zao Jiao* (Gleditsiae Sinensis, Fructus) also opens orifices both in the upper and lower body, enters the Stomach and Intestines to expel phlegm and damp, expels parasites and can moisten the bowels to treat constipation.

Wei Ling Xian (Clemetidis Chinensis, Radix)

Wei Ling Xian is pungent, dispersing and best at moving, with a warm opening nature, and enters all twelve channels, so it can disperse wind on the surface and also can transform interior damp, it can open the channels and also reach the collaterals, opening and leading out, and thus is an excellent herb for the treatment of painful wind conditions. The same qualities, though, suit it for phlegm treatments, and this has not been ignored by Classical authors. The *Ben Cao Jing Shu* notes: '*Wei Ling Xian* spreads, opens, and likes to move, and treats phlegm water in the heart region and the diaphragm, chronic accumulation leading to abdominal masses both movable and immovable, soft lumps and nodes in the flanks and chest, and knots of qi'. The *Yao Pin Hua Yi* says: '*Wei Ling Xian*, its nature is violent and rapid, "moving without staying",[23] and its primary areas of treatment are wind, damp, and phlegm building up and occluding the channels and collaterals'. The *Ben Cao Zheng Yi* remarks: '*Wei Ling Xian's* ability is to move, pierce, disperse, and overcome; it is appropriate for accumulated damp, halted phlegm, stagnant blood, and blocked qi'. Because of this ability to move, *Wei Ling Xian* (Clemetidis Chinensis, Radix) is very useful for treating limb problems, especially the legs, and especially pain and numbness. The sole problem is that its violent nature easily exhausts the zheng qi of the body, and so should not be used with weak patients.

Lian Qiao (Forsythiae Suspensae, Fructus)

Lian Qiao is a cooling anti-toxic herb that is rarely considered in the context of phlegm, despite its well-documented dispersing and penetrating abilities which have earned it the name of 'Sage of the Skin Ulcer Herbs'. Most modern texts will record that it can be used for 'dissipating nodules' but perhaps the only modern formula which employs its light dispersing abilities for hot-phlegm is Bao He Wan ('Preserve Harmony Pill', *Formulas and Strategies*, p. 455), where its use has been considered by some commentators to be a minor mystery. It is likewise able to promote urination and lead Heart fire out through the urine, according to the *Yao Xing Ben Cao*,[24] which again strengthens its ability to eliminate phlegm. Because heat resulting from obstructed qi and blood under the skin can also lead to phlegm-heat and eventually toxic-phlegm as the fluids from the blood and nutritive qi are boiled away, *Lian Qiao* (Forsythiae Suspensae, Fructus) must be kept in mind in such cases, or indeed any case of obstructed Lung heat or Heart fire affecting fluids.

Comparison with Jin Yin Hua (*Lonicerae Japonicae, Flos*). Both are cooling and anti-toxic, and both can vent heat through the surface while also cooling internal heat, and thus they are very often combined for these purposes. The difference is that *Jin Yin Hua* (Lonicerae) tends to disperse surface heat, it is sweet and so does not harm the Stomach; while *Lian Qiao* (Forsythiae Suspensae, Fructus) has a strong Heart fire cooling effect, and can disperse qi occluded at the blood level, and also treats difficult urinary syndrome ('lin zheng').

Xuan Shen (Scrophulariae Ningpoensis, Radix)

This is classed as a blood cooling herb which is sweet, bitter, salty and cold, with a moistening nature. It can enter the Lung, Stomach and Kidney channels. Its sweet-coldness nourishes yin, its bitter-coldness drains fire and eliminates toxins, and its salty-coldness softens hardness and moistens dry conditions. Because it is cool and moistening, *Xuan Shen* can nourish the Kidneys, controlling fire which is floating up. But it can also transform hot phlegm. Zhang Shan-Lei, in the *Ben Cao Zheng Yi*, describes this well: '*Xuan Shen* (Scrophulariae) has a bitter and sweet flavor: bitter can cool fire, sweet can nourish yin, and because of its sweet flavor, its descending nature is mild. The *Ben Cao* says that it only enters the Kidney channel, but [the writer] did not know that it especially enters the Lung zang organ, and therefore can relieve rootless floating fire, and disperse knots of phlegm and hot boils all around the body'. Due to its salty flavor, *Xuan Shen* is one of three herbs in the phlegm-nodule-removing formula Xiao Luo Wan ('Reduce Scrofula Pill', *Formulas and Strategies*, p. 441) which Professor Song Guang-Ji at the Zhejiang College of Traditional Chinese Medicine used for nodules and masses all around the body, not only the neck, with great effect. In my own practice I use it for breast lumps, ovarian cysts and uterine fibroids as a basic formula upon which to build, and the results are good.

Yu Jin (Curcumae, Tuber)

Yu Jin is pungent, bitter and cold, and enters the Heart and Liver channels at the blood level, and thus can drain Heart fire while cooling the blood and breaking up stagnation, and also can move qi at the blood level while dispersing obstructed Liver qi which has formed knots. This ability to remove obstruction has led to its name which, although sometimes translated 'Constrained Metal', should more probably be rendered 'Depression Gold' or 'Obstruction Gold', signifying its value in removing blocked qi. The removal of blocked qi is essential in the treatment of phlegm resulting from qi flow interruption, and *Yu Jin* is well-suited for this: 'Yu Jin is excellent to clear the qi and transform phlegm, and disperse stagnant blood; its nature is light and lifting, it is able to disperse oppressed blockages, and settle rebelling qi. It can reach up to the vertex, but moves best into the lower Jiao, and its most evident effects are in the treatment of obstruction from the failure of the qi, blood, fire, and phlegm to move' (*Ben Cao Hui Yan*). As Liver qi blockage from stress is a major etiological factor in the West, coupled with our propensity for phlegm production, *Yu Jin* would seem to merit some attention in this regard.

Bai Jie Zi (Sinapsis Albae, Semen)

White mustard seed is pungent, warm and dispersing, entering the Lungs and Stomach channels, with the special ability to penetrate the yin and restore yang movement. Zhu Dan-Xi said that

'Phlegm in the subcostal region, and between the skin and the membranes, cannot be reached without using *Bai Jie Zi*'. It enters the channels with the Lung qi and disperses cold phlegm occlusions causing pain in the joints, or yin-type ulcers, and can also reach the interior of the body to relieve pain in the epigastric and abdominal regions. As would be expected from its inclusion in San Zi Yang Qin Tang ('Three Seed Decoction to Nourish One's Parents', *Formulas and Strategies*, p. 445), *Bai Jie Zi* is also used for cold-phlegm oppressing the Lungs leading to wheeze and dyspnea. The usual dose is recorded at 3-9 g but doses of 15 g seem to get better results without causing any problems, although this should only be used with strong patients because the strong qi-moving warmth of *Bai Jie Zi* could injure the qi in a weak patient.

Comparison with Zi Su Zi **(Perillae Fructescentis, Fructus)**. Both herbs treat cold-phlegm cough and dyspnea but *Bai Jie Zi* is violently warm and parching, likes to move in the channels, and is best at moving qi and eradicating phlegm. *Zi Su Zi* is better at bringing qi down to settle dyspnea and disperse phlegm, which is its main indication, but is also moistening and therefore can be used for constipation.

Comparison with Dan Nan Xing **(Arisaemae cum Felle Bovis, Pulvis)**. Both move in the channels to treat 'broadly defined' phlegm but *Bai Jie Zi* promotes the flow of qi and eliminates knotted cold-phlegm causing joint pain, limitation of movement, and yin-type ulcers (yin ju). The *Dan Nan Xing* extinguishes wind and eradicates phlegm, and so is more suited to treating the spasms and cramps, or even hemiplegia, brought on by wind phlegm.

Mai Ya (Hordei Vulgaris Germinantus, Fructus)

This is usually classed under 'herbs that relieve food stagnation', which is indeed one of its major functions as it harmonizes the center, dispels accumulated food and brings down qi. This in itself would recommend it as an excellent root treatment for phlegm but *Mai Ya* has another ability which makes it even more useful in modern phlegm prescriptions: it can open Liver qi flow. The *Yao Pin Hua Yi* says: 'Large *Mai Ya*, when fried until fragrant, opens the Stomach, mainly treating both movable and immovable abdominal masses (zheng jia) and knotted qi, fullness and distension of the chest and diaphragm, and phlegm from qi obstruction.' The *Ben Cao Qiu Zhen*[25] notes:

> *Mai Ya*, with its fresh rising qi, promotes Liver to control Spleen Earth (ie, assist Spleen transport), and thus can disperse and lead [food into the Intestines]. Any qi obstruction causing severe epigastric distension or similar symptoms can be treated with *Mai Ya* to marvellous effect: people know that it eliminates food stagnation, but do not know that it also promotes Liver qi flow!

Thus *Mai Ya* is an excellent herb to use for weak patients with Liver and Spleen disharmony leading to loss of appetite and taste for food but again its functions can be extended beyond this. One of my lecturers in gynecology in China was Qiu Xiao-Mei, well-known throughout Hangzhou and the Jiangnan area of China for her expertise in the use of herbs for gynecological problems. In one lecture she mentioned that she often used *Mai Ya* (Hordei Vulgaris Germinantus, Fructus) in the standard way (fried, 60–120 g decocted and taken like tea) for reducing milk flow and breast discomfort in weaning but that she also extended this reasoning to apply it for breast lumps and distension, and again further for lumps in general such as ovarian cysts and even uterine fibroids. She would use 30–60 g of *Mai Ya* included in a standard formula for such a purpose, and found that in all of these cases she obtained better results. I have often used this approach in Melbourne, with equally good effect. This is consistent with the observation of the *Yao Pin Hua Yi* quoted above, that *Mai Ya* can be used for 'masses and knotted qi'. Because of its effect on lactation, however, it should be used carefully (or not at all) with breast-feeding mothers.

The following two essays discuss in detail the treatment of phlegm, describing the herbs which each author has found to be the most effective in different types of phlegm condition. The third short essay by Zhang Lu introduces a novel observation regarding the management of phlegm in the channels and collaterals.

The first is by Zhu Dan-Xi. People tend to think of him as only the originator of the 'tonify the yin' school; in fact Zhu Dan-Xi was a tremendously versatile physician in many areas. One of the most important, he believed, was the proper treatment of phlegm diseases.

Classical Essays

This essay is from Dan Xi Xin Fa ('Teachings of Dan Xi') 1481, 'Experiences in the treatment of phlegm'.

In general, when treating phlegm, if purging or diuretic herbs are used excessively, this will cause the Spleen qi to weaken, and phlegm will then be produced all the more easily.

For damp-phlegm use *Cang Zhu* (Atractylodis) and *Bai Zhu* (Atractylodis Macrocephalae); for hot-phlegm use *Qing Dai* (Indigo), *Huang Lian* (Coptidis), and *Huang Qin* (Scutellariae); for food stagnation use *Shen Qu* (Massa Fermentata), *Mai Ya* (Hordei Vulgaris Germinantus, Fructus), and *Shan Zha* (Crataegi). For wind-phlegm use *Dan Nan Xing* (Arisaemae cum Felle Bovis, Pulvis).

For old-phlegm use *Fu Hai Shi* (Pumice), *Ban Xia* (Pinelliae), *Quan Gua Lou* (Trichosanthis, Fructus et Pericarpium), *Xiang Fu* (Cyperi Rotundi), and *Wu Bei Zi* (Rhi Chinensis), taken together as a pill.

Phlegm above the diaphragm must be expelled through emesis,[26] draining here will not eliminate it.

Wind-phlegm usually produces strange symptoms; damp-phlegm usually produces lethargy, tiredness, and soft weakness.

Excess-qi type phlegm-heat knotted in the upper body, difficult to spit out: if it is clear phlegm, it will usually be cold. [This should be treated with] formulas like Er Chen Tang ('Two-Cured Decoction', *Formulas and Strategies*, p. 432); if the phlegm is thick, sticky, and turbid, emesis must be used.

Hot-phlegm with wind is most often encountered in exogenous invasions. If it is hot, it must be cooled; if there is food stagnation, it must be attacked, but if there is qi deficiency as well, [the attacking herbs] can be swallowed with the help of a qi tonifying decoction.

For phlegm rising into the upper body because of surging fire, treatment of the fire is primary, using herbs such as *Bai Zhu* (Atractylodis Macrocephalae), *Huang Qin* (Scutellariae), and *Shi Gao* (Gypsum).

Internal injury[27] with phlegm must be treated with herbs like *Ren Shen* (Ginseng), *Huang Qi* (Astragali), and *Bai Zhu*; using ginger juice to wash them down is a common approach. *Ban Xia* (Pinelliae) can also be added; if the deficiency is severe, add *Zhu Li* (Bambusae, Succus); if the middle Jiao qi is insufficient, increase *Ren Shen* and *Bai Zhu*.

Phlegm is such that it will follow the qi in its ascent and descent, and there is no limit to its compass. If Spleen is weak, then Spleen qi must be tonified, and the middle qi cleared, in order to transport phlegm downwards: Er Chen Tang ('Two-Cured Decoction') plus *Bai Zhu* is the type of method, with *Sheng Ma* (Cimicifugae, Rhizoma) used in conjunction to lift [the clear Spleen qi].

In cases where the disease is the result of middle Jiao phlegm plus food stagnation, [because] the Stomach also depends [on the middle Jiao] for its nourishment, attacking cannot be heedlessly employed. If attacked over-zealously, greater deficiency will result.

Phlegm which has lumped together, and cannot be coughed, vomited, or expectorated out: if found in qi blockage patients it will be very hard to treat.

Those with qi [obstruction], damp, phlegm, and heat together will also be very hard to treat.

Phlegm between the Stomach and Intestines can be cured by purging.

In the channels and collaterals, emesis must be used—but remember that the idea of 'spreading dispersal' is part of 'emesis'.

Epileptic disease can be brought on by a sudden fright, as fright causes the shen to abandon its abode (i.e. the Heart),[28] if the abode is empty then phlegm will be produced. Once phlegm enters the abode, the Heart shen will be refused entrance, and cannot return there.

If blood is damaged, ginger juice must be used to swallow the other herbs. *Huang Qin* (Scutellariae) treats hot phlegm, by borrowing its ability to bring down fire. *Zhu Li* (Bambusae, Succus) makes phlegm slippery, [but] without ginger juice it will not be able to enter the channels and collaterals. *Wu Bei Zi* (Rhi Chinensis) can treat old-phlegm, with the help of other herbs it is superb for treating stubborn phlegm.

Er Chen Tang ('Two-Cured Decoction') will take care of phlegm anywhere in the body. If you want it to move downward, add downward-leading herbs; if it is necessary for it to move upward, add upward-leading herbs.

Anytime emetic herbs are used, the qi should be lifted to ascend, and the vomiting will occur. For example, *Fang Feng* (Ledebouriellae), *Shan Zhi Zi* (Gardeniae), *Chuan Xiong* (Ligustici), *Jie Geng* (Platycodi), *Mai Cha* (grain tea), *Sheng Jiang* (raw ginger), and the juice of garlic, ginger, or leeks, or possibly Gua Di San ['Melon Pedicle Powder', *Formulas and Strategies*, p. 449] may be used.

Any wind-phlegm disease requires the use of wind-phlegm herbs, such as *Bai Fu Zi* (Typhonii Gigantei, Rhizoma seu Aconiti Coreani, Radix), *Tian Ma* (Gastrodiae), Xiong Huang (Realgar), *Niu Huang* (Bovis, Calculus), *Huang Qin* (Scutellariae), *Jiang Can* (Bombyx Batryticatus), and *Zhu Ya Zao Jiao* (Fructus Gleditsiae Abnormalis—abnormal fruit of Chinese Honeylocust).

Any lumps in the upper or lower body are usually phlegm. Ask the patient what they often crave to eat. Only after using emesis or a purge may other herbs be used.

Darkness around or under the eyes, as if blackened by smoke, is also phlegm.

Xu Xue-Shi[29] used Cang Zhu (Atractylodis, Rhizoma) to treat phlegm forming bubble-like nodes with great success. He says [that] these result from phlegm combining with stagnant blood.

Vertigo with indefinable epigastric discomfort[30] is fire shifting the phlegm. Use Er Chen Tang ('Two-Cured Decoction') plus herbs like *Shan Zhi Zi* (Gardeniae), *Huang Lian* (Coptidis), *Huang Qin* (Scutellariae). Belching with sour regurgitation is food which has become obstructed and produced heat leading fire qi to move upward. *Huang Qin* should be used as the chief herb, *Dan Nan Xing* (Arisaemae cum Felle Bovis, Pulvis) and *Ban Xia* (Pinelliae) as deputies, and *Ju Hong* (Citri Erythrocarpae, Pericarpium) as envoy. If heat is excessive, add *Qing Dai* (Indigo).

For phlegm under the lateral costal region, without the use of *Bai Jie Zi* (Sinapsis Albae, Semen) it cannot be reached. Phlegm between the skin and the membranes require ginger juice and *Zhu Li* (Bambusae, Succus) as guides. Phlegm in the limbs needs *Zhu Li* to open [the channels and collaterals].

Phlegm nodes knotted in the throat, so that dry things cannot be swallowed, should be treated using phlegm cutting herbs plus salty-softening flavours. *Gua Lou Ren* (Trichosanthes, Semen), *Xing Ren* (Pruni Armeniacae), *Hai Fu Shi* (Pumice), *Jie Geng* (Platycodi), and *Lian Qiao* (Forsythiae), with a small amount of *Mang Xiao* (Mirabilitum) as assistant, can be made into pills with ginger juice and honey, and dissolved in the mouth.

Hai Fen is *Hai Fu Shi* (Pumice), which can bring down hot-phlegm, parch damp-phlegm, soften knotted-phlegm, and disperse stubborn-phlegm. It can be included in pills or powders, but cannot be used in decoctions.

Zhi Shi (Citri seu Ponciri Immaturis, Fructus) drains phlegm, with the ability to charge blockades and break down barriers.

Xiao Wei Dan ('Little Stomach Pill')[31] treats all shoulder and arm pain from phlegm-heat above the diaphragm, wind-phlegm, and damp-phlegm, but it can damage Stomach qi: food accumulation and excess (shi) phlegm cases can use it, but not for too long.

Shen Yu Wan ('Added Evodia Pill')[32] can disperse phlegm.

A sensation of something in the throat which cannot be swallowed or coughed out is old-phlegm. If severe, emesis should be used; if mild, use *Quan Gua Lou* (Trichosanthis, Fructus et Pericarpium) as substitute. If the qi is shi (excess), *Jing Li* (Viticis Negundo, Succus) must be used.

Tian Hua Fen (Trichosanthis, Radix) is superb at bringing down hot-phlegm above the diaphragm. Phlegm within the confines of the diaphragm (i.e. in the vicinity of the Heart) can make people forgetful or cause mental disturbance. For this, and for wind-phlegm, *Zhu Li* (Bambusae, Succus) should be used, as it can also nourish blood; it has the same effect as *Jing Li* (Viticis Negundo, Succus). To treat somewhat more serious cases [of the above] who can still take in food, use both of these herbs, and the results will be rapid and safe. Both of these types of plant saps (i.e. the bamboo sap *Zhu Li* and the Vitex sap *Jing Li*) treat knotted-phlegm between the skin and the membranes, but they need ginger juice to do it.

Leek juice (i.e. juice of allium tuberosum) can treat blood which is obstructed and unable to move, and thin mucus in the middle Jiao. If several small cups of the natural juice are taken cold, there will initially be feelings of anxiety and restlessness in the chest, but afterwards they will be cured.

Anytime phlegm is involved in an illness, whether there is dyspnea, or cough, or vomiting, or loose stool, or vertigo and dizziness, or indefinable discomfort around the heart with palpitations, or chills, fever, and painful swellings, or stoppage (痞 pi: sensation of fullness but without pain) [preventing the normal flow of nutritive and protective qi, so that yin and yang undergo] separation, or blockage, or the sound of water moving within the chest and flanks, or a frequent feeling of cold in one area of the back, or numbness and loss of feeling in the limbs: all of these symptoms are the result of phlegm.

One who is good at the treatment of phlegm will not treat the phlegm, but will address the qi; once the qi flows smoothly, the jin and ye fluids of the whole body will follow the qi in effortless circulation.

Furthermore, Yan Yong-He (author of the *Yan Shi Ji Sheng Fang*, 1253) says: 'The most important thing for the qi in the body is to flow smoothly: if it is smooth, the fluids will flow openly, and there will be absolutely no problem with phlegm or thin mucus'.

The ancient formulas, in treating phlegm and thin mucus, used diaphoresis, emesis, purging, and warming methods; but in my humble opinion none is as important as smoothing the flow of qi, with separating and leading [downward] next.

Also [Wang] Yin-Jun's theory says: clear white phlegm is cold, thick turbid yellow is heat; did he not realize that in the beginning the phlegm will be clear and white, while after a period of time the phlegm will be yellow and turbid? Or that thin clear white phlegm will be that which is slippery and inundating the upper [part of the body], while the yellow turbid thick [phlegm] is stuck below? That which is easy to cough out will be the thin and white phlegm; while the hard-to-cough-out phlegm will be yellow, turbid and coalesced. In cases where the coughing and spitting have become chronic, [or] damp-heat creates obstruction, [or] both above and below have become sticky and knotted, in all of these situations there will be no white clear phlegm at all. In severe cases [the phlegm] will contain blood, if the blood becomes bad (bai) then the phlegm will become black, which is one of the variations of guan ge ('block and repulsion'); people generally do not realize this.

Moreover, clear white phlegm is bland in flavor, but after a long time it will gradually produce a bad taste: sour, pungent, scorched-putrid, or bitter: different in each case.

That most diseases will have some phlegm component is a fact that nobody recognizes. [For example] anytime the body has nodes which are not painful or red, and do not produce pus, this is a sign of phlegm.

Of the methods of treating phlegm, strengthening Spleen Earth and parching Spleen damp is the root therapy.[33]

[The following essay is from the *Yi Xue Zhuan Xin Lu* ('Record of the Transmission of the Heart of Medicine'), written by the Qing dynasty physician Liu Yi-Ren, and is based upon changes to Er Chen Tang ('Two-Cured Decoction', *Formulas and Strategies*, p. 432).]

Methods of addition to Er Chen Tang

Phlegm does not arise of itself, its production must have a reason: be it wind, or cold, or heat, or damp, or summerheat, or dryness, or excessive alcohol, or accumulation of food, or because of Spleen deficiency, or again because of Kidney weakness.

Nowadays those treating phlegm only know that *Dan Nan Xing* (Arisaemae) and *Ban Xia* (Pinelliae) are phlegm remedies; but they do not know how to treat the root of phlegm, and thus phlegm continues to worsen and the illness becomes hard to eradicate.

My limited knowledge notwithstanding, may I yet dare to describe the medicines that will treat the root?

Wind as a causative factor will produce frothy phlegm and saliva, the pulse will be floating and wiry, and the treatment should include herbs such as *Qian Hu* (Peucedani) and *Xuan Fu Hua* (Inulae).

Cold as a causative factor will produce clear cold phlegm and saliva, the pulse will be deep and slow, and the treatment should include herbs such as *Sheng Jiang* (Zingiberis), *Gui Zhi* (Cinnamomi Cassiae, Ramulus), and *Xi Xin* (Asari).

Heat as a causative factor will produce sticky yellow phlegm and saliva, the pulse will be tidal and rapid, and the treatment should include herbs such as *Huang Qin* (Scutellariae), *Huang Lian* (Coptidis), *Shan Zhi Zi* (Gardeniae), and *Shi Gao* (Gypsum).

Damp as a causative factor will produce jade-green phlegm and saliva, the pulse will be floating and languid, and the treatment should include herbs such as *Cang Zhu* (Atractylodis, Rhizoma), and *Fu Ling* (Poriae).

Summerheat as a causative factor will produce putrid-smelling phlegm and saliva, the pulse will be weak and indistinct, and the treatment should include herbs such as *Xiang Ru* (Elsholtziae), and *Bai Bian Dou* (Dolichos).

Dryness as a causative factor will produce string-like phlegm and saliva, or small pearl-like balls, or in some cases phlegm like glue or lacquer, and it will be difficult to cough out; the pulse will be slippery and rapid, and the treatment should include herbs such as *Gua Lou Ren* (Trichosanthes, Semen), *Tian Hua Fen* (Trichosanthis, Radix), and *Chuan Bei Mu* (Fritillariae Cirrhosae, Bulbus).

Alcohol accumulation as a causative factor will produce nausea, phlegm and saliva, with morning cough; the treatment should include herbs such as *Zhu Ling* (Polypori) and *Ge Hua* (Puerariae, Flos).

Food stagnation as a causative factor will produce peach-jelly-like phlegm and saliva, the chest and abdomen will feel stuffy and uncomfortable, and the treatment should include herbs such as *Xiang Fu* (Cyperi), *Zhi Shi* (Citri seu Ponciri Immaturis, Fructus), *Shen Qu* (Massa Fermentata), and *Mai Ya* (Hordei Vulgaris Germinantus, Fructus).

Spleen deficiency as a causative factor will produce frequent phlegm and saliva, with poor appetite and tiredness, and the treatment should include herbs such as *Bai Zhu* (Atractylodis Macrocephalae) and *Chen Pi* (Citri Reticulatae, Pericarpium).

If Kidney deficiency is the causative factor, when it does produce phlegm and saliva, it will be like a tidal flood, and will most often occur in the early hours of the morning. The treatment should include herbs such as *Tian Men Dong* (Asparagi), *Mai Men Dong* (Ophiopogonis), and *Wu Wei Zi* (Schisandrae).

It must be noted that all of the above are assistant and deputy herbs, while the chief and master formula is—Er Chen Tang (Two-Cured Decoction, *Formulas and Strategies*, p. 432). This cannot be done without.[34]

[This short selection from the *Zhang Shi Yi Tong* ('Comprehensive Medicine According to Master Zhang', 1695) by Zhang Lu (Early Qing, 1616?-1699, suggests a simple lifestyle change which may assist in the treatment of phlegm in the channels and collaterals.]

Since the phlegm in the body flows from the Stomach into the major channels (jing sui), the phlegm in the major channels must also of necessity return to the Stomach, and then can be either expelled from the mouth above, or led out through the Intestines below. It is only when the Spleen qi is quiet and resting that the phlegm can return like this. Thus those with phlegm conditions should eat breakfast and lunch, but after that allow the Spleen qi to rest quietly without moving, so as to give the phlegm in the channels a chance to return to the Stomach, and then follow the Stomach qi, as this only descends, rather than following the Spleen qi in its spread outward to the Four Extremities. This is the best. Try watching a patient with a mild phlegm condition: after lying quietly at night: the next morning [phlegm] can be brought up or passed out [below]. Those with serious phlegm conditions, having awakened from a coma, can then bring the phlegm up. Those passing it out below, is this not because they have not eaten, and the Spleen qi is quiet, so that phlegm has a route out of the body?

Case history: Phlegm obstructing the uterus causing recurrent miscarriages

Dr. Fang, female physician and 27 years of age, during her three years of marriage, had miscarried three times. All Western gynecological exams during this period were negative.

She reported that she often experienced mild lower backache and occasional dizziness. Leukorrhea was relatively profuse. The menstrual cycle, amount and colour were normal. While her energy and appetite were normal, she disliked greasy foods, and the stool was occasionally loose; her figure was solid and even slightly overweight. The complexion was slightly dark, the eyes were lackadaisical, the fingers short and the hands thick. The pulse was deep and slippery, the root of the tongue permanently greasy.

Since the first miscarriage she had been taking fetal-maintaining herbs, which obviously had not been effective.

As she was herself a doctor, her main concern was of some malignant pathology, and as a consequence tended to worry about this. She presented in Spring of 1972.

Comments

The most common causes of miscarriage are:

1. Kidney qi weakness with qi and blood deficiency, so that the fetus lacks nourishment and cannot be maintained. This usually results from either overwork, carrying heavy loads, or inappropriate sexual activity
2. Liver and Kidney yin deficiency so that xu-fire injures the fetus
3. Emotional distress or nervousness disturbing yin and yang, and interrupting the normal circulation of qi and blood, resulting in miscarriage.

But in the present case these factors did not appear.

The darkness of the complexion and the listlessness of the eye movement were not normal in such a young woman; they were signs of phlegm-damp obstructing the yang qi and preventing the Kidney jing-essence from rising to reach the eyes. The excessive weight, short fingers, and thick hands, plus the distaste for greasy foods, heavy leukorrhea, lower backache, deep slippery pulse and permanently greasy tongue coat at the root, when considered together, pointed to phlegm obstructing the uterus.

Treatment principle. Transform phlegm to secure the fetus, while also warming and nourishing Kidney qi.

Fu Ling	20 g	Poriae Cocos, Sclerotium
Mai Ya	20 g	Hordei Vulgaris Germinantus, Fructus
Yi Yi Ren	18 g	Coicis Lachryma-jobi, Semen
Du Zhong	15 g	Eucommiae Ulmoidis, Cortex
Bai Zhu	9 g	Atractylodis Macrocephalae, Rhizoma
Zhe Bei Mu	9 g	Fritillariae Thunbergii, Bulbus
Ju Hong	9 g	Citri Erythrocarpae, Pericarpium
Dang Gui	9 g	Angelica Polymorpha, Radix
Tu Si Zi	9 g	Cuscutae, Semen
He Shou Wu	15 g	Polygoni Multiflori, Radix
Huang Qin	3 g	Scutellariae Baicalensis, Radix
Zhi Gan Cao	3 g	Honey-fried Glycyrrhizae Uralensis, Radix

One bag to be taken every 3 to 5 days.

Explanation of prescription. The *Fu Ling* (Poriae), *Mai Ya* (Hordei) and *Yi Yi Ren* (Coicis) are not only able to strengthen Spleen's warmth and transformation, and thus prevent phlegm formation, but also can nourish Stomach qi and thus transform and disperse phlegm which has become obstructed within the channels and collaterals. Because of this mildness, there is no harm in long-term administration. There are instances in the Classical literature where *Yi Yi Ren* (Coicis) is described as contra-indicated during pregnancy, possibly because of its ability to open the collaterals which have become obstructed by damp, and because of its downward movement and diuresis. But these are exactly the qualities sought in this case. *Zhe Bei Mu* (Fritillariae) and *Ju Hong* (Citri Erythrocarpae, Pericarpium) are able to both cut phlegm and also move qi to remove blockage, in the spirit of the Classical statement 'One who is good at treating phlegm does not treat the phlegm, but moves the qi; when the qi circulates smoothly then all of the fluids in the body will follow smoothly.' *Mai Ya* (Hordei) has quite a lifting nature, and the effect of smoothing the Liver, as well as unbinding the Stomach and strengthening the Spleen, and is able to accomplish all of this without too much dispersing. When the Liver is relaxed and the Spleen strengthened, the fluids will circulate normally, and there should be no reason for phlegm-damp to build up.

Frequent miscarriages will necessarily injure Kidney qi, and thus this is taken into consideration with the additions of *He Shou Wu* (Polygoni), *Tu Si Zi* (Cuscutae), *Dang Gui* (Angelica) and prepared *Gan Cao* (Glycyrrhizae), which will warm and nourish Kidney qi. *Du Zhong* (Eucommiae) tonifies Kidneys, strengthens the tendons, and is also fetal-calming; with the addition of a small amount of *Huang Qin* (Scutellariae) the calming effect on future fetal movement is more complete.

The primary approach in this prescription is to transform phlegm, assisted by nourishing Kidneys, and supplemented with some qi moving and Liver relaxing herbs.

After taking the herbs for about three months she fell pregnant and after an uneventful pregnancy delivered a healthy baby boy. In the spring of 1980, Dr. Fang and her husband visited to express their gratitude, and the opportunity was taken to check up on her previous symptoms. Her eyes were now lively, the face rosy, and the fingers slender: the phlegm had dissipated without a trace.[35]

Case history: Phlegm-damp sinking downward causing ulceration of the legs

The patient named Cai, female, 24 years of age, was unmarried. She lived in Hubei, and Hubei in August is hot. With the blazing sun beating down in the steaming summer, everyone sheds their clothes in a vain attempt to escape the heat.

Ms. Cai, however, was different: she arrived at the clinic still dressed in her long army trousers. When asked her situation, she looked slightly embarrassed, blushingly drew up her trouser legs, and then we could see: ulcers as large as a hand covered the outside of both calves, in identical shapes.

Examination

On further questioning, she related that vaginal discharge was usually profuse, and her appetite was reduced, especially for greasy or rich meaty foods. Two years previously, the skin of the lateral aspects of her calves had, for some unknown reason, begun to thicken and become unbearably itchy and painful. No matter what time of year, the surface of the ulcerations ceaselessly exuded a thick sticky yellow fluid, even in the hottest summer weather. Everyone, when young, likes to look attractive and so, despite the suffering, she was unable to wear short pants: the distress this caused her showed on her face.

The tongue body was red, the root of the tongue had a firm full white greasy coat; the pulse was slippery and strong, the urine scanty and yellow. She presented on 5 August, 1981.

Comments

This case is one of phlegm-damp turning toxic, pouring down into the lower limbs, and producing ulcers.

The *Ci Yuan* dictionary contains the following definition of 'toxic': 'The basic meanings of toxic are three: one, harmful or malignant; two, painful or causing suffering; and three, substances which can injure people; all are termed toxic'. Anything which brings about injury to the organism, and continues to do so without relief, can be termed 'toxic'.

'Toxins' can be exogenous toxins: heat, fire, wind, damp, and phlegm can all build up and become toxic. In this instance we can assert that it is toxic-heat which has transformed into phlegm; the grounds for this assertion can be found in TCM theory but the proof is in the symptoms. The theory is in the *Nei Jing* Chapter 74: 'All painful itchy ulcerations belong to the Heart'.

The reason that ulcerations are the responsibility of the Heart is that the Heart controls fire and heat as well as the blood vessels; if the nutritive qi—part of the blood—does not flow well, and builds up inside the flesh, heat accumulates, blood degenerates (bai), the flesh rots, and ulcers form.[36]

All oozing fluids belong to damp, which is in the same class as phlegm, both being derived from pathogenic water. This case of ulcerations with continual secretion of thick sticky fluid is phlegm-damp in the extreme. The long-term leukorrhea, the coat of the tongue consistently firm white and greasy at the root, the deep and slippery pulse, the dislike for greasy rich meaty foods: symptom after symptom points to the crux of the matter—preponderance of phlegm-damp.

Due to the phlegm and damp failing to be eradicated in time, it spread rapidly, finally amassing in the lower body and forming ulcers. This is in line with Zhu Dan-Xi's dictum that 'Phlegm, in causing disease, follows the qi in its ascent and descent, and can reach everywhere in the body without exception.'

If this is not promptly dealt with, its influence can reach the degree mentioned in the *Wai Ke Zheng Zhi Quan Sheng Ji* ('The Complete Collection of Patterns and Treatments in External Medicine', 1740): 'Alternately itchy and painful; when broken, it secretes yellow fluid; when soaked to the limit it becomes a patch'. The general experience which traditional Chinese medicine has gathered in regard to the treatment of stubborn skin diseases can be summed up in the following way: hot burning pain with itching tends to be heat; itching that is particularly intense tends to be wind; if after scratching the area has a burning pain, this tends to be yin deficiency; and secretion of sticky greasy fluid tends to be phlegm. This has been shown over and over again to be accurate in practice, because treatments based on these postulates work. Turbid-phlegm with a sticky obstructive nature belongs to yin but the red tongue body, the secretion of sticky yellow fluid, and the scanty dark urine, give us the clue that the phlegm has transformed into heat, and thus the elimination of damp, the transformation of phlegm and the cooling of heat should all be combined in the treatment.

Because the patient was anxious to seek a cure, external as well as internal treatments were combined for faster results.

Internal Prescription

Yi Yi Ren	20 g	Coicis Lachryma-jobi, Semen
Che Qian Zi	30 g	Plantaginis, Semen
Yu Jin	10 g	Curcumae, Tuber
Xing Ren	10 g	Pruni Armeniacae, Semen
Mu Gua	15 g	Chaenomelis Lagenariae, Fructus
Wei Ling Xian	10 g	Clemetidis Chinensis, Radix
Pu Gong Ying	20 g	Taraxaci Mongolici cum Radice, Herba
Xuan Shen	15 g	Scrophulariae Ningpoensis, Radix
Wu Gong	1	Scolopendra Subspinipes
Sheng Gan Cao	10 g	Glycyrrhizae Uralensis, Radix
Five bags, to be taken as a decoction.		

External prescription

Ku Shen	30 g	Sophorae Flavescentis, Radix
Di Fu Zi	30 g	Kochiae Scopariae, Fructus
Tu Bei Mu	20 g	Bolbostemmae Paniculati, Rhizoma
Soak in 200 ml of 95% alcohol for five days, then dilute with distilled water to a 75% concentration, apply externally.		

The aim of this prescription is to cool heat, remove damp, transform phlegm, and open the collaterals. The *Yi Yi Ren* (Coicis) and *Che Qian Zi* (Plantaginis) remove damp and so prevent the formation of phlegm. The *Wei Ling Xian* (Clemetidis) and *Mu Gua*

(Chaenomelis) open the collaterals, disperse knots and transform phlegm. *Yu Jin* (Curcumae) and *Xing Ren* (Pruni) restore qi flow and so reduce qi blockage; both are pungent, which by dispersing can transform turbidity. *Xuan Shen* (Scrophulariae), *Gan Cao* (Glycyrrhizae) and *Pu Gong Ying* (Taraxaci) cool heat and relieve toxicity, so that the phlegm and damp dispersal action of the formula is contained within the primary goal of reducing the heat and the toxicity.

The *Wei Ling Xian* (Clemetidis) is chosen here to make use of its 'moving without staying … [nature] to open the channels and collaterals, and there is no blood or phlegm obstruction which is not immediately eradicated' (*Yao Pin Hua Yi*). The *Ben Cao Zheng Yi* also says: '*Wei Ling Xian* scatters and disperses: this is its ability; for accumulated damp, immobile phlegm, blood stagnation, blocked qi, or any excess, it is appropriate.'

Wu Gong (Scolopendra Subspinipes), although light in weight, has an effect that is equal to its task: it not only stops shock and opens the collaterals but also is good at transforming phlegm. Zhang Xi-Chun (1860–1933) remarks that its 'ability to move and disperse is unsurpassed in speed; whether within the zang-fu, or outside in the channels and collaterals, it is able to open any accumulated obstruction of qi and blood. Its nature is slightly toxic, but it in turn is excellent at reducing toxicity, so any and all toxins from ulcerations can be dispelled through its use.' Hence its use in this prescription. The beauty of it is that, with one substance, three effects are achieved: damp, phlegm and obstruction are all removed.

One of the special characteristics of the Chinese medicine treatment of open sores is that local phlegm is not only treated locally but rather the functioning of the whole organism is regulated. On the other hand, the local situation cannot be ignored, and thus externally applied herbs are used to cool heat, remove toxins and expel phlegm. When the herbs and the symptoms are in step, the results will naturally be good.

At the end of that year the patient, with joyful smiles, to express her gratitude brought to my home an expensive wall calender, which I politely refused. To change the subject I asked about her condition: after five packets of herbs (and the external lotion), the itching and pain of the ulcerations had ceased, and the exuded fluid was reduced in both amount and viscosity. However, because of the demands of work she could not spare time for more consultations, and so continued to use the original prescription. After ten or so more packets, the ulcerating had ceased, and the discharge and other symptoms also cleared up.[37]

NOTES

1. Instead of being regarded as just a cliche, the phrase should be employed as a useful reminder that both aspects must be covered in treatment. It is all too easy to simply try to 'vaporize' or 'flush away' phlegm. While this may indeed be necessary as part of a treatment, or constitute the first phase of a treatment strategy, the restoration of the healthy functioning of the body is essential for the disease to be completely cured. This concept of 'fu zheng' ('supporting the normal body functioning' or 'restoring the Correct') is a major strength of traditional Chinese medicine, and the lack of this concept is the number one major flaw in modern Western medicine and is a primary factor in its decline in popularity.

2. *Jing Yue Quan Shu* ('Complete Works of [Zhang] Jing Yue'), Shanghai Science and Technology Press, 1959, p. 530.

3. Such a list as this is simply a suggestion of a range of symptoms which could present in this condition: the fluids can be dried into phlegm anywhere, and the individual's symptoms will reflect this location. Also the focus of the yin deficiency will play an important role. For example, if Heart yin is deficient there will be Heart symptoms such as palpitations, insomnia, forgetfulness, and red tongue tip, and the focus of the body odor will be in the armpits; if Liver yin is deficient vertigo, tinnitus and red dry eyes with a sticky stretchy 'rubber-band-like' substance will be

reported; if phlegm is obstructing the surface tissues the patient will describe paradoxical feelings of cold on the skin but internal heat, or feeling chilly most of the time but heating up to an unbearable level very quickly; and so on. Treatment must take these variables into account.

4. *Jing Yue Quan Shu* ('Complete Works of [Zhang] Jing Yue'), Shanghai Science and Technology Press, 1959, p. 537.

5. *Ibid.*, p. 537.

6. For example, if the yin deficiency involves not only Kidneys but Lungs and Liver, Yi Guan Jian ('Linking Decoction', *Formulas and Strategies*, p. 271) could be chosen as a basis for alteration; if the yin deficiency is mild, involving the Lungs and Kidneys, and the phlegm visually apparent and relatively profuse, then Jin Shui Liu Jun Jian ('Six-Gentlemen of Metal and Water Decoction', *Formulas and Strategies*, p. 433) is more appropriate; and so on.

7. *Formulas and Strategies* attributes this formula to the *Dan Xi Xin Fa* ('Teachings of Dan Xi', Zhu Dan-Xi, 1481). But the formula is previously found attributed to the *Tai Ding Yang Sheng Zhu Lun* by Wang Gui in the fourth chapter of the fifty chapter work *Yu Ji Wei Yi* ('Subtle Meanings of the Jade Mechanism') begun by Xu Yong-Cheng (d. 1384) and completed by Liu Chun in 1396. Much of the rest of the *Yu Ji Wei Yi* is, however, influenced by Zhu Dan-Xi, who died in 1358—the *Dan Xi Xin Fa* being completed by his students. See note 19 in the Appendix on the development of phlegm disease theory in traditional Chinese medicine for more concerning Wang Yin-Jun.

8. Wiseman calls this 'rheum pattern', Maciocia calls yin 'Phlegm-Fluids', while *Formulas and Strategies* calls yin 'congested fluids'. 'Thin mucus' seems both straight-forward and accurate. See Chapter 6 (on thin mucus) for more information concerning differentiation and treatment.

9. Maciocia calls yi yin 'Phlegm-Fluids in the limbs', which describes the location; the Chinese literally means 'overflowing thin mucus'.

10. Zhang says 'with phlegm' because of course this prescription is also used for other conditions besides phlegm in the channels and collaterals, and the formula is described in a different section of the book from that discussing channel phlegm. The above quotes are from the *Jing Yue Quan Shu* ('Complete Works of [Zhang] Jing-Yue'), Shanghai Science and Technology Press, 1959, pp. 190-191. The formula Li Yin Jian is described in the same book pp. 999-1000.

11. The Chinese say 'Herbal weights are the Secret which is never transmitted' (zhong yao bu chuan zhi mi zai liang shang), a statement almost certain to grab the attention of the curious Westerner. The meaning, however, is not that herbal weights are a closely guarded secret; rather the idea is that one cannot transmit the knowledge required to accurately and consistently choose the appropriate weights for the herbs in a given prescription for a given patient: it is the result of long experience in the actual use of the herbs clinically. This is the reason that Chinese medicine cannot be applied from a book—or a computer program—with any hope of success beyond the occasional lucky hit. Most of us as students have had the experience of paging endlessly through books of symptoms or prescriptions looking for 'the one that suits my patient'. It is only later that we realize that it is never there! The strength of Chinese medicine is in its flexible ability to match the treatment exactly to the patient's pathological mechanisms, and this ability only comes to the practitioner who can understand and explain the cause and place of every symptom with which that patient presents. This understanding is based upon thorough familiarity with TCM physiology and pathology, and several years of thoughtful clinical practice. It is also the reason that the practice of traditional Chinese medicine is so much fun.

12. The quotes in this section, unless otherwise attributed, are found in the *Zhong Yi Tan Bing Xue* ('Study of TCM Phlegm Disease'), Zhu Ceng-Bo, Hubei Science and Technology Press, 1984, pp. 193-205.

13. *Ming Yi Bie Lu* ('Miscellaneous Records of Famous Physicians'), c. 500AD, by Tao Hong-Jing.

14. *Ben Cao Hui Yan* ('Treasury of Words on the Materia Medica'), Ming dynasty, by Ni Zhu-Mo.

15. *Tang Ye Ben Cao* ('Materia Medica for Decoctions'), 1306, by Wang Hao-Gu.

16. *Ben Cao Yan Yi Bu Yi* ('Supplement to the Extension of the Materia Medica'), c. 1347, by Zhu Dan-Xi.

17. *Shi Yi De Xiao Fang* ('Effective Formulas from Generations of Physicians'), by Wei Yi-Lin, 1345.

18. *Yi Yi Bing Shu* ('Book of Treatments for Doctors' Illnesses'), by Wu Ju-Tong, 1831; Jiangsu Science and Technology Press, 1985, p. 61. The meaning of the title is explained by a later commentator: 'If one wishes to relieve the illnesses of patients, the illnesses (mistakes) of the doctors must first be relieved. If one wishes to relieve the doctors' illnesses, then Wu's book is a must.' The book covers medical ethics, diagnosis, principles of treatment and the nature of certain common herbs.

19. Quoted in *Zhong Yao Ying Yong Jian Bie* ('Differentiations of Usage in Chinese Herbs'), Tianjin Science and Technology Press, 1984, p. 113.

20. Quoted in the *Zhong Yao Ying Yong Jian Bie* ('Differentiations of Usage in Chinese Herbs'), Tianjin Science and Technology Press, 1984, p. 100.

21. *Ri Hua Zi Ben Cao* ('Materia Medica of Ri Hua-Zi'), 713AD.

22. *Ben Jing Feng Yuan* ('Journey to the Origin of the Classic of Materia Medica'), by Zhang Lu, c. 1670.

23. 走而不守 'zou er bu shou'. 'Zou' means that a herb has a wide spectrum of use, and its effect occurs rapidly; 'shou' that it has a narrow application but the effect is prolonged. The phrase 'zou er bu shou' is in contradistinction to two

other phrases: 'neng zou neng shou' 能走能守, 'able to move, able to stay'; and 'shou er bu zou' 守而不走 'stays without moving'. For example, these phrases are classically used to differentiate the characteristics of raw ginger (*Sheng Jiang*), dried ginger (*Gan Jiang*) and quick-fried dried ginger (*Pao Jiang*). Raw ginger is pungent and warm, with a mild odor and flavor; it is used primarily to promote sweat and expel pathogenic influence; its effect is rapid, but does not last very long. Thus the *Yao Pin Hua Yi* says: 'Sheng Jiang mainly disperses'. Dried ginger is pungent and hot, with a strong odor but mild flavor; its texture is compact, and its predominant action is to move internally to warm the center and disperse internal cold. This effect is maintained somewhat longer than that of raw ginger, thus Xu Ling-Tai (1693-1771) says of it: '*Gan Jiang* disperses and can stay'. Quick-fried dried ginger is no longer pungent but has become bitter, its nature is warm and harmonious, and its primary action is warming the center and stopping diarrhea and bleeding. Because of this warming, consolidating and moderate effect, Zhang Yuan-Su (*c.* 1186) remarks: '*Pao Jiang* stops without shifting'.

Hence raw ginger 'moves without staying', dried ginger is 'able to move and able to stay', and quick-fried dried ginger 'stays without moving'.

24. *Yao Xing Ben Cao* ('Materia Medica of Medicinal Properties'), by Zhen Quan, c. 600AD.

25. *Ben Cao Qiu Zhen* ('Search for the Truth in the Materia Medica'), by Huang Gong-Xiu, 1773; Shanghai Science and Technology Press, 1979, p. 124.

26. Zhu Dan-Xi follows Zhang Zi-He in the idea that 'Emesis does not only include vomiting, but means causing sneezing, or lacrimation, or producing saliva; in short, anything that moves upward is part of the method of emesis'.

27. This usually refers to exhaustion: 'taxing' diseases.

28. *Ling Shu*, Chapter 80: 'The Heart is the abode of the shen (spirit)'.

29. Xu Shu-Wei, known as Xu Xue-Shi ('The Scholar Xu'), a famous Song dynasty physician and author, born about 1080, was noted for his expertise concerning the *Shang Han Lun* and his emphasis on 'eight principles' differentiation. Although the concept of differentiation by yin-yang, xu-shi, hot-cold and internal-external can be traced back to the *Nei Jing* and *Shang Han Lun*, it was not until the Ming dynasty that it became clarified into a separate and specific diagnostic technique. Furthermore, it may surprise some to know that the term 'Ba Gang'—eight guiding principles—was coined in the 1940s, and came into general usage in the 1950s. See *Zhong Yi Zhen Duan Xue* ('TCM Diagnostics'), by Deng Tie-Tao, People's Health Press, 1991, ISBN 7-117-00533-5/R.534, p. 268. For the circumstances under which Xu Xue-Shi used *Cang Zhu* 'with great success', see the case history concluding Chapter 6.

30. 'Cao za' 嘈杂, Wiseman calls this 'clamouring stomach'. The Chinese definition is 'an empty hot sensation as if of hunger, but not hunger; as if full, but not full; as if painful, but not painful.'

31. Xiao Wei Dan ('Little Stomach Pill') is one of Dan Xi's own formulas, from the *Dan Xi Xin Fa*. Its contents are:
    Yuan Hua 15 g (Daphne Genkwa, flos), soaked in vinegar overnight, then cooked black in a clay vessel without charring it.
    Gan Sui 15 g (Euphorbiae Kansui, Radix), wrapped with damp flour, then left in running water for six hours, then again washed and dried.
    Da Ji 15 g (Euphorbiae seu Knoxiae, Radix), boiled in water for two hours, then washed again with water and dried.
    Da Huang 45 g (Rhei, Rhizoma) wrapped in wet paper and baked, then sliced and baked dry but not charred, then moistened with wine and again fried until cooked and dried.
    Huang Bo 90 g (Phellodendri, Cortex), baked, then fried.
    The above herbs should be powdered, then formed into pills the size of cannabis seeds with rice paste. One dose is between 20-30 pills. If a purge is desired, they should be taken on an empty stomach.
    They are for the treatment of shoulder pain from wind phlegm, damp phlegm, or phlegm above the diaphragm.
    They should not be used for an extended period of time, or in large doses, as Stomach qi may be injured.

32. This is made up of Liu Yi San (Six-to-One Powder, *Formulas and Strategies*, p. 105) which is *Hua Shi* (Talc) and *Gan Cao* (Glycyrrhizae), plus *Wu Zhu Yu* (Evodiae Rutacarpae, Fructus).

33. *Dan Xi Xin Fa* ('Teachings of Dan Xi', 1481), quoted in *Zhong Yi Li Dai Yi Lun Xuan*, Jiangsu Science and Technology Press, 1983, pp. 410-412.

34. *Yi Xue Chuan Xin Lu*, ('Record of the Transmission of the Heart of Medicine') by Liu Yi-Ren, Qing dynasty, quoted in *Zhong Yi Li Dai Yi Lun Xuan*, Jiangsu Science and Technology Press, 1983, p. 413.

35. Case history taken from *Zhong Yi Tan Bing Xue* ('Study of TCM Phlegm Disease'), Zhu Ceng-Bo, Hubei Science and Technology Press, 1984, pp. 59-61.

36. See Appendix 2 on the history of phlegm theory development for more information on the development of ulcers as described by the *Nei Jing*.

37. Case history taken from *Zhong Yi Tan Bing Xue* ('Study of TCM Phlegm Disease'), Zhu Ceng-Bo, Hubei Science and Technology Press, 1984, pp. 89-91.

9

Damp: principles of treatment

One of the primary intentions of this book is to present material which is as yet unavailable in English. Damp, and also cold-damp, however, are subjects which have already been well-covered in a number of works in English,[1] perhaps due to the prevalence of these pathologies in acupuncture practice. Therefore only a brief recapitulation of damp and cold-damp pathology will be covered here, reserving the main part of the chapter for discussion of damp treatment principles and the herbs involved. Damp-heat, on the other hand, is an area as yet little touched upon in English, and thus Chapter 10 is devoted to investigating its etiology, pathology, symptomatology and treatment.

ETIOLOGY OF PATHOGENIC DAMP

Damp may arise from exogenous or endogenous sources. External invasion of damp can result from over-exposure to water, rain or damp living or working conditions, when the dampness of the external environment is more than can be dealt with by the body. Constitutional weakness or even temporarily lowered resistance is another factor that can allow a gradual encroachment of damp into the surface.

Endogenous damp may originate in irregular eating habits, such as over-consumption of cold, raw, greasy or sweet foods, or alcohol, or simple over-consumption itself, as this impedes digestion. Impeded digestion means that accumulation of semi-transformed food and fluids occurs, which becomes damp. Even without this over-consumption, accumulation can occur in the constitutionally weak Spleen and Stomach, where the function of digestion and distribution, particularly the latter, is weak or slow.

Nature of damp

The nature of damp may be summed up in seven points.

Damp is 'heavy' and 'turbid'

Damp is described as 'heavy' because the symptoms to which it gives rise usually include sinking, heavy and sore sensations, which often occur in the lower body;

while 'turbid' refers to the murky unpurified state of the substances that accumulate to form damp, demonstrated in signs like greasy tongue coat, cloudy urine, loose stool and leukorrhea.

Illnesses caused by damp tend to be chronic

This is because damp has a sticky, cloying nature which makes it difficult to completely eradicate, even when it is an exogenous pathogen located superficially in the surface tissues. One reason that this is so is that pathogenic damp tends to obstruct the very mechanisms which would normally act to resolve it: Spleen transformation and the flow of yang qi. Because of this, damp often quickly establishes a vicious cycle by which it grows ever stronger, and the processes opposing it become weaker, resulting in a frustratingly stubborn condition.[2]

The pathological development of damp disease is slow, but virulent and tenacious

The reasons for this are described above.

As a yin pathogen, damp harms yang and blocks the flow of qi

Damp 'harms' yang because it opposes its natural tendencies to expand and move, and thus consumes yang energy. Damp's sticky nature blocks the flow of qi, so that lethargy, lassitude, heaviness and distention appear.[3]

Damp can cause a wide range of problems involving all departments of medicine

Damp is intimately linked with Earth, and thus with the Spleen, the crucial activities of which affect every aspect of bodily functioning.

Damp tends to combine with other pathogens, especially wind, heat and cold

Again this is due to the 'sticky' nature of damp. Exogenous wind, which as a yang pathogen is spreading and dispersing, will often open the pores on the surface of the body and allow damp to slip in and lodge in the surface tissues. Damp then blocking the flow of defensive yang qi prevents the pores from acting normally, and the two pathogens can unite into 'wind-damp'.[4] This is one combination of a yin and a yang pathogen. Another example is damp-heat, the nature of which combination is thoroughly discussed in the next chapter. Cold, though, is a yin pathogen with a constricting nature that acts to intensify the sticky nature of damp; while the damp obstructs the flow of yang qi which would normally oppose the pathogenic cold: the two yin pathogens complement each other and so all too frequently combine to form 'cold-damp'.

Exogenous damp is a seasonal pathogen

This means that exogenous damp conditions tend to react to changes in the weather, and to be more prevalent in certain seasons.[5] Endogenous damp also responds, but in a less obvious manner.

Basic principles for expelling endogenous damp

While exogenous damp, in its early stages, can simply be expelled back through its route of entry—the surface—endogenous damp is more complicated.

Transformation of damp, parching damp and diuresis are the three fundamental principles in Chinese medicine for expelling endogenous damp. Selection of a particular principle depends on the location of the damp in the body. Generally speaking, if the upper Jiao is obstructed by damp, transformation is the basic principle; if the middle Jiao is blocked, then parching is employed; if damp pours down into the lower Jiao, then diuresis is used to expel it. This is expanded upon below.

Transformation

Because damp is a turbid sticky pathogen which easily obstructs the flow of qi, its nature must be 'changed' if the obstruction is to be removed. This is 'transformation', and the technique involves the use of herbs whose qualities are exactly the opposite of the heavy, sticky, turbid damp. Most of the herbs used for transformation of damp are pungent, fragrant and warm. The fragrance pierces the thick turbid-damp pathogen, the pungency breaks it up, and the warmth disperses it by promoting the normal flow of qi and blood through the previously obstructed area. Several methods of transformation will be described in the following pages.

Parching

This principle is often used for damp in the middle Jiao, to restore proper Spleen function. The Spleen is described in the Classical literature as 'liking a dry state and abhorring damp', meaning that Spleen's digestion and distribution functions will more easily be upset by a damp pathogen than will the functioning of other organs, and when this pathogen is eradicated, Spleen function is restored. Parching can be done with either pungent-warm parching herbs or with bitter-cold, depending on the nature of the pathogen: cold-damp, or damp-heat.

Diuresis

As will be seen, diuresis is a fundamental method of treatment for damp throughout the body but is especially useful for damp in the lower Jiao. Several methods of diuresis, such as sweet-bland diuresis and cooling-diuresis, will also be explained in the following pages. For the most part, diuretic herbs in Chinese medicine enter the Urinary Bladder, Lung or Spleen channels. The Lungs rule qi and are responsible for keeping the water metabolism regular and downward-flowing, so that when it reaches the Urinary Bladder it can be transformed into urine and excreted. The Spleen rules distribution. These functions are strengthened by diuretic herbs.

So each of the above principles can, from different locations and through different mechanisms, be used to eliminate pathogenic damp in the body. But it is clinically useful to remember that, with certain exceptions, diuresis holds a pre-eminent place in the treatment of damp, because of its action of direct expulsion. This is true to such an extent that a saying has it: 'Trying to treat damp without diuresis simply cannot be considered a proper treatment.'

In the following pages six methods based on the above three principles will be described. See Appendix 4 for an outline of the various forms damp can assume in the body and its clinical manifestations.

Six methods for the expulsion of damp

1. Sweet-bland expulsion of damp through diuresis to provide a route of exit for damp
2. Cooling diuresis to eradicate damp-heat
3. Fragrant transformation of damp to break up thick, turbid damp
4. Bitter-warm parching of damp to reinstate Spleen transformation and transportation
5. Wind-dispersing herbs to expel damp, to expel wind-damp in the surface tissues, and to assist the reinstatement of Spleen transport
6. Strengthening yang to transform damp, to promote yang warmth and movement to remove accumulated water and damp.

Discussion of damp treatment methods

Expulsion of damp with sweet and bland flavors

This diuretic method is fundamental to damp-expulsion prescriptions. It is based on the fact that many sweet and bland herbs like *Fu Ling* (Poriae Cocos, Sclerotium), *Zhu Ling* (Polypori Umbellati, Sclerotium), *Ze Xie* (Alismatis Plantago-aquaticae, Rhizoma), *Hua Shi* (Talc), *Tong Cao* (Tetrapanacis Papyriferi, Medulla) and *Yi Yi Ren* (Coicis Lachryma-jobi, Semen), for example, are potent diuretics; and as damp is considered heavy, viscous and sinking, diuresis provides an appropriate route of expulsion, which is in accordance with the Tai Ji Quan principle of 'leading the enemy by following the direction of flow', a principle that is also commonly used in Chinese medicine. Thus sweet-bland diuretics are fundamental herbs in the treatment of damp diseases.

Damp, however, can be on the surface, in the interior, or in the upper, middle or lower Jiao; and if damp remains for any length of time it can transform into, or link with, either heat or cold. So when these herbs are actually used in clinic they must be combined with other herbs in order to be appropriate. For example, sweet-bland herbs would have to be combined with bitter-warm herbs to treat cold-damp problems, with bitter-cold herbs to treat damp-heat, with fragrant herbs for heavy viscous damp, and with pungent-parching herbs for wind-damp diseases. This use of sweet-bland herbs as the major constituents of a prescription is most applicable in cases where damp itself is predominant;

the additions of the bitter-warm-fragrant, or pungent-parching herbs, are to stymie an early tendency of the damp to combine or change into a more complex pathogenic picture. If the condition has already become, say, a stubborn wind condition like rheumatism, then the primary constituents of the formula will have to be pungent-parching herbs, while the sweet-bland herbs will now assume an auxiliary role.

Remember, too, that 'damp', 'water' and 'thin mucus' all relate as products of disordered fluid metabolism: 'damp is the [general] overabundance of water, and thin mucus is the [local] accumulation of water'. For these reasons the diuretic effects of sweet-bland herbs are also used in the treatment of water and thin mucus, as described in the related chapters.

Examples of use. Tong Cao (Tetrapanacis Papyriferi, Medulla) and *Yi Yi Ren* (Coicis Lachryma-jobi, Semen) treat damp in the upper Jiao and promote the clearing and descending action of Lung qi. *Fu Ling* (Poriae Cocos, Sclerotium) and *Yi Yi Ren* expel damp from the middle Jiao and strengthen Spleen's transport function. *Zhu Ling* (Polypori Umbellati, Sclerotium) and *Ze Xie* (Alismatis Plantago-aquaticae, Rhizoma) open the flow from the Urinary Bladder and thereby expel damp from the lower Jiao. These herbs, like most sweet-bland herbs, work by improving the qi transformation function of the San Jiao which is responsible for both qi activity and fluid movement in fluid metabolism.

Subcutaneous edema of the face, limbs and abdomen resulting from weak Spleen damp-accumulation or the edema of pregnancy can be treated with *Fu Ling Pi* (Poriae Cocos, Cortex) and *Sang Bai Pi* (Mori Albae Radicis, Cortex) plus *Sheng Jiang Pi* (Zingiberis Officinalis Recens, Cortex), *Chen Pi* (Citri Reticulatae, Pericarpium) and *Da Fu Pi* (Arecae Catechu, Pericarpium). This is the famous 'Five-Peel Powder' (Wu Pi San) that combines qi-moving damp-expelling herbs—*Chen Pi, Sheng Jiang Pi* and *Da Fu Pi*—with the sweet-bland diuretics *Fu Ling* and *Sang Bai Pi*. The efficacy is further improved with the addition of another sweet-bland herb, *Dong Gua Pi* (Benincasae Hispidae, Cortex Fructus). For edema in pregnancy, the combination *Fu Ling* and *Dong Kui Zi* (Abutiloni seu Malvae, Semen) is recorded early on in the *Jin Gui Yao Lue* ('Golden Cabinet') but the formula

Bai Zhu San ('Atractylodes Powder') is more common nowadays for Spleen-xu type edema, as *Dong Kui Zi* must be used cautiously during pregnancy.

Formulas

Wu Pi San ('Five-Peel Powder')

Fu Ling Pi	Poriae Cocos, Cortex
Sang Bai Pi	Mori Albae Radicis, Cortex
Chen Pi	Citri Reticulatae, Pericarpium
Da Fu Pi	Arecae Catechu, Pericarpium
Sheng Jiang Pi	Zingiberis Officinalis Recens, Cortex

Source text: *Zhong Zang Jing* ('Treasury Classic') [*Formulas and Strategies*, p. 178]

For edema above the waist, add:

Zi Su Ye	Perillae Fructescentis, Folium
Qin Jiao	Gentianae Macrophyllae, Radix
Jing Jie	Schizonepetae Tenuifoliae, Herba et Flos
Ma Huang	Ephedrae, Herba

For edema below the waist, add:

Chi Xiao Dou	Phaseoli Calcarati, Semen
Ze Xie	Alismatis Plantago-aquaticae, Rhizoma
Che Qian Zi	Plantaginis, Semen

For constipation, add:

Da Huang	Rhei, Rhizoma
Zhi Shi	Citri seu Ponciri Immaturis, Fructus

For abdominal fullness and distention add:

Hou Po	Magnoliae Officinalis, Cortex
Qing Pi	Citri Reticulatae Viride, Pericarpium
Lai Fu Zi	Raphani Sativi, Semen

For qi-deficiency, add:

Dang Shen	Codonopsis Pilosulae, Radix
Huang Qi	Astragali, Radix
Bai Zhu	Atractylodis Macrocephalae, Rhizoma

Bai Zhu San ('Atractylodes Powder')

Bai Zhu	Atractylodis Macrocephalae, Rhizoma

Fu Ling Pi	Poriae Cocos, Cortex
Chen Pi	Citri Reticulatae, Pericarpium
Da Fu Pi	Arecae Catechu, Pericarpium
Sheng Jiang Pi	Zingiberis Officinalis Recens, Cortex

Source text: *Quan Sheng Zhi Mi Fang* ('Guiding Formulas for the Whole Life')

Bai Zhu San is made up of Wu Pi San ('Five-Peel Powder') with the exchange of *Bai Zhu* for *Sang Bai Pi*. This change is effected for two reasons: one, the formula aims at a warm dispersal of damp with the assistance of diuretic and qi moving herbs: *Bai Zhu* is warm, parching and strengthens the Spleen, while *Sang Bai Pi* is cold and diuretic, promoting the flow of Lung qi; two, *Bai Zhu* is an important herb for calming the fetus, while *Sang Bai Pi* does not have this property. It is for this latter reason that in the most common use of this prescription, the edema of pregnancy, the two herbs *Sha Ren* (Amomi, Fructus et Semen) and *Zi Su Geng* (Perillae Fructescentis, Herba) are added, both of which also warm the Spleen and calm the fetus.

The accumulation of water and thin mucus in the epigastric area can obstruct the proper flow of clear yang, leading eventually to dizziness as the pathogens are carried upward. This condition and its treatment are described in the *Jin Gui Yao Lue*, using the two-herb formula Ze Xie Tang ('Alisma Decoction'), composed of *Ze Xie* (Alismatis) and *Bai Zhu* (Atractylodis). *Ze Xie* is diuretic, leading the water and yin downwards to be excreted; *Bai Zhu* is parching and strengthens the Spleen, and so eliminates any remnant of the pathogens and restores the original rising flow of clear Spleen yang, so that the dizziness is relieved.

In Si Ling San ('Four-Ingredient Powder with Poria',) *Fu Ling, Zhu Ling, Ze Xie* and *Bai Zhu* combine to strengthen the Spleen and expel water to treat damp-heat diarrhea.[6] If *Gui Zhi* (Cinnamomi Cassiae, Ramulus)—which is sweet, pungent and warm—is added to make Wu Ling San ('Five-Ingredient Powder with Poria'), then the effect is to open the flow of yang and help qi transformation of fluids. This is used in the treatment of internal accumulation of water and yin, with symptoms like edema, anuria, vomiting and dizziness.

Both of the above prescriptions are based on *Fu Ling* and *Bai Zhu*, with additions and subtractions.

Formulas

Si Ling San ('Four Ingredient Powder with Poria')

Zhu Ling	Polypori Umbellati, Sclerotium
Fu Ling	Poriae Cocos, Sclerotium
Bai Zhu	Atractylodis Macrocephalae, Rhizoma
Ze Xie	Alismatis Plantago-aquaticae, Rhizoma

Source text: *Ming Yi Zhi Zhang* ('Displays of Enlightened Physicians', 16th Century) [*Formulas and Strategies*, p. 176]

Wu Ling San ('Five-Ingredient Powder with Poria')

Ze Xie	Alismatis Plantago-aquaticae, Rhizoma
Fu Ling	Poriae Cocos, Sclerotium
Zhu Ling	Polypori Umbellati, Sclerotium
Bai Zhu	Atractylodis Macrocephalae, Rhizoma
Gui Zhi	Cinnamomi Cassiae, Ramulus

Source text: *Shang Han Lun* ('Discussion of Cold-Induced Disorders') [*Formulas and Strategies*, p. 174]

Wu Ling San is a prescription originally found in the *Shang Han Lun* to be used in the treatment of incompletely eliminated surface pathogen which has attacked the Tai Yang channel, and through the channel has affected the qi transformation function of the Urinary Bladder itself, causing internal accumulation of water and damp. Later it was also found effective for several other related conditions: summertime cholera-like symptoms of vomiting and diarrhea; Spleen deficiency edema; and phlegm and thin mucus in the abdomen resulting from weak qi transformation in the Urinary Bladder. In all of these conditions, and whether there is an exogenous pathogen or not, the most important indications for the use of Wu Ling San are difficult or obstructed urination, white thick or greasy tongue coat, and a floating (or thready and languid) pulse. Each of the above conditions requires the same combination of Spleen-transportation-enhancing herbs and diuretic herbs, which together activate these two most powerful mechanisms for the elimination of damp. If there are heat symptoms,

Gui Zhi can be deleted. This again forms Si Ling San but lowers the diuretic effect somewhat.

In the treatment of painful urinary dysfunction (lin) syndrome, which includes all painful symptoms of urinary dysfunction (see Chapter Four), a variety of formulas is used to expel water and eliminate the urinary dysfunction. Although the effects of each formula will vary in accordance with the type of lin condition treated, still the basic principle is to use sweet-bland herbs to open the flow of urine.

Summary

Sweet-bland flavors help the qi transformation function of the San Jiao, allowing the uninhibited activity of the body's fluid metabolism. They can expel water and thin mucus, and also stop the progression of painful urinary dysfunction and other difficult urination conditions, and symptoms such as loose stool or diarrhea.

If, however, Spleen qi is weak and is not rising properly, or if yang is weak and damp starts to accumulate as a result, then it is best to use few if any diuretic herbs, as their action tends to be downward. What is needed in this case is warm restoration of Spleen and Stomach functioning to help the recovery of Spleen yang ascent. (See the section discussing 'bitter-warm parching of damp'.) Care is also required in cases of yin deficiency, as excessive diuresis can easily damage already weakened yin-fluids and, as Zhou Xue-Hai points out in his essay entitled 'On Promoting Urination' which concludes Chapter Five, excessive diuretics can also drain the yuan qi.

Cooling diuresis

This method uses bitter-cold cooling herbs and sweet-bland diuretic herbs in combination to treat diseases resulting from the interaction of damp with heat. This method, as well as other techniques and strategies for dealing with the peculiar nature of damp-heat, can be found described at length in the following chapter.

Fragrant transformation of damp

Internal blockage of turbid-damp, causing obstruction to the flow of qi, the rise of clear yang, and Spleen transportation, will cause symptoms such as fullness in the chest and abdomen, nausea, vomiting, sour regurgitation, loose stool, loss of appetite, heaviness of the limbs, excess salivation and a sweetish taste in the mouth. In these cases piercingly fragrant herbs will be used to penetrate and eliminate the turbid-damp, and to arouse the torpid Spleen to resume its proper functioning.

This method is also used with damp-phlegm, or even damp-heat or summerheat-damp (shu-shi) which can easily lead to turbidity.

In prescriptions the fragrant herbs are usually combined with sweet-bland diuretic herbs to provide an expulsion route for the now dispersed damp.

As we have seen above, however, damp often refuses to remain simply neutral but instead tends to combine with other pathogens such as heat or cold. If, for example, there are symptoms of damp-heat—yellow greasy tongue coat, dark yellow urine, fever, jaundice and restlessness, as well as the damp symptoms listed above—then the most commonly used herbs will include *Huo Xiang* (Agastaches seu Pogostemi, Herba), *Pei Lan* (Eupatorii Fortunei, Herba), *Bai Dou Kou* (Amomi Cardamomi, Fructus) and *Shi Chang Pu* (Acori Graminei, Rhizoma) for their fragrant damp-transformation qualities, and *Huang Qin* (Scutellariae Baicalensis, Radix), *Hua Shi* (Talc), *Mu Tong* (Mutong, Caulis), *Yin Chen Hao* (Artemesiae Capillaris, Herba) and *Lian Qiao* (Forsythiae Suspensae, Fructus) for their cooling diuresis.

If the tendency is towards cold-damp, with typical symptoms of obstructed qi flow such as headache, chills and fever, stuffy chest, abdominal and epigastric pain, nausea, borborygmus, diarrhea, and white greasy tongue coat, then the most commonly used herbs will be *Huo Xiang* (Agastaches seu Pogostemi, Herba), *Zi Su Ye* (Perillae Fructescentis, Folium), *Bai Zhi* (Angelicae, Radix), and *Shi Chang Pu* (Acori Graminei, Rhizoma) for their fragrance; combined with *Hou Po* (Magnoliae Officinalis, Cortex), *Da Fu Pi* (Arecae Catechu, Pericarpium), *Ban Xia* (Pinelliae Ternata, Rhizoma) and *Chen Pi* (Citri Reticulatae, Pericarpium) to dry the damp and harmonize the central Jiao.

The difference between the above two methods is that the former is primarily damp-heat at the qi-level, so bitter-cold and sweet-bland herbs are used to cool heat and expel the damp. This resembles the structure and mode of action of the prescription Gan Lu Xiao Du Dan ('Sweet Dew Special Pill to Eliminate Toxin').

In the latter method, the problem is primarily damp blockage of the Spleen and Stomach, so bitter-warm parching herbs are used. This is like the formula Huo Xiang Zheng Qi San ('Agastache Powder to Rectify the Qi').

In both of these examples, however, the utilization of the fragrant damp-transforming herbs is consistent.

Formulas

Gan Lu Xiao Du Dan ('Sweet Dew Special Pill to Eliminate Toxin')

Huo Xiang	Agastaches seu Pogostemi, Herba
Bai Dou Kou	Amomi Cardamomi, Fructus
Shi Chang Pu	Acori Graminei, Rhizoma
Bo He	Menthae, Herba
Huang Qin	Scutellariae Baicalensis, Radix
Lian Qiao	Forsythiae Suspensae, Fructus
Hua Shi	Talc
Mu Tong	Mutong, Caulis
Yin Chen Hao	Artemesiae Capillaris, Herba
Chuan Bei Mu	Fritillariae Cirrhosae, Bulbus
She Gan	Belamcandae Chinensis, Rhizoma

Source text: *Wen Re Jing Wei* ('Warp and Woof of Warm-febrile Diseases', 1852) [*Formulas and Strategies*, p. 187]

Gan Lu Xiao Du Dan is used in the early stages of infectious damp-heat febrile diseases with symptoms like fever and heavy lassitude, sore throat, swollen lymph glands, stuffy chest and abdominal distention, restlessness and no sweat (or if there is sweat the fever remains unrelieved), reddish urine, constipation, or impeded diarrhea, dysentery, jaundice, or other symptoms of damp-heat.

Huo Xiang Zheng Qi San ('Agastache Powder to Rectify the Qi')

Huo Xiang	Agastaches seu Pogostemi, Herba
Zi Su Ye	Perillae Fructescentis, Folium
Bai Zhi	Angelicae, Radix
Hou Po	Magnoliae Officianalis, Cortex
Da Fu Pi	Arecae Catechu, Pericarpium
Ban Xia	Pinelliae Ternata, Rhizoma
Chen Pi	Citri Reticulatae, Pericarpium
Jie Geng	Platycodi Grandiflori, Radix
Fu Ling	Poriae Cocos, Sclerotium
Bai Zhu	Atractylodis Macrocephalae, Rhizoma
Gan Cao	Glycyrrhizae Uralensis, Radix

Source text: *Tai Ping Hui Min He Ji Ju Fang* ('Imperial Grace Formulary of the Tai Ping Era', 1078-85) [*Formulas and Strategies*, p. 183]

A very common prescription in the summer months for common cold affecting the Stomach and Intestines, Huo Xiang Zheng Qi San is designed to treat wind-cold on the surface with headache, chills and fever, plus phlegm-damp blockage of the middle Jiao causing symptoms like stuffy chest, pain in the upper abdomen, nausea, vomiting and diarrhea.

Bitter-warm parching of damp

This method is used to treat damp resulting from weakness of the Spleen in digestion and distribution. As the name implies, bitter-warm herbs are used to parch damp with bitterness, and to support the Spleen's transport mechanism in order to promote the flow of qi, and thereby to eliminate the damp.

In this method, it should be noted, sweet-bland diuretic herbs are rarely if ever used in combination with the bitter-warm herbs. This is because the flow of Spleen qi is normally upward, and it is a result of the weakness of the qi and its consequent failure to rise properly that the pathogenic damp accumulated in the first place. So the emphasis in the selection of herbs should be placed on those that raise yang and assist Spleen transport. When Spleen qi can rise and the essence of food and fluids is distributed as it should be, then the normal flow of qi will gradually disperse the damp and the patient will be on the road to recovery. If, however, diuretic herbs are used, this will drag down the already weak and drooping Spleen qi: not only will the damp not be dispelled, but the distribution function of the Spleen will be further obstructed. Thus this situation is different from those covered under the statement 'Trying to treat damp without diuretics cannot be considered a proper treatment', and serves as a good example of the danger in the mechanical application of aphorisms.

When the Spleen is weak, damp accumulates which further blocks the flow of qi, causing symptoms like stuffy chest and epigastric area, loss of appetite, nausea, vomiting, sour regurgitation and belching; or in some cases headache, heaviness and lethargy, swollen painful joints, abdominal distention, diarrhea, and white greasy or even thick greasy tongue coat. One common selection of herbs to treat this would be *Bai Zhu* (Atractylodis Macrocephalae, Rhizoma) and *Cang Zhu* (Atractylodis, Rhizoma) to strengthen the Spleen's transport and parch damp, combined with *Hou Po* (Magnoliae Officinalis, Cortex), *Chen Pi* (Citri Reticulatae, Pericarpium) and *Huo Xiang* (Agastaches) to promote the flow of qi and thereby to eat away the damp. This resembles the structure of Classical prescriptions such as Ping Wei San ('Calm the Stomach Powder') and Bu Huan Jin Zheng Qi San ('Rectify the Qi Powder Worth More than Gold').

If the accumulation of damp is serious, and the consequent qi blockage severe, *Xiang Fu* (Cyperi Rotundi, Rhizoma), *Sha Ren* (Amomi, Fructus et Semen) and *Chuan Xiong* (Ligustici Wallichii, Radix) can be added to increase the movement of qi and so further assist damp removal. This is similar to Liu Yu Tang ('Six-Depression Decoction').

When the damp and qi blockage cause loose stool and a slightly obstructed flow of urine (which shows that because of the qi blockage, the differentiation of clear and turbid in the Spleen is affected), then herbs like *Ban Xia* (Pinelliae Ternata, Rhizoma), *Huo Xiang* (Agastaches seu Pogostemi, Herba) and *Fu Ling* (Poriae Cocos, Sclerotium) can be added to assist qi transformation and strengthen the Spleen's separation of clear and turbid. This resembles the formula Chu Shi Tang ('Expel Dampness Decoction').

Formulas

Ping Wei San ('Calm the Stomach Powder')

Cang Zhu	Atractylodis, Rhizoma
Hou Po	Magnoliae Officianalis, Cortex
Chen Pi	Citri Reticulatae, Pericarpium
Gan Cao	Glycyrrhizae Uralensis, Radix
Sheng Jiang	Zingiberis Officinalis Recens, Rhizoma
Da Zao	Zizyphi Jujubae, Fructus

Source text: *Tai Ping Hui Min He Ji Ju Fang* ('Imperial Grace Formulary of the Tai Ping Era', 1078-85) [*Formulas and Strategies*, p. 181]

Ping Wei San is a basic formula for the strengthening of Spleen and the parching of damp. The primary indications for its use are thick white greasy tongue coat, fullness in the epigastric region, lethargy, normal taste but no appetite, and no thirst. If the tongue coat is yellow and greasy, with a bitter taste in the mouth but no great thirst, these are the signs of damp-heat. Bitter-cold damp-expelling herbs like *Huang Qin* (Scutellariae Baicalensis, Radix) and *Huang Lian* (Coptidis, Rhizoma) should be added so that both damp and heat can be eradicated. If this is not done, it will be extremely difficult to effect a lasting cure. This is because the heat arises from the blockage caused by damp, and if the heat is removed but the damp is left, the heat will simply build up again in a short time. Likewise, once the heat has formed, it creates further damp and even phlegm, by drying normal body fluids which then join the mass of the pathogen. Prescriptions, for these reasons, must take both factors into account.

Bu Huan Jin Zheng Qi San ('Rectify the Qi Powder Worth More than Gold', *Formulas and Strategies* p. 182) is composed of Ping Wei San plus *Huo Xiang* and *Ban Xia*, which increase the formula's ability to open the blockage caused by damp.

Liu Yu Tang ('Six-Depression Decoction')

Xiang Fu	Cyperi Rotundi, Rhizoma
Cang Zhu	Atractylodis, Rhizoma
Shen Qu	Massa Fermentata
Shan Zhi Zi	Gardeniae Jasminoidis, Fructus
Lian Qiao	Forsythiae Suspensae, Fructus
Chen Pi	Citri Reticulatae, Pericarpium
Chuan Xiong	Ligustici Wallichii, Radix
Zhe Bei Mu	Fritillariae Thunbergii, Bulbus
Zhi Ke	Citri seu Ponciri, Fructus
Fu Ling	Poriae Cocos, Sclerotium
Zi Su Geng	Perillae Fructescentis, Herba
Gan Cao	Glycyrrhizae Uralensis, Radix

Source text: *Gu Jin Yi Jian* ('Medical Reflections Ancient and Modern', 1589)

Gong Ting-Xian, who edited and completed the *Gu Jin Yi Jian* for his father Gong Xin, records that the indications for the above formula are 'All blockages (yu)', and suggests the following additions:

If there is phlegm, add:

Dan Nan Xing	Arisaemae cum Felle Bovis, Pulvis
Ban Xia	Pinelliae Ternata, Rhizoma

If there is heat, add:

Chai Hu	Bupleuri, Radix
Huang Qin	Scutellariae Baicalensis, Radix

If there is blood stagnation, add:

Tao Ren	Persicae, Semen
Hong Hua	Carthami Tinctorii, Flos

If there is damp obstruction, add:

Bai Zhu	Atractylodis Macrocephalae, Rhizoma
Qiang Huo	Notopterygii, Rhizoma et Radix

If there is qi blockage, add:

Mu Xiang	Saussureae seu Vladimiriae, Radix
Bing Lang	Arecae Catechu, Semen

If there is food stagnation, add:

Shan Zha	Crataegi, Fructus
Sha Ren	Amomi, Fructus et Semen

Chu Shi Tang ('Expel Dampness Decoction')

Ban Xia	Pinelliae Ternata, Rhizoma
Hou Po	Magnoliae Officinalis, Cortex
Huo Xiang	Agastaches seu Pogostemi, Herba
Chen Pi	Citri Reticulatae, Pericarpium
Gan Cao	Glycyrrhizae Uralensis, Radix
Cang Zhu	Atractylodis, Rhizoma

Source text: *Shi Yi De Xiao Fang* ('Effective Formulas from Generations of Physicians', 1345)

The indications for this formula are heaviness of the whole body or alternatively vomiting and diarrhea resulting from the excessive consumption of cold or raw food.

The use of wind-dispersing herbs to expel damp

Expelling exogenous damp. The most common mechanism for the invasion of exogenous damp requires an initial attack of exogenous wind, which (as described above) because of its dispersing nature opens the pores and obstructs the protective circulation of protective qi. If the environment at that time is extremely damp, exogenous damp pathogenic factor is 'carried in' as it were with the wind, settling at any level from the superficial surface tissues to the muscles, tendons, bones or joints, depending on the weakness of the host and the virulence of the pathogen. If wind and damp are further involved with pathogenic cold, the resulting condition is the familiar bi-syndrome ('painful obstruction syndrome'), the treatment of which requires an understanding of the principles of wind-damp expulsion.

Briefly, there are two methods in the expulsion of wind-damp: the first is the diaphoretic dispersal of surface wind-damp, the second the dispersal of deep-set exogenous wind-damp by the use of wind-damp expelling and channel-qi moving herbs.

The first requires expulsion of the wind-damp with pungent-warm herbs to bring on mild sweating, with some movement of qi and blood. The sweating must be mild, not only to avoid damage to the qi and yin-fluids which could be carried out with the sweat, but also because a rapid profuse sweat would simply leave the heavy pathogenic damp behind in the surface tissues. The most common formula used in this situation is Qiang Huo Sheng Shi Tang ('Notopterygium Decoction to Overcome Dampness')

The second method requires the use of other herbs to promote the flow of qi and blood, encourage yang qi circulation, and tonify qi, blood, Liver and Kidneys. This is because when the flow of qi and blood is unobstructed and smooth the pathogenic factor is easily eradicated, hence the saying 'To treat wind, first treat the blood'. Encouragement of yang qi flow is both to restore its normal strength, since damp as a yin-pathogen strongly weakens yang, and because the warm flow of yang helps open the channels and carry away the pathogens. Tonification is important because the areas obstructed by the wind-damp have suffered a lack of qi and blood nourishment which should be redressed. The initial invasion of tendons and bones demonstrates a deficient condition of the Liver and Kidneys, which rule these areas (and the joints, which are composed primarily of tendon and bone). Therefore it is important to ascertain the status of the Liver and Kidneys when treating bi-syndrome or expelling wind-damp, so that they can be strengthened if necessary. A formula which deals with wind-damp expulsion, while also considering nourishment of qi and blood, and strengthening of the Liver and Kidneys, is Du Huo Ji Sheng Tang ('Angelica Pubescens and Sangjisheng Decoction').

Formulas

Qiang Huo Sheng Shi Tang ('Notopterygium Decoction to Overcome Dampness')

Qiang Huo	Notopterygii, Rhizoma et Radix
Du Huo	Duhuo, Radix
Gao Ben	Ligustici Sinensis, Radix
Fang Feng	Ledebouriellae Sesloidis, Radix
Chuan Xiong	Ligustici Wallichii, Radix
Man Jing Zi	Viticis, Fructus
Zhi Gan Cao	Honey-fried Glycyrrhizae Uralensis, Radix

Source text: *Nei Wai Shang Bian Huo Lun* ('Clarifying Doubts about Injury from Internal and External Causes', 1247) [*Formulas and Strategies*, p. 203]

Du Huo Ji Sheng Tang ('Angelica Pubescens and Sangjisheng Decoction')

Du Huo	Duhuo, Radix
Xi Xin	Asari cum Radice, Herba
Fang Feng	Ledebouriellae Sesloidis, Radix
Qin Jiao	Gentianae Macrophyllae, Radix
Sang Ji Sheng	Loranthi seu Visci, Ramus
Du Zhong	Eucommiae Ulmoidis, Cortex
Niu Xi	Achyranthis Bidentatae, Radix
Rou Gui	Cinnamomi Cassiae, Cortex
Dang Gui	Angelica Polymorpha, Radix
Chuan Xiong	Ligustici Wallichii, Radix
Sheng Di	Rehmannia Glutinosae, Radix
Bai Shao	Paeoniae Lactiflora, Radix
Ren Shen	Ginseng, Radix
Fu Ling	Poriae Cocos, Sclerotium
Zhi Gan Cao	Honey-fried Glycyrrhizae Uralensis, Radix

Source text: *Qian Jin Yao Fang* ('Thousand Ducat Formulas', 652AD) [*Formulas and Strategies*, p. 207]

Expelling endogenous damp conditions. This is actually a technique of lifting yang to eradicate damp. It is similar to bitter-warm parching in that it aims at damp resulting from Spleen deficiency but the herbs actually used differ in number, quantity and effect. In this method herbs are employed to remove endogenous damp which might otherwise be used to expel wind-damp from the tendons and bones, such as *Qiang Huo* (Notopterygii, Rhizoma et Radix), *Du Huo* (Duhuo, Radix), *Fang Feng* (Ledebouriellae Sesloidis, Radix) and *Gao Ben* (Ligustici Sinensis, Radix). These are all pungent, bitter and warm wind-expellers, which therefore are able to strengthen the spread and ascent of yang, and thus overcome the yin-natured pathogenic damp.

Another difference between bitter-warm parching and the use of wind-expelling herbs to remove damp is that the number of herbs used in the latter method is greater but with less amount of each herb. The idea is to employ their rising, pungent-dispersing qualities to induce normal clear yang qi to rise, thus restoring Spleen transport, which will in turn re-establish the descent of Stomach qi and thus allow turbid damp to descend and be transformed in the lower Jiao as usual. 'If ascent is desired, first descend; if descent is desired, first ascend' is the maxim.

It must be emphasized that these herbs are not at all intended to exercise a surface-opening diaphoretic effect (which would occur if fewer such herbs were used in greater amounts), but are intended only to restore normal ascending and descending action to the blocked qi mechanism of the middle Jiao.

At the same time herbs like *Cang Zhu* (Atractylodis, Rhizoma), *Bai Zhu* (Atractylodis Macrocephalae, Rhizoma), *Chen Pi* (Citri Reticulatae, Pericarpium) and *Shen Qu* (Massa Fermentata) are brought in to facilitate the distribution function that must deal with the now normally descending turbid damp. An example of a formula of this type is Sheng Yang Qu Shi Tang.

Formula

Sheng Yang Qu Shi Tang ('Lift Yang and Expel Dampness Decoction')

Qiang Huo	Notopterygii, Rhizoma et Radix
Fang Feng	Ledebouriellae Sesloidis, Radix
Sheng Ma	Cimicifugae, Rhizoma
Chai Hu	Bupleuri, Radix
Cang Zhu	Atractylodis, Rhizoma

Chen Pi	Citri Reticulatae, Pericarpium
Shen Qu	Massa Fermentata
Mai Ya	Hordei Vulgaris Germinantus, Fructus
Zhu Ling	Polypori Umbellati, Sclerotium
Ze Xie	Alismatis Plantago-aquaticae, Rhizoma
Zhi Gan Cao	Honey-fried Glycyrrhizae Uralensis, Radix

Source text: *Lan Shi Mi Cang* ('Secrets from the Orchid Chamber', 1336)

Strengthening yang to transform damp

This method is mainly used for cold-damp, phlegm and thin mucus (tan-yin) and edema, but if used skillfully it can be applied to the treatment of damp-heat as well. The use of the strengthening yang method in the treatment of cold-damp will be covered in this section; for information concerning its application in the treatment of phlegm, thin mucus, edema and damp-heat, please see the chapters relating to those pathologies.

The technique is characterized by the use of pungent-hot herbs to warm and open the flow of yang, assisted by precisely chosen diuretic herbs. The goal is to allow a strong flow of yang qi to transform pathogenic water and damp, which will then be carried out of the body. During application, the principle will remain the same while the actual herbs used will differ according to the organ involved. For example, to warm Spleen yang, *Wu Zhu Yu* (Evodiae Rutacarpae, Fructus), *Gan Jiang* (Zingiberis Officianalis, Rhizoma) and *Fu Ling* (Poriae Cocos, Sclerotium) could be used; while to warm and open the flow of Kidney and Urinary Bladder yang qi, *Gui Zhi* (Cinnamomi Cassiae, Ramulus) (or *Rou Gui* Cinnamomi Cassiae, Cortex), *Fu Zi* (Aconiti Carmichaeli Praeparata, Radix) and *Fu Ling* can be combined.

Different combinations—still based on the principle of strengthening yang to eliminate damp—will be used when the nature of the condition is complicated by different factors, as illustrated below.

Endogenous cold-damp. When cold predominates over damp, and the combined cold-damp has blocked the flow of yang qi, it can cause a wide variety of conditions. Most will share symptoms such as chills, general heaviness and aches, painful joints and aching lumbar area, all of which worsen in cold or damp weather, loose stool, a lack of sweating, languid (huan) and soft (ru) pulse, and a greasy white tongue coat. It is important to identify the primary source of weakness allowing the build-up of cold-damp, such as deficiency of Spleen yang or Kidney yang. This must be also be differentiated from bi-syndrome: pathogenic wind is not involved and, because the cold-damp accumulation is of endogenous origin, a different set of strategies apply than those used for exogenous wind-cold, even though the symptoms may appear similar.

Lower backache is a good example: a look at the role of endogenous cold-damp in the etiology of lower backache may serve to both illustrate the principles of cold-damp treatment, and be of most interest to us in the West, where we usually associate the condition solely with Kidney deficiency, 'arthritis' or sprain.

Endogenous damp and lower backache. Lower backache can result from a number of causes, such as Kidney yin or yang deficiency, trauma, exogenous wind-cold invasion, stagnant blood and even phlegm. Endogenous cold-damp is a less-well-known factor, especially in regard to the role that the Spleen can play.

Damp from any source can affect the Spleen, as both are Earth-natured, but if Spleen yang is deficient endogenous damp is an almost inevitable outcome. Pathogenic cold also developing from the Spleen deficiency can link with the damp to form a doubly yin-natured pathogenic factor that is both heavy and contracting, and thus extremely likely to lead to pain, especially in the lower body. In the condition under discussion, the primary sensation in the lower back will be one of heaviness and cold pain, with general lethargy, chills and other signs of Spleen involvement such as digestive disorders. In this type of lumbar pain, the cold-damp is not deep in the Kidney level but rather in the superficial musculature of the lumbar region and below. Here the already weak Spleen yang qi becomes obstructed through the yang-consuming dual influence of the pathogenic cold and damp which has settled to the lower body and set in at the muscular level: Spleen rules the flesh. Treatment is based on *Gan Jiang* (Zingiberis Officianalis, Rhizoma), *Fu Ling* (Poriae Cocos, Sclerotium) and *Bai Zhu* (Atractylodis Macrocephalae, Rhizoma) to warm Spleen yang and transform damp, expel cold and stop pain. A prescription specifically designed for this condition is Gan Cao Gan Jiang Fu Ling Bai Zhu Tang (otherwise known as Gan Jiang Ling Zhu Tang) from the *Jin Gui Yao Lue*.[7]

Gan Cao Gan Jiang Fu Ling Bai Zhu Tang ('Licorice, Ginger, Poria and Atractylodes Macrocephalae Decoction')

Gan Jiang	Zingiberis Officianalis, Rhizoma
Fu Ling	Poriae Cocos, Sclerotium
Bai Zhu	Atractylodis Macrocephalae, Rhizoma
Gan Cao	Glycyrrhizae Uralensis, Radix

Source text: *Jin Gui Yao Lue* ('Essentials from the Golden Cabinet') [*Formulas and Strategies*, p. 444]

This may be used as a foundation formula for this type of lower backache, as it treats the root of the problem, but there will usually be other additions to deal with the branch manifestations in order to achieve quick response. *Fu Zi* (Aconiti Carmichaeli Praeparata, Radix) and *Gui Zhi* (Cinnamomi Cassiae, Ramulus) can be added if the pathogenic cold is severe to warm and encourage the movement of yang. *Cang Zhu* (Atractylodis, Rhizoma) and *Yi Yi Ren* (Coicis Lachryma-jobi, Semen) can assist the removal of damp, through parching and diuresis respectively. *Mu Gua* (Chaenomelis Lagenariae, Fructus), *Gou Ji* (Cibotii Barometz, Rhizoma) and *Chuan Duan* (Dipsaci, Radix) can all be used to expel cold-damp from the muscles and tendons, and are specific for pain in the lower body, and particularly the lower back. If the condition has become chronic, the addition of one or two blood movers is necessary, such as *Ji Xue Teng* (Jixueteng, Radix et Caulis), *Dang Gui* (Angelica Polymorpha, Radix) or *Hong Hua* (Carthami Tinctorii, Flos).

If the cold-damp has developed as a result of Kidney yang deficiency failing to support lower Jiao transformation of fluids, there will be general aching and pain throughout the limbs and joints, as well as the lower back, and other symptoms indicating the pathogenic mechanism such as scanty but clear urination and reproductive system disorders. The pulse, it should be noted, may not be weak at the chi (proximal) position but this is not an indication of Kidney strength: it shows instead the presence of pathogenic cold-damp, and thus may be deep tight and wiry. The condition is treated with a combination of *Fu Zi* (Aconiti Carmichaeli Praeparata, Radix), *Fu Ling* (Poriae Cocos, Sclerotium) and *Bai Shao* (Paeoniae Lactiflora, Radix) to warm Kidney yang and transform damp, expel cold, and stop pain. The exact prescription for this is Fu Zi Tang ('Prepared Aconite Decoction') from the *Shang Han Lun*.

Fu Zi Tang ('Prepared Aconite Decoction')

Fu Zi	Aconiti Carmichaeli Praeparata, Radix
Ren Shen	Ginseng, Radix
Fu Ling	Poriae Cocos, Sclerotium
Bai Zhu	Atractylodis Macrocephalae, Rhizoma
Bai Shao	Paeoniae Lactiflora, Radix

Source text: *Shang Han Lun* ('Discussion of Cold-Induced Disorders') [*Formulas and Strategies*, p. 199]

This may appear similar to Zhen Wu Tang ('True Warrior Decoction', *Formulas and Strategies*, p. 197) which treats edema from Kidney yang deficiency, and indeed the pathologic mechanism is similar, but in Fu Zi Tang the emphasis is on warming tonification to eliminate cold-damp from the joints and limbs, while Zhen Wu Tang warms and disperses to eliminate internal accumulations of water resulting from the deficiency of Kidney yang. Again, additions may be necessary to speed response, such as *Du Zhong* (Eucommiae Ulmoidis, Cortex), *Gou Ji* (Cibotii Barometz, Rhizoma), *Niu Xi* (Achyranthis Bidentatae, Radix) and *Chuan Duan* (Dipsaci, Radix), all of which strengthen the Kidneys as well as benefiting the lower back.

Epigastric cold distention: blockage of qi by pathogenic cold-damp. This is another example of the pathogenic influence of cold-damp, which is quite common in clinic.

Yang deficiency allowing internal accumulation of cold-damp will occasionally result in a severe blockage in the flow of qi. This can give rise to a mixed excess and deficiency condition known in Chinese medicine as cold distention. The symptoms are an uncomfortable fullness around the chest and epigastric area, distention and pain in the upper abdomen, lethargy, loss of appetite, distention worse upon intake of food, cold hands and feet, general edema, deep slow pulse or deep wiry pulse, and a thick greasy moist tongue coat. The emphasis in treatment will depend on the mechanism involved.

Because cold is constricting, and damp is viscous and sticky, and both adversely affect yang qi, so the combination of cold and damp pathogens easily causes obstruction, accumulation and disturbance of the ascending and descending of the central Jiao qi mechanism. The *Ling Shu*, Chapter 35: 'Discussion of Distention' records: 'When cold-qi rebels upward, the True qi (zhen qi) and the pathogenic qi attack each other, and it is this mutual struggle that [obstructs the normal flow of qi and] causes distention.' In fact, clinical experience shows that a large percentage of distention cases can be traced to cold-damp blockage of qi. So when faced with symptoms such as painful distention that improves with pressure and warmth, white moist tongue coat, regurgitation of clear fluid and loose stool, then this is cold-distention in the middle Jiao, and the remedy is to warm the center, promote the flow of qi, eliminate cold and transform the damp.

Herbs to accomplish this include *Hou Po* (Magnoliae Officianalis, Cortex), *Chen Pi* (Citri Reticulatae, Pericarpium), *Mu Xiang* (Saussureae seu Vladimiriae, Radix) and *Cao Dou Kou* (Alpiniae Katsumadai, Semen) to warm the center and promote the normal flow of qi so that damp is eradicated. These will be combined with herbs like *Gan Jiang* (Zingiberis Officianalis, Rhizoma) and *Fu Ling* (Poriae Cocos, Sclerotium) to regulate the ascending and descending action of Spleen and Stomach, ensuring the rise of clear yang—through the warming action of *Gan Jiang*—and the descent of turbid yin-damp—by the sweet-bland diuresis of *Fu Ling*. This is like the prescription Hou Po Wen Zhong Tang ('Warm the Center Magnolia Bark Decoction').

If the damp blockage of qi is the result of a combined Spleen and Kidney yang deficiency, this is usually treated with *Fu Zi* (Aconiti Carmichaeli Praeparata, Radix), *Gan Jiang* (Zingiberis Officianalis, Rhizoma) and *Fu Ling* (Poriae Cocos, Sclerotium) as the main herbs, to warm yang and promote Spleen qi transformation. These will be combined with herbs like *Hou Po* (Magnoliae Officinalis, Cortex), *Bing Lang* (Arecae Catechu, Semen), *Mu Xiang* (Saussureae seu Vladimiriae, Radix) and *Cao Guo* (Amomi Tsao-ko, Fructus) to move the qi, break up the blockage, and thereby transform the damp. An example of this type of prescription is Shi Pi Yin ('Bolster the Spleen Decoction').

Formulas

Hou Po Wen Zhong Tang ('Warm the Center Magnolia Bark Decoction')

Hou Po	Magnoliae Officianalis, Cortex
Cao Dou Kou	Alpiniae Katsumadai, Semen
Gan Jiang	Zingiberis Officianalis, Rhizoma
Sheng Jiang	Zingiberis Officinalis Recens, Rhizoma
Mu Xiang	Saussureae seu Vladimiriae, Radix
Chen Pi	Citri Reticulatae, Pericarpium
Fu Ling	Poriae Cocos, Sclerotium
Zhi Gan Cao	Honey-fried Glycyrrhizae Uralensis, Radix

Source text: *Nei Wai Shang Bian Huo Lun* ('Clarifying Doubts about Injury from Internal and External Causes', 1231)

Shi Pi Yin ('Bolster the Spleen Decoction')

Fu Zi	Aconiti Carmichaeli Praeparata, Radix
Gan Jiang	Zingiberis Officianalis, Rhizoma
Fu Ling	Poriae Cocos, Sclerotium
Bai Zhu	Atractylodis Macrocephalae, Rhizoma
Mu Gua	Chaenomelis Lagenariae, Fructus
Hou Po	Magnoliae Officinalis, Cortex
Mu Xiang	Saussureae seu Vladimiriae, Radix
Da Fu Pi	Arecae Catechu, Pericarpium
Cao Guo	Amomi Tsao-ko, Fructus
Gan Cao	Glycyrrhizae Uralensis, Radix

Source text: *Shi Yi De Xiao Fang* ('Effective Formulas from Generations of Physicians', 1345) [*Formulas and Strategies*, p. 199]

Herbs to expel damp

As we have seen, pathogenic damp may result from either exogenous or endogenous factors.

Exogenous damp of recent onset is treated primarily with surface-opening herbs of a dispersing nature, discussed under 'Surface-opening Herbs'. Wind-damp is also of exogenous origin but of longer duration, having moved deeper into the tendons and bones. This is treated with 'Wind-damp Expelling Herbs'.

Herbs to expel wind-damp are usually pungent, bitter and warm and almost all enter the Liver channel. Liver rules tendons, where wind-damp most often sets in, so pungent-dispersing and bitter-draining herbs which directly enter the Liver channel can best expel the pathogenic damp from its seat in the tendons and bones. The pungency of these herbs dispels the wind, the bitterness parches and drains away the damp, and the warmth promotes the return of the normal flow of yang qi through the area, completing the expulsion of the pathogen, preventing its return and restoring nourishment to the site of the affliction.

Endogenous damp, depending on its location in the body, can be expelled by transformation, parching or diuresis. Transforming and parching herbs are usually fragrant-piercing, pungent-dispersing and warm, and most often enter the channels of the Spleen and Stomach. Diuretic herbs are of two types: sweet-bland diuretics and bitter-cold diuretics. Most enter the Urinary Bladder channel, while a few enter the channels of the Lungs or the Spleen.

The following is a brief list of the names, flavors, natures and properties of the herbs most commonly used to expel damp, as discussed in the sections above. The herbs in a given list all share the properties noted at the top (unless otherwise indicated), and thus these common properties are not included in the description of the qualities of an individual herb. What is included are the special qualities that each herb has in addition to their primary classification. The intention is to provide a quick reference for the differences between the herbs in a given class, in order to improve clinical precision in damp treatment herb selection. The list, however, should not be considered exhaustive.

Herbs to expel surface damp

These herbs are pungent and warm, open the surface and expel wind-cold.

Ma Huang (Ephedrae, Herba). Slightly bitter; enters the Lung and Urinary Bladder channels; promotes perspiration and the descent of Lung qi, and thus removes damp in two ways: through the surface; and by carrying fluids downward to the Urinary Bladder.

Gui Zhi (Cinnamomi Cassiae, Ramulus). Sweet; enters the Heart, Lung, and Urinary Bladder channels; promotes perspiration, opens flow of yang in the channels, and thus can treat damp in three ways: through the surface; by opening the flow of yang in the chest; and opening the flow of yang in the Urinary Bladder channel to assist Urinary Bladder qi transformation.

Zi Su Ye (Perillae Fructescentis, Folium). Enters the Lung and Spleen channels; promotes perspiration; promotes qi flow in the middle Jiao; fetal-calming; and thus can treat damp in two ways: through the surface; and by restoring Spleen and Stomach qi flow. Particularly indicated with pregnancy.

Xiang Ru (Elsholtziae Splendentis, Herba). Fragrant; enters the Lung and Stomach channels; promotes perspiration; transforms middle Jiao damp; diuretic; relieves Summerheat; and thus can treat damp in three ways: through the surface; in the middle Jiao; and through diuresis. Particularly indicated in Summerheat (shu) conditions.

Fang Feng (Ledebouriellae Sesloidis, Radix). Sweet; enters the Urinary Bladder, Liver and Spleen channels; promotes perspiration; expels wind-damp; stops diarrhea by lifting Spleen yang; and thus can treat damp in three ways: through the surface; in the tendons and bones; and in the middle Jiao.

Xi Xin (Asari cum Radice, Herba). Fragrant; enters the Heart, Lungs, Liver and Kidney channels; expels wind-cold; stops pain; warms Lungs to transform thin mucus; and thus can treat damp in four ways: through the surface; in the tendons and bones; fragrant-dispersal; and warm transformation of thin mucus in the upper Jiao.

Bai Zhi (Angelicae, Radix). Fragrant; enters the Lung and Stomach channels; promotes perspiration; stops pain; reduces swelling; pierces and parches damp; and thus can treat damp in three ways: through the surface; fragrant-dispersal; and warm-parching. Particularly indicated in damp headache and leukorrhea.

Gao Ben (Ligustici Sinensis, Radix). Enters the Urinary Bladder channel; promotes perspiration; dispels cold; stops pain; and thus can treat damp in two ways: through the surface; and opening yang qi flow internally. Particularly indicated in damp headache and cold-damp distention with diarrhea and abdominal pain.

Herbs to expel wind damp

These herbs all expel wind-damp from tendons and bones.

Du Huo (Duhuo, Radix). Pungent, bitter, slightly warm; enters the Kidney and Urinary Bladder channels; stops joint pain; and thus can treat damp in three ways: warming; bitter-parching; and pungent-dispersing. Particularly indicated for wind-cold-damp in the lower body.

Wei Ling Xian (Clemetidis Chinensis, Radix). Pungent, warm; enters the Urinary Bladder channel; strongly moving and piercing; opens all twelve channels; opens collaterals; transforms internal damp; and stops pain; and thus can treat damp in three ways: pungent-dispersal; warming; and piercing movement. Particularly indicated for wind-damp in the collaterals.

Qin Jiao (Gentianae Macrophyllae, Radix). Bitter, pungent, sweet; enters the Stomach, Liver and Gall Bladder channels; dispels wind-damp in the Liver channel; cools yin-deficient heat; relieves jaundice from damp-heat in the Stomach; and thus can treat damp in two ways: expelling wind-damp; and separating damp and heat in the middle Jiao. Particularly indicated in wind-damp with steaming bones from yin deficiency.

Mu Gua (Chaenomelis Lagenariae, Fructus). Fragrant, sour, warm; enters the Liver and Spleen channels; relaxes tendons; opens collaterals; harmonizes the Stomach; transforms damp; and thus can treat damp in three ways: fragrant transforming; wind-damp expelling; and calming the middle Jiao. Particularly indicated in lower body damp with impaired digestion.

Sang Ji Sheng (Loranthi seu Visci, Ramus). Bitter, neutral; enters the Liver and Kidney channels; tonifies Liver and Kidneys; expels wind-damp; fetal-calming. Particularly indicated in wind-damp conditions combined with Kidney deficiency or pregnancy.

Gou Ji (Cibotii Barometz, Rhizoma). Bitter, sweet, warm; enters the Liver and Kidney channels; tonifies Liver and Kidneys; strengthens bones and tendons; expels wind-damp. Particularly indicated in wind-damp coupled with Kidney deficiency, e.g. in older people.

Xi Xian Cao (Siegesbeckiae Orientalis, Herba). Pungent, bitter, cold; enters the Liver and Kidney channels; expels wind-damp; transforms and cools damp-heat; strengthens bones and tendons; expels wind and stops itch; and thus can treat damp in four ways: pungent-dispersal; bitter-draining; separating damp and heat; and expelling wind-damp-heat from the surface and thus stopping itch.

Diuretic herbs

Bland diuretics

These herbs are sweet and diuretic.

Fu Ling (Poriae Cocos, Sclerotium). Neutral; enters the Spleen, Stomach, Heart, Lung and Kidney channels; strengthens Spleen; harmonizes center; calms spirit; and thus can treat damp in two ways: restoring Spleen function; and diuresis.

Fu Ling Pi (Poriae Cocos, Cortex). Neutral; more diuretic than Fu Ling but less tonifying; moves on the surface to reduce subcutaneous edema.

Zhu Ling (Polypori Umbellati, Sclerotium). Neutral; enters the Kidney and Urinary Bladder channels. Stronger diuretic than Fu Ling; no tonifying action.

Ze Xie (Alismatis Plantago-aquaticae, Rhizoma). Cold; enters the Kidney and Urinary Bladder channels; drains damp-heat from the Kidneys and the Urinary Bladder; also relieves heat resulting from yin deficiency which has allowed the Kidneys' ministerial fire to flare.

Yi Yi Ren (Coicis Lachryma-jobi, Semen. Bland, slightly cold; enters the Lung, Spleen and Stomach channels; stops joint pain; clears Lung heat and pus; strengthens Spleen; stops diarrhea; and thus can treat damp in four ways: diuresis; Spleen tonification; expelling damp from the flesh; and preventing heat (especially in the Lungs) from drying body fluids into damp.

Che Qian Zi (Plantaginis, Semen). Cold; enters the Liver, Kidney, Small Intestine and Lung channels; relieves difficult-urination syndrome; stops diarrhea; brightens eyes; stops cough; and thus can treat damp in three ways: diuresis; promoting Small Intestine separation of clear and murky; and separating damp and heat.

Tong Cao (Tetrapanacis Papyriferi, Medulla). Bland, cold; enters the Lung and Stomach channels; cools heat; restores flow of milk; and thus can treat damp in three ways: opening the fluid pathways throughout the San Jiao; cooling heat; and diuresis.

Deng Xin Cao (Junci Effusi, Medulla). Bland, slightly cold; enters the Heart and the Small Intestine channels; clears Heart fire from Small Intestine; opens the fluid pathways of the San Jiao.

Dong Gua Pi (Benincasae Hispidae, Cortex Fructus). Sweet, slightly cold; enters the Spleen, Stomach, Large and Small Intestine channels; harmonious nature that does not harm the zheng qi.

Chi Xiao Dou (Phaseoli Calcarati, Semen). Sour, sweet, neutral or slightly cool; enters the Heart and Small Intestine channels; moves downward; enters the qi level to clear damp-heat or Summerheat through the urine; and enters the blood levels to eliminate toxic heat.

Hua Shi (Talc). Sweet, cold, slippery in nature; enters the Stomach and Urinary Bladder channels; harmonizes Stomach qi; promotes Urinary Bladder expulsion of urine by cooling obstructive heat and assisting fluid movement through its slipperiness; relieves damp-heat and Summerheat through diuresis.

Bitter-cold diuretics

These herbs are bitter cold, cooling and diuretic.

Mu Tong (Mutong, Caulis). Enters the Heart, Lung, Small Intestine and Urinary Bladder channels; takes Lung and Heart fire down and out through the urine; expels Urinary Bladder damp; promotes the flow of milk; and because of its relation with the Heart, can also promote the flow of blood.

Qu Mai (Dianthi, Herba). Slippery descending nature; enters the Heart and Small Intestine channels; moves blood; cools heat; relieves damp-heat lin-syndrome; and expels obstructed toxic heat.

Yin Chen Hao (Artemesiae Capillaris, Herba). Fragrant, only slightly cold; enters the Spleen, Stomach, Liver and Gall Bladder channels; clears damp-heat; relieves jaundice. Particularly indicated in jaundice (either yin-huang or yang-huang types of jaundice).

Bian Xu (Polygoni Avicularis, Herba). Neutral and downward moving; enters the Urinary Bladder channel; cools damp-heat; relieves lin-syndrome (painful urinary dysfunction).

Han Fang Ji (Stephaniae Tetrandrae, Radix). Pungent, very cold, downward moving; enters the Urinary Bladder and Lung channels; expels exterior pathogenic wind; eliminates internal damp-heat; especially good at eliminating lower Jiao blood level damp-heat; reduces swelling; stops pain. Particularly indicated in painful-obstruction syndrome combined with edema, but it easily damages zheng qi.

Herbs for fragrant transformation of damp

These herbs are fragrant and pungent, and transform damp.

Huo Xiang (Agastaches seu Pogostemi, Herba). Enters the Lung, Spleen and Stomach channels; promotes perspiration; transforms damp; harmonizes middle Jiao; moves qi; relieves Summerheat; and thus can treat damp in four ways: through the surface; fragrant-piercing; middle Jiao transformation; and moving qi.

Pei Lan (Eupatorii Fortunei, Herba). Neutral (i.e. not warm); fragrant; enters the Spleen and Stomach channels; transforms turbid-damp; harmonizes the middle Jiao; relieves Summerheat; and thus can treat damp in two ways: fragrant transformation; middle Jiao harmonization. Particularly indicated in halitosis, excessive saliva, and thirst from Spleen turbid-damp.

Bai Zhi (Angelicae, Radix). Fragrant; enters the Lung and Stomach channels; promotes perspiration; stops pain; reduces swelling; pierces and parches damp; and thus can treat damp in three ways: through the surface; fragrant-dispersal; and warm-parching. Particularly indicated in damp headache and leukorrhea.

Hou Po (Magnoliae Officianalis, Cortex). Bitter, warm, parching; enters the Spleen, Stomach, Lung, and Large Intestine channels; parches damp; moves qi; dispels fullness; helps Lung qi descend; warms the center; and transforms phlegm; and thus can treat damp in six ways: bitter parching; fragrant piercing; pungent dispersing; qi moving; opening the fluid pathways by helping Lung qi descent; assisting Spleen transformation of damp by warming the middle Jiao. This explains its frequent appearance in damp-treatment formulas of all descriptions.

Sha Ren (Amomi, Fructus et Semen). Warm, strongly fragrant; enters the Spleen, Stomach and Kidney channels; parches damp; awakens Spleen; moves middle Jiao qi; fetal-calming. Particularly indicated in the nausea of pregnancy.

Bai Dou Kou (Amomi Cardamomi, Fructus). Warm, lightly fragrant; enters the Lung, Spleen and Stomach channels; warms and opens the flow of qi throughout the San Jiao; calms Stomach; moves middle Jiao and Intestinal qi; breaks up food stagnation.

Shi Chang Pu (Acori Graminei, Rhizoma). Harmoniously warm; enters the Heart and Liver channels; transforms phlegm-damp; strengthens the Stomach; opens the orifices; promotes the harmonious activity of Heart shen.

Cao Dou Kou (Alpiniae Katsumadai, Semen). Warm; enters the Spleen and Stomach channels; parches damp; moves qi; strengthens Spleen; warms Stomach; stops nausea.

Parching herbs

Herbs for pungent-warm parching of damp

These herbs are pungent and warm, and all parch damp.

Cao Dou Kou (Alpiniae Katsumadai, Semen). Fragrant, warm; enters the Spleen and Stomach channels; moves qi; strengthens Spleen; warms Stomach; stops nausea.

Cang Zhu (Atractylodis, Rhizoma). Fragrant, pungent, bitter; enters the Spleen and Stomach channels; strengthens Spleen; promotes perspiration; expels wind-damp.

Cao Guo (Amomi Tsao-ko, Fructus). Strong characteristic odor, very pungent; enters the Spleen and Stomach channels; breaks up cold-damp obstruction lodged in the middle Jiao; expels phlegm; relieves malarial disorders.

Ban Xia (Pinelliae Ternata, Rhizoma). Slippery descending in nature; enters the Spleen and Stomach channels; moves qi downward; stops nausea; breaks up phlegm. Particularly indicated for thin clear phlegm-damp.

Herbs for bitter-cold parching of damp

These herbs are bitter and cold and all parch damp and cool heat.

Huang Qin (Scutellariae Baicalensis, Radix). Enters the Heart, Lungs, Gall Bladder, Large and Small Intestine channels; eliminates fire and toxic-heat, especially in the Lungs and Large Intestine; stops bleeding; fetal-calming. Particularly indicated in upper Jiao or Large Intestine damp.

Huang Lian (Coptidis, Rhizoma). Very bitter and very cold; enters the Heart, Liver, Gall Bladder, Stomach and Large Intestine channels; eliminates damp-heat, obstructed fire, and toxic heat. Particularly indicated in Heart and middle Jiao heat.

Huang Bo (Phellodendri, Cortex). Descending in nature; enters the Kidneys, Urinary Bladder and Large Intestine channels; especially good at draining Kidney fire and eliminating lower Jiao damp-heat. Particularly indicated in yin deficiency with fire flaring, and lower Jiao damp-heat and toxic heat.

Long Dan Cao (Gentianae Scabrae, Radix). Very bitter and very cold, with a descending nature; enters the Liver and Gall Bladder channels; eliminates fire in the Liver Channel; clears lower Jiao damp-heat.

Ku Shen (Sophorae Flavescentis, Radix). Very bitter and very cold, with a descending nature; expels wind; stops itching; promotes urination. Particularly indicated in lower Jiao damp-heat, and damp-heat itching of the skin.

Bai Xian Pi (Dictamni Dasycarpi Radicis, Cortex). Salty, with a moving nature that enters the tissues and the blood level; enters the Spleen, Stomach, Urinary Bladder and Small Intestine channels; expels wind-damp; relieves aching joints; promotes urination; takes heat out through the urine; and stops itching. Particularly indicated for lower Jiao damp-heat and itching damp-heat skin conditions.

NOTES

1. For a good example, see Giovanni Maciocia's *The Foundations of Chinese Medicine*, pp. 298-300.
2. The modern 'plague' of *Candida* is a common example.
3. One of the easiest mistakes to make in clinic is to confuse the manifestations of damp with the manifestations of qi deficiency: in both the Western patient often reports 'lack of energy'. Several questions will assist differentiation: 'When is the fatigue worse?' Actual qi deficiency will be worse later in the day, as energy is expended. Damp, conversely, will be worse in the morning after a night of quiet inactivity allows this yin pathogen to congeal. 'How do you actually feel?' When alerted, patients can often distinguish the heavy sensations of damp from the weakness of qi deficiency. 'How do they look?' and 'Are there any other signs of damp?' are questions which the practitioner can ask themselves as reminders. Often, however, both conditions will be mixed, and then the crux of differentiation will be on determining the relative degree of each. The proof, in the end, is always firmly in the pudding: if they did not improve on the first prescription, then that differentiation was incorrect. For this feedback to be useful, though, a 'testing' prescription should be heavily weighted in one direction—either to eliminate damp or to tonify qi. Otherwise a bad result shows only one thing: you were wrong.
4. It may be asked: 'Well, why doesn't the dispersing nature of wind disperse the damp?' The answer is, again, that a pathogen cannot perform a physiological function for the body.
5. It perhaps should be stressed that the basic theoretical seasonal relationship of pathogens in Chinese

Medicine is necessarily applicable only in China, or even more precisely, in those areas of China where that theory was initially developed. Many are the essays written by the more astute Chinese physicians disparaging those who mechanically applied precepts, theories or techniques purely 'by the book' without reference to their own situation or environment. An example of this is the article in section three of the *Zhen Jiu Ju Ying* ('Collection of the Essentials of Acupuncture and Moxibustion', 1529) discussing application of scarring-moxa to Dazhui (GV-14) on infants at birth, as is still performed today in Shandong Province to protect the baby from the extreme cold. In sultry Canton, however, this technique is not only useless, but deleterious: '...but nowadays people disregard the differences in climate between North and South, they just follow the prescription as written, to the harm of the infant.'

For this reason, practitioners are recommended to investigate the local environment and its predominant seasonal pathogen, e.g. cold, wind, parching-zao, and so on, and refer to the school of medicine in China that developed in an area climatically most similar to it, to reduce the confusion and inefficiency arising from the application of inappropriate theories.

6. The original indications for this formula are 'Treats internal injury from food and drink, with darkish scanty urine and loose stool'. *Ming Yi Zhi Zhang* ('Displays of Enlightened Physicians', 16th Century); People's Health Publishing, Beijing, 1982, p. 46.

7. See the *Jin Gui Yao Lue* ('Essentials from the Golden Cabinet', *c.* 210 AD), Chapter 11, Section 16.

Damp-heat 10

PATHOLOGY[1]

Damp-heat, a combination of the two single pathogens damp and heat, is both a cause and a result of pathological processes.

Taking the latter point first, some pathological mechanisms which can result in damp-heat are as follows:

1. A damp pathogen can invade the body, accumulate internally and produce heat which then combines with the damp to form damp-heat
2. Pathogenic fire or heat can build up and dry fluids into damp, which then combines with the heat to become damp-heat
3. Cold-damp can fail to be transformed by normal yang qi but rather becomes pent-up and turns to heat. The remaining damp then combines with the newly-formed heat to make damp-heat.

If the pathogenic damp-heat is not eliminated quickly, but instead gathers within the body, it can lead to a series of pathological changes and symptoms, and thus become a cause of disease.

Damp-heat is also a syndrome. Zhang Jing-Yue, in the *Jing Yue Quan Shu* ('The Complete Works of Jing Yue'), points out: 'Although damp syndromes are numerous, in the main they are two: differentiate first whether it is damp-heat, or whether it is cold-damp, and the rest will be clear.'

Special points in damp-heat diseases

There are many different types of damp-heat conditions but there will be some points in common.

Strong seasonal character

In seasons during which the temperature is hot and the earth damp, illnesses such as diarrhea and dysentery, sudden turmoil disorder (huo luan) and damp-warm disease are more frequently encountered clinically.

Other damp-heat conditions which already exist may simply be exacerbated at these times. Examples are damp-heat bi ('painful obstruction') syndrome, and damp-heat atrophy syndromes.

Ye Tian-Shi, in *Qing Dai Ming Yi Yi An Jing Hua*: Ye Tian Shi Yi An ('Best Cases of Famous Physicians of the Qing Dynasty: Cases of Ye Tian-Shi') says: 'Damp-warm disease is most common in the 'long summer' period, the steaming pent-up qi of the damp-heat enters through the nose and mouth, the upper Jiao is first affected and then it gradually spreads to the middle and lower Jiao.'[2]

Relatively prolonged course of disease

Damp has a sticky greasy nature which is gluey and hard to remove, when it comes into contact with heat.

The two pathogens tend to make each other worse: damp is dried and made more sticky by heat, and can even turn to phlegm. Heat, on the other hand, which as an uncombined pathogen is quite easily released through the surface or cooled, now becomes confined in the damp and very difficult to eradicate.

Whereas exogenous wind-cold is often curable with a single sweating, and an exogenous febrile disease can be dealt with by cooling or releasing, exogenous damp-heat is stubborn: often lingering within the body and becoming chronic.

Endogenous damp-heat has this tendency to linger as well, in all of its associated conditions, which can range as broadly as damp-heat bi ('painful obstruction') syndrome, atrophy syndrome, leukorrhea, edema, turbid urine, flank distention, abdominal distention, pain in the ribs, lower backache, or even enlargement of the liver.

Combination of damp and heat symptoms

Damp is a yin pathogen, heat is a yang pathogen, and when they combine to create illness, each manifests its special characteristics.

This can frequently lead to contradictory clinical pictures. There may be fever but the skin will not be hot to the touch, or the limbs will be cold instead of hot. Often, too, the patient will complain of sensitivity to cold but also report that in hot situations they warm up rapidly to an uncomfortable degree. There may be fever but no rapid pulse or red face, in fact the face could be pale yellow. Or there may be fever with no restlessness but, instead, a slow, dull-witted appearance. There may be thirst without much or any desire to drink;

and there may be intermittent mild sweating but only slight relief of the fever, which quickly returns. In the bowel it can lead to irregular stool: sometimes loose, sometimes constipated. Even the pulse can vary from thready, floating and weak, to rapid and slippery, or to deep and wiry, or to almost any combination of these.

Obvious obstruction of Spleen and Stomach function

Spleen controls middle Jiao transformation and transportation, likes dryness and hates damp; Stomach controls intake and acceptance of food and fluids. The most common area for endogenous damp formation is in the middle Jiao; but even exogenous damp-heat pathogens, because they usually enter through the mouth and thus have direct access to the Spleen and Stomach, can easily interfere with middle Jiao function. This will cause characteristic symptoms of poor appetite, epigastric fullness, abdominal distention, loose but sticky and difficult to pass stool, nausea, vomiting and heavy limbs. As Xue Sheng-Bai in the *Shi Re Tiao Pian* ('Systematic Differentiation of Damp-heat')[3] says 'Damp-heat diseases predominantly involve Yang Ming and Tai Yin channels. If the qi of the center is strong, the disease will be in Yang Ming. If the qi of the center is weak, the disease will be in Tai Yin.' This is confirmed by Zhang Xu-Gu, who explains that the qi of earth corresponds to the qi of damp, so that damp disease will always involve Spleen and Stomach, even if the damp pathogen is exogenous.

DAMP-HEAT ETIOLOGY AND PATHOLOGICAL MECHANISMS

Etiology of damp-heat disease

The occurrence of a damp-heat disease is determined by two factors: the strength of zheng qi and the strength of the pathogenic damp-heat.

The body's zheng qi is the crucial internal factor, and involves both sufficiency of the zheng qi itself and the functional balance between the various zang-fu.

For example, if the Lung qi spreads and descends properly, the fluid pathways (shui dao) remain open and regular. If the Spleen qi is strong, digestion and distribution is normal. If the Kidney qi is vigorous, and Kidney yin and yang balanced, Kidneys' control over fluid metabolism's opening and closing (kai he 开阖) is regular, and the amount of fluids retained or excreted is appropriate. If San Jiao is open and flowing, its function as the official in charge of irrigation can be executed as required. If the Urinary Bladder is transforming qi properly, urination is smooth and unimpeded.

In the above situation of harmony, internal damp has no starting place, and exogenous damp can usually be quickly eliminated. As the now lost Chapter 72 of the *Su Wen*, 'Discussion of Needling', is reported to have said: 'When the zheng qi exists internally, there can be no pathogenic disturbance'. If the body's qi is weak, the internal harmony of the zang fu is disrupted, pathogenic damp can easily develop, and the patient may also be susceptible to exogenous damp-heat invasion. Again, this is the situation described in the *Su Wen*, Chapter 33, in the famous quote 'For a pathogen to invade, the body must be weak'.

However, even in healthy patients, a strong exogenous damp-heat pathogen can occasionally overcome the ability of the body's resistance to prevent its invasion. When this happens, the Lungs can be closed off, the Spleen can be overcome, the Kidneys can be oppressed, and the San Jiao obstructed. This sets the scene for the creation of damp-heat disease.

Origins of damp-heat

As suggested above, the origins of damp-heat are four:

1. exogenous
2. endogenous
3. simultaneously endogenous and exogenous
4. damp and heat each contributing to the formation of damp-heat

Exogenous damp-heat

Exogenous pathogenic damp-heat is influenced by the following season, climate, geography, occupation and residence.

Season and climate. In China, early autumn is called the long summer (chang xia 长夏). The weather is hot and steamy and people easily succumb to damp-heat.

Alternatively, unrelieved damp weather can allow damp to gradually seep into the body, where the damp pathogen, because of its sticky nature, can resist expulsion through the surface or drainage out through the stool or the urine.

When this happens damp can become pent-up and produce heat, and the struggle between damp and heat is initiated. The *Wen Bing Tiao Bian* ('Systematic Differentiation of Epidemic Febrile Diseases', 1798) says: 'The season for warm-damp is the long summer and the beginning of autumn: the heat is produced from the midst of the damp.'

Geography. Areas such as China's Southeast, areas which have many rivers, lakes and even marshes, and copious rainfall, are by nature excessively damp. If the climate is also normally hot, by reason of latitude or other geographic peculiarities, the setting is perfect for producing damp-heat disease.

Physicians living in such areas, such as Zhu Dan-Xi, Ye Tian-Shi, Xue Sheng-Bai or Wu Ju-Tong, all of whom lived south of the Yang Zi river, tend to reflect this in their approach to medical theory.

Thus Zhu Dan-Xi proclaimed 'Damp-heat causes 80-90% of disease'; Ye Tian-Shi confirmed 'Damp pathogens cause the most widespread injuries'; and Xue Sheng-Bai wrote the specialist treatise on the topic of exogenous damp-heat disease: the *Shi Re Tiao Bian* ('Systematic Differentiation of Dampness and Heat').[4]

Exposure to rain, surface water and foggy mist can be a factor in developing a damp-heat condition. Any isolated episode of becoming thoroughly wet, if combined with weak zheng qi (even temporarily),[5] can cause an invasion of pathogenic damp. Usually it will be quickly expelled but if it is not, it can become pent-up and lead to damp-heat.

Residence and occupation. Residence in a damp house, or water-related occupations, are obvious factors in damp disease.

Case history: invasive nature of pathogenic damp

Two cases which I had within a short time after beginning practice in Australia illustrate the invasive nature of pathogenic damp, when it is offered the opportunity. Two young women had moved to a new residence shortly (in one case immediately) after they had undergone a termination of pregnancy. Each of them presented six months or so after the termination complaining of amenorrhea, which had never been a problem previously. Examination revealed obvious signs of damp and phlegm, and upon questioning each admitted that their new residence was quite damp inside: one to the extent that the walls actually dripped water. They were both treated with similar prescriptions, based upon Ye Tian-Shi's Cang Fu Dao Tan Tang ('Guide Out Phlegm Decoction with Atractylodes and Cyperus'):

Cang Zhu	Atractylodis, Rhizoma
Xiang Fu	Cyperi Rotundi, Rhizoma
Bai Zhu	Atractylodis Macrocephalae, Rhizoma
Ban Xia	Pinelliae Ternata, Rhizoma
Chen Pi	Citri Reticulatae, Pericarpium
Fu Ling	Poriae Cocos, Sclerotium
Dan Nan Xing	Arisaemae cum Felle Bovis, Pulvis
Zhi Ke	Citri seu Ponciri, Fructus
Gan Cao	Glycyrrhizae Uralensis, Radix

to which I added:

Chuan Xiong	Ligustici Wallichii, Radix
Dang Gui	Angelica Polymorpha, Radix

Within several weeks of beginning these herbs, each had a menstrual period. The treatment was consolidated with Ba Zhen Wan ('Eight Treasure Pill', *Formulas and Strategies*, p. 259) and a warning that they should consider moving again. Both did, and later consultations on other matters revealed no recurrence of the amenorrhea. This was clearly a case of damp opportunistically invading an open and vulnerable uterus and obstructing the uterine vessels (bao mai), preventing the normal flow of menstrual blood.

But sometimes the cause is more subtle: for example, heavy work with perspiration soaking the clothes which can allow a damp invasion which, again, if not expelled can develop into heat.

Water-related occupations include not only sailors, fisherman and scuba divers but also rice-paddy farmers and dishwashers who only expose certain areas of the anatomy to repeated wetness.

Endogenous damp-heat

Endogenous damp can develop in many ways and in many locations but the following are the most common: Spleen qi deficiency; Liver qi overcoming Spleen, with qi failing to move fluids, and qi blockage turning to heat; and lower Jiao damp-heat.

Spleen qi deficiency. Spleen deficiency in its functions of transformation will lead to damp which,

if transport also fails, can accumulate and turn to heat. One way that transformation and transportation can be diminished is through frequent excessive consumption of heavy, rich, sweet or greasy foods, often together with alcohol. This can lead to middle Jiao congestion suppressing Spleen and Stomach, and soon damp, which then produces heat. Another way to injure Spleen qi is through irregular eating habits, or eating raw, cold or unclean foods, or overwork or continual worry. Weak Spleen qi means that Spleen's ability to absorb, transform and distribute is reduced, so that the residue, which is neither transformed nor eliminated through normal methods, accumulates as damp. If at the time when weak Spleen has allowed damp to build up, Stomach has also accumulated heat, or spicy pungent food is consumed, or alcohol imbibed in excess or there is emotional upset, then heat as well as damp will be produced, and the two pathogens then lock together.

Thus the *Jing Yue Quan Shu* ('Complete Works of Jing Yue', 1624) says: 'Damp conforming with yin becomes cold-damp, damp conforming with yang becomes damp-heat.'

Liver Qi affecting Spleen. Frustration and stress can lead to Liver qi obstruction, and Liver qi will then fail to assist Spleen transport, which will result in damp accumulation internally.

If in addition qi backs up and turns to heat, damp steams and heat becomes locked in the damp, the two pathogens become linked together in a struggle that can cause numerous pathological changes all around the body. This is the explanation of Kong Bo-Hua's (1885-1955) statement that 'The origin of damp-heat is none other than Liver lording it over a weak Spleen, so that the bandits (i.e. damp and heat) are brought into existence by Liver taking advantage of a defeated Spleen.'

Lower Jiao damp-heat. Lower Jiao damp-heat most often appears in the Urinary Bladder, the Dai channel or the Liver channel, and will be the result of middle Jiao damp pouring downwards and accumulating in these areas, then producing heat. In the Urinary Bladder, damp-heat will manifest as urinary discomfort, frequency, scantiness or murkiness; in the Dai channel it will manifest as yellowish vaginal discharge; and in the Liver channel it will produce genital irritation and even suppurative ulcerations. Lower Jiao damp-heat can also be the result of exogenous invasion of damp-heat, similar to the bio-medical categories of sexually transmitted disease or urinary tract infection.[6]

Endogenous and exogenous factors combined

As so far described, damp-heat can be a result of exogenous invasion or of internal production. But the most common clinical origin of damp-heat disease is an initial Spleen qi deficiency leading to damp-heat internally, then followed by an invasion of exogenous damp-heat which stirs the endogenous damp-heat, creating a complex and difficult situation. Xue Sheng Bai describes the situation like this:

> Internal injury to Tai Yin with retention of accumulated damp and thin mucus, followed by the arrival of an exogenous pathogen, will link the endogenous and exogenous conditions together and thus produce damp-heat disease.

This is entirely a case of initial internal injury, and then a secondary exposure to an exogenous pathogenic influence, and does not come from the zang or the fu organs. If the damp-heat syndrome does not involve internal injury, so that the middle qi is strong, the disease will always be mild. On the other hand, there may be an initial condition brought on by [exogenous] damp, followed by overwork or excessive hunger leading to disease; this is also internal injury combined with [exogenous] damp [although the order of exposure is reversed]. As far as branch and root are concerned, they are the same illness. Thus overwork, exhaustion and injury to the Spleen are all deficiencies; while damp and thin mucus halted and accumulating are excess: which is more and which is less, which strong and which weak, these are the issues that must be weighed in clinic.

Damp and heat produce each other

Damp accumulating to form heat. Damp's nature is sticky and obstructive, adhesive and hard to eliminate. If a damp pathogen either invades or accumulates internally, and the normal physiological mechanisms for dealing with it fail, it will accumulate in quantity and influence, and will eventually transform into heat. The normal physiological mechanisms referred to are unrestricted qi transformation, freely circulating transportation, and unobstructed elimination through urination.

This concept of 'damp building up and producing heat' was already present in the *Nei Jing*. For example, the *Su Wen*, Chapter 74, says: 'Damp rises excessively and becomes heat: treat with bitter-warm [flavors], assisted by sweet and pungent.' In the same chapter is another statement: 'The control of damp is in Earth [but if] heat conversely overcomes it, the treatment requires bitter-cool [herbs].' And again: 'The ascendancy of Tai Yin, with fire qi pent-up internally, will cause boils in the center which will then spread to the exterior. The disease is in the flanks and ribs, when severe, it can cause pain in the heart area and nauseous heat.' Liu Wan-Su (*c.* 1120-1200) clearly declared: 'Accumulated damp produces heat', which was supported by the statement in the *Yi Xue Zheng Chuan* ('True Lineage of Medicine', by Yu Tian-Min, 1515): 'Damp obstruction produces heat.'

This process requires certain conditions, however. The most crucial is lack of movement or transport, so that the damp pathogen is pent-up; exactly like a pile of compost will heat up and give off steam.

A second important factor is the over-consumption of pungent-spicy flavors, or excessive emotional activity, both of which can speed the transformation to heat.

Beyond this, the process of damp turning to heat depends on the patient's constitution. A body type that is excessively yin will not easily turn hot but will more readily turn cold and form cold-damp. A body that has yang predominating will turn hot as soon as damp presents itself. So the *Lin Zheng Zhi Nan Yi An* ('Medical Records as a Guide to Diagnosis', 1766), says: 'When their color is greyish red, and their flesh is firm and compact, this type of body is yang, and an exposure to an exogenous damp pathogen will easily turn hot'.

Pent-up heat leading to damp. Pathogenic heat obstructed internally and prevented from either being cooled or drained away is left without an escape route. If this goes on for a long time, the obstruction will affect the flow of fluids, which will then build up into damp. Liu Wan–Su, in the section on damp in his *Xuan Ming Fang Lun* ('Clear and Open Discussion of Formulas', 1172), actually explains this according to the Wu Xing theory, saying: 'Damp is the qi of Earth, which is capable of being produced by fire and heat'. He later goes into greater detail in describing the process by which this occurs:

Damp diseases by nature do not follow the xiang sheng cycle [since the xiang sheng—production—cycle is normally a physiological mechanism, not pathological]. It is because of the obstruction of fire and heat pathogens that water and fluids fail to move freely, become halted, and produce damp. Therefore instances of damp disease are frequently the culmination of heat, which often is combined with other pathological symptoms. This should, therefore, be spoken of as damp-heat.

Zhu Dan-Xi in the *Ge Zhi Yu Lun* ('Inquiries into the Properties of Things', 1347) says: 'When heat has remained for a long time, its qi can transform into damp. Damp and heat produce each other.'

Li Chan, in the *Yi Xue Ru Men* ('Introduction to Medicine', 1575) also says: 'Damp-heat results from damp producing heat, or from heat producing damp; any diarrhea or dysentery is always brought on by damp-heat pouring downward.'

PATHOLOGY OF DAMP-HEAT DISEASE

Damp-heat pathogens most often enter the body through the mouth

Before the Ming dynasty, the idea was that exogenous pathogens mainly invaded through the skin.

It was Wu You-Ke in the *Wen Yi Lun* ('Discussion of Epidemic Warm Diseases', 1642) who first suggested that 'pathogens can enter through the nose and mouth', an important breakthrough for traditional Chinese medicine, especially the febrile disease specialists who were making great advances at the time.

Xue Sheng-Bai, after observation and clinical experience, pointed out in his *Shi Re Tiao Bian* ('Systematic Differentiation of Dampness and Heat'): 'In pathogenic damp-heat, invasion through the surface accounts for one or two out of ten, while entry through the mouth and nose accounts for the other eight or nine.'

Clinical observation by other physicians supports this, especially in diseases such as warm-damp (shi wen), dysentery, jaundice, diarrhea, and sudden turmoil disorder (huo luan). 'Entering through the mouth' most often refers to damp-heat disease which results from the consumption of contaminated vegetables and food, or polluted drink.

Damp-heat pathogens also can enter through the skin, such as in damp-heat bi (painful obstruction) syndrome, damp-heat atrophy syndrome, damp-heat lower backache, damp-heat headache and so on. These problems are principally the result of residing for a considerable period in a damp place, or getting rain-soaked or wet with dew, so that damp enters the skin and builds up internally, turning to heat.

Further, there is the possibility of invasions from other channels, which occurs in damp-heat difficult urination syndrome, murky urine or damp-heat leukorrhea. While these diseases can be caused by zang-fu damp-heat pouring down, more often poor genital hygiene allows pathogenic damp-heat to invade the local channels and spread throughout the area.

Pathogenic damp-heat is frequently toxic

Infectious diseases were, in ancient Chinese medicine, usually termed epidemic toxins[7] or toxic qi, epidemic qi, heteropathic qi and so on. As the *Su Wen*, Chapter 72 (now lost), is reported to have said: 'When the Five Epidemics arrive, all easily infect each other: old and young alike have similar symptoms, and there is no way to treat them successfully. How can one not have the disease passed on to oneself? Qi Bo replied: The reason that some do not contract the disease is that their zheng qi [still] exists internally, and the pathogen cannot disturb them, and thus the toxic qi is averted'. In the *Yi Lun Pian* it also records: 'If it is contagious, it is termed toxic'. Clinical experience confirms that many damp-heat diseases are obviously contagious, such as warm-damp, dysentery, jaundice, diarrhea, cholera and the like. These are not just common damp-heat diseases, however, but 'damp-heat epidemic toxins'.

In other cases, an exogenous damp-heat pathogen itself may not be infectious but can still become toxic through the process of invasion and failing to be eliminated, so that damp and heat work each other into an extreme state—damp enclosing heat until it transforms into fire, heat concentrating damp even further—until they become toxic. Wang Meng-Ying in the *Wen Re Jing Wei* ('An Outline of Epidemic Febrile Diseases', 1852) says: 'Damp-heat, obstructed, often becomes toxic'. In the *Qing Dai Ming Yi Yi An Jing Hua*: Chen Lian-Fang Yi An ('Best Cases of Famous Physicians of the Qing Dynasty: Cases of Chen Lian-Fang') it says: 'When damp and heat are mixed, fire is produced from damp, and the fire becomes toxic'. Once damp and heat become toxic, the power of the now intense fire not only scorches the fluids but can enter the ying and blood levels to disturb the Heart and even stir up pathogenic wind. The *Shi Re Tiao Bian* ('Systematic Differentiation of Dampness and Heat') notes an example of this:

> Damp-heat syndrome: when there is loss of blood in the upper or lower body, or sweating of blood, the toxic pathogen has entered deep into the ying (nutritive qi) level. This must be

drained away using a large prescription with *Xi Jiao* (Rhinoceri, Cornu), *Sheng Di* (Rehmannia Glutinosae, Radix), *Chi Shao* (Paeoniae Rubra, Radix), *Mu Dan Pi* (Moutan Radicis, Cortex), *Lian Qiao* (Forsythiae Suspensae, Fructus), *Zi Cao* (Lithospermi seu Arnebiae, Radix), *Qian Cao* (Rubiae Cordifoliae, Herba), *Jin Yin Hua* (Lonicerae Japonicae, Flos) and similar herbs.

Damp-heat easily damages the Spleen and Stomach

Stomach primarily holds food, as it is 'the Sea of Food and Fluids' (shui gu zhi hai); the Stomach orifice is the mouth, which is where most damp-heat pathogens enter the body.

Spleen chiefly transforms and transports, prefers dry and is disturbed by damp. But because Earth and damp have an integral relationship, like calls to like, and thus damp-heat easily injures Spleen and Stomach. As the *Shi Re Tiao Pian* ('Systematic Differentiation of Dampness and Heat') says: 'Yang Ming is the Sea of Food and Fluids, Tai Yin is the organ of damp Earth, and thus it is Yang Ming and Tai Yin which suffer [damp-heat] disease', and 'Most damp-heat illnesses belong to Yang Ming and Tai Yin. If the middle qi is strong, the illness will be in Yang Ming, if the middle qi is weak, the illness will be in Tai Yin.'

Damp-heat easily blocks the qi mechanism

The *Nan Jing*, in the Sixty-sixth Difficulty, says: 'The function of the San Jiao is to make the yuan qi separate [and perform its various functions]. It is responsible for the passage of the three qi through the five zang and six fu'.[8] The three qi are the zong qi of the chest from inspired air, the gu qi of the middle Jiao from food, and the activated constitutional jing qi of the lower Jiao.

The *Ling Shu*, Chapter 36, says:

> Of that qi emerging from the San Jiao: that which warms the muscles and the flesh, and fills out the skin, is the jin-fluid; while that which flows without moving is the ye-fluid (i.e. the thick and viscous fluids of the joints and bones, which 'flows' but does not 'move'). When the weather is warm, or the clothing thick, the surface tissues open, and thus sweat emerges … When the weather is cold the surface

tissues close, the fluids [on the surface], (literally 'qi' and 'damp') do not move, and water flows downward to the Urinary Bladder, there to become urine or qi.

The *Nan Jing*, in the Thirty-first Difficulty, says: 'San Jiao is the road of water and foods, the beginning and the end of qi'.

From the above statements we can see that San Jiao is not only the pathway for yang qi transport but is also the route for the ascent and the descent of the qi movement, controlling qi transformation for the whole body, and indeed determining exactly where in the body the yuan qi will be distributed.

Damp-heat being sticky by nature, once pathogenic damp-heat invades the body, it most easily seeps into the San Jiao, which then becomes blocked with the damp-heat so that qi transformation fails to occur, the qi mechanism is impaired, the clear yang does not rise and murky yin does not descend.

One result of clear yang not rising is the obstruction of yang qi in the chest (xiong bi, thoracic bi) leading to pain. Murky yin not descending from the upper or middle Jiao can lead to scanty or impeded urination, and constipation. Unaroused middle yang may lead to epigastric fullness and lack of appetite. Failed Urinary Bladder qi transformation in the lower Jiao causes difficult urination. All of the above are the result of damp-heat obstructing the qi mechanism.

Damp-heat easily influences fluid metabolism

The *Ling Shu*, Chapter 36, says:

> If San Jiao does not drain, and the jin and ye fluids are not created by transformation, then food and fluids will together move into the midst of the Intestines and Stomach; the murky waste cannot return to the Colon [for expulsion] but remains in the San Jiao unable to seep into the Urinary Bladder. Then the lower Jiao becomes distended, the fluids flood and become edema.

The *Su Wen* is even more clear in Chapter 8: 'The San Jiao is the Official in charge of Irrigation: the place where fluid pathways emerge.'

These statements indicate the function of San Jiao as being the controller of the fluid metabolism. If damp-heat obstructs this function, then:

a) a disadvantaged upper Jiao loses its spreading transforming ability and cannot 'open and regulate the fluid pathways, sending downward to the Urinary Bladder'
b) the middle Jiao is dazed by the damp-heat, the yang is blocked, and the Spleen's power of digestion and distribution is lost, so that even more water and damp accumulate
c) damp-heat in the lower Jiao results in Kidneys losing the strength to vaporize and transform fluids into either urine or reusable qi. This results in uncontrolled or frequent urination, or conversely fluid retention and scanty urination, as the Kidneys' ability to control 'opening and closing' (kai he) of the various excretory routes for fluids is lost.

If water and damp halt in the upper Jiao, it becomes thin mucus or phlegm; if they collect in the middle, it will lead to fullness and abdominal distention; if the pathogens move downward into the lower Jiao, the result can be diarrhea, or murky urine, or leukorrhea; if it seeps outward, it will cause edema. As Liu Wan-Su (1110-1200) remarks in the *Su Wen Xuan Ji Yuan Bing Shi* ('Examination of the Original Patterns of Disease from the Mysterious Mechanisms of the *Su Wen*'): 'When damp and heat struggle, the struggle leads to obstruction, the obstruction disturbs normal urination, and there will be edema'.[9]

Damp-heat entering the blood easily obstructs the channels and collaterals (mai luo)

Blood is led by the qi, and if qi is obstructed the blood will stagnate. As previously noted, pathogenic damp-heat very easily blocks the flow of qi; when this happens, the vessels lose their impetus, and the blood in turn will stagnate.

If pathogenic damp-heat enters deep into the blood level, the heat will simmer the nutritive qi and blood, causing redundant blood-heat stagnation. The *Jin Gui Yao Lue*, Chapter 22 notes: 'If heat is excessive, blood can be coagulated and blocked.' The *Yi Lin Gai Cuo* ('Corrections of Errors Among Physicians', 1830, by Wang Qing-Ren) confirms: 'When blood suffers heat, it simmers and forms clots'.

In another type of situation, a seasonal epidemic damp-heat pathogen can penetrate deep into the ying (nutritive qi) and blood levels, leading to blood-heat and often bleeding, as was noted under the discussion of 'toxin' above.

Damp-heat easily creates phlegm

The mechanisms of how this can occur should be very clear to those who have read the chapters on phlegm elsewhere in this book. Pathogenic damp is often a precursor of phlegm, which itself is often nothing but thickened damp. When the element of pathogenic heat is added, a potent factor for thickening the damp is available. If in this pregnant situation we also find that the flow of qi has been obstructed, so that even normal fluids slow, the eventual delivery of phlegm is virtually assured. As Wu Cheng in his *Bu Ju Ji* ('Anthology of Up-To-Date Prescriptions', 1739) points out: 'Damp and heat coagulate into knots and produce phlegm'.

Symptoms of damp-heat

Low grade fever

Damp is a yin pathogen, heat is a yang pathogen. When they combine, the heat is pent-up within the damp and is prevented from reaching the surface where it could otherwise disperse itself. The heat then collects at the qi level, leading to fever which never becomes high or raging. Some other characteristics of this type of fever are that, despite the heat, the face is not red, and may even be sallow; and that the skin does not feel hot to the touch but may even feel cold, until after prolonged contact the sensation of heat gradually increases until it finally feels burning to the examining hand. With the fever, there will be little of the restlessness which typifies a purely yang excess but instead a slow, dull-witted appearance, as the ascent of clear yang to the head is slowed by the heavy damp.

These are all signs that the damp is blocking the surface tissues, so that normal protective qi cannot reach the surface (especially of the limbs) and thus they are cold, but the same obstruction of the surface means that pathogenic heat cannot be dissipated and so there is fever. The pathogenic damp, locking in the heat, prevents heat from rising to the face so that it does not become red. Damp also prevents the rise of normal qi and blood so that the face appears sallow.

During this time, there may be intermittent mild sweating but only slight abating of the fever, which quickly returns. This shows that the pathogenic heat is being held in by the damp pathogen and so cannot be completely dissipated through the surface; as soon as the sweating stops the heat builds up again. The sweat in this case will also be distinctive: because of the drying effect of the heat the perspired fluid will be greasy and odorous.

The mouth may be dry but there will be little desire to drink; there will also be lethargy and possible sensation of fullness in the chest.

Fever from damp-heat is different from the fever of exogenous wind-cold which is often curable with a single sweating, or the fever of exogenous febrile disease which will respond to cooling or allowing heat to be released through the surface. Exogenous damp-heat fever is often a long and drawn out affair, as it is difficult to treat and can become chronic.

Afternoon fever

In exogenous damp-heat disease, the fever is usually most apparent in the afternoon. Because the heat is blocked by damp from reaching the exterior, most of the time the fever will be low grade, as described above. The afternoon, however, is under the influence of the Yang Ming channels, which have 'abundant qi and abundant blood' by virtue of their connection with the digestive system where qi and blood are supplemented. Thus in the afternoon the battle between the body's defences (the zheng qi, now reinforced by the beneficial influences of the Yang Ming channels) and the pathogenic damp and heat becomes more fierce, and the heat gradually builds into fever which is more apparent than at other times.

It can be quite easy to confuse this afternoon fever with the flushing found with the heat resulting from yin deficiency with fire flaring, which can also begin in the late afternoon and evening, but the nature of the condition is fundamentally different.

The heat from deficient fire flaring will be most intense in the palms and soles, and the force of the heat seems to emanate from within the bones. It will usually be accompanied by restlessness, flushed red face, insomnia, bad dreams, night sweats, spermatorrhea and so on, and have the tongue and pulse signs which typify yin deficiency with fire flaring: red tongue with little coat and a rapid thready pulse.

The patient with afternoon fever from exogenous damp-heat on the other hand will usually present with a sallow face and dulled expression, poor appetite, little or no thirst, white greasy tongue coat and a pulse which is floating thready and weak (ru).

Wu Ju-Tong, in his *Wen Bing Tiao Bian* ('Systematic Differentiation of Warm Diseases', 1798) encapsulates all of this in one quote: 'Headache, chills, aching body, tongue white without thirst, pulse wiry thready floating and weak, sallow face, stuffy chest and poor appetite, afternoon fever which resembles yin deficiency, and the condition is chronic: this is called damp-heat.'

Chest obstruction—xiong bi (thoracic bi)

Xiong bi means obstruction in the chest with a feeling of stuffiness as if the qi is blocked internally, or something has collected and is causing pressure. There is no pain or dyspnea but the sensation has been present for an extended period of time. This is the result of damp and heat obstructing the San Jiao and blocking the flow of yang qi in the chest, causing phlegm to coalesce and preventing the smooth flow of Lung qi.

Thoracic bi is a classic symptom of damp-heat, according to Xue Sheng-Bai in his *Shi Re Tiao Bian* ('Systematic Differentiation of Dampness and Heat'): 'Damp occludes clear yang causing chest obstruction … chest obstruction is a consistent sign of damp-heat.'

Thirst without desire to drink

This is another common symptom of damp-heat. There is thirst because normal fluids are somewhat parched by the heat, and the damp obstructs the rise of normal jin and ye fluids of the Stomach so that they cannot reach and moisten the throat and mouth. If pathogenic damp dominates the situation, however, the excessive build up of pathological fluids internally makes the thought of further fluid intake unattractive. If both damp and heat are equally strong, the drying of the fluids will be somewhat more pronounced and there will be slightly more desire to drink. The amount of fluid intake will be small however, again because of the internal presence of damp. The patient may even feel like only rinsing the mouth without swallowing.

When the heat is stronger than the damp, however, the damage to the fluids is more extensive and the amount of fluid intake correspondingly increases. Even in this situation the amount of fluid taken will not be comparable to the level one would expect if the heat were the sole pathogen.

Lack of appetite and ability to eat

Damp-heat gathers internally and dampens the middle region, the yang of the middle Jiao cannot spread and so the movement of qi is disrupted. When this happens the Stomach ability to accept food and the Spleen function of transport suffer, so that even after one or two days without eating there is no sensation of hunger, and food does not appear or smell appetizing. If the patient is forced to eat, the epigastric area becomes full and uncomfortable. This combination of circumstances leads to the Chinese phrase 'bu ji bu na': 'neither hungry, nor (able to) take in'.

Heaviness of head and body

The head is the meeting place for all the yang qi. With damp-heat, though, the clear yang cannot rise and reach the head and turbid-damp cannot descend, and thus the head feels heavy and hard to hold up, and also feels tight as if wrapped with a band. On cloudy overcast days these feelings will be noticeably worse. This symptom was mentioned as early as the *Su Wen*, Chapter 3: 'Because of damp, the head will feel as if wrapped'.

Damp's nature is sticky, turbid and heavy with a sinking tendency, so that it very easily obstructs its almost perfect opposite: the clear yang. The consequence is that the whole body feels heavy and lethargic.[10]

Spleen influences the limbs because of its identity with the flesh; therefore damp oppressing Spleen yang will lead to restless aching of the muscles of the limbs, especially of the legs, which will also feel heavy. Again, this is because damp tends to sink.

Scanty, dark, difficult urination

As we know from the *Su Wen*, Chapter 8, the San Jiao is the fluid pathway for the body. Damp-heat is the pathogenic influence which most easily blocks the San Jiao function; when the damp cannot be transformed it will sink into the lower body and accumulate. Such an accumulation in the Urinary Bladder will prevent it from vaporizing fluids to recover the reusable qi and expel unredeemable fluids as urine and thus urine production declines. The pathogenic heat cannot take the place of Urinary Bladder's physiological warmth: it cannot promote qi transformation, for example, but can only parch the fluids which are there and thus the urine is dark, and may even feel burning. Pathogenic heat, again, is another factor in the reduction of urine volume in that it also dries up normal fluids in the body. The degree of darkness and burning of the urine is the measure of the degree of heat existing together with the damp; the cloudiness of the urine indicates, similarly, the degree of damp present.

Loose but difficult passage of stool

Damp-heat accumulation blocks qi flow, as we have seen, anywhere in the body: the Large Intestine is no exception. If the qi movement in the colon is blocked, passing stool becomes difficult: an urge is felt but only a small amount of stool is passed, leaving an 'incomplete' feeling—and a persisting urge to move the bowels.

If damp is dominant, the stool will be loose but still with the sensation of incompleteness. If the damp and the heat are equally strong, the heat dries the damp while the damp clutches the heat, and this produces a gluey tar-like stool, sticky and hard to pass. When the heat is strongest, there will be constipation—but never with really hard dry stool.

Nausea and vomiting

This is a very common symptom of damp-heat, because the pathogens not only interfere with the rise of Spleen yang but also with the Stomach's attempt to carry turbid waste downward into the Intestines. Thus Stomach qi is unable to descend normally and instead pushes upward leading to nausea and vomiting. Dry retching with a bitter taste in the mouth indicates internal retention of damp-heat with Wood fire rebelling upward: Liver and Gall Bladder qi obstruction has turned to fire and, instead of assisting Spleen transport, has encouraged the pathological rise of Stomach qi, which is already

hampered in its descent by the damp-heat. The same result can occur if the damp-heat itself obstructs the Liver and Gall Bladder qi.

Dry retching with a glossy mirror-like tongue shows that damp-heat has produced fire which has then severely injured the Stomach fluids.

If there is vomiting of clear fluids but other signs of damp-heat, this indicates chronic retention of thin mucus and phlegm, with a secondary damp-heat condition.

Abdominal distention

If the clear yang cannot rise nor the turbid yin descend because of damp-heat interference in the qi movement through the San Jiao, then clear yang and turbid yin will intermix and become a substantial obstruction to the flow of qi through the body. This will be especially noticeable in the abdomen because of the heavy sinking nature of damp. As the *Su Wen*, Chapter 2, states: 'Turbid qi above will then produce distention'.

Signs of damp-heat

Thick greasy tongue coat

'The tongue coating is the product of the Stomach steaming; the Qi of the five Yin Organs is derived from the Stomach, and therefore one can diagnose the Cold or Hot and Deficiency or Excess condition of the Yin Organs from the tongue coating' says the *Xing Se Wai Zhen Jian Mo* ('Simple Study of Diagnosis from Body Forms and Facial Color', 1894, by Zhou Xue-Hai).[11]

Damp-heat, for example, causes a thick greasy tongue coat because the heat steams the murky damp to rise and coat the tongue. This thick greasy coat is like cottage cheese thinly spread over the whole tongue: if it is scraped off it simply returns.

In damp-heat conditions, if the coat is white thick and greasy, this means that damp is greater than heat. If it is white thick greasy and dry, this means that damp dominates and heat is pent-up. If the coat is white thick and greasy, covered with a film of sticky murky fluid, this shows that middle Jiao damp is predominating over heat, and obstructing the Spleen transformation of fluids (this type of tongue coat will be found in the 'vomiting of clear fluids with other signs of damp-heat' mentioned under 'nausea and vomiting' above).

If the coat is yellow slippery and moist, like raw egg yolk spread over the tongue, this is damp-heat and also water and thin mucus, with the heat somewhat stronger than the damp. If the tongue coat is darkish yellow, dirty, thick and murky, this shows a preponderance of dirty turbid pathogenic damp-heat in the interior. Yellow thick greasy and sticky indicates heat exceeding damp, with the tendency to dry damp into phlegm. Yellow thick and dry shows that heat is stronger than damp, with the possibility that heat can produce fire and even become toxic. If the edge of the yellow coating is greasy black, this too is pent-up heat in the interior.

No specific pulse

Because of the variety of combinations in the degrees of damp and heat pathogens, there is no specific pulse that will appear in all damp-heat conditions.

Generally, though, if damp exceeds heat, the pulse will be languid (huan, 缓) and floating-weak-thready (ru, 濡). If heat exceeds damp, the pulse is often rapid. If damp and heat are pent-up internally, turning to fire and becoming toxic, the pulse will be tidal and big. Otherwise the variations in pulse will reflect the zang-fu organ pathology brought about by the damp-heat, for example, in damp-heat jaundice the pulse is usually slow or languid; while in damp-heat bi (painful obstruction) syndrome, the pulse will be rapid, wiry and slippery. Thus Xue Sheng-Bai in his *Shi Re Tiao Bian* ('Systematic Differentiation of Dampness and Heat') concludes: 'Damp-heat conditions have no standard pulse: it may be tidal, or languid (huan), or thready, or hidden (fu); it will vary according to the condition'.

Miliaria crystallina (bai pei, 'white vesicles')

'Miliaria' means prickly heat, which is often associated with tiny itchy vesicular eruptions of the skin when sweat fails to reach the surface and is trapped in the surface tissues. These little blisters will contain clear or sometimes white fluid. After the vesicle itself recedes, a thin layer of skin will peel off the location. They are usually found on the neck, in the armpits or on the chest and abdomen, and are rarely seen on the face or limbs. The vesicles appear with perspiration: a group of them will appear each time the patient sweats.

Their etiological mechanism is damp obstructing the surface, so that sweat cannot be thoroughly cleared; or damp-heat at the qi level, pent-up and unable to move, so that the heat steams the damp toward the surface tissues, resulting in the eruption of these tiny blisters. They can also be a sign of incorrect treatment: the damp-heat may have been mistakenly treated with greasy yin tonics, which further obstructs the damp, and then the heat steams it toward the surface as above.

The appearance of these vesicles can indicate the state of growth or decline of the pathogen and the strength of the normal zheng qi. Because pathogenic damp-heat is sticky and stubborn, a single occasion of heat steaming the damp outward will not eliminate the problem; on the contrary, the vesicles will tend to occur anytime the patient sweats or even becomes overheated. Thus they can be used to judge the state of the damp-heat.

Symptoms of impending miliary eruption. Besides the usual damp-heat symptoms the patient has always had, they will begin to feel stuffy in the chest and hot, as if just about to perspire. This is a sign that damp and heat obstruction is intensifying, building up into a sweat, after which a portion of the pathogen will hopefully be released.

Adverse and favorable vesicular appearance. If the vesicles are raised, translucent and glistening, full-to-bursting, and well-defined; and the if patient feels happier with a lessening of the stuffy sensation in the chest and a reduction of the heat, these signal that the zheng qi is overcoming the pathogen: damp and the heat are moving outward through the surface, and the body's own jin and ye fluids are still strong.

If the vesicles do not appear full, and are not glistening, and the patient is hot but only raises a slight sweat, with a dry mouth and thirst, this means that the pathogen is overcoming the zheng qi: the heat is strong but the body fluids are exhausted.

If the vesicles appear empty, with a white 'dried-bone' or greyish color, and the patient is confused or irrational, this is an unfavorable signal that the pathogenic toxin is sinking deeper into the body, and that both the qi and the fluids are exhausted.

Thus although these miliary vesicles in general are a good sign that the damp and heat are moving toward the surface, if they do not clear up in time the qi and fluids can be exhausted. Therefore they should never be ignored in clinic.

The situation is clearly described by Ye Tian-Shi:

Again, there is a tiny blister which looks like a crystal. This is damp-heat injuring the Lungs: although the pathogen has been expelled, the qi and fluids are depleted. Thus [in the early stages, the condition] requires tonification with sweet herbs, or before long the injury will extend [not only to the Lungs but also] to the qi and fluids. The blisters are caused by damp-heat in the wei (protective qi) level, so that sweat is unable to be thoroughly expelled. One should regulate the qi level to expel the pathogen. If the blisters are white like dried bone, this is a very bad sign: it shows exhaustion of the qi and fluids.

Principles of damp-heat treatment

Differentiate which pathogen is mild and which serious, then expel damp and cool heat

In damp-heat disease, heat is contained within the damp which by enveloping it prevents it from escaping, while the heat steams and moves the damp. Like oil mixed into flour, they are very hard to separate. Simply cooling pathogenic heat will not work, as the heat itself can be created by the damp obstruction; over-use of cooling herbs, too, can injure the yang qi in the body. Similarly, over-use of diuretic or parching herbs in an attempt to eliminate damp can injure the normal yin fluids. Thus Wu Ju-Tong points out: 'Simply cooling heat will not remove the damp; simply expelling damp will cause heat to burn even more.'

Thus the treatment should be adjusted to match the relative strengths of the damp and the heat pathogens:

When the damp exceeds the heat. In this case removal of damp is primary and cooling heat secondary, because removal of the damp will eliminate the barrier preventing the heat from escaping. It will also eliminate the original source of the heat, in the case of damp obstruction producing heat in the first place. Thus the key in damp-heat treatment is to first separate the two pathogens, and in this way isolate the heat; the key to separating the two pathogens lies in effectively eradicating damp. So Ye Tian-Shi says: 'Heat arises from within the damp: without expelling damp, heat will never depart.' There are a number of methods for expelling damp, as outlined in the chapter on principles of damp treatment and in the section following: such as promoting Lung fluid metabolism, strengthening Spleen to parch damp, fragrant transformation of damp, bland diuresis, and opening the flow of yang qi to increase urination and remove damp.

When the pathogenic heat exceeds the damp. Cooling heat is primary and expelling damp is secondary, because in this case it is the obstruction of pathogenic heat which is blocking the circulation of fluids, resulting in damp; and the heat is also drying the body fluids to produce damp. The more powerful the pathogenic heat, the more damp will be created. This vicious cycle can only be broken by reducing the power of the heat, after which the damp will lessen. Zhang Jing-Yue, in the Damp Syndromes section of his *Jing Yue Quan Shu* ('Complete Works of Jing Yue', 1624), says: 'In damp-heat, both cooling and moving should be used; when the heat goes, the damp goes too'. He also points out: 'If the heat is most severe, cooling fire is the most important, assisted by promotion of the [Urinary Bladder function of] separation [into clear qi and murky excreteable fluids] and diuresis … if the heat is mild, then separation and diuresis is most important, assisted by cooling fire.' Otherwise, if one ignores the heat despite its predominance and only tries to eliminate damp with diuresis or fragrant parching herbs, the heat will gain in power, and could even become toxic.

If damp and heat are equal in strength. Here the two pathogens should be dealt with equally: cooling heat while removing damp with the most appropriate method.

Carefully distinguish the location of the problem, and then choose the most appropriate method to deal with it

When treating damp-heat, one must not only distinguish their relative strengths but also identify the pathogenic locus: whether on the surface or deep in the interior, whether in the upper body or in the lower, whether in the zang or in the fu organs.

Mild damp-heat on the surface. This should be dispersed with fragrance: a gradual light sweat can release the pathogen through the exterior of the body.

Damp-heat blocking the upper Jiao obstructing Lung qi. The flow of nutritive and protective qi through the surface tissues is interrupted and the ascent and descent of all the qi in the body becomes abnormal. By going to the original location of the problem and lightly lifting and opening Lung qi, the whole situation can be rectified. As Wu Ju-Tong, in his *Wen Bing Tiao Bian* ('Systematic Differentiation of Warm Diseases', 1798), suggests: 'Because the Lungs rule the qi of the whole body, if the qi can be transformed [in the Lungs], then the damp will also be transformed.'

Damp-heat blocking the middle Jiao. Spleen qi is prevented from rising and the Stomach qi from descending. Pathogenic water and damp are then retained internally and the movement of qi will be disrupted. In this case bitter-cold herbs should be used to both drain heat and parch damp, while also awakening the Spleen and assisting Spleen transport.

Damp-heat in the lower Jiao obstructing Kidney yang. Urinary Bladder qi transformation cannot proceed normally and so urine is reduced. The treatment here is the use of bland diuretics. When the turbid-damp is drained away through the urine, the yang qi flow will be restored and the pathogenic heat cleared away.

Open San Jiao qi movement

San Jiao is the pathway for the body's yang qi to ascend and descend, and is thus the source of all qi transformation; it is also the pathway for fluids to be moved about the body by the qi. Any treatment of damp-heat disease must necessarily open San Jiao, so that yang qi flows smoothly and qi transformation occurs normally, after which the fluid metabolism will be regular and harmonious and pathogenic damp will have no place to exist. With no damp to hold it in, any heat will disperse as it is formed. Ye Tian-Shi makes an interesting point about the nature of the two pathogens in a quote from the *Qing Dai Ming Yi Yi An Jing Hua*: Ye Tian-Shi Yi An ('Best Cases of Famous Physicians of the Qing Dynasty: Cases of Ye Tian-Shi'):

> Damp and heat—both are qi. They can cloud and oppress the qi all over the body but have no substantial nature which can be attacked.

From upper failure to clear and regulate, [damp and heat] spread to the middle and lower Jiao. This is different from the Six Channel transmission system in Cold Injury (Shang Han). The idea is that of Liu He-Jian whose method was, specifically, to ensure the openness of the San Jiao. In the Ming dynasty, Zhang Si-Nong also treated [this condition] primarily with bitter pungent and cold. Both were based upon promoting movement at the qi level: when the qi flows openly the damp is dispersed.

The first step in opening the flow of San Jiao qi is to promote the spreading and descent of the Lungs. The Lungs form the protective covering (hua gai, 华盖) for all of the other organs in the body and have the uppermost position in the trunk, with control over opening and spreading, contracting and descending. If damp-heat is flourishing and affects the upper Jiao, the Lung qi will be blocked, as mentioned before. By restoring proper Lung qi activity, the qi transformation will return to normal: externally the surface circulation will be reinstated, internally the fluid pathways reopen and fluids can reach the Urinary Bladder so that the pathogen can have a route of expulsion. Simply by opening Lungs, the pathogen will often expel itself through the urine. As the *Lin Zheng Zhi Nan Yi An* ('Medical Records as a Guide to Diagnosis', 1766), says: 'When the Lungs' Metal-natured clear and contracting qi can descend, the Urinary Bladder's qi transformation will be open and unobstructed, and naturally there will be no illnesses such as damp-fire or heat, or summer-heat and damp.' In the *Yi Yuan* ('Origin of Medicine', 1861, by Shi Shou-Tang) it says: 'That the Lungs should be [a primary focus of] treatment in damp-heat disease has been a settled point of discussion since high antiquity.'

In order to open the flow of Lung qi, pungent fragrant herbs should be used for fragrant transformation: light, lifting and bringing to the surface, which is the action Wu Ju-Tong described when he said 'Treating the upper Jiao is like the [working of] a feather: if it is not light, it will not lift.'

The second step in opening San Jiao qi flow is to strengthen Spleen. The rising and falling of the body's zheng qi is determined by the middle Jiao, because when Spleen is healthy it can rise normally, while Stomach qi descends. When the rise of qi is normal the Heart and Lungs can promote the flow of protective and nutritive qi to nourish the exterior, while in the lower body the Liver and the Kidneys can nourish the bones and tendons to solidify the physical substratum. In the middle the Spleen and Stomach supply the essential qi to nourish the four limbs. If all of this proceeds normally, there will be no disease. But if damp-heat blocks the center, the mechanism of ascent and descent becomes ponderous, clear qi does not rise, turbid qi does not descend, qi transformation fails and San Jiao is blocked. To remedy the situation, one should use pungent-warm and bitter-warm herbs, as pungent opens and bitter parches and drains. This will dry and transform pathogenic damp, and stimulate Spleen qi so that it transports energetically. Once this occurs, the ascending-descending axis will swing into action again, transforming qi—and therefore the damp—and allowing damp to be expelled from the body through the urine. Zhang Xu-Gu puts it this way: 'The ascent and descent of the qi in the San Jiao is motivated by the Spleen. If the middle Jiao is harmonious, then the upper and lower Jiao work smoothly.'

The third step is diuresis. Damp, as a yin pathogen with a heavy occluding nature, easily blocks yang qi, and so Zhang Zhong-Jing said: 'use warm herbs to harmonize'. With damp-heat however the situation is somewhat different: within the damp is heat, and so the over-use of pungent-warm herbs will exacerbate the heat, and the effects of the heat from the herbs and the pathogenic heat will combine to injure the yin fluids. Diuresis must be used so that only a small amount of pungent-warm herbs is necessary to disperse the damp obstruction, after which the San Jiao qi movement can carry the damp in its dispersed state to the Urinary Bladder in the lower Jiao to be excreted through the urine. The more damp is eliminated, the better the now less-obstructed movement of San Jiao can circulate the yang qi, which will have the effect of moving pathogenic heat outwards to the surface through which it can be dispersed. Hence the saying: 'Treatment of damp without diuresis is no treatment at all.'[12]

To treat the root, seek the source: harmonize the central region

The most common source of damp is failed Spleen transformation, followed by failed Spleen transport.

Even if damp is not the result of Spleen malfunction, damp-heat diseases will almost always have some impact on the middle Jiao due to the affinity of Earth and damp. Another reason that the middle Jiao is important in damp-heat treatment is, again, the pivotal role it plays in the ascending and descending of San Jiao qi movement. Using pungent herbs to lift and disperse, combined with bitter herbs to parch and descend, will restore harmony to the middle Jiao and so balance this rising and falling mechanism. In yet another aspect, Stomach controls the intake of food, holding and warming it while the Spleen extracts the essence and distributes it. Interference with Stomach function will lead to loss of appetite and reduced ability to take in food, and also cause loose stool and diarrhea due to failure of the food to be held long enough for the Spleen to act upon it. Even if the focus of the damp-heat treatment is elsewhere than the Spleen and Stomach, the healthy functioning of the middle Jiao must be kept in mind and protected, so that, for example, not too many bitter-cold herbs are used to cool; purging is not pursued too vigorously; and descending diuretics are used cautiously if Spleen qi's ability to lift is impaired. Even when parching herbs are used, care must be taken to protect the Stomach yin, because, as a yang organ, 'Stomach prefers moisture and abhors dryness.' When cooling heat, too, the excessive use of cold herbs can actually augment the yin-congealing nature of the pathogenic damp, and thus make it even more difficult to eradicate.

One of the cheapest and most effective ways of reducing the middle Jiao damp-heat is through diet and eating habits. Eating until only 50-60% full ensures sufficient Spleen qi to accomplish transformation of the amount consumed—even if the patient eats much more frequently. Avoiding rich, sweet, greasy, raw or cold foods will reduce damage to the Spleen yang, while care with spicy, hot foods and alcohol will prevent continued reinforcement of pathogenic heat.

Fundamental methods and herbs used in damp-heat treatment

Promoting Lung qi flow to transform damp

The rationale behind this approach has been explained above. There are actually three aspects to this method:

Opening the Lungs to assist the pathogenic influence to reach the surface and disperse. This is used for exogenous damp-heat, which most often enters through the nose and mouth: the orifice of the Lungs is, of course, the nose; and thus Lung surface symptoms will often be the first noticeable signs of damp-heat invasion. These will be chills and mild fever with little or no perspiration, tight chest, lower backache, heaviness and lethargy, heavy aching head, white, greasy tongue coat and languid (huan) floating thready weak pulse. Pungent fragrant dispersing herbs should be used to open the Lungs and assist the pathogen to exit through the surface:

Huo Xiang	Agastaches seu Pogostemi, Herba
Pei Lan	Eupatorii Fortunei, Herba
Dan Dou Chi	Sojae Praeparatum, Semen
Xing Ren	Pruni Armeniacae, Semen
Zi Su Geng	Perillae Fructescentis, Herba
Xiang Ru	Elsholtziae Splendentis, Herba
Niu Bang Zi	Arctii Lappae, Fructus
Bo He	Menthae, Herba

If there is internal Summerheat and damp, with exogenous cold on the surface, such as could occur with electric fans or air conditioning, then a formula such as Xin Jia Xiang Ru Yin ('Newly Augmented Elsholtzia Decoction', *Formulas and Strategies*, p. 43) can be used.

Opening the Lungs to transform damp and allow heat to escape through the surface. This can be used for either exogenous damp-heat which has moved to the interior and is affecting the Spleen, or linked with already present internal damp; and also for internal damp-heat. The symptoms will be low grade fever unrelieved by sweating, sensations of stuffiness in the chest and fullness in the epigastric area, nausea, no thirst or thirst without much desire to drink, murky urine, loose stool, white greasy tongue coat, pulse languid floating thready and weak. The method should be to lightly open the Lung qi in the upper Jiao to assist qi transformation of damp, while assisting pathogenic heat to reach the surface and disperse:

Xing Ren	Pruni Armeniacae, Semen
Bai Kou Ren	Amomi Cardamomi, Fructus
Yi Yi Ren	Coicis Lachryma-jobi, Semen
Hou Po	Magnoliae Officinalis, Cortex
Huo Xiang	Agastaches seu Pogostemi, Herba
Jie Geng	Platycodi Grandiflori, Radix

Gua Lou Pi	Trichosanthes, Pericarpium

This is similar to the action of *San Ren Tang* ('Three Nut Decoction', *Formulas and Strategies*, p. 186).

If the heat is more obvious, one can add:

Shan Zhi Zi	Gardeniae Jasminoidis, Fructus
Dan Dou Chi	Sojae Praeparatum, Semen

in order to increase the light bitter draining effect, as described by Ye Tian-Shi: 'Light bitter and mild pungency both are things which assist movement and flow'.

Opening Lungs to promote fluid metabolism. When damp-heat is pent-up internally, and the qi movement is obstructed, the urine will become scanty and dark, or even cease altogether; there will be a steamy hot distended feeling in the head, thirst without much intake of fluids and a sticky greasy tongue coat. This is what is known as 'Lung qi not transforming above, leading to urine not flowing below.' Once the Lung qi transformation is restored, the fluid metabolism can begin to work again, as Wu Ju-Tong confirms: 'Lungs, through regulation of the fluid pathways, can cause fluids to reach the Urinary Bladder; once the obstruction in the Lungs is opened, the Urinary Bladder will open as well.' The *Yi Yuan* ('Origin of Medicine', 1861, by Shi Shou–Tang) is very precise:

> One should use pungent herbs which are light in weight to treat this; the pungent herbs are those such as *Xing Ren* (Pruni Armeniacae, Semen), *Bai Kou Ren* (Amomi Cardamomi, Fructus), *Ban Xia* (Pinelliae Ternata, Rhizoma), *Hou Po* (Magnoliae Officinalis, Cortex) and *Zi Su Geng* (Perillae Fructescentis, Herba). Bland herbs should also be used [for diuresis], such as *Yi Yi Ren* (Coicis Lachryma-jobi, Semen), *Tong Cao* (Tetrapanacis Papyriferi, Medulla), *Fu Ling* (Poriae Cocos, Sclerotium), *Zhu Ling* (Polypori Umbellati, Sclerotium) and *Ze Xie* (Alismatis Plantago-aquaticae, Rhizoma). When the sluice gate is unlocked above, and the lower stream opened, damp is led downward and given a route out.

These methods of opening Lung qi to deal with damp-heat predominantly aim at transforming damp and allowing heat to disperse through the surface; there is not much here to actually cool heat itself. Therefore this approach is best if the damp-heat is in the upper Jiao, with the pathogens in the wei (protective qi), or qi levels; or if damp predominates, even if it is in the middle or lower Jiao. If heat is stronger than damp, trying to allow it to disperse through the surface will not be sufficiently effective: bitter-cold herbs to cool heat must be added.

In general, some of the most common herbs to open Lung qi and transform damp are:

Xing Ren	Pruni Armeniacae, Semen
Pi Pa Ye	Eriobotryae Japonicae, Folium
Qian Hu	Peucedani, Radix
Zi Su Geng	Perillae Fructescentis, Herba
Dan Dou Chi	Sojae Praeparatum, Semen
Jie Geng	Platycodi Grandiflori, Radix

Of these, the first four can not only spread Lung qi and open the surface but also help Lung qi to descend, and transform phlegm, which is exactly suited to the physiological actions of the Lungs, and so they are very commonly employed in clinic. *Jie Geng* is pungent and thus dispersing, bitter and so draining, and through its rising nature can help lift the other herbs in a prescription to act in the Lungs, and so it is often used as a guiding herb. *Dan Dou Chi* is a mild surface opener which disperses through the surface pent-up heat in the Lungs or the Stomach. It is often used for the sensations of stuffy chest and irritability which can result from damp-heat obstructed in the upper Jiao.

Combining pungent flavors to open, and bitter flavors to bring down

'Treating the middle Jiao is like poising a balance bar: if it is not in equilibrium, it is unstable.' The combined use of pungent and bitter herbs is a way to restore equilibrium to the ascent of Spleen qi and the descent of Stomach qi, if they have been upset by the pathogenic influence of damp-heat.

If, in the middle Jiao, the damp exceeds the heat, then pungent-warm and bitter-warm herbs should be combined, so that warmth and pungency can disperse obstruction, while the warmth and bitterness can parch the damp. A yang-natured flavor such as pungency lifts, expands and opens so that Spleen is relieved of damp oppression and Spleen yang is enabled to rise. Bitter descends, drains and parches, so that the pathogenic damp which has been dispersed by the pungent flavor can be drained away and the rest of the damp parched; the bitterness will also assist the Stomach qi to descend

properly. The effects will not stop at the middle Jiao, however: as mentioned previously, the middle Jiao is the pivot for San Jiao qi movement and thus the key to qi transformation generally. Restoration of balanced middle Jiao functioning will have beneficial ramifications throughout the body. Two formulas which combine pungent-warmth and bitter-warmth are San Ren Tang ('Three-Nut Decoction', *Formulas and Strategies*, p. 186) and Huo Po Xia Ling Tang ('Agastache, Magnolia Bark, Pinellia and Poria Decoction', *Formulas and Strategies*, p. 187). In each of these, *Ban Xia* (Pinelliae Ternata, Rhizoma) and *Bai Kou Ren* (Amomi Cardamomi, Fructus) are warm and pungent, while *Hou Po* (Magnoliae Officinalis, Cortex) and *Xing Ren* (Pruni Armeniacae, Semen) are warm and bitter. Similarly, in Huo Xiang Zheng Qi San ('Agastache Powder to Rectify the Qi', *Formulas and Strategies*, p. 183) the warm and pungent *Ban Xia* and *Chen Pi* (Citri Reticulatae, Pericarpium, which is itself slightly bitter) are combined with the warm and bitter *Hou Po* to achieve the same results. A third example is Yi Jia Jian Zheng Qi San ('First Modification to Rectify the Qi Powder', *Formulas and Strategies*, p. 184), in which pungent-warm *Da Fu Pi* (Arecae Catechu, Pericarpium) is used with *Chen Pi* and *Hou Po*.

If the damp and heat in the middle Jiao are equally strong and hard to separate, the best approach is to simultaneously dry damp and cool heat, by using herbs that are pungent-warm and bitter-warm with herbs that are bitter-cold. This is the method adopted in the formula Lian Po Yin ('Coptis and Magnolia Bark Decoction', *Formulas and Strategies*, p. 189), which has the coldness of *Huang Lian* (Coptidis, Rhizoma) and *Shan Zhi Zi* (Gardeniae Jasminoidis, Fructus) to cool heat, while also using their bitterness to drain and parch damp; combined with bitter-warm herbs like *Hou Po* to dry and drain, and pungent-warm herbs like *Ban Xia* and the fragrant *Shi Chang Pu* (Acori Graminei, Rhizoma) to disperse. A number of formulas designed for middle Jiao damp-heat use the bitter-cold of *Huang Qin* (Scutellariae Baicalensis, Radix) and *Huang Lian* to bring rebelling qi down, break the knot of heat at the qi level and also parch turbid-damp, while simultaneously using the pungency of *Zhi Shi* (Citri seu Ponciri Immaturis, Fructus) and *Ban Xia* to open the knot of damp at the qi level, and thus together restore movement to the San Jiao qi mechanism. Occasionally the pungent-warm *Sheng Jiang* (Zingiberis Officinalis Recens, Rhizoma) is used to settle rebelling Stomach qi.

If pathogenic heat exceeds the damp, see section on bitter-cold to cool heat and dry damp, p. 263.

Using bland flavors to promote urination and leach out damp

Diuresis is not only used for lower Jiao damp-heat causing edema; or urination that is difficult, burning, scanty, frequent or turbid; or leukorrhea. It is also used to provide a route of escape for damp-heat pathogens which have been expelled or drained from other parts of the body, and so it is an indispensable part of any damp-heat treatment. The most common herbs to promote urination and leach out dampness are sweet and bland in flavor, such as:

Fu Ling	Poriae Cocos, Sclerotium
Tong Cao	Tetrapanacis Papyriferi, Medulla
Yi Yi Ren	Coicis Lachryma-jobi, Semen
Hua Shi	Talc
Ze Xie	Alismatis Plantago-aquaticae, Rhizoma
Che Qian Zi	Plantaginis, Semen
Jin Qian Cao	Jinqiancao, Herba
Dong Kui Zi	Abutiloni seu Malvae, Semen
Yu Mi Xu	Zeae Mays, Stylus

Of these, *Hua Shi* is sweet, bland and cold: the bland flavor leaches out damp, the sweet protects and harmonizes Stomach qi and stops insatiable thirst and the cold cools heat. It is also slippery in nature (hence the Chinese name 'slippery stone'), and thus it can benefit lower orifices and promote dispersal of obstructions. It is often used for Summerheat and damp with urinary obstruction. As Zhang Xi-Chun says: 'For urinary difficulty from heat, *Hua Shi* is the most important herb.' Thus it is used in at least nine standard formulas for damp-heat.

Tong Cao is sweet bland and cold and enters the Lungs and Stomach, and so can drain heat obstruction in the Lungs downward, and promote the movement of the fluid pathways so that heat is carried down and out through the urine. Because it enters the Stomach, it can promote the flow of breast milk. One of the special characteristics of *Tong Cao* is its ability to both rise and descend. The *Ben Cao*

Gang Mu explains this, after describing the above actions, by saying: 'Its qi (nature) is cold, thus it descends; its flavor is bland, and so it ascends.' Anyone doubting this would be reassured by the extreme lightness of the herb itself: it almost floats on air. *Tong Cao* is often combined with *Hua Shi* in the treatment of damp-heat, as for example in such formulas as San Ren Tang ('Three-Nut Decoction', *Formulas and Strategies*, p. 186), Huang Qin Hua Shi Tang ('Scutellaria and Talcum Decoction', *Formulas and Strategies*, p. 187), Xing Ren Hua Shi Tang ('Apricot Kernel and Talcum Decoction', *Formulas and Strategies*, p. 187) and several others.

Fu Ling is also commonly used, both for its diuretic and also its Spleen qi strengthening effects; *Chi Fu Ling* (Poriae, Cocos Rubrae, Sclerotium) though, is somewhat better at separating the damp pathogen from the heat pathogen, while *Fu Ling Pi* (Poriae Cocos, Cortex) is a better diuretic, although less Spleen strengthening.

Ze Xie is sweet and cold, with its primary actions in the lower Jiao because it enters the Kidney and Urinary Bladder channels. One of its special characteristics is the ability to drain excessive ministerial fire in the Kidney channel, which is the main reason for its inclusion in the formula Liu Wei Di Huang Wan ('Six-Ingredient Pill with Rehmannia', *Formulas and Strategies*, p. 263). But promotion of urination can have far-reaching effects in the other parts of the body as well, and so the importance of *Ze Xie* is not limited to the lower Jiao. Hence the *Ben Cao Gang Mu* says: 'Damp-heat in the Spleen and Stomach can cause heaviness of the head, blurry vision and tinnitus; *Ze Xie* can leach away this damp and the heat will soon follow.'

There is a further class of diuretic herbs which are also used in the treatment of damp-heat disease; they are not bland, however, but rather bitter and cold. These include:

Mu Tong	Mutong, Caulis
Qu Mai	Dianthi, Herba
Yin Chen Hao	Artemesiae Capillaris, Herba
Bian Xu	Polygoni Avicularis, Herba
Shi Wei	Pyrrosiae, Folium

Each of these, again, has its special uses. *Mu Tong*, besides its urine promoting effect, can lead heat out through the urine like *Tong Cao* but, because it is bitter, *Mu Tong* can also directly act to cool Heart fire. *Qu Mai* and *Bian Xu* are often combined for urinary discomfort in damp-heat conditions affecting the Urinary Bladder. The difference between them is that *Qu Mai* enters the Heart channel blood level and breaks up blood stagnation, while also entering the Small Intestine and promoting fluid separation, and thus is better suited to conditions where heat exceeds damp. *Bian Xu* acts directly on the Urinary Bladder to eliminate damp-heat through the urine, and is thus more appropriate for conditions where damp is predominant. *Yin Chen Hao* is bitter, slightly cold and fragrant and is specific for damp-heat obstructing the Liver and Gall Bladder leading to jaundice. *Shi Wei* acts both on the Lungs and on the Urinary Bladder, so dealing with both the uppermost and the lowermost aspects of the fluid metabolism. It can also cool the blood and stop bleeding.

Using fragrance to transform damp

Fragrance is very yang because of its light rising expanding nature. Clinically, patients with turbid-damp will often report that odors such as perfumes and petrol make them nauseous or give them headaches.[13]

This occurs because the extreme yang nature of the fragrance can pierce the turbid-damp and break it up, and then, through the lifting action of the fragrance, cause it to rise to the head. At the same time it also acts on the normal qi of the Stomach, which has been blocked from descending by the damp, and this qi rises as well, leading to nausea. Therapeutically, this activity can be turned to advantage by using precise amounts of fragrant herbs to pierce and disperse turbid-damp overwhelming the Spleen. The degree of fragrance applied should be just enough to break up the damp and revive the Spleen qi, without excessively lifting. In fact, some of the best fragrant herbs also stop nausea, either because by dispersing the damp they restore normal ascent of Spleen and also descent of the Stomach qi, or because they are both fragrant and also bitter and so directly assist Stomach qi descent.

The most common fragrant herbs are:

Huo Xiang	Agastaches seu Pogostemi, Herba
Pei Lan	Eupatorii Fortunei, Herba
Bai Kou Ren	Amomi Cardamomi, Fructus
Sha Ren	Amomi, Fructus et Semen
Shi Chang Pu	Acori Graminei, Rhizoma

Huo Xiang and *Pei Lan* are frequently used together to break up heavy damp oppression of the Spleen. But *Huo Xiang*'s strong point is in its ability to stop nausea, while *Pei Lan* is better at eliminating old rotten turbidity, and thus is used in cases where bad breath and a sweet metallic taste in the mouth are prominent features. *Sha Ren* and *Bai Kou Ren* are similar in both nature and flavor, in that they both use fragrance to transform damp, and both move qi to open the central region. But *Bai Kou Ren* has a fragrance which is clear and light, with a relatively mild warming and parching effect; it can also open the flow of Lung qi, and thus it is used for damp-phlegm obstructing the Lungs causing sensations of stuffy chest, and for milder cases of middle Jiao damp. *Sha Ren*, in contrast, has a stronger fragrance, is very warming and parching, moves qi more strongly and acts specifically on the Spleen and Stomach to break up more severe damp obstruction. Because it has a stronger warming effect, *Sha Ren* will be used more often for cold-damp than for damp-heat; whereas *Bai Kou Ren*, being milder in warmth, is frequently used in damp-heat formulas. *Shi Chang Pu* is also warm but its warmth is harmonious, with a light spreading action that allows it to enter the middle Jiao and lightly disperse turbid-damp to revive the Spleen and reopen the Stomach, and assist the rise of clear yang. It is this last effect which is the special ability of *Shi Chang Pu*, and thus it can 'lift the clear yang, excite the spirit, open the orifice of the Heart, sharpen the hearing, and strengthen the brain'.

Strengthening Spleen to parch damp

Weakness of Spleen transport is a fundamental source of endogenous damp, and thus strengthening Spleen is an equally fundamental method of treatment. It can be used in damp-heat conditions when damp exceeds heat, or in the later stages of the affliction when Spleen has been weakened by prolonged damp oppression, and some pathogenic damp still remains. The most common herbs are:

Cang Zhu	Atractylodis, Rhizoma
Bai Zhu	Atractylodis Macrocephalae, Rhizoma
Bai Bian Dou	Dolichos Lablab, Semen
Cao Dou Kou	Alpiniae Katsumadai, Semen

Cang Zhu is one of the strongest fragrant parching herbs, because it is not only fragrant but also pungent, bitter and warm, being able to strengthen Spleen, dry damp, disperse obstruction and expel turbid filth. Zhu Dan–Xi described *Cang Zhu* as being of the first importance in the treatment of damp:

> *Cang Zhu* treats damp, and can be used in the upper, middle or lower body ... if ascent and descent has become abnormal through improper transformation, the disease is in the middle Jiao. Thus any herbs used must both lift and descend: if one wishes to lift, one must first cause descent; if one desires descent, one must begin with lifting. Therefore *Cang Zhu*, as a Foot Yang Ming channel herb with a harsh-pungent nature and flavor, can strengthen the Stomach and Spleen, release the energy from food, and cause all other herbs to enter [the middle Jiao] to open and drain the damp in Yang Ming, and remove constriction.

The *Ben Cao Zheng Yi* says that 'without the harshness of *Cang Zhu*' heavy damp oppressing the Spleen and causing lethargy and lassitude with continual desire to lie down, aching limbs, stuffy chest, abdominal distention and thick greasy tongue coat 'cannot be opened'. It also mentions that for Summerheat and damp, or in damp-warm disease, the fragrance of herbs such as *Cang Zhu* and *Huo Xiang* should be used together to awaken the Spleen. However, when *Cang Zhu* is used in damp-heat treatments it will usually be combined with a bitter-cold herb to balance its yang nature and avoid exacerbating pathogenic heat, as in Er Miao San ('Two-Marvel Powder', *Formulas and Strategies*, p. 195) where it is used with *Huang Bo* (Phellodendri, Cortex). It should be noted, however, that it is often avoided in damp-heat formulas for this very reason. *Bai Zhu* is less harsh than *Cang Zhu* but is much more tonifying of Spleen qi, while still retaining the ability to parch damp. *Bai Bian Dou* is mildly fragrant and transforms damp without being too

drying. In fact, when used in its raw state, it cools Summerheat and damp; in order to parch damp and strengthen Spleen, it should be fried or baked.

Opening the flow of yang qi to transform damp

A vicious cycle can occur in which damp-heat obstructing the flow of yang qi results in a series of disruptions to the qi transformation functions around the body, leading to increased retention of damp. To break this cycle, and restore the flow of yang qi, the original damp-heat blockage must be eliminated. But it comes back to the old problem: if one uses only warm herbs to transform damp and promote yang qi, the pathogenic heat will get worse; if one employs cold herbs for the heat, the damp will thicken. If, in desperation, one tries to promote urination, this too will fail: obstruction of the yang qi movement will mean that not enough yang qi will be available to the Urinary Bladder to accomplish its qi transformation, and thus urine will remain scanty. It was probably a clinical impasse such as this which prompted Ye Tian-Shi to comment, dryly: 'Opening the flow of yang qi is most difficult.'

In this situation, the only recourse is to open Tai Yang to promote San Jiao, and open the Lung qi to clear the fluid metabolism. In other words, one must simultaneously:

1. use spreading dispersing herbs to promote the flow of yang qi and restore qi transformation
2. use warm-pungent and warm-bitter herbs to restore San Jiao qi movement, as the San Jiao is both the pathway for yang qi and also the pathway for fluids
3. use bland herbs to promote urination, as once the urine can flow, the major obstruction to the movement of yang qi will disappear, and so Ye Tian-Shi observed: 'Opening the flow of yang qi is not achieved through warmth but rather through promoting urination.'

Only by employing all three aspects together, in a measured fashion, and working slowly but steadily, can one hope to gradually open the yang qi flow and restore normality to the fluid metabolism. The study of one of Wu Ju-Tong's formulas can aid the understanding of this principle: his Cao Guo Yin Chen Tang ('Amomum and Capillaris Decoction').

Cao Guo Yin Chen Tang ('Amomum and Capillaris Decoction')

Cao Guo	Amomi Tsao-ko, Fructus
Yin Chen Hao	Artemesiae Capillaris, Herba
Chen Pi	Citri Reticulatae, Pericarpium
Da Fu Pi	Arecae Catechu, Pericarpium
Hou Po	Magnoliae Officinalis, Cortex
Fu Ling Pi	Poriae Cocos, Cortex
Zhu Ling	Polypori Umbellati, Sclerotium
Ze Xie	Alismatis Plantago-aquaticae, Rhizoma

In this formula, Wu Ju-Tong uses *Fu Ling Pi*, *Zhu Ling* and *Ze Xie* to promote urination; with *Chen Pi*, *Da Fu Pi* and *Hou Po* to parch damp and move the qi, thus opening the San Jiao. *Cao Guo* is warm and assists Urinary Bladder's qi transformation, while the *Yin Chen Hao* cools and leads the heat downward, and then out of the body.

Using bitter-cold flavors to clear heat and dry damp

Cold-natured herbs clear heat, bitter flavors dry damp, and so herbs with both of these attributes are well suited to damp-heat conditions in which heat exceeds damp. If damp and heat are equal, the method should be to use pungent-warm and bitter-warm together with bitter-cold herbs, as mentioned previously. If damp exceeds heat, bitter-cold herbs must be used cautiously: one or two bitter-cold herbs can be used in small amounts in a prescription of predominantly pungent-warm and bitter-warm herbs. Otherwise, not only will the damp not be expelled but the cold contraction will instead thicken the damp, leading to a worsening of the condition. The most commonly used bitter-cold herbs are:

Huang Qin	Scutellariae Baicalensis, Radix
Huang Lian	Coptidis, Rhizoma
Huang Bo	Phellodendri, Cortex
Shan Zhi Zi	Gardeniae Jasminoidis, Fructus
Long Dan Cao	Gentianae Scabrae, Radix
Ku Shen	Sophorae Flavescentis, Radix

The first three herbs are extremely cold and bitter, and not only clear heat and parch damp but also drain fire and relieve toxicity. As a general rule of thumb, *Huang Qin* acts to clear upper Jiao damp-heat, while also cooling the blood; *Huang Lian* clears and parches middle Jiao damp-heat, while also cooling Heart fire; and *Huang Bo* clears lower Jiao damp-heat, while also bringing down flaring fire from yin deficiency. In clinic, however, they are often used in combination, as for example in Huang Lian Jie Du Tang ('Coptis Decoction to Relieve Toxicity', *Formulas and Strategies*, p. 78) where all three are used together, or Xie Xin Tang ('Drain the Epigastrium Decoction', *Formulas and Strategies*, p. 79), Xing Ren Hua Shi Tang ('Apricot Kernel and Talcum Decoction', *Formulas and Strategies*, p. 187), Ge Gen Qin Lian Tang ('Kudzu, Coptis and Scutellaria Decoction', *Formulas and Strategies*, p. 60), and Qin Lian Er Chen Tang ('Two-Cured Decoction with Coptis and Scutellaria', which is just as its name describes), all of which combine *Huang Qin* and *Huang Lian*. Again, in Bai Tou Weng Tang ('Pulsatilla Decoction', *Formulas and Strategies*, p. 99), *Huang Lian* and *Huang Bo* are combined.

Long Dan Cao, *Shan Zhi Zi* and *Ku Shen* can all clear and drain damp-heat, promote Gall Bladder function and relieve jaundice. *Long Dan Cao* is especially able to enter and clear Liver channel damp-heat leading to swelling, while also expelling Urinary Bladder fire, as can be seen in its eponymous formula, Long Dan Xie Gan Tang ('Gentiana Longdancao Decoction to Drain the Liver', *Formulas and Strategies*, p. 96), in which *Shan Zhi Zi* is also used to drain heat out through the urine and relieve irritable discomfort in the chest. *Ku Shen*, besides clearing heat and drying damp, also expels wind and destroys parasites, and is commonly used for both itchy skin conditions and hot dysentery.

Clearing heat and relieving toxicity

This method is an essential component in the treatment of either exogenous epidemic toxic damp-heat, or endogenous damp-heat which has produced fire and thus become toxic; otherwise, the therapy will have little effect. Of course, as in all of the methods, differentiation of the relative degree of pathogenic influence exerted by each of the two factors, damp and heat, will be the key to proper herb selection. The most commonly used cooling antitoxic herbs are:

Jin Yin Hua	Lonicerae Japonicae, Flos
Lian Qiao	Forsythiae Suspensae, Fructus

Ban Lan Gen	Isatidis seu Baphicadanthi, Radix
Da Qing Ye	Daqingye, Folium
Bai Tou Weng	Pulsatilla Chinensis, Radix
Tu Fu Ling	Smilacis Glabrae, Rhizoma

Jin Yin Hua and *Lian Qiao* are certainly the most frequently used of the above, as they also are light and thus have the ability to encourage the pathogen to reach and be expelled through the surface. Gan Lu Xiao Du Dan ('Sweet Dew Special Pill to Eliminate Toxin', *Formulas and Strategies*, p. 187), Chang Pu Yu Jin Tang ('Acorus and Curcuma Decoction') and Yi Yi Zhu Ye San ('Coix and Bamboo Leaf Powder') all use *Lian Qiao*; while Qing Luo Yin ('Clear the Collaterals Decoction', *Formulas and Strategies*, p. 104) uses *Jin Yin Hua*. At present, the use of these two herbs has broadened to include acute epidemic dysentery, acute jaundice, damp-heat lin ('difficult urination') syndrome and even damp-heat edema. *Ban Lan Gen* and *Da Qing Ye* are very bitter and cold and thus cool heat and clear toxicity, cool the blood and sooth the throat, and so are important herbs for the treatment of damp-heat jaundice. *Bai Tou Weng* clears heat and relieves toxicity, cools the blood and stops diarrhea and is the first choice in the treatment of damp-heat dysentery. *Tu Fu Ling*, because of its cooling antitoxic diuretic actions, is often used for difficult or turbid urination from damp-heat, and also damp-heat leukorrhea, or even damp-heat spermatorrhea. Because it is specific for the lower Jiao, and yet is not overly bitter or cold while still being effective for toxic-heat, it was a favorite herb of one of my teachers, Qiu Xiao-Mei in Hangzhou.

Cooling and moving the blood

'Heat entering the blood chamber' (re ru xue shi, 热入血室) is a concept familiar to most students of the *Shang Han Lun* and the febrile disease schools but is less well known in the context of damp-heat.

In exogenous damp-heat disease, the pathogenic damp can become parching and enter deep into the nutritive qi (ying) and blood levels. At this point herbs to cool and drain heat from the nutritive qi and the blood must be used, often in conjunction with herbs that disperse blood, because the heat can dry blood, forming clots and causing stagnation. The following quote from Xue Sheng-Bai's *Shi Re*

Tiao Bian ('Systematic Differentiation of Dampness and Heat') describes the situation:

> Damp-heat syndrome. The menstrual period has just arrived, there is high fever, thirst, irrationality with confusion, pain in the chest and abdomen, the tongue is possibly without a coat, the pulse is slippery and rapid. The pathogen has sunk into the nutritive qi level; one should use a large prescription with herbs such as *Xi Jiao* (Rhinoceri, Cornu), *Zi Cao* (Lithospermi seu Arnebiae, Radix), *Qian Cao Gen* (Rubiae Cordifoliae, Radix), *Guan Zhong* (Dryopteridis Crassirhizomae, Rhizoma), *Lian Qiao* (Forsythiae Suspensae, Fructus), fresh *Shi Chang Pu* (Acori Graminei, Rhizoma) and *Jin Yin Hua* (Lonicerae Japonicae, Flos).

A second quote outlines a similar situation:

> Damp-heat syndrome: when there is loss of blood in the upper or lower body, or sweating of blood, the toxic pathogen has entered deep into the ying (nutritive qi) level. This must be drained away using a large prescription with *Xi Jiao* (Rhinoceri, Cornu), *Sheng Di* (Rehmannia Glutinosae, Radix), *Chi Shao* (Paeoniae Rubra, Radix), *Mu Dan Pi* (Moutan Radicis, Cortex), *Lian Qiao* (Forsythiae Suspensae, Fructus), *Zi Cao* (Lithospermi seu Arnebiae, Radix), *Qian Cao* (Rubiae Cordifoliae, Herba), *Jin Yin Hua* (Lonicerae Japonicae, Flos) and similar herbs.

In endogenous damp-heat disease, when the damp and heat have become chronic, and gradually invaded the nutritive qi and blood levels, one should also add herbs that cool and disperse blood. For example, nosebleeds or bleeding gums with damp-heat jaundice; blood in the urine with damp-heat lin (painful urinary dysfunction) syndrome; and blood in the stool with damp-heat dysentery: all are symptoms of heat in the blood with possible blood stagnation, and all should have blood-cooling and dispersing herbs added to the basic prescription designed to deal with these problems. Some of the most common herbs used in this way are:

Shui Niu Jiao	Bubali, Cornu
Chi Shao	Paeoniae Rubra, Radix
Mu Dan Pi	Moutan Radicis, Cortex

Bai Mao Gen	Imperatae Cylindricae, Rhizoma
Sheng Di	Rehmannia Glutinosae, Radix
Qian Cao Gen	Rubiae Cordifoliae, Radix

Shui Niu Jiao is a substitute for the (now endangered) rhinoceros.[14] Water buffalo horn (*Shui Niu Jiao*) works just as well, in larger doses, to cool the blood, stop bleeding and reduce toxicity. *Mu Dan Pi* and *Chi Shao* both cool and move the blood, the main difference being that *Mu Dan Pi* cools heat from yin deficiency as well as heat from pathogenic excess (shi heat), while *Chi Shao* only cools excess heat but is better at stopping pain than *Mu Dan Pi*. One of the concerns when using cold herbs to cool heat in the blood is that the very coldness of the herbs will tend to slow and stagnate the blood flow. This is not a problem with *Chi Shao* and *Mu Dan Pi* however, because as well as cooling the blood, they also move blood and remove stagnation. *Qian Cao Gen* does both of these things and also stops bleeding. *Bai Mao Gen* not only cools blood and stops bleeding but is also a cooling, bland-flavored diuretic to remove damp, and so is often used in damp-heat conditions with bleeding.

Nourishing yin while cooling heat and promoting urination

Yin deficiency can occur in conjunction with damp-heat disease in two situations: either the patient is constitutionally yin deficient and has also developed pathogenic damp-heat through either exogenous invasion or endogenous creation; or during the course of treatment for the damp-heat there has been excessive use of herbs which can damage yin, such as fragrant parchers, or diuretics, or purging herbs, or even bitter-cold herbs.[15] The treatment of yin deficiency combined with damp-heat can be very tricky, because to nourish yin one requires cool moistening herbs which tend to encourage damp, while to eliminate damp-heat one often requires drying or bitter herbs which can also injure the normal yin fluids. The only solution is precision in the choice of herbs to match the exact degree of deficiency and excess in the individual patient, and to choose herbs which are neither too greasy (in yin tonification) nor too pungent or parching (in the removal of damp). One of the earliest formulas designed to deal with this problem was Zhu Ling

Tang ('Polyporus Decoction', *Formulas and Strategies*, p. 176) from the *Shang Han Lun*.

Some herbs which nourish yin without being excessively greasy and damp promoting are:

Sha Shen	Glehniae Littoralis, Radix
Yu Zhu	Polygonati Odorati, Rhizoma
Shi Hu	Dendrobii, Herba
Lu Gen	Phragmitis Communis, Rhizoma
Nu Zhen Zi	Ligustri Lucidi, Fructus
Han Lian Cao	Ecliptae Prostratae, Herba
Tian Hua Fen	Trichosanthis, Radix
Bai He	Lilii, Bulbus
Gui Ban	Testudinis, Plastrum
Bie Jia	Amydae Sinensis, Carapax

Some herbs which can treat damp without overly damaging yin, by lightly spreading and opening, or mildly cooling, transforming and promoting urination are:

Xing Ren	Pruni Armeniacae, Semen
Yi Yi Ren	Coicis Lachryma-jobi, Semen
Chuan Bei Mu	Fritillariae Cirrhosae, Bulbus
Fu Ling	Poriae Cocos, Sclerotium
Shan Yao	Dioscoreae Oppositae, Radix
Lian Qiao	Forsythiae Suspensae, Fructus
Hua Shi	Talc

In a prescription composed of herbs from these two groups, a small amount of one or two bitter-parching and pungent-dispersing herbs can be added, such as:

Xuan Fu Hua	Inulae, Flos
He Ye	Nelumbinis Nuciferae, Folium
Pei Lan	Eupatorii Fortunei, Herba

Contraindications in the treatment of damp-heat disease

Pungent-warm diaphoresis

In the early stages of an exogenous damp-heat invasion, the pathogenic damp-heat obstructs the surface tissues, causing fever and aversion to cold, headaches and little or no sweating, all of which are very similar to an exogenous wind-cold attack. The method of treatment should be to use fragrant herbs to spread and open Lung qi, to allow the pathogen to be dispersed through the surface with a very mild and gradual perspiration. If the condition is mistakenly diagnosed as wind-cold and very pungent and warm herbs such as *Ma Huang* (Ephedrae, Herba) and *Gui Zhi* (Cinnamomi Cassiae, Ramulus) are used to disperse constricting pathogenic cold, the result will often be a heavier sweat than necessary. This will not only not expel a damp pathogen but will also exacerbate the pathogenic heat. Damp tends to be cloying and difficult to move quickly and so, in the above situation, the sweat will indeed pour out but it will leave the pathogenic damp behind, and instead carry off the patient's protective qi which will flow out of the open pores with the sweat. Worse, the pungent warm lifting action of the wind-cold expelling herbs can carry the influence of the damp-heat pathogen upward, not out through the surface which is still blocked by damp but instead into the head where the pathogenic influence can obstruct the clear orifice of the mind, leading to vertigo, blurry vision, tinnitus, deafness and even fainting and difficult speech. Thus Wu Ju-Tong, in his *Wen Bing Tiao Bian* ('Systematic Differentiation of Warm Diseases', 1798), says: 'Causing [this type of patient] to sweat will lead to fainting and deafness, and in severe conditions blurry vision and reluctance to speak.'

Bitter-cold purging

In the course of a damp-heat disease, if the damp-heat pathogen obstructs the qi flow through the Stomach and Intestines so that descent is disrupted, this causes abdominal distention, flatulence, thickening of the tongue coat at the root, and slippery floating weak and thready pulse. The method of treatment should be to clear heat, parch damp and open the normal flow of Stomach and Intestinal qi, with possibly a mild qi-moving laxative component. If the symptoms show that the middle Jiao is more involved, for example with epigastric as well as abdominal distention, loss of appetite and ability to eat, difficult defecation or constipation, then this indicates that damp exceeds heat and the damp is oppressing the Spleen so that the ascent and descent of qi is disrupted. Here the method of treatment should be to transform damp and revive the Spleen, regulate qi flow, and restore Spleen transportation.

Under either of these circumstances, one cannot use violent purging bitter-cold herbs such as *Da*

Huang (Rhei, Rhizoma) and *Mang Xiao* (Mirabilitum): because of the sticky nature of damp, a quick strong bitter-cold purge will not be effective by itself but will in fact succeed only in damaging Spleen yang and dragging it downward, resulting in continuous diarrhea.

Moist greasy tonics

As discussed briefly above, the fever in damp-heat disease is often most prominent in the afternoon, and is also accompanied by dryness of the mouth, and so could easily be confused with yin deficiency with fire flaring unless the possibility is recognized and care taken with differentiation. The method of treatment is to clear heat and transform damp. Mistaken differentiation as yin deficiency, followed by the prescription of moist greasy yin tonics such as *Sheng Di* (Rehmannia Glutinosae, Radix), *Shan Zhu Yu* (Corni Officinalis, Fructus), *Mai Men Dong* (Ophiopogonis Japonici, Tuber) or *Tian Men Dong* (Asparagi Cochinchinensis, Tuber), will add to the damp obstruction and thereby increase the heat, prolonging the condition and making it very difficult to cure. Thus the *Wen Bing Tiao Bian* ('Systematic Differentiation of Warm Diseases', 1798) remarks: 'Moistening [this type of patient] will lead the disease to deepen without relief.'

Sweet-warm obstructing tonics

Damp is a yin pathogen which easily blocks the flow of yang qi, and therefore patients will occasionally present with symptoms of cold limbs, facial pallor, lethargy and tiredness. The method of treatment should be to combine the three approaches, described above on page 262 under 'Fundamental methods of damp treatment', of opening the flow of yang qi, restoring normal qi movement through the San Jiao and promoting urination with sweet-bland diuretics. This will restore yang circulation and transform damp, thus freeing the heat for dispersal.

If, though, the condition is mistakenly diagnosed as insufficiency of yang qi leading to cold, and sweet-warm tonics such as *Dang Shen* (Codonopsis Pilosulae, Radix) or *Huang Qi* (Astragali, Radix) are employed, this will both add to the pathogenic heat, and also further obstruct the damp and prevent its transformation.

Dietary contraindications

Spleen function is often the first casualty of damp-heat disease, as discussed at length previously: its ability to transform is reduced, and so the amount of food it can deal with is smaller; it cannot transport well, and so food tends to sit in the epigastric area; the Stomach becomes affected to the extent that it cannot accept any more food and thus both appetite and the ability to eat are impaired. If the impairment extends to the ascent and descent of qi through the San Jiao, then nausea will show the tendency of Stomach qi to rise instead of descending, and loose stool will demonstrate the failure of Spleen qi to lift, allowing instead the half-digested food and damp to pour down through the Intestines, to exit as loose stool.

Therefore diet is an essential part of damp-heat treatment. Patients should be advised not to eat to satiety, giving the Spleen qi more 'room' to accomplish its task of transforming, which would be weighed down by a full Stomach, and completely overburdened if the patient overeats. Bland foods should also be recommended, both because they tend to be lighter and easier to digest but also because the bland flavor itself assists diuresis, and thus the treatment. Heavy greasy rich foods tend to be difficult to digest and will readily form phlegm and damp; while hot spicy foods can add to the heat. Cold and raw foods, despite the New Age 'received wisdom' that they 'have more Life Energy', actually require the body to expend Spleen and Stomach yang energy to warm them up prior to digestion. Even then the digestion of these cold and raw foods will still be far more difficult than with cooked foods.

NOTES

1. Most of this chapter is based on translations from the first half of the *Shi Re Lun* ('Discussions of Damp-heat'), written by Jiang Shen, a Chinese traditional doctor of twenty years experience in dealing with damp-heat problems in clinic. The *Shi Re Lun* was published by the Joint Publishing Company, Hong Kong, 1989. All quotes in this chapter, unless otherwise attributed, derive from this source.

2. This will of course be different in other countries and climates. A practitioner should be familiar enough with the local conditions to recognize the effects of the weather on patients. A period of study in China during the extremely oppressive heat of the 'long summer', without a breath of wind to stir the air, is an unforgettable, but quite valuable, experience.

3. The *Shi Re Tiao Pian* ('Systematic Differentiation of Damp-heat') was not published as a separate work but rather found amalgamated into a number of the Febrile Disease school texts and attributed to Xue Sheng-Bai (1681-1770). See *Zhong Guo Yi Xue Shi*, 'History of Chinese Medical Studies' by Pei Chi-Liu, published by Hwa Kang Press, Taiwan, 1974, pp. 522-524, and the note on page 629.

4. Students of traditional Chinese medicine in the West often fail to take advantage of one of the greatest strengths of TCM: the recorded clinical experience of over twenty centuries. One of the best ways to begin to use this experience in one's own clinic, as mentioned before, is to discover which famous Chinese doctors of the past lived in climatic situations similar to one's own, and to study their works first. For the dangers of failing to do this, see note 5 in Chapter 9.

5. Zheng qi can become temporarily weak if one is exhausted or stressed or recovering from a previous illness. Another situation occurs when one's pores are open to exogenous influence, for example after bathing or after exertion. This could be termed 'temporary local weakness of zheng—here especially the protective—qi'.

6. Not all 'urinary tract infections' as diagnosed by Western medicine will be exogenous damp-heat, as many will be the result of internal production of damp. The patient's history (such as recent change of sexual partner) will provide important clues in differentiation.

7. The words 'toxic' and 'toxin', to Western minds, carry implications of uncleanliness, as in the rather vague idea in naturopathy of 'toxins in the blood' which must be removed with 'blood cleansers'; or patients who say 'I feel very toxic' or 'Will these herbs clear away all my toxins and clean me out?' But the Chinese word 'du' 毒, for all of its various meanings, never implies dirt or filth—this is one of our own preoccupations. 'Toxin' in Chinese, as has been noted in *Formulas and Strategies* (p. 78) 'can mean different things depending upon the context. It may refer to the cause of a disease, the pathological mechanism of a disease, or the toxicity of a substance, and is sometimes used interchangeably with the term for pathogenic influence (xie). ... Chinese medicine also differentiates between yin and yang toxin.' The basic idea behind something toxic is that it is harmful to the body, with the connotation in Chinese of severity. Thus, pathogenic fire is harmful but only when it reaches an intense degree does it become 'toxic fire'. This is an example of a yang toxin. Pathogenic damp, too, is harmful but will only become 'toxic damp' if extreme. This is an example of a yin toxin. One way that a pathogenic factor can become extreme is by

being limited in its ability to spread—and so unable to dilute itself, as it were—and thus most cases of 'toxic' pathogens are those that have built up to an intense degree in a local area, often leading to eruptions on the skin or ulcers on the tongue and mouth. Another way to be extremely harmful is to affect a large number of people, and thus highly contagious diseases are often termed 'toxic', as in the *Shang Han Lun*: 'Injury by cold becomes toxic when its qi becomes most lethal and contagiously virulent'.

8. 'Bie shi' 別使. The complete quote is 'san jiao zhe, yuan qi zhi bie shi' 三焦者, 原气之别使 See note 25 in Chapter 1 on fluid metabolism relating to the San Jiao and its description in the *Nan Jing*.

9. *Su Wen Xuan Ji Yuan Bing Shi* ('Examination of the Original Patterns of Disease from the Mysterious Mechanisms of the Su Wen'), by Liu Wan-Su (1110-1200); Zhejiang Science and Technology Press, 1984, annotated by Fan Yong-Sheng, p. 66.

10. Western patients are likely to say, simply, 'I feel tired'; it is the responsibility of the practitioner to elicit the information which will enable the differentiation to be made between actual lack of energy and heaviness from damp which is suppressing the otherwise quite normal level of energy.

11. Translation from Maciocia, *Tongue Diagnosis in Chinese Medicine*, 1987, Eastland Press, Seattle, p. 19.

12. As noted previously, there is one situation in which diuresis should be used cautiously, and that is when Spleen qi is deficient and unable to rise normally. This, of course, also gives rise to damp, and so the temptation to use diuresis is strong. But the downward moving tendency of many diuretics, while necessary to carry damp to the lower Jiao, can also drag the Spleen qi downward, further weakening it, and thus complicating an already difficult situation.

The answer, as outlined in the chapter on the treatment of damp, is to use bitter-warm herbs which parch damp but also strengthen Spleen qi: a good example is *Bai Zhu* (Atractylodis Macrocephalae, Rhizoma).

13. This can also occur if a patient has a tendency to yang qi rising excessively, as the lifting nature of the fragrance will add to this ascent. But the symptom picture will usually be very different from that of a patient with turbid-damp.

14. The rhinoceros was formerly indigenous to China.

15. That bitter-cold herbs can damage yin is a fact which, I find, often surprises students. One can easily accept that yang-natured herbs such as *Cang Zhu* (Atractylodis, Rhizoma) will also dry normal fluids; or that excessive diuretics can push through fluids which would otherwise be recovered by the Urinary Bladder, and so damage yin; or that the fragrance of herbs such as *Xiang Fu* (Cyperi Rotundi, Rhizoma) can disperse and thus injure normal fluids; but bitter is itself yin-natured, and so is cold—so why would these cause yin deficiency? The key is in the actions: bitter drains and descends, and this action will occur whether the subject of the action is physiological or pathological, and thus normal yin fluids can be drained as well as pathological fluids. Excessive use of cold herbs will congeal normal fluids and prevent smooth flow, thus taking them out of normal circulation at least, and creating cold-damp or phlegm at worst. In either case the yin does not benefit. Thus the treatment for heat from yin deficiency is not cooling heat—this is used for heat from pathogenic excess (shi heat). The treatment for heat from yin deficiency is to remove the deficiency by tonifying yin, and the heat, which is after all only physiological heat uncontrolled by the weak yin, will soon be restored to balance.

Origin and development of phlegm theory in traditional Chinese medicine

---

INTRODUCTION

So little has been written on phlegm theory in English that it appears worthwhile to describe its historical development over the centuries during which traditional Chinese medicine has become what it is today. Often, knowing who said what, in what context, allows one to determine exactly how much weight to give a statement, and to realise whether the concept or technique has been superseded by another more fitting or effective.

Of course, it is not possible to record everything ever written upon the subject of phlegm in Chinese medicine. What will be attempted in the course of this chapter is to introduce some of the major contributions to the development of phlegm theory, to note relevant influences, and to emphasize the introduction of new concepts. At the end of this chapter will be selections of famous essays on phlegm, translated in full. I hope that comparisons between these and the historical period of the writers can help to provide a deeper understanding of how historical investigation can assist clinical effectiveness. Perhaps this will bear out the Chinese saying that traditional Chinese medicine is not an exact science but rather a literary endeavor.[1]

HUANG DI NEI JING

The *Nei Jing* does not actually contain the word 'phlegm' (tan 痰) but its pathophysiology is discussed in the *Nei Jing* under the category thin mucus (yin 饮) and damp. For example, in Chapter 71 of the *Su Wen* it says: 'The arrival of Tai Yin produces accumulated thin mucus which obstructs the diaphragm'. Other references indicate that phlegm-dispersing herbs had been used since at least the fifth century BC.[2]

The first mention of phlegm as such and its relationship to other fluid pathologies is found in the *Jin Gui Yao Lue* under the categories 'tan-yin' (phlegm and thin mucus 痰饮), 'shui-qi' (water-qi 水气) and 'cough'.

JIN GUI YAO LUE

The point to remember about the *Jin Gui Yao Lue* ('Essentials from the Golden Cabinet', c. 210 AD) in relation to the development of phlegm theory is that, like the *Nei Jing*, water and thin mucus are the primary focus, while phlegm is simply a further progression of thin mucus pathology. For example, phlegm (tan) is considered only one of the four 'yin' (thin mucus) diseases: xuan yin 悬饮 is thin mucus accumulating in the ribs and flanks, yi yin 溢饮 is thin mucus in the limbs, zhi yin 支饮 is thin mucus in the epigastric area, and tan yin 痰饮 is phlegm and thin mucus in the Stomach and Intestines.

In the *Jin Gui*, Chapter 12, entitled 'Tan Yin Ke Sou Bing Mai Zheng Bing Zhi'—the chapter on phlegm, thin mucus and cough—the discussion is in fact more involved with the pathology of water in the Five Zang as the following examples display:

- 'Water beneath the Heart (i.e. in the epigastric area) will cause a sensation of hardness, discomfort, difficulty breathing, with an aversion to water and no desire to drink.'
- 'Water in the Lungs, [will cause] vomiting of frothy fluid.'
- 'Thin people with palpitations below the umbilicus, with vomiting of frothy fluid and vertigo; this is water.'
- 'When the water goes, the vomiting will cease.'

The formulas which are advanced to deal with these conditions are also—from a modern perspective—clearly designed to eliminate water and very thin mucus, rather than phlegm of any viscosity.

On the other hand, some of TCM phlegm theory's most enduring quotes originate in this chapter, such as 'Those afflicted with tan yin should be harmonized with warm herbs',[3] and the first reference to 'cold on the back the size of a hand' is found here, although in this work it is attributed to thin mucus under the Heart rather than to phlegm.

ZHU BING YUAN HOU LUN

The earliest clear differentiation between 'tan' (phlegm) and 'yin' (thin mucus) comes in the Sui Dynasty text *Zhu Bing Yuan Hou Lun* ('General Treatise on the Etiology and Symptomatology of Disease', 610 AD) by Chao Yuan-Fang.[4] He said, for example: 'If the pulse is more wiry, it is phlegm; floating and thin means yin (thin mucus)'. He went on to describe hot-phlegm, cold-phlegm, knotted-

phlegm and so on, and proceeded to make the first description of a headache from phlegm: 'Yin-qi rebels upward and combines with wind and phlegm to strike at the head, thus making the head painful.'

From this point on in the history of traditional Chinese medicine, medical information proliferated rapidly. As doctors began recording their individual experiences with different illnesses, under different environmental conditions, and as seen through the understanding of their teaching lineages, schools of medical thought came into being. This activity, naturally, furthered phlegm theory development.

QIAN JIN YAO FANG

For example, the Tang Dynasty *Qian Jin Yao Fang* ('Thousand Ducat Formulas', 652AD) by Sun Si-Miao (c. 581-682) brings together not only the basic medical theory up to the Tang dynasty but also combines it with a system of approach and specified methods of using herbs. In Chapter 18, section 6, it describes the use of *Chang Shan* (Dichorae Febrifugae) and *Cong Bai* (Allii Fistulosi) in the treatment of combined hot and cold-phlegm in the diaphragm area and phlegm headache; the use of *Zao Jiao* (Gleditsiae Sinensis), *Ba Dou* (Croton), and *Ban Xia* (Pinelliae Ternata) to treat 'accumulated firm mass' which would now be called stubborn phlegm accumulation; and also introduces specific formulas for the treatment of phlegm in the chest, sour regurgitation from phlegm, nausea and vomiting of phlegm, and so on.[5]

This is a step beyond simply differentiating phlegm and thin mucus, as was done in the *Zhu Bing Yuan Hou Lun*, to basing therapy on the distinction.

The *Qian Jin Yi Fang* ('Supplement to the Thousand Ducat Formulas'), also by Sun Si-Miao, c. 682 AD, Chapter 18, besides recording the material in the *Jin Gui Yao Lue's* chapter on phlegm, thin mucus and cough, goes on to list more than twenty formulas of use in phlegm therapy, some of which are still in clinical use today.

SHI LIAO BEN CAO

The Tang dynasty *Shi Liao Ben Cao* ('Materia Medica of Food Therapy', c. 713 AD), besides mentioning the use of common phlegm-transforming herbs, notes that 'the flesh of the pig can bring out phlegm: those with malarial disease are definitely forbidden to eat it';[6] and 'winter melon seeds mainly benefit qi and prevent aging, expel sensations of fullness in the chest from qi, disperse phlegm and stop restlessness.'[7]

SHENG JI ZONG LU

The *Sheng Ji Zong Lu* ('Comprehensive Recording of the Sages' Benefits', *c.* 1112), two hundred volumes compiled by Imperial order, containing around 20 000 formulas, also—as may be expected—includes a rich section entitled 'Phlegm Symptoms', where it says, among many other things: 'Interference with the qi of the San Jiao will block the channels (mai dao), then water and fluids will slow and obstruct; without the ability to spread and move, they will accumulate into phlegm and thin mucus, causing diseases without number … Those best at treating these diseases will first open the pathways of the qi.'[8]

SAN YIN JI YI BING ZHENG FANG LUN

The *San Yin Ji Yi Bing Zheng Fang Lun* ('Discussion of Illnesses, Patterns, and Formulas Related to the Unification of the Three Etiologies', 1174) by Chen Yan (zi-name Wu Zu) goes a bit further than above, noting that:

> Internally, the seven emotions cause havoc, the zang-organ qi cannot move, it stops and produces thickened fluid, which in turn produces thin mucus. This is the internal reason. Externally, the six pathogens invade, the pores cannot open, and sweating cannot take place when it should: it gathers into thin mucus. This is the external reason. Or injury from eating and drinking, gluttony without measure, claiming tiredness so that no exercise is taken: here the jin-ye fluids cannot move, they accumulate, and become phlegm and thin mucus. This is neither internal nor external. The product of these three sources will give many different symptoms.

and a symptom list follows.[9]

YAN YONG-HE

Yan Yong-He, the author of the *Yan Shi Ji Sheng Fang* ('Formulas to Aid the Living', 1253), and the *Ji Sheng Xu Fang* ('More Formulas to Aid the Living' 1267), was the originator of the well-loved Gui Pi Tang formula ('Restore the Spleen Decoction', *Formulas and Strategies*, p. 255), as well as Qing Pi Tang ('Clear the Spleen Decoction', *Formulas and Strategies*, p. 144) and Si Mo Tang ('Four Milled-Herb Decoction', *Formulas and Strategies*, p. 301). In regards to phlegm pathogenesis, Yan observed:

> A person's qi pathway is meant to operate smoothly, as then the fluids can flow openly, with no chance of phlegm (tan yin) disorder; [but] if this regularity is upset, the qi pathway closes off, water and thin mucus occlude in and around the chest and diaphragm, collect, and become phlegm. In this type of illness, the symptoms can vary: there may be dyspnea, or cough, or vomiting, or diarrhea, or vertigo, or palpitations, or sadness and dread, chills and fever, or pain, or swelling, fullness, cramps and knots in the muscles, or anuria, or epigastric obstruction, all caused by nothing other than phlegm.

He also quoted Pang An-Shi[10] who said in his *Shang Han Zong Bing Lun* ('Discussion of Shang Han and General Diseases'): 'The body does not have phlegm moving upward [by itself, just as] no river under Heaven moves backward', which indicates the importance of the flow of qi in carrying phlegm around the body.

Yan Yong-He is notable in that, for his time, he had a remarkably deep grasp of the mechanisms and variety of symptoms for which phlegm could be responsible. If we consider his statements from a Western point of view, we can see that phlegm is recognized as influencing Western bio-medical systems as varied as the respiratory, the digestive, the circulatory, nervous and urinary systems. His observations still retain their validity and usefulness for the modern practitioner of traditional Chinese medicine, over seven hundred years later. Despite the complexity of phlegm diseases and symptoms (for example, that phlegm illnesses are not limited to chronic conditions but may be acute as well), he was able even in those times to introduce his own viewpoint of their mechanism and treatment, based upon his rich and extended medical experience. Especially noteworthy is his proposal of the now routine method of 'expediting the flow of qi as the foremost approach' in the treatment of phlegm.

Zhu Ceng-Bo comments, however:

Nonetheless he was still hampered by certain concepts from the earlier classics, as evidenced in statements such as:

'A mistake with warming or diuresis need not be harmful; wrongly purging or sweating [the patient, however] will cause more than superficial damage.'

This idea derives from the *Jin Gui Yao Lue*, Chapter 12, which insists:

'Those afflicted with tan yin should be harmonized with warm herbs'.

Purging, however, (continues Zhu Ceng–Bo) is not only an allowable phlegm treatment, it can actually achieve quite remarkable results with severe cases of stubborn phlegm, old phlegm, or hot phlegm leading to collapse or stroke.

We can learn from the ancients, but need not blindly copy them.[11]

ZHANG ZI-HE

Zhang Cong-Zheng (zi-name Zi He)[12] not only differentiated phlegm into wind-phlegm, hot-phlegm, damp-phlegm and food-phlegm but was also responsible for the introduction of the concept of 'phlegm misting the Heart', and was the initiator of the use of phlegm theory to explain and treat emotional and mental disorders, as Li Chan, the author of the Qing dynasty *Yi Xue Ru Men*, 1575, later agreed: 'Qi-phlegm is formed by repression of the seven emotions'.[13]

This is an historical example of the Chinese medical viewpoint that what Westerners would call 'mental disorders' are very often precipitated by organic imbalance.[14]

ZHU GONG

Zhu Gong, the Song dynasty author of the *Nan Yang Huo Ren Shu* ('The Nan Yang Book to Safeguard Life'), 1108, a work in the *Shang Han Lun* tradition, observed:

Phlegm in the epigastric area (Zhong Wan, CV-12) can also cause chills and fever, aversion to

wind, spontaneous perspiration, fullness and obstruction of the chest and diaphragm, just like an attack by exogenous cold, but the head will not ache and the neck will not be stiff, which is the distinction ... the pulse will be floating and slippery but will not be floating and tight.[15]

Li Chan (mentioned above) describes a similar situation, saying:

In the early stages of a phlegm condition there may be headache and fever, very much like the surface symptoms of an exogenous attack. After a period of time there will be hot flushes worsening at night, which again will resemble 'yin fire'.[16]

What these two authors are describing is the phlegm obstruction of the normal flow of nutritive and protective qi, creating a non-exogenous surface disharmony which can lead to symptoms of chills and fever, spontaneous perspiration and so on. Their medical experience (and that of others which confirm this: see Ye Tian-Shi's notes on the same phenomenon later in this chapter) has taught them that an apparently obvious diagnosis—an attack by cold, for example—must still be carefully differentiated, as it may not be such at all but something else: here, surface phlegm obstruction.

ZHU DAN-XI

Zhu Dan Xi (1281-1358) is one of the most famous of the Yuan dynasty medical authors, with a number of major works to his credit, the best known being *Dan Xi Xin Fa* ('Teachings of Zhu Dan Xi'), *Jin Gui Gou Xuan* ('Scythe of Mysteries from the Golden Cabinet') and *Ju Fang Fa Hui* ('Exposition of the Formulas from the Imperial Grace Formulary'). He is considered the originator of the 'Nourish the Yin' school, because of his statement that 'there is often a surplus of yang but yin is usually deficient'. In truth, he was a very well-rounded physician, famed for his skill in the treatment of a wide variety of illnesses, for which he would use yang-warming as often as yin-nourishing herbs. The subject of phlegm did not escape his attention.

Each of his books contains descriptions of phlegm illness, treatments and formulas. In the *Ju Fang Fa Hui* ('Exposition of the Formulas from the

Imperial Grace Formulary') for example, he mentions that when 'qi accumulates to become phlegm', the symptoms follow a pattern: 'either fortnightly, or monthly, the previous symptoms will reappear', pointing out a characteristic of phlegm diseases: that if they are not thoroughly eliminated, they can relapse more frequently than other types of illness.

Zhu Dan-Xi points out that the concept of 'qi accumulation leading to phlegm' reflects the influence of Liu Wan-Su (1120-1200), who emphasized the importance of qi and fire in his works, with which of course Dan Xi was familiar.[17] But Dan Xi reminds us that in fact phlegm can be formed through the processes of qi deficiency, qi blockage or qi in counter-flow, and goes on to describe in detail their symptoms and treatment.

In his book *Jin Gui Gou Xuan* ('Scythe of Mysteries from the Golden Cabinet'), of one hundred and thirty-nine topics (usually based on a symptom), the possible phlegm etiology and treatment is discussed in fifty-three, without counting the topical section specifically devoted to phlegm itself. His description of the symptom patterns is detailed, and the treatment methods are safe yet effective. Not only are vertigo, headaches, counter-flowing qi and leukorrhea described as being 'predominantly produced by phlegm', but a phlegm treatment approach is outlined for conditions such as urinary tract disorders, hernia, impotence, abdominal pain, pain in the costal regions and infertility. His discussion of wind-stroke is noteworthy in that Dan Xi says 'this cannot be treated as wind' but instead one should 'strongly tonify qi and blood, and then treat the phlegm'.

Zhu Dan-Xi's chief pupil Dai Si–Gong (1324-1405) was able to build on his teacher's ideas, and even surpass them in certain areas.

For example, Zhu Dan-Xi says:

> In any treatment for phlegm, if diuretic herbs are used excessively, this will cause the Spleen qi to weaken and be drawn downwards. If this happens, phlegm will be all the more easily produced, and in greater measure.

Dai Si-Gong comments upon this, remarking:

> In all humility, I must point out that phlegm can originate not only in the Spleen and Stomach but also in the [process of pathogenic influence in] Six Channels: the origin

is different. Here, however, the statement appears to say that the pathogenic influence and the formation of the illness [in the Spleen] are the same! As to treatment, it is necessary to first allay the source of the pathogen, which afterwards will extend to the cessation of the illness.[18]

The meaning being that some phlegm does not originate from Spleen weakness, and in these cases the use of diuretic herbs does not constitute a problem.

WANG GUI

Wang Gui, known as Wang Yin-Jun, was a Yuan dynasty physician, alchemist and recluse in the Lu Shan mountains (which is the origin of his second name, meaning 'Gentleman Hermit'). His major work, the *Tai Ding Yang Sheng Zhu Lun* ('Treatises on the Calm and Settled Nourishment of the Director of Life', 1338),[19] describes his alchemical and medical theories, among which are very detailed descriptions of tan-yin and water pathologies.

Wang Yin-Jun is the true originator of the famous 'Gun Tan Wan' ('Vaporize Phlegm Pill', *Formulas and Strategies*, p. 424) to treat the various consequences of a combination of phlegm fire and stubborn phlegm; a remarkably effective remedy that is still in wide use today.

He says:

> The nature of phlegm as a substance is that it follows the qi in its ascent and descent, and there is no place which it does not reach, causing dyspnea, cough, nausea, diarrhea, dizziness and discomfort in the region of the Heart, palpitations, chills and fevers with swelling and pain, fullness and obstruction. There may be the thunderous sound of phlegm seeping through the chest and flanks, a habitual crawling sensation over the whole body, nodes which are neither red nor swollen, a mass in the neck which is not scrofulous but similar, or a plug in the throat like a plumstone, or the production through coughing or expectorating of a substance resembling peach paste, or a knotted feeling in the chest as if two types of qi were coupling, or a frequent awareness of a spot of cold in the center of the back, or a red

swelling like fire within the skin, or a cold pain like ice under the heart. One limb may be swollen hard and numb, or the tips of the ribs may form protrusions, or the bones of the joints may suffer unusual stabbing pain, or the lower back and legs may become aching sore and weak, or there may be vomiting of cold liquid, green water or black fluid, or there may be a sudden break-out of dreams of fires or swords and halberds. There could be pus in the stool and urine, or failure to pass either. The throat may become suddenly occluded, or the teeth ache, or the ears ring. [Phlegm] can lead to exhaustion, epilepsy, aphonia, hemiplegia, amenorrhea, leukorrhea, children's terrors and convulsions, and even actions such as scheming and plotting without reason like an evil spirit; all can be categorized as symptoms of phlegm.[20]

These descriptions by Wang Yin-Jun of the extreme variety of the possible symptoms of phlegm did much to expand the field of TCM phlegm theory into every branch of medicine, and formed an early echo of the notion that 'bizarre illnesses can be blamed on phlegm' and 'the Hundred Afflictions are all the bane of phlegm'.

ZHANG JING-YUE

One of the most famous of the Ming dynasty authors is Zhang Jie-Bin (1563-1640, zi-name Jing Yue), whose works include the *Lei Jing* ('Systematic Categorization of the *Nei Jing*'), the *Lei Jing Tu Yi* ('Illustrated Wings to the *Lei Jing*'), the *Zhi Yi Lun* ('Record of Questions and Doubt') and the *Jing Yue Quan Shu* ('The Complete Works of Jing Yue').

Zhang in his early years was greatly influenced by the works of Zhu Dan-Xi and Liu Wan-Su, but later came to dispute the emphasis given by Zhu Dan-Xi on the frequency of yang excess and yin deficiency. Zhang felt that yin could not do without yang: without qi, the form of the body could not be maintained, while without yin-substance there was no physical basis for the action of qi. Therefore, he re-emphasized the position of the *Nei Jing* that material is produced from yang but completed in yin.

With his comprehensive grasp of Chinese medical literature up to his time, Zhang Jie-Bin also made extensive contributions to TCM phlegm theory.

Perhaps the most important of these were the twin concepts of phlegm arising from deficiency, and phlegm treatment necessarily addressing the root. He says:

Phlegm is simply the body's fluids, which are themselves nothing but transformations from food and fluids. Since this phlegm is also a transformed substance, it cannot then be classified as 'untransformed' (i.e. as thin mucus is untransformed by the Spleen and Stomach). But transformation, if normal, produces a strong body with flourishing nutritive and protective qi; in this case, [what would in a pathological situation be] phlegm is [still normal] blood and qi.

On the other hand, if transformation proceeds abnormally, then the zang fu become diseased, the body fluids fail (bai), and qi and blood then produce phlegm. This is exactly like robbers and thieves creating chaos in society: who are they but [otherwise] good people in a troubled world? The rise of brigands, however, must of necessity be the consequence of malady in the governance of the country, just as the appearance of phlegm must result from infirmity of the yuan qi.

Zhang also says:

Phlegm around the body leads to difficult-to-fathom illnesses ... Any phlegm in the channels and collaterals is generally transformed from the jin-fluids or the blood. If it transpires that nutritive and protective qi are harmonious, then jin-fluid acts as jin, and blood acts as blood; where could phlegm exist?

It is only if there is damage to the yuan yang, or attenuation in the activity of the shen, that there will then be a lack of qi amidst the water, jin will coalesce and blood fail [to move] and go bad, both of which can transform into phlegm!

This yield of phlegm, or [the converse] production of jing-essence and blood, how could it be external to the jing and blood, from some unrelated pathogenic phlegm?

Because Zhang Jing-Yue has observed that phlegm may be formed from jin-fluids and blood, he rightly emphasizes that phlegm treatment must of necessity seek the root. He continues:

Strong people can eat and drink whatever they like, in whatever quantities, and everything they eat is duly transformed. We never see it becoming phlegm.... It can be seen that hardly any of the phlegm under Heaven is 'excess' phlegm, and also that hardly any phlegm should be attacked.... [To treat phlegm, we should] treat the root. By gradually replenishing the basic root, phlegm will—without [direct] treatment—eliminate itself... Therefore anyone who wants to treat phlegm, but does not know its source, is simply groping blindly in the dark!

Zhang Jing-Yue's view is that in dealing with phlegm one must seek the root, and that simply addressing the phlegm is insufficient. This is especially realistic in terms of deficient cases or those who have become deficient through chronic phlegm, where he vividly portrays the futility and danger involved in continually attempting to eliminate phlegm that is actually arising from the deficiency itself! He also emphasizes that phlegm is not a primary pathogen but rather a secondary product of a primary disease process, which may in turn instigate further problems. This issue of primary—which he terms the 'root'—and secondary—the 'branch'—is crucial to the accurate diagnosis and treatment of phlegm disease.

ZHAO XIAN-KE

Zhao Xian-Ke was the famous Ming dynasty author of the *Yi Guan* ('The Pervading Link of Medicine')[21] which was published in 1617. The 'pervading link' was the concept of Mingmen fire, from which angle Zhao considered all medical questions. Phlegm was no exception, and for that time it provided a completely new approach in phlegm treatment. Zhao says:

Wang Lun (zi-name Jie-Zhai, author of the *Ben Cao Ji Yao*, 1496) said: The basis of phlegm is water, and its source is the Kidneys. Here Jie Zhai is the first to state that the basis of phlegm is in the Kidneys, which is expressing that which none before had expressed—what a pity that he did not follow through! All of the formulas that he designed to treat phlegm treated the branch only.

Zhao went on to explain:

The term phlegm indicates pathology: phlegm is not something originally present within the body. If phlegm is not the result of water flooding, then it will be the result of water boiled by fire. All that is necessary is to differentiate whether fire is present or not.

Thus if Kidneys are deficient and unable to control water so that it cannot return to its spring-point, it will rebel upwards and the inundation will produce phlegm. This phlegm, though, is pure water—no fire is involved. Zhao Xian-Ke would use Fu Gui Ba Wei Wan ('Kidney Pill from the *Golden Cabinet*', *Formulas and Strategies*, p. 275) in order to restore Kidney fire.

Yin-deficiency leading to fire flaring and boiling the water was slightly more complicated, however. If the fire flared from the Kidneys 'like dragon fire (long huo) arising from the sea', the water would be carried upward in a rush with the flaring of the fire. If the fire flared from the Liver 'like thunder fire (lei huo) springing from the earth, the rapid wind brings on rain, and the torrents produce phlegm'. This type of phlegm will be thick and frothy, due to the involvement of fire. Zhao would use Liu Wei Di Huang Wan ('Six Ingredient Pill with Rehmannia', *Formulas and Strategies*, p. 263) to complement—and thus control—the excessive fire with strengthened Kidney water. Once the fire was controlled, the phlegm would disappear for lack of sustenance.

These approaches are all aimed at the root of the phlegm, and not at the branch manifestations. One who is expert at phlegm treatment, Zhao tells us, will first strengthen the Kidneys, supplementing fire or water as necessary with Fu Gui Ba Wei Wan or Liu Wei Di Huang Wan, after which Si Jun Zi Tang ('Four-Gentlemen Decoction', *Formulas and Strategies*, p. 236) or Liu Jun Zi Tang ('Six-Gentlemen Decoction', *Formulas and Strategies*, p. 238) will be used to strengthen the Spleen to control water.

If the Spleen is constitutionally weak, then these formulas—or similar appropriate formulas such as Bu Zhong Yi Qi Tang ('Tonify the Middle and Augment the Qi Decoction', *Formulas and Strategies*, p. 241) or Li Zhong Wan ('Settle the Middle Pill', *Formulas and Strategies*, p. 219)—should be used first, and then followed with the Liu Wei or Ba Wei formulas.

GONG JU-ZHONG

The Ming dynasty physician Gong Ju-Zhong, in his work *Hong Lu Dian Xue* ('A Spot of Snow on a Red Hot Stove'),[22] provides an extremely valuable work for the study of the symptomatology and treatment of phlegm-fire, as it describes in great detail the mechanisms of pathology and the possible mistakes in differentiation and treatment of this condition. Suggested formulas and other therapeutic approaches such as moxibustion are given. Ten different categories of lifestyle 'taboo' for phlegm patients are laid out. They include reducing the desire for wine, for sex, for gluttony, and for profit and power; diminishing anger, volubility and melancholy; and being cautious with eating and regularity of living.

His comments on the undesirability of superfluous speech are interesting:

Qi vibrates the throat to produce sound. Feelings stimulate the Heart to create speech. Thus it is said: Sound is the concordance of the Lungs, Speech is the sound of the Heart. Also fire causes disease because injury to Water allows it to flare up and scorch Lung Metal, impairing its production and transformation. The mother (Metal) makes the son (Water) even more deficient, thus creating a vicious cycle whereby Water is more and more feeble and fire increasingly strong, the Lungs incrementally injured and Metal as a result intensifying in heat. The approach should be to nourish the yin and bring down the fire, so that Metal's contraction is restored.

If there is a great deal of speech or the talk becomes excited, the vibration injures the orifice of the Lungs and this leads to cough or hoarseness. In addition, because during speech the exhalation is more than the inhalation, this disturbs the evenness of the breath and the circulation of the qi of the Five Zang is similarly delayed.

This is what is meant by 'If the Lungs require filling (shi), first harmonize the breathing'.[23]

He points out that 'most bland foods are tonifying', and warns us that 'only thinking of gratifying the taste buds will conversely damage the Spleen: bland foods themselves contain tonification, … in the midst of bland foods is True Qi.'

Gong Ju-Zhong's outline of symptoms and treatment is noteworthy for its clarity and practicality, and also for its individuality. For example, under 'Lower Back Pain' he says:

The Classics state: 'The Lumbar area and below all belongs to the Kidneys'. The main [causes of lower back pain are] damp-heat, Kidney deficiency, stagnant blood, accumulated phlegm and sprain.

A big pulse shows Kidney deficiency, for which herbs such as *Du Zhong* (Eucommiae), *Gui Ban* (Testudinis, Plastrum), *Huang Bo* (Phellodendri), *Zhi Mu* (Anemarrhenae), *Gou Qi Zi* (Lycii Chinensis, Fructus) and *Wu Wei Zi* (Schisandrae) should be powdered, and made into pills using pork spine marrow as an adhesive.

A choppy pulse means stagnant blood, for which Bu Yin Wan (another name for Hu Qian Wan, 'Hidden Tiger Pill', *Formulas and Strategies*, p. 268) with added *Tao Ren* (Persicae) and *Hong Hua* (Carthami) should be used.

A languid[24] pulse indicates damp-heat. Use herbs such as *Cang Zhu* (grey Atractylodis), *Du Zhong* (Eucommiae), *Huang Bo* (Phellodendri) and *Chuan Xiong* (Ligustici).

For lower backache from phlegm accumulation, use Er Chen Wan ('Two-Cured Decoction', *Formulas and Strategies* p. 432) plus *Dan Nan Xing* (Arisaemae cum Felle Bovis, Pulvis) and increased *Ban Xia* (Pinelliae).

Any of the conditions which involve fire cannot be harshly treated with [bitter] cold herbs. For lower back pain, *Lu Jiao Jiao* (Cervi Colla Cornu) is a must.[25]

Gong's individuality is in the casting of phlegm as a factor in lower back pain, and his straightforward method of treatment.

He also notes that pain in the right costal region with a slippery pulse means that phlegm has moved into the area, and proposes moving qi to open repression and disperse nodes.

Gong remarks that while spermatorrhea with dreams does indicate 'breakdown of communication between Heart and Kidney, with Water and Fire failing to benefit each other, it really implies the onset of phlegm-fire', and suggests treating this with phlegm-cutting, fire-draining and Heart-calming herbs such as *Fu Shen* (Poriae Cocos Paradicis, Sclerotium), *Yuan Zhi* (Polygalae), *Shan Yao* (Dioscoreae) and *Qian Shi* (Euryales).

Gong Ju-Zhong is also unusual in that he strongly supports the use of moxa in the treatment of phlegm-fire:

> The ancients established their methods thus:
>
> Mild illnesses could be restored to harmony through the use of pills, powders, drinks or decoctions.
>
> Deep and stubborn conditions could not be eliminated without the use of needles and moxa, because needles have a scourging effect. The needling techniques nowadays, though, only rarely achieve remarkable effects, and even consistently good results are infrequent. In those of delicate constitution, cases of needles causing sudden demise are not unheard-of.
>
> The [good] effects of moxa, on the other hand, are hard to enumerate. It is ever effective in all categories of illness, whether cold or hot, excess or deficient, mild or severe, distal or local.
>
> In cold diseases, [this physiological] fire disperses, like a hot sun melts ice, which is the concept of cold dissipating from warmth.
>
> Heat diseases are dispelled by moxa, like a heat-wave being followed by a cold spell, which is the concept of venting pent-up fire.
>
> Deficient conditions are strengthened by moxa, like fire forcing the qi within water to rise (i.e. as in evaporation). This is the concept of warm tonification.
>
> Excess conditions are broken up with moxa, just as fire consumes materials, which is the concept of draining excess.
>
> Phlegm diseases are banished by moxa, because with heat the qi moves, and the fluids are then able to flow smoothly.
>
> So moxa will never lead to weakness or deficiency. ... In old chronic diseases, for which the strength of herbal treatment is inadequate, one must utilise the strength of fire to force it out by the roots.
>
> In phlegm-fire-caused steaming bones exhaustion, spermatorrhea, nightsweats and fatigue, or similar situations, one should moxa the following points:

Si Hua	M-BW-4
Ge Shu	BL-17
Shen Shu	Bl-23
Fei Shu	BL-13
Zu San Li	ST-36
He Gu	LI-4

The single point Tan Zhong (CV-17) may also be added.

> If these points are located accurately, the results are invariably effective.[26]

The efforts of the above mentioned authors, Chao Yuan-Fang, Yan Yong-He, Zhang Cong-Zheng, Li Chan, Zhu Dan-Xi, Wang Gui, Zhang Jie-Bin, Zhao Xian-Ke and Gong Ju-Zhong, are much more detailed and explicit in describing phlegm mechanisms and symptomatology than the undeveloped *Nei Jing* theory that thin mucus is formed through accumulation of body fluids, and are also a great advancement on Zhang Zhong-Jing's descriptions in the *Jing Gui Yao Lue*. By the later half of the Ming dynasty, TCM theories of phlegm pathology were relatively well-developed.

LI SHI-ZHEN

One Ming dynasty physician, well known even in the West, is Li Shi-Zhen (1518-1593), author of a great many works, among the most famous of which are the *Ben Cao Gang Mu* (the great Materia Medica), *Bin Hu Mai Xue* (on pulse), and the *Qi Jing Ba Mai Kao* (on the 8 extra channels).

Li Shi-Zhen included a tremendous amount of collected material relating to phlegm diagnosis and treatment in his books but was himself expert in the treatment of stubborn phlegm diseases. He records one case in the *Ba Dou* (Croton) section of the *Ben Cao Gang Mu*: an old woman of sixty had suffered from diarrhea for five years, and any consumption of meat, raw foods or oil would lead to pain. She had tried Spleen regulators, lifting formulas and astringent diarrhea-stopping herbs, all without success: in fact, each time the diarrhea would get worse. She then came to Li Shi-Zhen. He found the pulse was deep and slippery, and so recognized it as 'long term injury to Spleen and Stomach with accumulated cold obstruction', and said 'the method should be to use a warm purge, so that the cold could be expelled and the diarrhea halted'. He designed small Croton pills covered with wax to allow passage through to the bowel. She took about fifty of them. On the second day, 'there was no pain or diarrhea, and she was cured'. One of the effects of Croton is to strongly expel cold-phlegm accumulation, and thus Li Shi-Zhen could use it to instantaneously cure a stubborn diarrhea case of five years standing. This is the more amazing in that the patient was already sixty years old: only an expert would have been daring enough to use such a potentially dangerous maneuver! He goes on to comment on the effectiveness of this treatment, and to warn of the dangers of inappropriate use:

> Since that time, I have used this treatment successfully in close to one hundred cases of diarrhea and dysentery from obstruction. All were cured without a purging effect. The key is in the exact matching of illness and treatment: if this treatment is used inappropriately, then this contravenes the law against using yin damaging herbs in mild cases.[27]

In the *Ben Cao Gang Mu*, Li Shi-Zhen records over three hundred formulas to treat phlegm, not including individual herbs used in phlegm therapy, which constitutes the largest collection of formulae for any disease or symptom in the book. This, of course, was a great contribution to the progress of phlegm theory at the time, and continues to be useful right up to the present. The book outlines eight distinct categories of phlegm treatment, including:

- Parching damp to cut phlegm
- Cooling heat to cut phlegm
- Warming transformation to cut phlegm
- Moistening dryness to cut phlegm
- Dispelling food stagnation to cut phlegm
- Moving qi to cut phlegm
- Phlegm and blood stagnation treated together
- External treatments to expel phlegm.

GONG XIN

Gong Xin in his *Gu Jin Yi Jian* ('Medical Reflections Ancient and Modern', 1589), in the chapter on tan-yin, went further in describing the changes which phlegm can undergo, pointing out:

> Phlegm is transformed from jin and ye fluids, and this may be a result of exposure to wind, cold, damp, or heat pathogens, or injury from the seven emotions or food; these cause the qi

to rebel and the fluids to thicken and change into phlegm and thin mucus. This can then be coughed or vomited up, or become stuck in and obstruct the chest and diaphragm, or remain accumulated in the Intestines and Stomach, or flow into the channels and collaterals of the four limbs, following the rise and fall of the qi, reaching everywhere in the body without exception.

In terms of the diseases which it can cause, it can become wheeze, or cough, it can bring on nausea or vomiting; it can occlude the diaphragm leading to the extraordinary condition of 'guan ge' (in which food is vomited as soon as it is taken, while the bowels and urine become blocked);[28] it can bring on diarrhea, or vertigo, or indefinable epigastric discomfort (cao za); it can cause palpitations, insanity, chills and fever, or pain. Phlegm can be the source of watery sounds in the chest and costal regions, or a spot of icy cold on the back, or numbness of the limbs, or a hundred other afflictions, all of which may be associated with phlegm.

In the process of enumerating symptoms of phlegm, the ancient physicians—like Gong Xin, Wang Yin-Jun, and Zhu Gong—are also setting out the parameters and definitions of phlegm diseases, quantifying and qualifying the conditions which create and maintain phlegm. Li Yong-Cui, writing in the Qing dynasty work *Zheng Zhi Hui Bu* ('A Supplement to Diagnosis and Treatment'), explains in more detail how emotions cause phlegm:

> When the jin and ye fluids flow smoothly, how can there be phlegm? If there is an invasion of wind or cold or dryness or damp from the exterior, or interior disturbance from shock, fury, anxiety, or concentration, or from over-work and overeating, or untempered consumption of wine and sexual activity, [then] the nutritive and protective qi will not be clear, the qi and blood become murky, toxic, and fail to function (bai),[29] the body fluids brew and this is how phlegm is produced.

ZHEN JIU DA CHENG

The *Zhen Jiu Da Cheng* ('Great Compendium of Acupuncture and Moxibustion', 1601) does not theorize in any depth about the pathological mechanisms of phlegm development, but the extent to which its author Yang Ji-Zhou was influenced by developments in the field can be assessed by reading between the lines of his indications for acupuncture points.

For example, Feng Long (ST-40) is mentioned as a major point for wind-phlegm headache, as would be expected of a Yang Ming channel point which is also the Luo-connecting point for the Spleen and Stomach;[30] Ge Shu (BL-17) is important for 'Stomach and diaphragm cold-phlegm';[31] Pi Shu (BL-20) can be used for 'phlegm causing malaria-like recurring chills and fever';[32] and Shang Wan (CV-13) is indicated in cases of 'profuse phlegm and vomiting of saliva-like liquid'.[33]

Now these are more or less what would be expected, even with the simplest conceptions of phlegm and phlegm production: points related to the Spleen and Stomach, or located in the area around the middle Jiao, will naturally suggest themselves as suitable for phlegm treatment. The mention of the 'malaria-like recurring chills and fever from phlegm' evidences a deeper understanding of the mechanisms involved (see below) but it is the next point which shows beyond doubt that Yang Ji-Zhou was thoroughly familiar with the complexities of phlegm theory, and utilized this understanding in clinical practice. His indications for Tai Xi (KI-3), the Shu-stream point on the Kidney channel, include the following: 'wheeze and dyspnea, nausea and vomiting, phlegm excess (tan shi), gluey feeling in the mouth'.[34] Without a clear grasp of the Kidneys' role in phlegm production, these indications would seem completely out of character for a Kidney channel point. Furthermore, in his discussion of herbs which act on the Kidney channel, Yang includes Yuan Zhi (Polygalae Tenuifoliae, Radix) as an essential herb in the re-establishment of Heart and Kidney relations: Yuan Zhi is a major phlegm dispelling and Spirit calming herb.[35]

In the Great Compendium chapter 'Essentials of Treatments', sections 72-76, and the following discussion, Yang Ji-Zhou describes the treatment and pathogenesis of malarial disorders (nue, 疟):

72. Spleen cold bringing on malaria:
Hou Xi (SI-3), Jian Shi (PC-5), Da Zhui (GV-14), Shen Zhu (GV-12), Zu San Li (ST-36), Jue Gu (GB-39), He Gu (LI-4), Gao Huang (BL-43).
73. Malaria, first chills, then fever:
Jue Gu (GB-39), Bai Hui (GV-20), Gao Huang (BL-43), He Gu (LI-4).
74. Malaria, first fever, then chills:
Qu Chi (LI-11), first tonify and then reduce; Jue Gu (GB-39), first reduce and then tonify; Gao Huang (BL-43); Bai Lao (M-HN-30).
75. More fever than chills:
Hou Xi (SI-3), Jian Shi (PC-5), Bai Lao (M-HN-30), Qu Chi (LI-11).
76. More chills than fever:
Hou Xi (SI-3), Bai Lao (M-HN-30), Qu Chi (LI-11).

Question: What is the source of this condition?

Answer: All are from Spleen and Stomach weakness, with over-exposure during the mid-Summer months to shu-Summerheat, by the Autumn it will produce malaria. The symptoms can present as fever more than chills, or only chills, or only fever: if the qi dominates then there will be more fever; if phlegm predominates then there will be more chills. This is all caused from phlegm and thin mucus immobility and obstruction, qi and blood exhaustion and dispersal, Spleen and Stomach weakness and failure, and unregulated sexual activity. In some patients, attacks will occur once per day; in others, every other day; and again in some attacks will occur every three days. In the long term, without treatment, it becomes a major problem: after the malaria, edema can develop, or exhaustion, or diarrhea, or abdominal distension, or excessive thin mucus and water. For those with swelling under the ribs following chronic malaria, it is necessary to regulate the Spleen, enhance the appetite, and transform phlegm and thin mucus. The point selection in treatment should be according to that described above.[36]

YU CHANG

The famous Qing dynasty physician Yu Chang (c. 1585-1664) was born in the Ming and died in the early years of the Qing at the age of eighty. He was the originator of the well-known formula Qing Zao Jiu Fei Tang ('Eliminate Dryness and Rescue the

Lungs Decoction', *Formulas and Strategies*, p. 160), was exceptionally experienced, and had his own views on the management and pulse indications of phlegm. He said 'The pulse descriptions for tan-yin listed in the *Jin Gui Yao Lue* have been extrapolated in several ways, which are hard to thoroughly grasp'. He goes on to explain:

> Phlegm and thin mucus coalescing in the middle Jiao interfere with the opening and closing mechanism [of the Stomach], and so the pulse because of this turns deep wiry, or urgent wiry, or somewhat wiry, or wiry tight, or again hidden and imperceptible. Without rapidly eliminating the tan-yin, how can the pulse be restored to normal? If it is shallow, the treatment should be shallow; if deep, treat deeply; if neither shallow nor deep, aim for the appropriate depth in your treatment. Immobile phlegm can be attacked, hardened phlegm can be whittled away'.[37]

Yu Chang remarks that wiry and deep pulses are frequently encountered in phlegm diseases. His comments on 'treating deeply', 'treating shallowly', and 'treating at the appropriate depth' mean that a long-term phlegm disease, in an old or weak person, will be likely to be deep-set and hard to eradicate, and so one should aim at the root. A recent phlegm disease, in a strong patient with good qi, is 'shallow' and so should be treated as the acute symptoms dictate, to eliminate the phlegm as soon as possible. A phlegm condition which is somewhat established— 'neither shallow nor deep'—in a patient who is neither weak nor yet very strong, or a weak patient with an excess condition on the surface, will require an appropriately crafted approach designed to eliminate the existing phlegm while supporting the normal qi.

As befitting the title of his book, *Yi Men Fa Lu* ('Precepts for Physicians'), Yu Chang sets out twelve rules of 'Forbidden Uses of Herbs' in phlegm treatments. For example:

> Carelessly using Er Chen Tang ('Two-Cured Decoction', *Formulas and Strategies*, p. 432) in cases of yin deficiency and parched conditions
>
> Carelessly using either of the Qing Long Tangs ('Major or Minor Blue-Green Dragon Decoction', *Formulas and Strategies* p. 34 and p. 38 respectively) in cases of yang deficiency with profuse sweating

> Carelessly using pungent-dispersing herbs in cases of Heart deficiency with un-rooted shen
>
> Carelessly using bitter purges in cases of weak Lungs and little qi
>
> Carelessly using Gun Tan Wan ('Vaporize Phlegm Pill', *Formulas and Strategies*, p. 424) in cases of Spleen deficiency edema.'[38]

Yu Chang also puts forth laws, such as:

> Any time hot-phlegm has ridden wind-fire upwards to enter [the upper part of the body, with] blurry vision and tinnitus—seemingly a deficient condition—and warm tonifiers are mistakenly used, this will weld the phlegm and remove any route of elimination. The doctor is culpable.[39]

YE TIAN-SHI

Ye Tian-Shi (1667-1746), in the Qing dynasty, is best known for his major contributions to the febrile disease theory in his book *Wen Re Lun* ('Discussion of Warmth and Heat'), but he was also an expert at phlegm treatment. He says:

> Phlegm is transformed from food and fluids. Some phlegm is the result of obstruction by the six exogenous pathogens, causing the mechanism of ascent and descent of the Spleen, Lungs, and Stomach to become abnormal, so that fluids and foods cannot be transformed and transported as clear substances but instead produce phlegm. Some phlegm is a consequence of obstruction, so that qi and fire cannot move freely, and instead steam [the fluids] to change [and which then turn to phlegm]. Some is from excessive consumption of sweet, greasy, fatty or foul foods, or too much tea or alcohol, leading to phlegm production. Some occurs with constitutional yang deficiency of the Spleen and Stomach allowing turbid-damp to coalesce; and some, too, is from Kidney deficiency allowing water to flood and become phlegm. In addition, there is taxation from yin deficiency: the ministerial dragon (i.e. Kidney) fire rises and inflames the Lungs, and causes phlegm.

Ye Tian-Shi's case histories are very interesting for their exact and parsimonious use of herbs, as well as their subtlety of diagnosis. The following two case studies (involving the same patient) are taken, in order, from the book *Ye Shi Yi An Cun Zhen Shu Zhu* ('Annotated True Cases of Ye Tian-Shi'), which is based upon a sheaf of Ye's cases passed down through his family, then annotated at one level in the 1930s by Li Qi–Xian, then again recently by Peng Xian-Zhang.[40]

Case studies of Ye Tian–Shi

CASE SEVEN

Title. Light rising and spreading to promote upper contraction [and descent], as a method for treating wind-warmth plus pathogenic thin mucus floating upwards: cough worse with lying flat.

Original wording. Name: Wu. The upper body subjected to wind-warmth, thin mucus floating upward, when lying flat the cough is worse. Yin (thin mucus) is classified as yin (i.e. not yang). First use light rising and spreading to restore contracting descent above, then move to regulate thin mucus.

Jie Geng	Platycodi Grandiflori, Radix
Ma Dou Ling	Aristolochiae, Fructus
Yi Yi Ren	Coicis Lachryma-jobi, Semen
Fu Ling	Poriae Cocos, Sclerotium
Tong Cao	Tetrapanacis Papyriferi, Medulla
Chuan Bei Mu	Fritillariae Cirrhosae, Bulbus
Cook over high flame. Take one dose.	

Commentary (by Li Qi-Xian). The treatment of an unadulterated illness is relatively simple but treating a mixed one is more difficult. Wind-warmth as an illness is comparatively easy to treat but admixed with pathogenic thin mucus it is harder.

Because wind-warmth is a yang pathogen, and thin mucus is a yin pathogen, they will struggle with each other. If the treatment is not up to scratch, it can cause the illness to become chronic and hard to cure.

If one vainly tries to use pungent-coolers for the wind-warmth [as one normally would], then the influence of the thin mucus will be broadened.

If one fruitlessly attempts to use warm herbs to regulate the thin mucus internally, this, conversely, will encourage fire to support the power of the wind.

So this is why the treatment of this case is rather difficult.

But here, this initial use of light lifting and spreading to restore normal descent and contraction above, thereafter dealing with the thin mucus, is actually a remarkable technique!

The use of light lifting and spreading herbs causes the Lungs' contracting descent to recover, and because Lungs are contiguous with the skin, so the wind pathogen on the exterior will naturally be expelled. Lungs rule the opening and harmonization of the water pathways, so the thin mucus in the interior will no longer well upwards [because Lung qi now descends normally].

Once the wind-warmth has already been expelled, even if some pathogenic thin mucus still remains, dealing with it afterwards is legitimate.

This is why, when Chinese doctors treat disease, the sequence of mild, urgent, primary and secondary is essential to understand.

Explanation of prescription (by Pang Xian-Zhang). These are all Hand Tai Yin channel herbs.

Jie Geng (Platycodi Grandiflori, Radix) is bitter, pungent and neutral, entering Lungs and draining heat, while also expelling surface pathogens.

Ma Dou Ling (Aristolochiae, Fructus) is bitter, pungent and cold, settling Lungs and leading qi downward, while also able to clear Lung heat and restore Lung contraction.

Yi Yi Ren (Coicis Lachryma-jobi, Semen) is sweet and bland, clearing the Lungs, helping qi, and also has the effect of tonifying Spleen while eliminating damp through diuresis.

Fu Ling (Poriae Cocos, Sclerotium) is sweet and neutral, draining Lungs and stopping cough, while also having the function of benefiting Spleen and opening orifices.

Tong Cao (Tetrapanacis Papyriferi, Medulla) is bland and cold, entering the Lungs to lead heat downwards.

Chuan Bei Mu (Fritillariae Cirrhosae, Bulbus) is pungent and bitter, entering the Lungs to disperse nodes and dispel phlegm.

All the herbs are chosen on the basis of their lightness and lifting; the herb flavours are all bitter [which drains], pungent [which disperses], sweet [which tonifies and harmonizes], and bland [which is diuretic].

How could this, an exposure to wind-warmth with pathogenic thin mucus leading to severe cough when lying flat, not be cured?

CASE EIGHT

Title. The method of nourishing yin, moistening the Lungs, calming Liver, and dispersing phlegm, to treat severe cough brought on by spasms around the left flank.

Original wording. The same patient again. 'Light can expel excess' is exactly appropriate for upper body wind warmth but here spasms on the left flank brings on severe cough. The Classics say that if the left ascent is excessive, the descent on the right will be inadequate. This is not Liver Wood excess; Spring Wood sprouts, qi ascends and pushes upward. This is entirely scarcity of blood fluid, not controlling its spouse.

Sweet Xing Ren	Pruni Armeniacae, Semen
Yu Zhu	Polygonati Odorati, Rhizoma
Gan Cao	Glycyrrhizae Uralensis, Radix
Tao Ren	Persicae, Semen
Chao Huo Ma Ren	Cannabis Sativae, Semen, fried

Commentary (by Li Qi-Xian). 'Light can expel excess'[41] refers to the method in the previous case, where light rising spreading herbs were used first to treat wind-warmth, and the thin mucus was dealt with subsequently.

But here, the wind-warmth has been cured [in this patient] but there is still cough brought on by left flank spasm. Is it that Liver qi is excessively pathogenic? or is thin mucus bringing on this movement of Liver qi?

Ye Tian-Shi does not approach the problem in this way but instead maintains that the cause is as follows: In early Spring the qi of Wood begins to push upward [in the Jue Yin channel][42] and that its excessive rising [which is affecting the normal descent of the Lung qi and thus leading to cough] is due to the scarcity of Liver blood which 'is not controlling its spouse' (i.e. Liver qi).

We can see that the main etiology here is in the substance of the Liver, not in its function.[43] Liver qi ascends on the left, and Lung qi descends on the right;[44] here the Liver blood is deficient so that Liver has no nourishment, thus the ascent of Liver qi on the left is excessive; Lung yin is deficient, as its yin-natured activities of contraction and descent have lost power, thus the Lung qi descent on the right is inadequate.

This is why, in the early Spring season, when Spring Wood sprouts and moves, qi will ascend and push upward, the left flank will have tightness causing severe cough. If this is treated as a simple case of Liver qi excess, it would conversely damage Liver qi. In the original wording of the case, although Ye Tian-Shi does not mention the exact treatment principle, it is implied in the words 'This is entirely scarcity of blood fluid, not controlling its spouse.'

Explanation of prescription (by Pang Xian–Zhang). These are Hand Tai Yin and Foot Jue Yin channel herbs.

Sweet Xing Ren (Pruni Armeniacae, Semen) is bitter, sweet and warm, moistening the Lungs and bringing down phlegm.

Tao Ren (Persicae, Semen) is bitter, neutral, and slightly sweet, calming and moderating the Liver and moving blood.

Yu Zhu (Polygonati Odorati, Rhizoma) is sweet and neutral, moistening dryness.

Huo Ma Ren (Cannabis Sativae, Semen) is sweet, neutral, and nourishes yin.

Gan Cao (Glycyrrhizae Uralensis, Radix) is sweet and neutral, and can nourish yin if combined with other moistening herbs.

The *Hou Ma Ren* (Cannabis seeds) are fried ('chao') to elicit their moistening effects while eliminating any purging action.

The purpose of tonifying yin is to ensure that blood is not parched, and Liver can obtain nourishment. Once the Liver is nourished, its excesses will be moderated, qi will not ascend excessively, the movement on the flanks will cease: how could the cough fail to be cured? Although in the preceding consultation with this patient Ye had announced the intention of subsequently regulating the thin mucus, since the symptoms had changed because of seasonal influence, why should he not change the treatment as the symptoms indicate?[45]

More from Ye Tian-Shi

Ye Tian-Shi gives another example of his proficiency with phlegm conditions in his book *Yi Xiao Mi Chuan* ('Secret Transmissions of Medical Efficacy'), in the section entitled 'Four Conditions Resembling Shang Han (Injury from Cold)'. Under the first, 'Phlegm Conditions', he describes how:

Phlegm is transformed from the body fluids. In general, if wind harms the Lungs, the Lung qi can not clear and phlegm is produced. If damp injures the Spleen, Spleen qi coalesces, becomes turbid and phlegm is produced. The person can then similarly (i.e. similar to exogenous injury from wind) exhibit trembling chills, high fever, aversion to wind, and spontaneous sweating. But the pathogenic fullness of the chest and diaphragm, with qi rushing up into the throat [so that the person] cannot breathe, are both from the discomfiture of the Lung qi.

Therefore, although resembling [exogenous] injury from cold, yet the head does not ache, the neck is not stiff, and the pulses may be either floating and slippery at the cun (distal) position, or deep and hidden. These are the differences.[46]

HE MENG-YAO

He Meng-Yao (1694-1764) was a well-rounded scholar, being an official and a poet as well as a physician. His literary training plus his extensive clinical experience combined to produce a peculiar flexibility of mind, as evidenced in his numerous books, such as *Fu Ke Liang Fang* ('Prescriptions for Gynecology'), *Yi Bian* ('Fundamentals of Medicine'), and *You Ke Liang Fang* ('Prescriptions for Pediatrics'), among others.

In the *Yi Bian* he records:

Phlegm is originally the body's fluids, and follows the qi in its movements. If the qi is harmonious, the jin-fluids flow and the ye-fluids are distributed so that the Hundred Articulations receive their moisture, what could cause the production of phlegm to lead to illness? If qi loses its clear descent, and becomes over-heated, then the fluids are subjected to the sweltering effect of fire, and turn thick and turbid; if qi loses its warm harmony, and becomes over-chilled, then fluids accumulate from the cold and gradually turn tacky and bunch up, forming phlegm.

Thus although phlegm is a single substance, it can result from heat or from cold; its source is different, can its treatment be identical?

The method of differentiation from the ancients is that thick and yellow phlegm is from heat, while thin and clear is from cold. This, however, only refers to the general situation, and should not be taken as gospel.

Let me try to discuss this in terms of exogenous invasion: once I myself had this experience with cough from exposure to wind. The cough was continual, the phlegm profuse and easy to cough out, and its color was thin and clear. I mistakenly treated it as cold but afterwards became very tired and lethargic. Following this, I realized the explanation, and only then knew that it was caused by extreme heat. What had happened was that fire had become quite compressed and was compelling [me to cough repeatedly], and the frequent cough was constantly expelling the phlegm so that it had no chance to remain long enough to turn thick and yellow. Once the fire had been exhausted and the qi became more settled, the cough gradually subsided. The phlegm that came out then—about once every six hours—was conversely thick and yellow: the fire was not then forcing it up, phlegm was able to stay inside longer, and became yellow and thick because it was subjected to the heat. The illness thereafter soon cleared up.

It was only following this experience that I knew that thick yellow phlegm [shows] that the force of the fire is still rather moderate and mild; thin clear phlegm, on the other hand, could be from powerful fire, urgent and on the ascend-ant. In these cases, pungent-cooling openers and dispersers should always be used, and warming hot herbs are not appropriate.

Again, discussing this from the point of view of internal injury: weakened Kidney fire with water flooding and becoming phlegm that is thin and clear should be treated with warmth and heat, which consolidates [the water and prevents its upward flooding]. But even if Kidney fire is intense, so that water boils and becomes phlegm, the phlegm can still be clear and thin. Just like the movement of dragon thunder which precipitates a rain storm, there will be a sudden up-rushing, so that although the phlegm may be slightly turbid and bubbly, it could not really be called thick and yellow. Likewise, this should be treated with sweet cold Water-strengtheners, and warming hot herbs are inappropriate. Who can [now] say that thin clear phlegm must be cold?! ... These things need to be finely discriminated; it is even more obvious that the pulse must be used as reference.'[47]

CHEN XIU-YUAN

Chen Nian-Zu (zi-name Xiu–Yuan, 1753-1826) was the author of over fifteen books on medicine, including *Yi Xue San Zi Jing* ('The Three Character Classic of Medicine'), *Nu Ke Yao Zhi* ('Important Pointers on Gynecology'), and *Yi Xue Shi Zai Yi* ('The Study of Medicine is Actually Easy').

It says in the introduction to the latter work:

This book has assembled the essence of works such as the *Shen Nong Ben Jing, Nei Jing, Nan Jing, Qian Jin, Wai Tai, Sheng Ji* and *Huo Ren,* and all of the major writings of the Yuan and Ming dynasty sages, sifting and selecting only the pure and unadulterated aspects, encom-passing over 100,000 words, and expressing them in simple modern terminology, so that everyone can understand. Even those who have never studied medicine, should they occasion-ally become sick, need only to use the herbs according to the symptoms, and they will not be wrong by so much as a hair. The wonderful thing is it is so easy to understand!

Those who are already experts in the field, once they have this book, can use it to draw together all other medical writings ... deriving, from the difficult, the simple principles.[48]

One of the simple principles Chen proposed in the treatment of phlegm is well worth extracting, for its balance and moderation. He says, in the same book:

> Any time tan-yin is not yet excessive, or although excessive, is not yet hardened and stubborn, one cannot attack it but only dissolve and then lead [it into the Intestines for elimination].[49] That [phlegm] which is not reduced and eliminated by dissolution can be led [into the Intestines] and expelled.'[50]

This approach, which avoids excessive measures while remaining effective, can have great clinical significance if used appropriately, and also clearly points out the importance of thoroughly differentiating the nature of the pathogen before selecting treatment. To attack phlegm which has not hardened is futile because the attack has no solid substance upon which to take effect. While dispersing phlegm would not be sufficient for hardened phlegm, it is perfect for merely lightly congealed phlegm. Once dispersed, it is led out through the Intestines.

ZHOU XUE-HAI

Zhou Xue-Hai, in his 1898 work *Du Yi Sui Bi* ('Informal Notes while Reading Medicine', 1898) discusses the necessary difference between the treatments of thin mucus and phlegm (see this section translated in full at the end of this chapter). His most cogent points are that while tonification of fire and diuresis are essential to the treatment of thin mucus, these are completely inappropriate for phlegm:

> In the treatment of phlegm (i.e. as opposed to thin mucus) one must not tonify fire, and even more emphatically must not promote urination; with tonification of fire and diuresis, even if it is damp-phlegm (i.e. not parched-phlegm) it will still be brewed by the fire, jelling into an ever more sticky and stubborn state, until it finally cannot be uprooted.

He also emphasizes the need for auxiliary promotion of normal body fluids during any phlegm

treatment, 'as only in this way will phlegm have something upon which to be carried out.'

WU SHANG-XIAN

Wu Shang-Xian (*c.* 1806-1886) was one of the greatest modern exponents of external therapy, using not only herbs but hydrotherapy, moxibustion and breathing therapy, pointing out that it was not only very effective but also highly affordable for those who could not otherwise pay for expensive decoctions. In his book, the *Li Yue Pian Wen* ('A Rhyming Discourse on New Therapeutics', 1864) he describes the use of such herbs as *Ru Xiang* (Olibanum, Gummi), *Mo Yao* (Myrrha), *Hong Hua* (Carthami Tinctorii, Flos), *Tao Ren* (Persicae, Semen) and *Jiang Huang* (Curcumea, Rhizoma) to move blood, combining them into a plaster with phlegm-cutting herbs like *Bai Jie Zi* (Sinapsis Albae, Semen) and *Dan Nan Xing* (Arisaemae cum Felle Bovis, Pulvis) to treat combined phlegm and blood stagnation.

TANG RONG-CHUAN

The *Xue Zheng Lun* ('Discussion of Blood Conditions') by Tang Rong–Chuan (1851-1908) has become a modern classic in the treatment of bleeding. It is not just a book of symptoms and matched formulas, however. Tang explains in great detail the mechanisms of pathology involved, and does not shrink from amplifying an aspect almost to the point of caricature if he feels that it has been hitherto under-emphasized, for example where he states assertively in the very first lines of his book: 'The whole body is nothing more than yin and yang; these two characters 'yin' and 'yang' are just water and fire; 'water' and 'fire' are just qi and blood. Water transforms into qi; fire transforms into blood'.

Accustomed to thinking of the identity of fire and qi, and the similarity of water and blood, these lines can appear rather shocking at first glance but Tang goes on to explain his reasoning.

The 'water' refers principally to the water of the Kidneys and the Urinary Bladder. Because both are located below the navel, in the 'Dan Tian' (Cinnabar Field), they constitute the home to which all of the water and jing-essence of the body must return. But this water cannot of itself transform into qi: it relies upon the 'Yang of Heaven' inhaled through the Lungs to lead the Heart fire downwards, linking to the Dan Tian and heating the Water Zang and the Water Fu, before it is transformed into yuan qi and protective qi. This is why he says 'water transforms into qi', and also 'the qi of the whole body is produced from the midst of the Dan Tian Sea of Qi below the navel.' If the qi is weak, water and fluids cannot surge upwards nor be carried downwards to nourish the body. Furthermore, if water comes to a standstill and does not transform, qi itself can become impeded and fail to warm the body.

Tang summarizes this relationship as 'qi is produced from water so it can transform into water; water is transformed through qi but it can also harm qi.'

His 'fire' mainly refers to Heart fire as the source of heat throughout the whole body. Tang points out that the warmth of the limbs and body, and the activity of the body's functions, rely completely upon the effect of heat. It is only through the influence of this heat that the Spleen and Stomach are able to separate, convert and absorb the essence of food and fluids, which then by the action of Heart fire can be changed into blood fluid. In this way, if fire is not extreme, it is intrinsically able to produce blood; if fire is intemperate, however, not only will blood not be produced it will, conversely, be damaged. This connection is summarized as 'fire is controlled by the Heart, it can transform and produce blood fluid, and can warm the whole body' and 'excessive transformation by fire will conversely result in failure of transformation.'

Therefore it is clear that qi is produced from Kidney water and blood is formed through Heart fire. Only if Heart fire descends can Kidney water convert into qi; only if Kidney yang ascends can food and fluids ripen, and Heart fire produce blood. In this way, the Heart and the Kidneys, one yin and one yang, one rising the other sinking, in mutual assistance and benefit, ensure the continuous and unimpaired production of qi and blood for the body.

Tang Rong-Chuan also notes that the pivot for this ascent and descent of Heart and Kidneys is the Spleen, saying: 'Blood is produced from Heart fire and is stored below in the Liver; qi is produced from Kidney water and is controlled above by the Lungs; in between, the activator of this rising and falling is

the Spleen.' This is very similar to Li Dong-Yuan's emphasis of the importance of the Spleen and Stomach, except that Li stressed the importance of lifting Spleen yang (as he was addressing mainly internal deficiency conditions in his book the *Pi Wei Lun*), whereas because Tang is writing about bleeding, he emphasizes Spleen yin moistening and protection.

In terms of phlegm theory, Tang Rong-Chuan described both the pathology and the treatment for the stubborn combination of stagnant blood and phlegm coalescing to form immovable abdominal mass (zheng 癥).

> The definition of 'zheng' (as opposed to 'jia', movable abdominal mass) is its constancy and failure to disperse; blood is the major component [of the stagnant mass], qi the lesser factor, and because the qi cannot overcome the blood it will not disperse. The mass may be made up completely of blood, or the mass of stagnant blood may within it hold water; again, the blood may accumulate for a period of time and itself become phlegm and water ... With weak patients and chronic accumulation, it is not suitable to attack only, but rather a combined attack and support treatment must be implemented if the enemy is to be overcome. ... To attack phlegm and water [accumulation], Shi Zao Tang ('Ten Jujube Decoction', *Formulas and Strategies*, p. 128) should be used.[51]

SUMMARY

From the spare beginnings in the *Nei-Jing*, where the focus was on thin mucus in such sayings as 'thin mucus develops in the middle' and 'accumulated thin mucus: angina', rudimentary phlegm theory received its first serious attention in the *Jin Gui Yao Lue*, where Zhang Zhong-Jing gave a relatively detailed account of how both cold-phlegm and hot-phlegm could affect the chest, and how phlegm could obstruct chest yang. The *Zhu Bing Yuan Hou Lun* not only listed numerous types of phlegm but also clearly differentiated phlegm from thin mucus for the first time, and described the symptoms and mechanism for 'tan jue tou tong'—headache with cold limbs, caused by phlegm. The *Sheng Ji Zong Lu* contained a section exclusively devoted to a very extensive discussion of phlegm.

Zhang Cong-Zheng was the first to introduce the concept of 'phlegm misting the Heart', and initiated phlegm-removal as a method for treating emotional and mental disorders.

Zhu Dan-Xi pointed out that phlegm symptoms can occur at regular intervals, and can be very stubborn with frequent relapses; and together with Pang An-Shi stressed that 'in order to treat phlegm, first address the qi'.

Wang Yin-Jun designed the Gun Tan Wan ('Vaporize Phlegm Pill', *Formulas and Strategies*, p. 424), a formula used throughout the centuries for the aggressive treatment of hot and stubborn phlegm, as well as advancing the concept of phlegm as a pathogenic agent with a very broad reach, and detailing the symptoms which it could cause. It was Wang Yin-Jun's influence that gave currency to the idea that 'bizarre illnesses can be blamed on phlegm'.

Zhang Jing-Yue (Zhang Jie-Bin), because of his encyclopedic scholarship in classical Chinese medicine, is really in a class of his own. His incisive observations of the often heavy-handed phlegm-removing treatments used before and during his time are both instructive and entertaining, as well as subtle in the extreme. Several of his essays on phlegm are translated at the end of this chapter. If one were to attempt to single out the most important concepts in this wealth of information, they could well be the idea that phlegm could arise from deficiency, and that simply eliminating phlegm will almost never be effective, because the underlying mechanism must be discovered and rectified, in short 'treating the root'. This by itself is not new but the idea that tonification of qi—or even blood—could eliminate phlegm is certainly arresting. This works, he says, because if there is 'a lack of qi amidst the water, jin will coalesce and blood fail [to move] and go bad, both of which can transform into phlegm!' In this condition, the phlegm is not created outside of the blood and then mixed with it, he says, so if you try to remove all of the phlegm which is being created from the blood, it will only work— he remarks dryly—if you eliminate all of the blood! Tonification is the only answer. 'If it transpires that nutritive and protective qi are harmonious, then jin-fluid acts as jin, and blood acts as blood; where could phlegm exist?'

Zhao Xian-Ke emphasized the importance of Kidney yin and yang as the foundation of the body.

A root treatment of phlegm must, he said, balance Kidney yin and yang, while also harmonizing the Kidneys and Spleen.

Gong Ju-Zhong elaborated the theory and treatment of phlegm-fire, extending even to the use of moxa and rules for changing one's lifestyle.

Li Shi-Zhen's famous *Ben Cao Gang Mu* contains a great deal of material related to phlegm and its treatment; in fact, he records over three hundred formulas to treat phlegm, constituting the largest collection of formulae for any disease or symptom in the book.

By the Qing dynasty, phlegm theory had reached the stage where standardized phlegm treatments for many specific conditions were recognized. These were codified by Yu Chang in his book *Yi Men Fa Lu* ('Precepts for Physicians'), as were the consequences of mistaken treatments and even the conditions that constituted malpractice. As Yu says: 'Any time hot-phlegm has ridden wind-fire upwards to enter [the upper part of the body, with] blurry vision and tinnitus—seemingly a deficient condition—and warm tonifiers are mistakenly used, this will weld the phlegm and remove any route of elimination. The doctor is culpable.'

Tang Rong-Chuan built upon the earlier suggestion of Zhu Dan-Xi—that phlegm and stagnant blood could mix—and went further, describing concretely how it could occur clinically and its treatment. Wu Shang-Xian developed external therapy for the same problem, using blood movers combined with such phlegm-cutting herbs as *Bai Jie Zi* (Sinapsis Albae, Semen) and *Dan Nan Xing* (Arisaemae cum Felle Bovis, Pulvis).

Now that traditional Chinese medicine has moved into the West, we will undoubtedly be seeing further developments in TCM phlegm theory resulting from the impact of the different lifestyles in the West upon the traditional clinical approaches used in China. Developing effective clinical strategies is one thing, but it is important that Western practitioners thoroughly understand the depth and subtlety of traditional Chinese medicine before we claim to be able to 'adapt Chinese medicine for the West'.

Understanding the slow process of development, the repeated testing and checking, the presenting of viewpoints for peer review, the sheer cautious tentativeness, during the course of a medical theory's development, will possibly give us in the West a little more of the humility which may lead to wisdom.

In case anyone thinks that the study of the historical development of phlegm theory in Chinese medicine is only of academic interest, or that the 'presenting of viewpoints for peer review' has lessened in modern times, I would like to include a short article from the 'Journal of Chinese Medicine' 1991, vol. 32, No. 12, which arrived in the mail as this chapter was being completed. It exemplifies how historical studies can increase clinical effectiveness, describes how the fruits of such research are used in a modern setting and invites peer comment.

Contemporary Essay

The following essay is a discussion of the treatment of dyspnea from yin deficiency and excess phlegm by Jiang Xi-Quan, Chongqing City, Jiangjin District People's Hospital.

The treatment of dyspnea from yin deficiency and excess (shi) phlegm has always been a difficult area for doctors throughout the ages. The major approaches employed in the past are introduced below.

Zhang Jing–Yue designed Jin Shui Liu Jun Jian ('Six Gentlemen of Metal and Water Decoction', *Formulas and Strategies*, p. 433), which uses the powder of Er Chen Tang ('Two-Cured Decoction', *Formulas and Strategies*, p. 432) plus *Shou Di* (Rehmanniae) and *Dang Gui* (Angelica Polymorpha), to be washed down with a decoction of raw ginger and red dates. This achieves the effect of transforming phlegm while nourishing yin, regulates both dryness and moisture and treats both Metal and Water. It has proven quite effective in the treatment of dyspnea from yin deficiency allowing water to flood, causing excess phlegm that has a salty taste.

The *Xing Xuan Yi An* (1817) uses this formula as a basis upon which to add *Shan Zhi Zi* (Gardeniae), *Dan Dou Chi* (Sojae Praeparatum, Semen), *Hai Fu Shi* (Pumice) and *Jin Fu Cao* (Inulae, Herba). This increases the phlegm dispersing and fire descending effects of the formula.

Li Shi-Cai (1667) uses a decoction of the Lung-opening and phlegm-transforming herbs *Jie Geng* (Platycodi), *Ban Xia* (Pinelliae), *Zhi Ke* (Citri seu Ponciri, Fructus), and *Gan Cao* (Glycyrrhizae) to wash down Liu Wei Di Huang Wan ('Six-Ingredient Pill with Rehmannia', *Formulas and Strategies*, p. 263), combining decoction and pills to treat upper body excess phlegm with lower body deficiency of yin.

Wang Xu-Gao (1798) copied this idea when he used Su Zi Jiang Qi Tang ('Perilla Fruit Decoction for Directing the Qi Downward', *Formulas and Strategies*, p. 299) removing the *Rou Gui* (Cinnamomi Cassiae, Cortex) to wash down Du Qi Wan ('Capital Qi Pill', *Formulas and Strategies*, p. 264).

Ye Tian-Shi, when treating upper body Lung heat excess with lower body yin deficiency, had the patient take the yin nourishing lower Jiao replenishing herbs in the morning, and the upper Jiao cooling and spreading herbs in the evening.

Yu Chang employed an 'encasing' technique. He added *Huai Niu Xi* (Achyranthis Bidentatae, Radix), *Ci Shi* (Magnetitum), and *Rou Gui* (Cinnamomi Cassiae, Cortex) to Du Qi Wan ('Capital Qi Pill', *Formulas and Strategies*, p. 264), powdering all the herbs and mixing them with toffied honey into small glossy pills. When these were half dried, he would then use finely powdered *Ban Xia* (Pinelliae), *Chen Pi* (Citri Reticulatae, Pericarpium) and *Zhi Gan Cao* (Glycyrrhizae) to cover them. The patient was instructed to take the pills in the morning. In the Stomach, the outer coating of the pills would work to expel phlegm and thin mucus, while the inner pill's yin nourishing herbs would be absorbed later, in the lower Jiao, where the effect was needed to tonify Kidneys.

Shou Di (Rehmanniae Glutinosae Conquitae, Radix) is the major herb to nourish Kidney yin and jing-essence but all the Materia Medica describe its greasy Stomach-disturbing nature; it is particularly contraindicated for those with weak digestion. Thus a number of doctors advocate that it be charred. The problem is, how much of the yin nourishing effect then remains? Wang Xu-Gao went into the problem of yin deficiency with phlegm quite thoroughly, and his treatments were very carefully considered. When he used Jin Shui Liu Jun Jian ('Six Gentlemen of Metal and Water Decoction', *Formulas and Strategies*, p. 433), he fried the *Shou Di* with *Sha Ren* (Amomi) until it was flaky, then added it after the other herbs in the Six Gentlemen were cooked, bringing the decoction to the boil once or twice more only. He noted: 'This is imitating the 'thin decoction boiling method' (yin zi jian fa, where the resulting decoction is of thin consistency rather than thick as is usual), in which turbid herbs are delivered in a clear form, in order that yin can be nourished without further obstruction of the turbid phlegm.'

Wang Meng-Shi (1808-1867, a famous Febrile Disease school author) noticed that dyspnea with yin deficiency in the lower body and excess phlegm in the upper body would have a wiry slippery pulse in the right cun and guan (distal and median) positions and a thready rapid pulse in the left guan and chi (median and proximal) positions. He often used *Xing Ren* (Pruni Armeniacae, Semen), *Chuan Bei Mu* (Fritillariae Cirrhosae), *Zhu Ru* (Bambusae in Taeniis, Caulis), *Xuan Fu Hua* (Inulae, Flos), *Hai Fu Shi* (Pumice), *Ge Ke* (Cyclinae Sinensis, Concha), *Tian Hua Fen* (Trichosanthis, Radix), *Lu Gen* (Phragmitis Communis, Rhizoma) and *Dong Gua Ren* (Benincasae Hispidae, Semen) as a formula cooked with water in which 15-30 g of *Shou Di* (Rehmanniae) had been soaked. He remarked: 'Turbid herbs delivered lightly can cool the upper body and strengthen the lower body: killing two birds with one stone.' Shi Nian-Zu comments on this, saying 'In this formula, all of the herbs besides *Shou Di* are phlegm-expelling herbs that assist Lung descent; when the *Shou Di* broth is used to decoct them, the yin is restored and then the qi moves. Once the qi moves then the phlegm heat in the upper body will descend. This is not only [Wang] Meng-Ying's invention: anyone who has tried this method to treat yin deficiency with excess phlegm has had 100% success.'

Shou Di which has not been fried retains all of its yin nourishing effects, and because the above method is very simple, it is quite popular. Over the last ten years, anytime I have a case of dyspnea from yin deficiency with excess phlegm, I tell the patient to soak the *Shou Di* for thirty minutes in water which has just been boiled, then remove the *Shou Di* and use the liquid to boil the other herbs without adding any more water. This seems to get good results.

Over the last few years, with acute cases of yin deficient and phlegm excess type of bronchial asthma or acute bronchitis with wheezing, I have used Ma Xing Shi Gan Tang ('Ephedra, Apricot Kernel, Gypsum and Licorice', *Formulas and Strategies*, p. 88), adding *Huang Qin* (Scutellariae), *Ting Li Zi* (Tinglizi, Semen), *Zi Su Zi* (Perillae Fructescentis, Fructus), *Di Long* (Lumbricus), *She Gan* (Belamcandae Chinensis, Rhizoma), *Zi Wan* (Asteris Tatarici, Radix) and *Yu Xing Cao* (Houttuyniae Cordatae, Herba); if there is constipation I often add *Da Huang* (Rhei, Rhizoma). This gets good results.

When the patient's pathogen is 60-70% eliminated, and the cough and dyspnea reduced without the illness developing further, I continue the above prescription because the pathogen—although reduced—has not been completely eradicated. The heat, while less, is still accumulated; the phlegm, despite its scantiness, still exists: in the channels and collaterals of the Lungs and Stomach, stubborn phlegm has jelled into an enduring 'root' from which the illness can recur. Under the tyranny of long-standing pathogenic heat, the jin-ye fluids are reduced day by day, and Lung yin is similarly damaged, but a yin nourishing formula will only block the epigastric area and produce phlegm. Under these circumstances, if *Wu Wei Zi* (Schisandrae Chinensis, Fructus) 8-10g is added to the above formula, one can often achieve unexpectedly good results.

Similarly, with old or weak patients, or those with recurring exogenous invasions, who have pathogenic heat injuring yin and the resulting wheeze or rough breathing, one can add a little bit of *Wu Wei Zi* [which is sour-constricting] to their prescription [which is otherwise designed] to open the Lungs, expel the pathogen, cool heat and eliminate phlegm. This can be done even in the midst of pathogenic dominance, and still gets good results, [despite the contracting action of the *Wu Wei Zi*].

The *Shen Nong Ben Cao Jing* ('Shen Nong's Materia Medica') records that *Wu Wei Zi* 'strengthens the yin and benefits the jing-essence'. The *Lei Gong Pao Zhi Yao Xing Jie* ('Lei Gong's Description of Herbal Natures and Preparations') says that *Wu Wei Zi* 'enters the Lung and Kidney channels, replenishing Kidney channel's insufficient Water, constricting Lung qi's scattered Metal'. It is 'an important herb for producing jin-fluids, a marvellous prescription for closing and contracting'. Used together with *Ma Huang* (Ephedrae, Herba), the effects are both dispersing and contracting, one opens and one closes: the yin is nourished without retaining the pathogen, the pathogen is attacked without damaging the zheng qi.

Again, *Wu Wei Zi* can be used simultaneously with *Shi Gao* (Gypsum). The *Shi Gao* controls the warm astringency of the *Wu Wei Zi*; the *Wu Wei Zi* moderates the heaviness of *Shi Gao*. The two herbs together can provide a strong restorative for the yin and jin-fluids. However, *Wu Wei Zi* is after all an astringent herb: in cases such as we are discussing, where pathogenic phlegm is built up and dominant, the amounts should not be excessive. 8-12g is about right.[52]

The Zhu Bing Yuan Hou Lun: 'The Symptoms of Phlegm and Thin Mucus Diseases'

The *Zhu Bing Yuan Hou Lun* ('General Treatise on the Etiology and Symptomatology of Diseases') was written by Chao Yuan–Fang in 610AD).

Phlegm and thin mucus symptoms

Phlegm and thin mucus disease is a result of weak yang qi failing to maintain open pathways for qi, so that the body fluids are unable to transit smoothly. The qi of water and thin mucus stops in the chest-repository, congeals and becomes phlegm. Also, in those cases where a once fleshy person is now thin, with borborygmus from the sound of water and fluids coursing through the Intestines, this is likewise called tan-yin. The symptoms of phlegm and thin mucus disease are a sensation of fullness and distension of the chest and flanks, [which is the consequence of] inability to digest food and fluids so that they turn into water and thin mucus, and cease to flow in the abdomen or the flanks.

Water and thin mucus enter the Intestines and the Stomach, making a sound with their movement. The body feels heavy, there is copious saliva, shortness of breath, sleepiness, and pain in the chest and the upper back. In severe cases the shortness of breath leads to cough and inability to lie flat, and the person must sit up; the body will look swollen.

When the pulse is taken, if one hand is wiry, this is phlegm; if floating and slippery,[53] this is thin mucus.

Phlegm and thin mucus with inability to digest food

Phlegm and thin mucus patients who are unable to digest food are thus because phlegm and water have accumulated between the chest-repository and the Urinary Bladder. As the pathogen remains for a prolonged time, it flows into and damages the Spleen and Stomach. Spleen abhors damp, and as it is overcome by water, distention will result, and thereafter digestion will fail. There may be possible weak-type distention of the abdomen, or food and fluids undigested, or occasional nausea and vomiting: these are all symptoms of phlegm and thin mucus disease.

Symptoms of hot-phlegm

Hot-phlegm is the term referring to that which is caused by a long term build-up of water and thin mucus. Because of this build-up, the qi of yin and yang cannot circulate smoothly, the upper Jiao blockage produces heat which then struggles with the phlegm and thin mucus, coalescing and not dispersing. This can cause deficient heat (xu-heat) in the body, interfering with eating and drinking, and causing symptoms such as a mild heat in the face and head. For this reason it is known as 'hot-phlegm'.

Symptoms of cold-phlegm

Cold-phlegm is the result of weakness in the Spleen and Stomach with inability to transform and transport food and fluids, leading to accumulation of phlegm and water which encumbers the area between the chest and the diaphragm, hampers the yang qi, and leads to sour regurgitation and up-rushing qi, blueness of the extremities, and inability to eat and drink.

Symptoms of solid knotted-phlegm

The symptoms of solid knotted-phlegm result from phlegm and water accumulating in the area of the chest and diaphragm and struggling with hot and cold qi, so that they congeal and do not disperse. This obstructs the qi flow, and thus leads to sensations of blockage and fullness in the epigastric area and abdomen, difficult breathing, vertigo, blurry vision, and frequent nausea. For this reason it is known as 'solid knotted-phlegm'.

Symptoms of headache from phlegm at the diaphragm and uprushing wind[54]

The term 'phlegm at the diaphragm' refers to phlegm and thin mucus which has collected above the diaphragm in the chest, and subsequently been subjected to great cold. This prevents yang qi from moving [normally], leads the phlegm and water to collect and knot without dispersal, so that yin qi conversely rises, connects with wind-phlegm, and rushes up to the head. This causes pain in the head which may persist for several years unabated; after a long period of time it may link with the brain, causing deeper pain. Thus it is called 'headache from diaphragm phlegm and uprushing wind'. If the patient has sensations of cold in the extremities, and the sensations reach the elbows and knees, the prognosis is poor.

General phlegm symptoms

Phlegm diseases all result from obstruction of the qi in the blood vessels causing water and thin mucus to accumulate without dispersing, thus becoming phlegm. This [phlegm] may be cold, or hot, or may form solid knots, or prevent food from being digested, or may cause sensations of fullness in the chest and abdomen, or shortness of breath and sleepiness: the [possible] symptoms are not uniform, and thus it is termed 'general phlegm'.[55]

Classical Essays

Zhang's comments on the mechanisms and differentiation of phlegm

From the *Jing Yue Quan Shu*, 'The Complete Works of [Zhang] Jing-Yue', written by Zhang Jie-Bin in 1624. ('Jing Yue' is Zhang Jie-Bin's 'zi': a self-selected alternative name.)

Tan-yin (phlegm and thin mucus) as a symptom, in the *Nei Jing*, is only mentioned as 'accumulated thin mucus', and phlegm is not individually designated.

The reason that the *Nei Jing* does not emphasize phlegm can be understood if we consider the following:

The designation 'phlegm' began with Zhang Zhong-Jing, and later generations passed it on, without regard for whether it was really phlegm or not; some would unthinkingly pronounce 'phlegm-fire', some would quote 'strange diseases come from phlegm', or say 'phlegm is the Mother of the Hundred Afflictions', as if phlegm were overwhelming—so why did the *Nei Jing* ignore it?

They do not know that for phlegm to become pathological there must be a cause, for example, wind or fire producing phlegm. If one treats the wind or fire, though, and the wind or fire is extinguished, then the phlegm will be cleared in and of itself. If the phlegm is the result of deficiency or excess, then curing the deficiency or excess will naturally calm the phlegm.

One will never hear of wind or fire being self-extinguished simply by treating the phlegm which results from it, nor that excess or deficiency will be relieved spontaneously through eradicating phlegm.

The reason for this is that phlegm is necessarily a product of disease, not disease a product of phlegm.

This is why the *Nei Jing* never mentions phlegm individually: it is because phlegm is not the root of illness but instead is the later manifestation (branch).

Nowadays the medical profession, universally, knows a hundred stratagems for attacking phlegm, and that this is treating disease; but surprisingly does not know the reason for the phlegm, or why it has arisen. Have they then discarded the reasoning which reminds us that to move the finger, we activate the arm? or that to fill the leaf, we must save the root?

Once the branch and the root are mixed up, one's own judgement becomes inaccurate; trying to effect a cure then becomes difficult.

Phlegm and thin mucus, although they can be spoken of as being in a similar category, in fact have some differences. Thin mucus is a type of watery fluid, and symptoms such as vomiting of clear fluid with bloating and fullness of the chest and abdomen, sour regurgitation, foul belching and watery-sounding borborygmus are all the result of residue from food and fluids, accumulated and not moving, and this is what is called yin (thin mucus).

The difference between phlegm and thin mucus is that thin mucus is clear and limpid, while phlegm is turbid and murky; thin mucus affects primarily the Stomach and Intestines, while phlegm reaches everywhere. Food and fluids, untransformed, stay to become thin mucus; the condition comes completely from the Spleen and Stomach.

Phlegm, which is ubiquitous and formed anywhere, can stem from injury to any of the Five Zang. Thus, to treat these, one should know the differences, and not forego investigation into the root of the problem.

Phlegm is simply the body's fluids, which are themselves nothing but the result of transformation from food and fluids. Since this phlegm is also a transformed substance, it cannot then be classified as 'untransformed' (i.e. as thin mucus is untransformed by the Spleen and Stomach). But transformation, if normal, results in a strong body with flourishing nutritive and protective qi; in this case, [what would in a pathological situation be] phlegm is [still normal] blood and qi.

On the other hand, if transformation proceeds abnormally, then the zang fu become diseased, the body fluids fail (bai), and qi and blood then produce phlegm. This is exactly like robbers and thieves creating chaos in society: who are they but [otherwise] good people in a troubled world? The rise of brigands, however, must of necessity be the consequence of malady in the governance of the country, just as the appearance of phlegm must result from infirmity of the yuan qi.

I once heard Li Zhai's[56] statement that 'Once the qi and blood have been made to thrive, what phlegm can there be?'. In my youth I doubted this assertion, thinking 'does he mean to say there is no such thing as shi-phlegm?' But now that I have more accurate cognisance, I have begun to believe that it is in fact so. Why do we hold this view?

The fact is, the transformation of phlegm is based on fluids and food, and if the Spleen is strong and the Stomach healthy like that of a young person's, then whatever is eaten will be transformed, and it all becomes qi and blood; where could retention occur to become phlegm?

It is only when there is incomplete transformation, where one or two parts out of ten are retained, that those one or two parts become phlegm. If three or four parts are retained, then those three or four parts become phlegm. In the worst cases, the retention reaches seven or eight parts, and in these cases the qi and blood become daily more weakened, while the phlegm day by day increases.

That is the rationale: precisely because the yuan qi is unable to transform and transport, the more deficiency there is then the more will phlegm thrive.

Therefore Li Zhai's statement: is it not a product of repeated observation?

Nowadays, we see those who treat phlegm all saying 'How can illnesses from phlegm be cured without expelling it?' They do not know that if the zheng qi 正气 does not move, then xu-phlegm will accumulate. Using all the means at one's disposal will not only not eliminate it but will in fact add to the deficiency. So the result will be either a patient brought to the brink of collapse by attack, or an occasional temporary relief with an even worse deficiency appearing at some other day. Both are the outcome of misguided attack. What they should know is that the type of phlegm which can be attacked is rare, while that which should not be attacked is abundant. Those treating phlegm are obliged to first distinguish excess or deficiency.

There is 'deficient phlegm' and 'excess phlegm': these must be differentiated. People may ask: if there is an excess amount of phlegm, how can there be this difference between excess and deficiency? The fact is that the words 'xu' deficiency, and 'shi' excess both have meaning only in regard to the yuan qi. That which can be attacked is 'excess' phlegm, while that which may not be attacked is 'deficient' phlegm.

How do we know which phlegm is 'that which can be attacked'? From the youth and still abundant vigor [of the patient], and the undamaged blood; they may have overeaten sweet rich foods, or there may be excessive [environmental] damp and heat, or wind-cold may have closed the skin, or rebelling qi may have entangled the Liver and diaphragm internally, any of which could have led to sudden formation of phlegm or thin mucus. One must still check the energy of both the body and the energy of the disease, and only if both are strong will this be 'excess' phlegm. Why 'excess' phlegm? Because the yuan qi is still 'shi' (abundant). In this case one should commence an eliminative strike, and there is nothing wrong with solely aiming to eradicate the phlegm.

How do we know which phlegm is 'that which may not be attacked'? This can be recognised from the debilitated figure and the lack of vigor [of the patient], when age has begun to take its toll; this will be 'deficient' phlegm. There may have been a long history of illness, or overwork, or worry, alcohol and sex, any of these factors causing weakness that is not a result of wind[-stroke] or collapse: this will also be 'deficient' phlegm. There may be a thready rapid pulse without pathogenic yang in the organs, with symptoms like occasional nausea, diarrhea, shortness of breath, and hoarseness. One must still check the energy of both the body and the energy of the disease, and if there is no sign of excess this will be 'deficient' phlegm. Why 'deficient' phlegm? Because the yuan qi is already inadequate. In this case one should merely seek to harmonize and tonify; an attack would be courting disaster.

Furthermore, 'excess' phlegm is rare, and while it comes on suddenly, its departure is equally quick, and so the illness it causes is easily treated. Why is this? Because the root of the disease is not deep.

So 'excess' phlegm is not worth worrying about—the most to be feared is 'deficient' phlegm!

In short, the treatment of phlegm is none other than making the yuan qi day by day stronger, and the phlegm daily less, until only a little is left, which in tiny amounts is not a problem, and in fact this can assist Stomach qi [as Stomach abhors dryness].[57]

If yuan qi grows weaker day by day, then the food, fluids, jin and ye, all become nothing but phlegm! If you expel it, it simply reduplicates. That there is a method for attacking phlegm in a way that eliminates it completely, while preserving the yuan qi from any damage, I do not believe.

Therefore, those adept at treating phlegm simply bar it from being produced, which is the only means for tonifying Heaven (i.e. xian tian 'prenatal constitution'; and hou tian 'acquired constitution').

But those in practice now treating phlegm do not bother to differentiate xu and shi but blithely attack it all generally. One such is Wang Yin–Jun with his idea that 'internally and externally, the Hundred Diseases are all born of phlegm', and his exclusive use of Gun Tan Wan ('Vaporize Phlegm Pill', *Formulas and Strategies*, p. 424) and similar formulas. People like this only think of the present situation and never perceive the damaging consequences later.

The Five Zang, it is true, can all contribute to the production of phlegm but it is also true that this takes place only through the Spleen and Kidneys.

This is because Spleen controls damp, if damp is stirred it becomes phlegm; Kidneys control water, if water floods, it too becomes phlegm.

Thus the transformation of phlegm is no place other than the Spleen, while the root of phlegm is nowhere but the Kidneys. So any phlegm condition can be traced, if not to the one, then to the other—these two organs will definitely be implicated.

However, the phlegm in Spleen patients can be either 'deficient' or 'excess'. For example, if damp obstruction has become extreme, this is the 'excess' condition of the Spleen. If Earth is too weak to control Water, this is Spleen 'deficiency'.

The phlegm in Kidney patients, though, is never anything but 'deficient'. This is because [Kidney] Fire cannot support and produce Earth, and also cannot control Water. Yang not controlling yin must result in water rebelliously invading Spleen. All of this is the result of fire within yin being weak. If fire flares and scorches the Lungs, then jing-essence is not conserved; jin-fluids become parched, and ye-fluids desiccated, with Metal and Water both injured: this is the weakness of Water within yin.

These are the differences between excess and deficiency in the Spleen and the Kidneys, and it is this which requires differentiation.

Again, although our ancestors described categories such as damp-phlegm, [qi-]blocked-phlegm, cold-phlegm, and hot-phlegm, and although it may be located in the upper part of the body, or the lower, or be hot or cold, and each is [admittedly] different, nonetheless in terms of origin of transformation and production, how could it be other than these two organs?

For example, cold-phlegm and damp-phlegm are basically Spleen patient problems, but is not the production of cold-damp originally related to the Kidneys (i.e. in failing to warm Spleen)? Wood obstruction produces wind, but the phlegm of Liver patients—with a strong Wood oppressing Earth—could it not be related to Spleen? Flaring fire overcomes Metal, with phlegm in the Lungs, but the pathogenic fire flaring up: if it does not come from the middle and lower Jiao, then where is it from?

Therefore anyone who wants to treat phlegm, but does not know its source, is simply groping blindly in the dark![58]

Zhang Jing-Yue discusses pathogenic phlegm in the channels and collaterals

Phlegm around the body leads to difficult-to-fathom illnesses: paralysis, convulsions and cramps, hemiplegia, all are such due to deep-lying phlegm obstruction. Given this, how can phlegm not be in the same category as other pathogens? Without expelling pathogenic phlegm, how can the illness be cured? To this I say: do you know phlegm's origin and behavior? Any phlegm in the channels and collaterals is generally transformed from the jin-fluids or the blood. If it transpires that nutritive and protective qi are harmonious, then jin-fluid acts as jin-fluid [should act], and blood acts as blood; where could phlegm exist?

It is only if there is damage to the yuan yang (original or primal yang), or attenuation in the activity of the Heart shen, will there then be a lack of qi amidst the water, jin-fluids will coalesce and blood fail [to move] and go bad, both of which can transform into phlegm!

This yield of phlegm, or [the converse] production of jing-essence and blood, how could it be external to the jing and blood, from some unrelated pathogenic phlegm?

If it is said that phlegm in the channels must be attacked in order to be eradicated, then the jing-essence and the blood must also be completely eliminated before that would be possible. Otherwise how could the phlegm by itself be attacked, without stirring the jing and blood?

Repeated injury to the jin-fluids and the blood, exhausting the yuan qi ever further, leads to the situation that the more that is lost, the more phlegm is created, necessarily worsening the problem; this is why the treatment of phlegm would never cease—what will cease is the yuan qi!

Again, where there is no independent pathogenic phlegm but rash attempts to attack it as such are made: how profound is their ignorance!

Therefore, anytime phlegm-dispelling herbs are used, such as those in formulas like Gun Tan Wan ('Vaporize Phlegm Pill', *Formulas and Strategies*, p. 424) or Sou Feng Shun Qi Wan[59] then it must be certain that the yuan qi is not damaged.

The occasional obstruction, or some slight phlegm that is not abated, can be cleared away—who would say that this is not effective? But if the illness has involved the yuan qi, and the only conception is to treat the branch, then there will be nothing but a daily weakening with each day of use.[60]

Zhang Jing-Yue comments on treating the root of phlegm

Most of the phlegm in people is all from a weak middle Jiao. But since phlegm is actually Water, its root is in the Kidneys, and its branch (later manifestations) is in the Spleen.

That which is from Kidneys derives from water not returning normally to its source but rather flooding and becoming phlegm.

That which is from Spleen derives from food and fluids not properly transforming, i.e. Earth not controlling Water.

Has it not been observed how strong people can eat and drink whatever they like, in whatever quantities, and how everything they eat or drink is duly transformed? We never see it becoming phlegm.

It is those who cannot eat, on the other hand, who do produce phlegm. This is weak Spleen unable to transform food, and the food itself then becomes phlegm.

Thus anyone suffering from a deficiency illness (xu lao)[61] will necessarily have excessive phlegm; as the illness reaches the danger stage, the phlegm will become even worse. This is simply because the Spleen is even more impaired, and completely unable to transform: water and fluids turn altogether to phlegm.

In that case, what of the relationship between phlegm and illness? Is the illness from the phlegm, or the phlegm a result of the illness? Is it not that phlegm must be from the illness?

It can thus be seen that hardly any of the phlegm under Heaven is 'excess' phlegm, and also that hardly any phlegm should be attacked.

Therefore the treatment of phlegm needs the warming of Spleen and the strengthening of Kidneys in order to treat the root of phlegm. By gradually replenishing the basic root, phlegm will—without [direct] treatment—eliminate itself.[62]

Zhou Xue–Hai on the need to treat phlegm and thin mucus separately

The following essay is from *Du Yi Sui Bi*, 'Informal Notes while Reading Medicine', 1898.

The nature of yin (thin mucus) is Water, clear and not sticky, and it will not be produced if water is transformed into sweat or urine [as is normal].

The nature of tan (phlegm) is thick and very sticky, and it will not be produced if the qi transformations into ye-fluid and blood are normal.

Thin mucus is produced when the qi transformation in the San Jiao fails to transport. This failure of transport comes from insufficient Mingmen fire.

The Classics say: San Jiao is the official in charge of waterways, where water moves. The Urinary Bladder is the official of lakes, where water is stored; it can be moved from here through qi transformation.

Generally, when water enters the Stomach, the Spleen disperses the essence, carrying it up to the Lungs, and this becomes jin-fluids. The dregs are poured into the San Jiao, [carried to the Urinary Bladder] and steamed by the warm qi; what is not turned into urine is flushed outward as sweat, which is why if sweat is profuse, urine is reduced.

That which travels downward into the Urinary Bladder, because Urinary Bladder has only an upper outlet and no lower outlet[63], must rely on the qi transformation of the San Jiao before it can begin to come out.

The reason that it is called 'water' in the San Jiao, while in the Urinary Bladder it is called 'jin-ye', is because the water in the San Jiao has a clear nature and a bland flavour; [but] when it is drained outward as sweat its flavour is salty, and when it is drained downward as urine the odour is meaty and foul: both have undergone changes by the person's qi, and do not change back into the original nature of water.

Thus sweat and urine can both be termed jin-ye [in the Classical quote]; in fact both are [the same:] water.

If the force of fire does not transport, water builds up in the middle Jiao, and is shot up into the Lungs. To treat this, tonify fire and regulate qi: this is treating the root. Bringing on sweat and promoting urination will treat the branch.

Phlegm, on the other hand, no matter whether it is dry-phlegm or damp-phlegm, is all formed through the insufficiency of Spleen qi, unable to soundly transport. Normally, the essence of food and fluids, through the converting transformation of the Spleen qi, can reach the muscles to produce blood[64] in order to moisten dryness; and is able to reach the tendons and bones where this essence becomes ye-fluids, to ease bending and stretching. Here, though, Spleen qi is weak, Earth cannot produce Metal, Shan Zhong[65] becomes weak-willed and timid, and this essence lacks the strength required to reach the muscles; instead it remains in the Stomach and Intestines, accumulates, and becomes phlegm. That which has already arrived at the skin and the [inner] membranes[66] also lacks the strength to reach the tendons and bones, and thus becomes phlegm between the skin and the subcutaneous tissues.

There is another reason that those with much phlegm will have trouble with stretching and bending [the limbs], which is that as phlegm increases, the blood necessarily is reduced.

The method of treatment for this will be to strengthen the Spleen while promoting orderly San Jiao movement, to expedite the San Jiao's ascent and descent of qi, and the various qi transformative processes [supported thereby]. This is the treatment of the root; opening obstruction and busting stagnation will treat the branch. Treatment for parched-phlegm must also use [the methods of] cooling heat and producing jin-fluids, as only in this way will phlegm have something upon which to be carried out. The reason that stagnation busting must be used is that phlegm is in the same category as blood (i.e. both are yin), and stuck phlegm and stagnant blood are treated together.

In the treatment of phlegm (i.e. as opposed to thin mucus) one must not tonify fire, and even more emphatically must not promote urination; with tonification of fire and diuresis, even if it is damp-phlegm (i.e. and not parched-phlegm) it will also be brewed by the fire, jelling into an ever more sticky and stubborn state, until it finally cannot be uprooted.

This is the main difference between the treatment of thin mucus and the treatment of phlegm.

As to those patients suffering thin mucus, of course this will also be accompanied by some phlegm; and those with phlegm will also have some thin mucus. The two conditions are almost always found together, and this is why the ancients did not differentiate between them. But every illness has its root, and every condition has its priority. Those suffering from thin mucus with some phlegm can have the thin mucus treated and the phlegm will naturally eliminate itself; if the phlegm is quite bad, though, the use of some phlegm treatment in conjunction with the primary thin mucus treatment is suitable. Those who have developed thin mucus as the result of a primary phlegm disease can have the phlegm treated and the thin mucus will go of itself; if the thin mucus is quite bad, though, some supplemental treatment for this may be needed.[67]

Lin Pei–Qin on pathological mechanisms and treatment of phlegm and thin mucus

From the *Lei Zheng Zhi Cai* ('Tailored Treatments Arranged According to Pattern') by Lin Pei-Qin, died 1839.

Phlegm and thin mucus are both transformed from jin-ye fluids: phlegm is thick and murky, thin mucus is clear; phlegm arises from fire, thin mucus is the result of damp.

Phlegm is produced in the Spleen, when damp dominates and the food essence is no longer transported; it then congeals and knots up, and either obstructs the Lung orifice, or flows into the channels.

The gathering of thin mucus in the Stomach occurs when cold exists: the watery fluids cease movement, then flood, and no matter whether the mucus sits beneath the Heart in the epigastric region, or seeps into the Intestines, both are the result of Spleen and Stomach water and damp congealing into thin mucus. Yang qi is required for healthy transport, so that murky yin can descend: like having a fierce sun in an empty sky causing the clouds to disperse, the treatment should be the regulation of the Spleen so that damp is expelled.

If Kidney yang is deficient, Fire will lose control of Water, which can then accumulate and become phlegm, or thin mucus which rushes upward. [Because it is from yang deficiency] the phlegm or thin mucus will be clear, and the treatment should be to open the flow of yang and drain away damp. On no account should greasy yin tonics such as Si Wu Tang ('Four Substance Decoction', *Formulas and Strategies*, p. 248) or Liu Wei Di Huang Wan ('Six-Ingredient Pill with Rehmannia', *Formulas and Strategies*, p. 263) be used.

If Kidney yin is deficient, Fire will certainly scorch Metal, fire will knot into phlegm, and become phlegm-fire ascending so that the phlegm will be turbid and thick. The treatment should be to nourish yin, clear the heat and moisten fluids. Under no circumstances should warming and parching formulas such as Er Chen Tang ('Two-Cured Decoction', *Formulas and Strategies*, p. 432) or Liu Jun Zi Tang ('Six-Gentlemen Decoction', *Formulas and Strategies*, p. 238) be used: treatments must be differentiated!

As a rule, clear and thin is yin, thick and turbid is phlegm. The yin accumulates only in the Stomach and Intestines, while phlegm can follow the rise and fall of the qi to reach anywhere in the body:

in the Lungs, cough;
in the Stomach, nausea;
in the Heart, palpitations;
in the head, vertigo;
in the back, coldness;

in the chest, tightness;
in the flanks, distention;
in the guts, diarrhea;
in the jing luo, swelling;
in the limbs, pain.

The changes are endless. This is what they meant in former times when it was said strange diseases are mainly from phlegm, sudden diseases are mainly from fire.

In the same vein, the dictum 'If there is phlegm do not just treat phlegm' means that the root must be sought in treatment.

Otherwise the fear is that, in concentrating upon the eliminating the last vestige of phlegm, the Stomach qi will be further weakened, and [the problem] inadvertently multiplied! ...[68]

NOTES

1. Much of this chapter is based on the work of Zhu Ceng–Bo, who is undoubtedly the most prolific modern writer on the subject of TCM phlegm theory, its clinical application and its history. From his books *Zhong Yi Tan Bing Xue* ('TCM Phlegm Disease Studies'), Hubei Science and Technology Press, 1984, p. 9; and *Lun Zhong Yi Tan Bing Xue Shuo* ('Discussions on TCM Phlegm Theory'), Hubei People's Press, 1981; and his article 'Superficial Discussion of the Formation and Development of TCM Phlegm Disease Studies', Journal of Traditional Chinese Medicine, Beijing, 1983, 10, pp. 59-61.

2. The *Book of Songs*, for example, mentions the collection of *Bei Mu* (Fritillariae), a common phlegm-transforming herb; and the *Wu Shi Er Bing Fang*, excavated from the Ma Wang Dui archeological dig in Changsha, Hunan, in 1973, lists more than ten other herbs commonly used in the treatment of phlegm diseases, including *Ban Xia* (Pinelliae), *Fu Ling* (Poriae), *Bai Fu Zi* (Typhonii Gigantei, Rhizoma seu Aconiti Coreani, Radix), *Xing Ren* (Pruni Armeniacae), and so on.

3. Bing tanyin zhe, dang yi wen yao he zhi. 病痰饮者，当以温药和之.

4. See the translation of his section on phlegm diagnosis at the end of this chapter.

5. *Qian Jin Yao Fang* ('Thousand Ducat Formulas', 652AD) by Sun Si Miao (c. 581-682), People's Health Publishing, Beijing, 1982, pp. 331-335.

6. *Shi Liao Ben Cao*, ('Materia Medica of Food Therapy', c. 713 AD), People's Health Publishing, Beijing, 1984, p. 74.

7. *ibid*. p. 132.

8. *Sheng Ji Zong Lu*, in two volumes, ordered by Zhao Ji, 1112AD (Southern Song Dynasty); Beijing, People's Health Publishing, 1992, vol. 1, p. 1154.

9. *San Yin Ji Yi Bing Zheng Fang Lun* ('Discussion of Illnesses, Patterns and Formulas Related to the Unification of the Three Etiologies', by Chen Yan, 1174), People's Health Press, Beijing, 1983, p. 174.

10. Pang An-Shi (1042-1099) was a famous Song dynasty physician (especially talented in acupuncture) and author of the *Shang Han Zong Bing Lun* ('Discussion of Shang Han and General Diseases'). *Cf. Zhong Guo Yi Xue Shi* ('History of Chinese Medical Studies') by Pei Chi-Liu, published by Hwa Kang Press, Taiwan, 1974, pp. 294-295.

11. *Zhong Yi Tan Bing Xue* ('TCM Phlegm Disease Studies'), Hubei Science and Technology Press, 1984, p. 9.

12. Zhang Cong-Zheng, (1156-1228), was a native of Henan and the author of the *Ru Men Shi Qin* ('Confucians' Duties to their Parents'), a book which is a later compilation of ten other shorter works. The original *Ru Men Shi Qin* had only three chapters, and it is possible that some of the material in the larger work originated with Zi He's students. Zhang, of course, is the outstanding representative of the 'Purge the Pathogen School' (Gong Xie Pai). While he was strongly influenced by Liu Wan-Su, Zhang in his turn influenced not only Zhu Dan-Xi but also the later Febrile Disease school advocates.

13. *Yi Xue Ru Men* ('Introduction to Medicine' 1575), by Li Chan; Jiangxi Science and Technology Press, 1988, p. 733.

14. The Western insistence upon the mind-body dichotomy can give rise to such diverting sights as European commentators expressing incredulity at 'the Chinese tendency to somaticize their mental illnesses'. They are apparently unable to imagine the possibility that it is the Chinese who are clear-thinking enough to be able to discriminate between a disorder precipitated by emotions, and emotions precipitated by a physical disorder. As I heard one patient in China remark, 'I have all of the symptoms of anxiety: tightness of the chest and throat, queasy stomach, and restlessness;

but I have nothing to be anxious about! There must be some internal imbalance. Can you give me some herbs?' Westerners, on the other hand, tend to label this group of symptoms (and many others!) as 'anxiety', and then cast about until they can find something about which to be anxious. Needless to say, in the current climate of 'self-help' workshops and 'spiritual psychologies' which emphasize the excitation of emotions to fever pitch, such ideas as just expressed are unlikely to be popular. Still, it must be said that the Chinese idea of 'mental hygiene'—refusing to give unnecessary time to disturbing thoughts—is a concept we desperately need.

15. Quoted in *Zhong Yi Tan Bing Xue*, Zhu Ceng-Bo, Hubei Science and Technology Press, 1984, p. 9. This book is called 'Nan Yang' because Zhang Zhong-Jing, author of the *Shang Han Lun*, was from Nan Yang; he added 'Huo Ren' (i.e. to safeguard life) because Hua Tuo reputedly utilized this phrase in all his book titles. Originally it had been relatively straightforward 'Wu Qiu Zi's One Hundred Questions on Cold Injury'; *Wu Qiu Zi Shang Han Bai Wen*. Wu Qiu Zi means '(he who) seeks no sons': Zhu Gong's self-selected nickname.

16. *Yi Xue Ru Men* ('Introduction to Medicine', 1575), by Li Chan; Jiangxi Science and Technology Press, 1988, p. 732.

17. As he acknowledges in his prologue to *Ge Zhi Yu Lun* ('Enquiries into the Properties of Things', Jiangsu Science and Technology Press, 1985, pp. 4-5) where Dan Xi describes his own experiences in learning medicine.

18. This is not to say that Dan Xi's point is not valid: Spleen qi must be able to rise but most diuretic herbs have a downward action which would be counterproductive in the case of a weak Spleen qi barely able to lift itself. The approach in a case like this must be to promote Spleen transformation and transport, instead of simply trying to eliminate the excess damp, phlegm and thin mucus through the urine.

19. Wang Yin-Jun's book is named after two selections from the *Zhuang Zi*: The name of Chapter 3 'The Nourishment of the Director of Life' (i.e. the Dao) and a phrase from Chapter 23 in the 'Mixed Chapters': 'When the rebellious self is calmed, the person shines with the Celestial Light'.

20. Quoted in *Zhong Yi Tan Bing Xue* ('TCM Phlegm Disease Studies'), Zhu Ceng-Bo, Hubei Science and Technology Press, 1984, p. 11, and attributed to 'Treatises of Wang Yin-Jun' from the *Yi Shu* ('Techniques of Medicine', 1817, by Cheng Wen-You).

21. *Yi Guan* ('The Pervading Link of Medicine'), 1687, by Zhao Xian-Ke; People's Health Publishing, 1982, pp. 59-60.

22. *Hong Lu Dian Xue* ('A Spot of Snow on a Red Hot Stove'), 1630, by Gong Ju-Zhong, (?-1646), Ming Dynasty, Shanghai Science and Technology Press, 1982. The intriguing title of the book refers to the effect on Lung yin of vigorous fire. Gong was particularly expert in the treatment of 'Fei lao' ('Pulmonary Consumption Disorder').

23. *ibid.*, p. 125.

24. huan 缓 Wiseman translates 'moderate'.

25. *ibid.*, pp. 81-82.

26. *ibid.*, pp. 113-115.

27. *Ben Cao Gang Mu*, People's Health Publishing, 1978, vol. 3, p. 2054.

28. Wiseman calls guan ge 关格 'block and repulsion'.

29. 'Bai 败) means 'failed', 'bad', 'rotted', or 'unfresh' but its use in TCM carries with it the connotations of one of its early classical appearances, in the *Su Wen*, Chapter 58, 'Discussion of Qi Points':

> Qi Bo said: The meeting places between two strands of muscle may be large or small: the large are called valleys (gu) and the small are called streams (xi). So we say that between the muscles are valleys and streams, [which are where the protective and nutritive qi flow]. If a pathogen occupies this area, its interaction with the normal qi will lead to obstruction and then heat in the vessels (mai). When the heat is extreme, the flesh will rot (bai) from the effect of both the heat and the lack of nourishment, and the end result of this combined with the arrested flow of ying (nutritive) and wei (protective) qi will be the formation of pus. The heat will gradually intensify, eating away the flesh internally, while externally a large pustule will become evident. If this occurs around a joint, the very marrow of the joint will itself become pus, and in the end the joint will be destroyed (bai). *Huang Di Nei Jing Su Wen Shi Jie*, Le Qun Publishing, Taipei, 1976, p. 420.

30. *Zhen Jiu Da Cheng* ('The Great Compendium of Acupuncture'), People's Health Press, Beijing, 1984, p. 774.

31. *ibid.*, p. 833.

32. *ibid.*, p. 836.

33. *ibid.*, p. 959.

34. *ibid.*, p. 868.

35. *ibid.*, p. 862.

36. *ibid.*, pp. 1151-1152.

37. *Yi Men Fa Lu*, Shanghai Science and Technology Press, 1983, p. 182-183.

38. *ibid*, p. 189.

39. *ibid*, p. 189.

40. *Ye Shi Yi An Cun Zhen Shu Zhu* ('Annotated True Cases of Ye Tian–Shi'), Sichuan Science and Technology Press, 1984.

41. (轻可去实 'Qing ke qu shi'). 'Light' refers to the use of herbs with a mild qi spreading action, or light-weight herbs, or few herbs in tiny amounts; 'excess' means a pathogenic excess or excess from internal imbalance. So the method uses 'light' to overcome 'excess'.

Its potential area of application is very broad but in practice it is most commonly applied in upper Jiao pathologies.

For example, a surface excess from pathogenic wind-cold invasion can be treated with light pungent-warm surface openers such as *Ma Huang* (Ephedrae, Herba) and *Gui Zhi* (Cinnamomi Cassiae, Ramulus), combined with *Xing Ren* (Pruni Armeniacae, Semen) and *Gan Cao* (Glycyrrhizae Uralensis, Radix), to open the Lung qi so that the wind-cold is dispersed with the perspiration, and the 'excess' on the surface is eliminated.

Or pathogenic wind can affect the Lungs directly, closing them off and causing symptoms of sore throat, hoarseness and a sensation of tightness in the throat. The pungent flavor can be used to disperse the pathogen, with bitter to drain qi downwards; for example *Niu Bang Zi* (Arctii Lappae, Fructus), *Bo He* (Menthae, Herba), *Ma Bo* (Lasiosphaerae, Fructificatio), *Jin Yin Hua* (Lonicera Japonica, Flos), *She Gan* (Belamcandae Chinensis, Rhizoma), *Shan Dou Gen* (Sophorae Subprostratae, Radix), combined with *Xing Ren* (Pruni Armeniacae, Semen) and *Jie Geng* (Platycodi Grandiflori, Radix).

Ye Tian-Shi often said that 'formless pathogens can be inhaled through the mouth and the nose, and close off the upper orifice: one can only lightly clear and open Lung qi. If one tries to cool heat, cold descends, and [the effect] goes directly into the Stomach and Intestines, without relating in any way [with the problem] in the throat.'

One can also use the method in the case of anger leading to rebelling qi and the consequent loss of smooth Liver circulation affecting Lung contraction and descent. Then both Lungs and Liver are in 'excess' due to internal disharmony, and all of the body's qi is rebelling upward. The symptoms will be rapid breathing, dyspnea and wheeze, with distention of the chest and flanks; both urine and stool will be impeded. This condition is sometimes called 'Liver qi interfering with Lungs'. Light clearing openers and mild descending herbs can be used, such as *Pi Pa Ye* (Eriobotryae Japonicae, Folium), *Xuan Fu Hua* (Inulae, Flos), *Sang Bai Pi* (Mori Albae Radicis, Cortex), *Gua Lou Pi* (Trichosanthes, Pericarpium), *Xing Ren* (Pruni Armeniacae, Semen), *Chuan Bei Mu* (Fritillariae Cirrhosae, Bulbus) and *Zi Su Zi* (Perillae Fructescentis, Fructus). Several of these can be selected and combined to restore Liver movement and bring down Lung qi. The wheeze and dyspnea will be calmed and the chest and flank's comfort restored; and both stool and urine flow returned to normal.

Ye Tian-Shi was probably the most skilled of all in the agile use of this technique, which can regulate qi by simply mediating the qi mechanism, without the problems of excessive fragrance leading to dryness associated with most herbs in the 'qi-moving' class.

42. The Febrile Disease school, of which Ye Tian-Shi was a founding member, placed great emphasis upon the theory of the 'Five Movements and the Six Qi'. Wu Ju-Tong (1758-1836), a later authority in this area,

said 'The definition of wind-warmth is that in the early Spring yang qi begins to open, under the command of Jue Yin, and wind combines with warmth'. Ye Tian-Shi is pointing out that this patient's condition is a result, not only of his internal disharmonies, but of those disharmonies in relation to the seasonal changes in his environment.

43. 'The substance of Liver is yin, while its function is yang' is a quote from Tang Rong-Chuan (1862-1918) in the *Xue Zheng Lun* ('Discussion of Blood Syndromes', 1884), Shanghai Science and Technology Press, 1977, p. 163. An influential 'modern' classic, it is extensively quoted. The meaning is that Liver blood (its yin-natured 'substance') is essential for the proper movement of Liver qi (its yang-natured 'function').

44. *Su Wen*, Chapter 52: 'The vital concerns of the zang must be scrupulously observed: the Liver produces (sheng) on the left, Lungs store (cang) on the right'. (See also the chapter on fluid metabolism.) Statements such as this are often glossed by Western commentators as evidence of the faulty anatomical knowledge of the ancient Chinese. As should be abundantly clear by now, Chinese medicine is little concerned with anatomy as such but very greatly concerned indeed with the functional relationships within the body, and between the body and the external environment. To understand this statement, we must remember, as introduced earlier in this book, that the Chinese compass placed the South at the top, which was also the direction which the Emperor always faced on his throne, and to which houses were ideally oriented. Therefore, facing South, the morning sun would appear on the left, and the setting sun on the right. The rising growth of Wood energy, then, ascends on the left; the declining contraction of Metal (with its associations of evening and autumn quiet settling) descends on the right. As in the Heavens, so in the body.

45. *Ye Shi Yi An Cun Zhen Shu Zhu* ('Annotated True Cases of Ye Tian-Shi'), Sichuan Science and Technology Press, 1984, pp. 10-12.

46. *Yi Xiao Mi Chuan* ('Secret Transmissions of Medical Efficacy'), Qing dynasty, by Ye Tian-Shi; Zhong Hua Bookstore, Hong Kong Press, 1975, p. 27.

47. *Yi Bian* ('Fundamentals of Medicine'), Shanghai Science and Technology Press, 1982, pp. 115-116.

48. *Yi Xue Shi Zai Yi* ('The Study of Medicine is Actually Easy'), Fujian Science and Technology Press, pp. 5-6.

49. Wiseman has 'abduct' for 'dao' in his glossary, which means, in both modern and Classical Chinese, to 'lead', to 'guide', or, occasionally, to 'flow'. I agree that 'we should not fear an obscure term if it better suits our needs' but this seems to be stretching it.

50. *ibid.*, p. 91.

51. *Xue Zheng Lun* ('Discussion of Blood Syndromes', 1884), People's Health Publishing, Beijing, 1986, p. 176.

52. Jiang Xi-Quan, Chongqing City, Jiangjin District People's Hospital, in *Zhong Yi Za Zhi* ('Journal of Traditional Chinese Medicine'), Beijing, 1991, vol. 32, No. 12, p. 51, (in Chinese).

53. The equivalent passage in the *Jin Gui Yao Lue* ('Golden Cabinet') has 'floating and thready slippery'. See *Jin Gui Yao Lue*, Chapter 12, Section 20.

54. The word here translated as uprushing is 'jue' 厥, which Wiseman has as 'inversion', i.e. of the normal direction of energy. 'Jue' has at least seven different uses in Classical literature, from 'sudden collapse' to 'cold extremities' to 'uprushing' (e.g. as in 'jue yang' which means extreme yang, rising up without descent, unbalanced by yin). See the discussion by Porkert of the meaning of 'jue' on p. 38 of his *Theoretical Foundations of Chinese Medicine*, MIT Press, 1974.

55. *Zhu Bing Yuan Hou Lun Jiao Shi* ('Annotated Explanation of the Generalized Treatise on the Etiology and Symptomatolgy of Disease'), annotated by the Nanjing College of TCM, People's Health Publishing, 1983, pp. 607-611.

56. Li Zhai is better known as Xue Ji, 1488-1558, author of *Nu Ke Cuo Yao* ('Essentials of Gynecology and Obstetrics', 1548) and other works.

57. Wang Ang, in the *Ben Cao Bei Yao* ('Essentials of the Materia Medica', 1751), in his discussion of *Chen Pi* (Citri Reticulatae, Pericarpium) quotes Zhu Dan-Xi as saying that 'Stomach qi also depends upon phlegm for nourishment (Wei lai tan yi yang), so that it should not be completely eradicated, because if it is the deficiency will become worse'. (*Ben Cao Bei Yao*, Taichong, Taiwan, Chao Ren Publishing, 1980, p. 270.) Wang Ang is incorrect here in two points, however. The first is in suggesting that the Stomach qi depends upon phlegm, which is by definition pathological. The second is in his quote itself. Dan Xi says, in both the *Dan Xi Xin Fa* and the parallel passage in the *Dan Xi Zhi Fa Xin Yao*, 'If there is phlegm in the middle Jiao, which the Stomach also relies upon for support, then one cannot attack unrestrainedly, otherwise it will cause deficiency'. This is Zhang's point too: excessive drying of phlegm will damage Stomach functioning, through parching yin and through removing the substances which the Stomach, as a Fu-organ, must pass on.

58. *Jing Yue Quan Shu* ('Complete Works of Jing Yue', 1624) Shanghai Science and Technology Press, 1959, pp. 530-532.

59. Here I suspect Zhang Jing-Yue did not mean the formula from the *Yi Fan Lei Ju*, which is aimed at moving qi and moistening the bowel, but meant rather Zhu Dan-Xi's Sou Feng Hua Tan Wan ('Seek the Wind and Cut the Phlegm Pill') which is made up of:

Ren Shen	30 g	Ginseng, Radix
Jiang Can	30 g	Bombyx Batryticatus
Bai Fan	30 g	Alum
Chen Pi	30 g	Citri Reticulatae, Pericarpium
Tian Ma	30 g	Gastrodiae Elatae, Rhizoma
Jing Jie	30 g	Schizonepetae Tenuifoliae, Herba et Flos
Huai Jiao Zi	30 g	Sophora Japonicae, Semen
Ban Xia	120 g	Pinelliae Ternata, Rhizoma
Chen Sha	15 g	Cinnabaris

60. *Jing Yue Quan Shu* ('Complete Works of Jing Yue', 1624), Shanghai Science and Technology Press, 1959, pp. 190.

61. Xu lao 虚劳 Wiseman translates as 'vacuity taxation'.

62. *ibid.*, p. 190.

63. A modern note to this says: 'Due to poor anatomical expertise, the ancients had this inaccurate statement'. But it seems to me that it is the modern commentators themselves who have failed to grasp that 'the ancients' are not talking anatomy at all but rather functional activity. (Nonetheless, it is coming to light that previous conceptions of the supposedly meagre anatomical knowledge of the ancient Chinese have undervalued their achievements in this field.) This is explained clearly in the very next line: 'it must rely on the qi transformation of the San Jiao before it can begin to come out'. In other words, the Urinary Bladder can accept fluids freely but it cannot expel fluids by itself (hence 'no lower outlet'), relying for this upon the San Jiao qi transformation and, ultimately, the power of Kidney yang.

64. See Chapter 1 under Blood and jin and ye fluids for the classical quote describing this process.

65. 膻中 Shan Zhong, the 'Upper Sea of Qi', not the point of the same name. The qi in this upper sea is the zong ('gathering') qi so necessary for channel qi movement.

66. 'Mo yuan'. This concept is described as the internal equivalent of the subcutaneous 'cou li' (crevices of the surface tissues), where the San Jiao movement of yuan qi occurs.

67. *Du Yi Sui Bi* ('Random Notes while Reading Medicine'), 1898, by Zhou Xue-Hai, Jiangsu Science and Technology Press, 1983, pp. 114-115.

68. From the *Lei Zheng Zhi Cai* ('Tailored Treatments Arranged According to Pattern') by Lin Pei-Qin, d.1839, quoted in the *Zhong Yi Li Dai Yi Lun Xuan* ('Selected Medical Essays by Traditional Chinese Doctors of Past Generations'), 1983, edited by Wang Xin-Hua, published by the Jiangsu Science and Technology Press, 1983, p. 400.

Major contributors to phlegm theory

Date	Origin	Aspect introduced
475 BC	*Huang Di Nei Jing* Chapter 71	Thin mucus (yin) first mentioned
210 AD (Han Dynasty)	*Jin Gui Yao Lue* , by **Zhang Zhong-Jing** : Chapters on Tan-yin, Shui Qi, and Cough	Phlegm and thin mucus first mentioned
610 AD (Sui Dynasty)	*Zhu Bing Yuan Hou Lun* ('General Treatise on the Etiology and Symptomatology of Disease') by **Chao Yuan-Fang**	First clear differentiation between phlegm and thin mucus. Description of hot-phlegm, cold-phlegm, knotted-phlegm and other phlegm types
652 AD (Tang Dynasty)	*Qian Jin Yao Fang* ('Thousand Ducat Formulas') by **Sun Si-Miao** (c. 581-682)	Assigns specific treatment approaches to certain phlegm categories
1112 (Southern Song Dynasty)	*Sheng Ji Zong Lu* ('Comprehensive Recording of the Sages' Benefits') ordered by the emperor **Zhao Ji**	Lists 96 formulas divided among eight categories of phlegm and thin mucus
1174 (Southern Song Dynasty)	*San Yin Ji Yi Bing Zheng Fang Lun* ('Discussion of Illnesses, Patterns, and Formulas Related to the Unification of the Three Etiologies') by **Chen Yan**	Describes the origins of phlegm from internal factors (e.g. emotions), external factors (e.g. weather) and other factors (e.g. diet)
1156 –1228 (Jin Dynasty)	**Zhang Cong-Zheng** (zi-name **Zi-He**), author of the *Ru Men Shi Qin* ('Confucians' Duties to their Parents')	Differentiates phlegm into wind-phlegm, hot-phlegm, damp-phlegm, and food-phlegm, introduces concept of 'phlegm misting the Heart'
1281–1358 (Yuan Dynasty)	**Zhu Dan-Xi** , author of *Dan Xi Xin Fa* ('Teachings of Zhu Dan-Xi'), *Jin Gui Gou Xuan* ('Scythe of Mysteries from the Golden Cabinet') and *Ju Fang Fa Hui* ('Exposition of the Formulas from the Imperial Grace Formulary')	Describes phlegm tendency to gather and disperse; notes that phlegm can be formed through qi deficiency, qi blockage or qi in counter-flow
(Yuan Dynasty)	**Wang Gui** (**Wang Yin-Jun**), author of the *Tai Ding Yang Sheng Zhu Lun* ('Treatises on the Calm and Settled Nourishment of the Director of Life', 1338)	Originator of the famous 'Gun Tan Wan' ('Vaporize Phlegm Pill'). Describes the extremely varied symptomatic manifestations of phlegm
1518–1593 (Ming Dynasty)	**Li Shi-Zhen** , author of the *Ben Cao Gang Mu* (the great Materia Medica), *Bin Hu Mai Xue* (on pulse), and the *Qi Jing Ba Mai Kao* (on the eight extra channels)	The *Ben Cao Gang Mu* records over three hundred formulas to treat phlegm, and outlines eight distinct categories of phlegm treatment
(Ming Dynasty)	**Zhao Xian-Ke**, author of the *Yi Guan* ('The Pervading Link of Medicine', 1617)	Famous exponent of the Mingmen School; also expert *I Jing* scholar; emphasizes the importance of the Kidneys in phlegm treatment
1563–1640 (Ming Dynasty)	**Zhang Jie-Bin** (zi-name *Jing-Yue*), whose works include the *Lei Jing* ('Systematic Categorization of the *Nei Jing* '), the *Lei Jing Tu Yi* ('Illustrated Wing to the *Lei Jing* '), the *Zhi Yi Lun* ('Record of Questions and Doubt') and the *Jing Yue Quan Shu* ('The Complete Works of Jing Yue')	Explains phlegm pathology in great detail, with particular regard to Mingmen; describes phlegm arising from deficiency, criticizes currently prevalent phlegm treatments, and emphasizes that phlegm treatment must necessarily address the root
1601 (Ming Dynasty)	**Yang Ji-Zhou**, author of the *Zhen Jiu Da Cheng* ('Great Compendium of Acupuncture and Moxibustion')	While not discussing phlegm phenomena in depth, individual point indications and point selections for illnesses reveal a sophisticated grasp of phlegm mechanisms in pathology
?–1646 (Ming Dynasty)	**Gong Ju-Zhong**, author of *Hong Lu Dian Xue* ('A Spot of Snow on a Red Hot Stove', 1630)	Studies the symptomatology and treatment of phlegm-fire, and describes in great detail the mechanisms of pathology and the possible mistakes in differentiation and treatment of this condition
c. 1585–1664 (Ming and Qing Dynasties)	**Yu Chang** , author of the *Yi Men Fa Lu* ('Precepts for Physicians', 1658)	Sets out twelve rules of 'Forbidden Uses of Herbs' in phlegm treatments
1667–1746	**Ye Tian-Shi** , author of the *Wen Re Lun* ('Discussion of Warmth and Heat')	Contributes to phlegm theory development both discursively and through recorded case histories with comments on practical treatment approaches
1694–1764 (Qing Dynasty)	**He Meng-Yao**, author of *Fu Ke Liang Fang* ('Prescriptions for Gynecology'), *Yi Bian* ('Fundamentals of Medicine'), and *You Ke Liang Fang* ('Prescriptions for Pediatrics'), among others	Refines certain aspects of phlegm diagnosis, pointing out, for example, that thick yellow phlegm may indicate cold, and thin clear mucus can indicate intense heat

Type of phlegm	Location of phlegm	Primary factors in diagnosis			Biomedical examples (with TCM conditions)
		Phlegm appearance	Major symptoms (other symptoms)	Tongue and tongue coat	
Exogenous wind-phlegm	Lungs	White, thin, and a bit frothy	Recent cough (chills, fever and tickle in the throat)	Thin white tongue coat	Acute bronchitis (wind-phlegm invading Lungs)
Qi-phlegm	Channels and collaterals, Liver, or Heart	(Phlegm may not be visibly evident)	Soft painless nodes in the neck, breast, or inguinal region without changes in skin color; (plum-stone throat; stuffy chest; mood swings; apathy; poor concentration)	Thin greasy tongue coat	Thyroid enlargement, or swollen lymph glands (qi-phlegm forming nodes) Depression (qi-phlegm oppressing the Spirit)
Hot-phlegm or Phlegm-fire	Lungs	Thick, sticky (or yellow with pus; or streaks of blood)	Red face, thirst (possibly fever)	Yellow greasy tongue coat	Pneumonia (hot-phlegm pent up in the Lungs)
	Heart and/or Liver	(Phlegm may not be visibly evident)	Anxious restless feeling in the chest, nightmares, bitter taste and dry mouth (fury or other loss of mental equilibrium, red eyes, sound of phlegm in the throat, stroke, or even coma)	Tongue body red	Neurasthenia (phlegm-fire disturbing the Heart) Mania and Hysteria (phlegm-fire overwhelming the Heart) CVA (phlegm-fire inciting internal wind)
Endogenous wind- phlegm	Liver	Thick, profuse (or if not visibly evident, may yet be heard in voice)	Hemiplegia, facial paralysis, cramps, epilepsy and difficulty swallowing, sound of phlegm in the throat	Thin white or thin greasy tongue coat	Cerebral thrombosis or embolism (wind-phlegm entering the collaterals) Epilepsy (intermittent wind-phlegm obstruction)
Damp-phlegm	Lungs	Profuse white sticky and easy-to-expectorate; thick phlegmy-sounding cough	Tightness in the chest, loss of appetite and possibly loose stool	Tongue coat greasy white	Chronic bronchitis (damp-phlegm obstructing Lungs)
	Liver, Heart, Spleen and Stomach, Intestines	(Phlegm may not be visibly evident, or if in the Spleen, Stomach or Intestines there may be vomiting of watery fluid or phlegm)	Excessive weight gain, dizziness, heaviness of the head as if wrapped, excessive saliva, fullness in the chest, poor concentration, reduced appetite, borborygmus		Vertigo, hypertension (turbid-phlegm welling upward) Irritable Bowel Syndrome (thin mucus in the Intestines)
Blood stagnation-phlegm	Heart	(Phlegm may not be visibly evident)	Tightness in the chest, occasional chest pain	Tongue coat greasy white	Coronary heart disease, angina (stagnation-phlegm in chest)
	Liver	(Phlegm may not be visibly evident, but heard in throat)	Numbness of the limbs, stiff tongue with difficult speech	Tongue body dark purple	Sequela of stroke (internal wind and stagnation-phlegm)
	Channels and collaterals	(Phlegm may not be visibly evident, except as swelling)	Joint pain and swelling with restricted movement and deformity of the joints		Chronic rheumatism or arthritis (stagnation-phlegm bi-syndrome)
	Spleen and Stomach	Vomiting of phlegm and/or dark blood	Chest or epigastric pain, difficulty swallowing		Gastric ulcer, gastric carcinoma (qi-blockage and stagnation-phlegm)
Parched- phlegm	Lungs	A slight amount of sticky stretchy phlegm, difficult to cough out	Dry cough, dry nose and throat, dry mouth, dry stool, scanty urine, dry skin and possible fever	Tongue coat thin white and dry, may be red tip to the tongue	Acute laryngitis, pharyngitis, or bronchitis (parched-phlegm disturbing Lungs)
Cold-phlegm	Lungs	Profuse white thin and very frothy.	Pallor, aversion to cold, dyspnea.	Tongue coat white and slippery; tongue body pale	Chronic bronchitis (cold-phlegm hidden in Lungs)
	Channels and collaterals	May not be visibly evident)	Sore aching joints with local swelling but no change in skin color and no local heat		Nodules of the joints (congealed cold-phlegm obstruction)

Type of damp		Clinical manifestations
Exogenous damp	Surface damp	Aversion to cold, low-grade fever, tight aching head, heavy lethargy, malaise, tiredness, stuffy chest, lack of thirst, tongue coat thin white slippery, pulse floating soft and languid
	Cold damp	Generalized aching of the body, heavy painful joints restricting movement, edema of the limbs, lack of sweating, loose stool, tongue coat white greasy, pulse floating soft and slow
	Summerheat damp	Vomiting and diarrhea, fever with sweating, sensations of fullness in the chest and abdomen, loss of appetite, tongue coat white and slippery, pulse floating soft and weak
	Warm damp	Headache, chills and fever, sallow pale hue, generalized heaviness and aching, apathy, stuffy chest, no thirst or hunger, tongue coat white, pulse wiry thready or floating and soft
Endogenous damp	Damp obstructing the upper Jiao	Heavy head, dizziness, stuffy fullness of the chest and epigastric area, loss of taste, poor appetite, white greasy tongue coat
	Damp obstructing the middle Jiao	Abdominal distention and fullness, protracted epigastric fullness after eating, nausea, weak heavy limbs, loose stool and diarrhea, thick white greasy tongue coat
	Damp pouring down to the lower Jiao	Edema of the feet, murky difficult urination, loose stool, leukorrhea in women, scrotal sweating or eczema in men, genital itching
	Damp heat ascending	Redness and swelling of the eyes and lids with exudation, ulceration of the oral cavity and tongue
	Damp heat moving into and blocking the surface tissues	Eczema, boils and weeping lesions of the skin
	Damp heat pouring into the joints	Redness, pain and swelling of the joints
	Wind damp blocking the bones and joints	Wandering pain in the joints
	Cold damp obstructing the channels and collaterals	Localized numbness or loss of sensation

Major Writers

Cao Xiao-Zhong, Song Dynasty	曹孝忠
Chao Yuan-Fang, Sui Dynasty	巢元方
Chen Lian-Fang, 1840-1914	陈莲舫
Chen Meng-Lei, ?-1741	陈梦雷
Chen Nian-Zu, 1753-1823 Zi-name: Chen Xiu-Yuan	陈念祖 陈修圆
Chen Shi-Duo, Qing Dynasty	陈士铎
Chen Shi-Gong, 1555-1636	陈实功
Chen Shi-Wen, Song Dynasty	陈师文
Chen Shu-Yu, Qing Dynasty	陈树玉
Chen Wu-Zi (see Chen Yan)	
Chen Xiu-Yuan (see Chen Nian-Zu)	
Chen Yan, Southern Song Dynasty Zi-name: Chen Wu-Ze	陈言 陈无择
Chen Zi-Ming, 1190-1270	陈自明
Cheng Guo-Peng, 1679-? Zi-name: Cheng Zhong-Ling	程国彭 程钟龄
Cheng Wen-You, Qing Dynasty	程文囿
Cheng Wu-Ji, 1066-c.1156	成无己
Cheng Zhong-Ling (see Cheng Guo-Peng)	
Da Ming (see Ri Hua-Zi)	大明
Dai Si-Gong (see Dai Yuan-Li)	
Dai Yuan-Li, 1324-1405 Zi-name: Dai Si-Gong	戴原礼 戴思恭

306

Deng Tie-Tao, 20th Century	邓鉄涛
Dong Su, Ming Dynasty	董宿
Dou Mo, 1196-1280	窦默
Fang Xian, Ming Dynasty	方贤
Fu Ren-Yu, Qing Dynasty Zi-name: Fu Yun-Ke	傅仁宇 傅允科
Fu Yun-Ke (see Fu Ren-Yu)	
Gao Wu, Ming Dynasty	高武
Ge Hong, 283-343	葛洪
Gong Ju-Zhong, ?-1646 Zi-name: Gong Ying-Yuan	龚居中 龚应圆
Gong Ting-Xian, Ming Dynasty Zi-name: Gong Zi-Cai	龚廷贤 龚子才
Gong Wen-De, 20th Century	龚文德
Gong Xin, Ming Dynasty Zi-name: Gong Rui-Zhi	龚信 龚瑞芝
Guo Ai-Chun, 20th Century	郭爱春
Guo Qian-Heng, 20th Century	郭谦亨
Han Mao, Ming Dynasty	韩蚤
He Meng-Yao, 1694-1764	何梦瑶
He Xi-Ting, 20th Century	何熹廷
Ho Peng Yoke, 20th Century	
Hong Ji, Ming Dynasty Zi-name: Hong Jiu-You	洪基 洪九有
Hu Xiang-Ji, 20th Century	胡洋吉
Hua Tuo, ?-c.203	华佗
Huang Fu-Zhong, Ming Dynasty Zi-name: Huang Yun-Zhou	皇甫中 皇云洲
Huang Gong-Xiu, Qing Dynasty	黄宫绣
Huang Yuan-Yu, 1705-1758 Also known as Huang Yu-Lu	黄元御 黄玉路
Jia Suo-Xue, Late Ming Dynasty Zi-name: Jia Jiu-Ru	贾所学 贾九如
Jiang Sen, 20th Century	蒋森
Jiang Xi-Quan, 20th Century	江锡权
Kong Bo-Hua, 1885-1955	孔伯华

Kou Zong-Shi, c.-1117	寇宗奭
Li Chan, 1120-1200 Zi-name: Li Jian-Zhai	李梴 李健斋
Li Cong-Fu, 20th Century	李聪甫
Li Dong-Yuan (see Li Gao)	
Li Gao, 1180-1251 Zi-name: Li Dong-Yuan	李杲 李东垣
Li Shi-Zhen, 1518-1593	李时珍
Li Qi-xian 20th Century	李启贤
Li Yong-Cui, Early Qing Dynasty Zi-name: Li Xiu-Zhi	李用粹 李修之
Li Zhai (See Xue Ji)	立斋
Li Zhen-Tong, Qing Dynasty	李珍同
Li Zhong-Zi, 1588-1655 Zi-name: Li Shi-Cai	李中梓 李士才
Lin Pei-Qin, 1772-1839 Zi-name: Li Yun-He	林佩琴 林云和
Liu Chun, Ming Dynasty	刘纯
Liu Pei-Chi, 20th Century	刘伯骥
Liu Wan-Su, 1120-1200 Zi-name: Liu Shou-Zhen	刘完素 刘守真
Lou Ying, 1320-1389	楼英
Maciocia, Giovanni, 20th Century	
Meng Shen, 621-713	孟詵
Ni Zhu-Mo, Late Ming Dynasty	倪朱谟
Pang An-Shi, 1042-1099	庞安时
Pei-Chi Liu (See Liu Pei-Chi)	
Peng Xian-Zhang, 20th Century	彭宪彰
Porkert, Manfred, 20th Century	
Qian Yi, 1035-1117 Zi-name: Qian Zhong-Yang	钱乙 钱仲阳
Qin Bo-Wei, 1901-1970	秦伯未
Qin Zhi-Zhen, Qing Dynasty Zi-name: Qin Huang-Shi	秦之桢 秦皇士
Ri Hua Zi, Tang Dynasty Also known as Da Ming	日华子 大明

Said, Edward, 1935-

Shen Jin-Ao, 1717-1776 沈金鳌

Shi Fei-Nan, Qing Dynasty 石芾南
Zi-name: Shi Shou-Tang 石寿棠

Shi Shi-Sheng, 20th Century 施士生

Shi Shou-Tang (see Shi Fei-Nan)

Sun Ren-Cun, Song Dynasty 孙仁存

Sun Si-Miao, c.581-622AD 孙思邈

Tang Rong-Chuan (see Tang Zong-Hai)

Tang Zong-Hai, 1862-1918 唐宗海
Zi-name: Tang Rong-Chuan 唐容川

Tao Hong-Jing, 452-536AD 陶弘景

Unschuld, Paul, 20th Century

Wang Ang, 1615-c.1695 汪昂

Wang Gui, Yuan Dynasty 王桂
Also known as Wang Yin-Jun 王隐君

Wang Hao-Gu, 1200-1308 王好古

Wang Hong-Xu, Qing Dynasty 王洪绪
Zi-name: Wang Wei-De 王维德

Wang Ken-Tang, 1549-1613 王肯堂
Zi-name: Wang Yu-Tai 王宇泰

Wang Meng-Ying (see Wang Shi-Xiong)

Wang Qing-Ren, 1768-1831 王清任

Wang Ru-Kun, 20th Century 王汝琨

Wang Shi-Xiong, 1808-1868 王士雄
Zi-name: Wang Meng-Ying 王梦英

Wang Shu-He, Wei-Jin Period 王叔和

Wang Tao, 670-755 王焘

Wang Wei-De (see Wang Hong-Xu)

Wang Xin-Hua, 20th Century 王新华

Wang Yin-Jun (see Wang Gui)

Wei Yi-Lin, 1277-1347 危亦林

Wei Zhi-Xiu, 1722-1772 魏之琇
Hao-name: Liu Zhou 柳洲

Weng Wei-Jian, 20th Century 翁维健

Wu Cheng, Early Qing Dynasty	吴澄
Wu Chun-Fu, Ming Dynasty	吴春甫
Wu Ju-Tong (see Wu Tang)	
Wu Kun, 1552-c.1620	吴崑
Wu Min, Ming Dynasty Zi-name: Wu Jin-Shan	吴旻 吴进山
Wu Qian, Qing Dynasty	吴谦
Wu Qiu-Zi (see Zhu Gong)	
Wu Shang-Xian, c.1806-1886 Zi-name: Wu Shi-Ji	吴尚先 吴师机
Wu Shi-Ji (see Wu Shang-Xian)	
Wu Shi-Kai, Qing Dynasty	吴世铠
Wu Song-Kang, 20th Century	吴颂康
Wu Tang, 1758-1836 Zi-name: Wu Ju-Tong	吴瑭 吴鞠通
Wu You-Ke, Ming Dynasty Zi-name: Wu You-Xing	吴又可 吴有性
Xiu-Yuan (see Chen Nian-Zu)	
Xu Shu-Wei, 1079-c.1154 Also known as Xu Xue-Shi	许叔微 许学士
Xu Xue-Shi "The Scholar Xu" (see Xu Shu-Wei)	
Xu Yan-Chun, ?-1384 Zi-name: Xu Yong-Cheng,	徐彦纯 徐用诚
Xu Yong-Cheng (see Xu Yan-Chun)	
Xue Ji, 1487-1559 Hao-name: Li Zhai	薛己 立斋
Xue Sheng-Bai (see Xue Xue)	
Xue Xue, 1681-1770 Zi-name: Xue Sheng Bai	薛雪 薛生白
Yan Yong-He, c.1206-1268	严用和
Yang Ji Zhou, 1522-1620	杨继洲
Ye Gui, 1667-1746 Zi-name: Ye Tian-Shi	叶桂 叶天士
Ye Lin, 1862-1908	叶霖
Ye Tian-Shi (see Ye Gui)	
Ye Xi-Chun, 1881-1968	叶熙春

You Yi, ?-1749	尤怡
Yu Bo, 1438-c.1517 Zi-name: Yu Tian-Min	虞搏 虞天民
Yu Chang, c.1585-1664	喻昌
Yu Gen-Chu, 1734-1799	俞根初
Yu Ying-Tai, Ming Dynasty	俞应泰
Zhang Cong-Zheng, 1156-1228 Zi-name: Zhang Zi-He	张从正 张子和
Zhang Jie-Bin, 1563-1640 Zi-name: Zhang Jing-Yue	张介宾 张景岳
Zhang Jing-Yue (see Zhang Jie-Bin)	
Zhang Lu, 1617-1699 Zi-name: Zhang Lu-Yu	张璐 张璐玉
Zhang Nan, Qing Dynasty Zi-name: Zhang Xu-Gu	章楠 章虚谷
Zhang Shan-Lei, 1873-1934	张山雷
Zhang Shou-Kong, Ming Dynasty Zi-name: Zhang Xin-Ru	张受孔 张心如
Zhang Xi-Chun, 1860-1933	张锡纯
Zhang Xu-Gu (see Zhang Nan)	
Zhang Yin-An (see Zhang Zhi-Cong)	
Zhang Zhi-Cong, 1610-1674 Zi-name: Zhang Yin-An	张志聪 张隐庵
Zhang Zi-He (see Zhang Cong-Zheng)	
Zhao Fen-Zhu, 20th Century	赵棻主
Zhao Ji, 1082-1135 (Song Emperor, ordered compilation of the Sheng Ji Zong Lu by Cao Xiao Zhong)	赵佶
Zhao Jin-Duo, 20th Century	赵金铎
Zhao Xian-Ke, Ming Dynasty	赵献可
Zhen Li-Yan, 542-627AD	甄立言
Zheng Xian-Li, 20th Century	郑显理
Zhou Shen-Zhai (see Zhou Zhi-Gan)	
Zhou Xue-Hai, 1856-1906	周学海
Zhu Ceng-Bo, 20th Century	朱曾柏
Zhu Dan-Xi (see Zhu Zhen-Heng)	

Zhu Gong, Ming Dynasty
Hao-name: Wu Qiu-Zi

朱肱
无求子

Zhu Zhen-Heng, 1282-1358
Also known as Zhu Dan-Xi

朱震亨
朱丹溪

Zhou Zhi-Gan, c.1508-1586
Hao-name: Zhou Shen-Zhai

周之幹
周慎斋

Bibliography

Ba Shi Yi Nan Jing Ji Jie
(Collected Explanations of the Classic of Eighty-One Difficulties), ed. by Guo Ai-Chun and Guo Hong-Tu, Tianjin Science and Technology Press, 1984.

《八十一难经集解》，郭爱春等

Ben Cao Bei Yao
(Essentials of the Materia Medica), Wang Ang, 1664; Taichung, Taiwan, Chao Ren Publishing, 1980.

《本草备要》，汪昂

Ben Cao Gang Mu
(The Great Materia Medica), Li Shi-Zhen, 1596; People's Health Publishing, Beijing, 1978.

《本草纲目》，李时珍

Ben Cao Hui Yan
(Treasury of Words on the Materia Medica), Ni Zhu-Mo, 1624.

《本草汇言》，倪朱谟

Ben Cao Jing Shu Ji Yao
(Abstracts of the Essential Commentaries on the Materia Medica), Wu Shi-Kai, 1809.

《本草经疏辑要》，吴世铠

Ben Cao Qiu Zhen
(Search for Truth in the Materia Medica), Huang Gong-Xiu, 1773; Shanghai Science and Technology Press, 1979.

《本草求真》，黄宫绣

Ben Cao Yao Yi
(Extension of the Materia Medica), Kou Zong-Shi, 1116.

《本草衍义》，寇宗奭

Ben Cao Yan Yi Bu Yi
(Supplement to the Extension of the Materia Medica), Zhu Dan-Xi, c. 1347.

《本草衍义补遗》，朱丹溪

Ben Cao Yue Yan
(Survey of the Materia Medica), Xue Ji, c. 1550.

《本草约言》，薛己

Ben Cao Zheng Yi
(The Rectified Materia Medica), Zhang Shan-Lei,
1917.

《本草正义》，张山雷

Ben Jing Feng Yuan
(Journey to the Origin of the Materia Medica
Classic), Zhang Lu, 1695.

《本经逢原》，张璐

Bian Zheng Lu
(Records of Differentiation of Symptoms),
Chen Shi-Duo, 1687.

《辨证录》，陈士铎

Bin Hu Mai Xue
(The Pulse Studies of Bin Hu), Li Shi-Zhen, 1564.

《濒湖脉学》，李时珍

Bin Hu Mai Xue Xin Shi
(New Explanation of the Pulse Studies of Bin
Hu), Wang Ru-Kun; Henan Science and
Technology Press, 1983.

《濒湖脉学新释》，王泅琨

Bu Ju Ji
(Anthology of Up-to-Date Prescriptions),
Wu Cheng, 1739.

《不居集》，吴澄

Chong Ding Tong Su Shang Han Lun
(Revised Popular Guide to the Discussion of
Cold-induced Disorders), Yu Gen-Chu, 1776.

《重订通俗伤寒论》，俞根初

Dan Xi Xin Fa
(Teachings of Dan Xi), Zhu Dan-Xi, 1481.

《丹溪心法》，朱丹溪

Dan Xi Zhi Fa Xin Yao
(Essentials from the Teachings of Dan Xi);
Shandong Science and Technology Press, 1985.

《丹溪治法心要》，朱丹溪

Du Yi Sui Bi
(Random Notes While Reading Medicine), Zhou
Xue-Hai, 1898; Jiangsu Science and Technology
Press, 1985.

《读医随笔》，周学海

Forgotten Traditions of Ancient Chinese
Medicine, Paul Unschuld, Paradigm Publications,
1990.

Formulas and Strategies: Chinese Herbal
Medicine, Dan Bensky and Randall Barolet,
Eastland Press, 1990.

Fu Ke Liang Fang
(Prescriptions for Gynecology), He Meng-Yao,
c. 1755.

《妇科良方》，何梦瑶

Fu Ren Da Quan Liang Fang
(The Complete Fine Formulas for Women), Chen
Zi-Ming, 1237; Jiangxi People's Publishing, 1983.

《妇人大全良方》，陈自明

Fu Ren Gui
(Standards of Gynecology), Zhang Jing-Yue,
1636; Guangdong Science and Technology Press,
1984.

《妇人规》，张景岳

Fu Shou Jing Fang
(Exquisite Formulas for Fostering Longevity), Wu
Min, 1534.

《扶寿精方》，吴旻

Ge Zhi Yu Lun
(Inquiries into the Properties of Things),
Zhu Dan-Xi, 1347; Jiangsu Science and
Technology Press, 1985.

《格致余论》，朱丹溪

Gu Jin Tu Shu Ji Cheng: Yi Bu Quan Lu
(Collection of Books and Illustrations Past and
Present: Complete Records of the Medical
Section), Chen Meng-Lei et al., 1725;
People's Health Publishing, 1988.

《古今图书集成
医部全录》，
陈梦雷

Gu Jin Yi Jian
(Medical Reflections Ancient and Modern), Gong
Xin, 1589.

《古今医鉴》，龚信

Gu Jin Yi Tong
(Unification of Medicine Past and Present),
Xu Chun-Fu, 1556.

《古今医统》，徐春甫

Han Shi Yi Tong
(Comprehensive Medicine According to Master
Han), Han Mao, 1522; Jiangsu Science and
Technology Press, 1985.

《韩氏医通》，韩悉

Hong Lu Dian Xue
(A Spot of Snow on a Red Hot Stove), Gong Ju-
Zhong, 1630; Shanghai Science and Technology
Press, 1982.

《红炉点雪》，龚居中

Huang Di Nei Jing Su Wen Ji Zhu
(Collected Annotations to the Su Wen), Zhang
Yin-An, 1670; Shanghai Science and Technology
Press, 1980.

《黄帝内经素问集注》，张隐庵

I Ching
(Book of Changes), Wilhelm/Baynes edition,
Routledge and Keegan Paul, London, 1971.

《易经》

Ji Sheng Fang
(Formulas to Aid the Living), Yan Yong-He, 1253.

《济生方》，严用和

Ji Sheng Xu Fang
(More Formulas to Aid the Living),
Yan Yong-He, 1267.

《济生续方》，严用和

Jin Gui Gou Xuan
(Scythe of Mysteries of the Golden Cabinet),
Zhu Dan-Xi, Yuan Dynasty.

《金匮钩玄》，朱丹溪

Jin Gui Yi
(Supplement to the Golden Cabinet), You Yi,
1768.

《金匮翼》，尤怡

Jing Yue Quan Shu
(The Complete Works of Jing-Yue), Zhang Jing-
Yue, 1624; Shanghai Science and Technology
Press, 1959.

《景岳全书》，张景岳

Ju Fang Fa Hui
(Expositions of the Formulas from the Imperial
Grace Formulary), Zhu Dan-Xi, Yuan Dynasty.

《局方发挥》，朱丹溪

Lan Shi Mi Cang
(Secrets from the Orchid Chamber),
Li Dong-Yuan, 1336.

《兰室秘藏》，李东垣

Lei Jing
(Systematic Categorization of the Nei Jing),
Zhang Jing-Yue, 1624; People's Health
Publishing, 1982.

《类经》，张景岳

Lei Jing Tu Yi
(Illustrated Wings to the Systematic
Categorization of the Nei Jing), Zhang Jing-Yue,
1624; People's Health Publishing, 1982.

《类经图翼》，张景岳

Lei Zheng Pu Ji Ben Shi Fang
(Classified Formulas of Universal Benefit from my
Practice), Xu Shu-Wei, 1150.

《类证普济本事方》，许叔微

Lei Zheng Zhi Cai
(Tailored Treatments According to Pattern),
Lin Pei-Qin, 1839.

《类证治裁》，林珮琴

Li, Qi and Shu: An Introduction to Science and
Civilization in China, Ho Peng Yoke, Hong Kong
University Press, 1985.

Li Yue Pian Wen
(A Rhyming Discourse on New Therapeutics), Wu
Shi-Ji, 1864; People's Health Publishing, 1984.

《理瀹骈文》，吴师机

Lin Zheng Zhi Nan Yi An
(Medical Records as a Guide to Clinical Patterns),
Ye Tian-Shi, 1766; Shanghai Science and
Technology, 1991.

《临证指南医案》，叶天士

Ling Shu Jing Jiao Shi (2 vols.)
(Comparative Explanation of the Ling Shu),
Hebei Medical Institute; People's Health
Publishing, 1982.

《灵枢经校释》，河北医学院

Lu Shan Tang Lei Bian
(Catalogued Differentiations from Lu Shan Hall),
Zhang Zhi-Cong, 1670; Jiangsu Science and
Technology Press, 1982.

《侣山堂类辨》，张志聪

Lun Zhong Yi Tan Bing Xue Shuo
(Discussion on TCM Phlegm Theory),
Zhu Ceng-Bo; Hubei People's Press, 1981.

《论中医痰病学说》，朱曾柏

Mai Jing
(Pulse Classic), Wang Shu-He, 242AD;
People's Health Publishing, 1984.

《脉经》，王叔和

Ming Yi Bie Lu
(Miscellaneous Records of Famous Physicians),
Tao Hong-Jing, c. 500AD.

《名医别录》，陶弘景

Ming Yi Zhi Zhang
(Displays of Enlightened Physicians), Huang Fu-
Zhong, 16th Century; People's Health Publishing,
1982.

《明医指掌》，皇甫中

Nei Ke Zhai Yao
(Summary of Internal Medicine), Yu Ying-Tai,
mid-19th Century.

《内科摘要》，俞应泰

Nan Jing Zheng Yi
(The Correct Meaning of the Nan Jing), Ye Lin,
1895; Shanghai Science and Technology Press
(undated).

《难经正义》，叶霖

Nan Yang Huo Ren Shu
(The Nanyang Book to Safeguard Life),
Zhu Gong, 1111.

《南阳活人书》，朱肱

Nei Wai Shange Bian Huo Lun
(Clarifying Doubts about Injury from Internal and
External Causes), Li Dong-Yuan, 1231; Jiangsu
Science and Technology Press, 1982.

《内外伤辨惑论》，李东垣

Nu Ke Cuo Yao
(Essentials of Gynecology), Xue Ji, 1548.

《女科撮要》，薛己

Nu Ke Yao Zhi
(Essential Advice on Gynecology), Chen Xiu-
Yuan, Qing Dynasty; Fujian Science and
Technology Press, 1982.

《女科要旨》，陈修园

Orientalism
Edward Said; Routledge and Keegan Paul,
London, 1978.

Pi Wei Lun
(Discussion of the Spleen and Stomach),
Li Dong-Yuan, 1249.

《脾胃论》，李东垣

Pi Wei Lun Zuan Yao
(A Compilation of Essential Discussions on the
Spleen and Stomach), Shaanxi TCM College;
Shaanxi Science and Technology Press, 1986.

《脾胃论纂要》
陕西中医学院

Pu Ji Ben Shi Fang
(Formulas of Universal Benefit from my Practice),
Xu Shu-Wei, 1150.
(Shortened name of Lei Zheng Pu Ji Ben Shi
Fang.)

《普济本事方》，许叔微

Qi Jing Ba Mai Kao
(On the Extraordinary Channels), Li Shi-Zhen,
1577.

《奇经八脉考》，李时珍

Qi Xiao Liang Fang
(Remarkably Effective Fine Formulas), Dong Su
and Fang Xian, 1470.

《奇效良方》：董宿，方贤

Qian Jin Yao Fang
(Thousand Ducat Formulas), Sun Si-Miao,
652AD; People's Health Publishing, 1982.

《千金要方》，孙思邈

Qian Jin Yi Fang
(Supplement to the Thousand Ducat Formulas),
Sun Si-Miao, 682AD.

《千金翼方》，孙思邈

Qing Dai Ming Yi Yi An Jing Hua
(Best Cases of Famous Physicians of the Qing
Dynasty), Qin Bo-Wei, 1928.

《清代名医医案精华》
秦伯未

Quan Guo Gao Deng Yi Yao Yuan Xiao Shi Youg
Jiao Cai
(National Provisional Teaching Material for
Higher Medical Education Institutions), Shanghai
Science and Technology Press, 1984.

《全国高等医药院校使用教材》

Quan Sheng Zhi Mi Fang
(Guiding Formulas for the Whole Life),
Sun Ren-Cun, Song Dynasty.

《全生指迷方》，孙仁存

Ri Hua Zi Zhu Jia Ben Cao
(The Collated Materia Medica of Ri Hua Zi),
Ri Hua Zi, (also known as Da Ming), c. 970

《日华子诸家本草》，日华子
（或称大明）

Ru Men Shi Qin
(Confucians' Duties to their Parents), Zhang
Cong-Zheng, 1228.

《儒门事亲》，张从正

San Yin Ji Yi Bing Zheng Fang Lun
(Discussion of Illnesses, Patterns and Formulas

《三因极一病证方论》，陈言

Related to the Unification of the Three
Etiologies), Chen Yan, 1174; People's Health
Publishing, Beijing, 1983.

Shang Han Lun
(Discussion of Cold-induced Disorders), Zhang
Zhong-Jing, 210AD; People's Health Publishing,
1987.

《伤寒论》，张仲景

Shang Han Jiu Shi Lun
(Ninety Discussions on the Shang Han Lun),
Xu Shu-Wei, 1132.

《伤寒九十论》，许叔微

Shang Han Ming Li Lun
(Clarification of the Theory of Cold-induced
Disorders), Cheng Wu-Ji, 1142.

《伤寒明理论》，成无己

Shang Han Zong Bing Lun
(Discussion of Shang Han and General Diseases),
Pang An-Shi, 1100; Hubei Science and
Technology Press, 1987.

《伤寒总病论》，庞安时

She Sheng Mi Pou
(Secret Investigations into Obtaining Health);
Hong Ji, 1638.

《摄生秘剖》，洪基

Shen Shi Yao Han
(Scrutiny of the Precious Jade Case), Fu Yun-Ke,
1644. Also known as the Yan Ke Da Quan
(A Complete Work on Opthalmology.)

《审视瑶函》，傅允科
《眼科大全》

Shen Shi Zun Sheng Shu
(Master Shen's Book for Recovering Life),
Shen Jin-Ao, 1773.

《沈氏尊生书》，沈金鳌

Sheng Ji Zong Lu
(Comprehensive Recording of the Sages'
Benefits), compiled by the Song Dynasty Tai Yi
Medical College, c. 1111-1117, edited by Cao
Xiao-Zhong et al.; People's Health Publishing,
Beijing, 1984 (2 vols.)

《圣济总录》，曹孝忠

Shi Liao Ben Cao
(Materia Medica of Food Therapy), Meng Shen,
c. 713; People's Health Publishing, Beijing, 1984.

《食疗本草》，孟诜

Shi Re Lun
(Discussion of Damp Heat), Jiang Sen, 1989;
Joint Publishing Company, Hong Kong.

《湿热论》，蒋森

Shi Re Tiao Bian
(Systematic Differentiation of Damp Heat),
Xue Sheng-Bai, Qing Dynasty.

《湿热条辨》，薛生白

Shi Shi Mi Lu
(Secret Records of the Stone Chamber),
Chen Shi-Duo, 1687.

《石室秘录》，陈士铎

Shi Yi De Xiao Fang
(Effective Formulas from Generations of
Physicians), Wei Yi-Lin, 1345.

《世医得效方》，危亦林

Si Sheng Xin Yuan
(Secret Sources of the Four Masters), Huang
Yuan-Yu, 1753.

《四圣心源》，黄元御

Su Wen Xuan Ji Yuan Bing Shi
(Examination of the Original Patterns of Disease
from the Mysterious Mechanisms of the Su Wen),
Liu Wan-Su, 1182; Zhejiang Science and
Technology Press, 1984.

《素问玄机原病式》，刘完素

Tai Ding Yang Sheng Zhu Lun
(Treatise on the Calm and Settled Nourishment of
the Director of Life), Wang Gui, 1338.

《泰定养生主论》，王桂

Tai Ping Hui Min He Ji Ju Fang
(Imperial Grace Formulary of the Tai Ping Era),
1107-1110; edited by Chen Shi-Wen, Imperial
Medical Department. Also known as He Ji Ju
Fang.

《太平惠民和剂局方》，
    陈师文等

    《和剂局方》

Tan He Tan Zheng
(Phlegm and Phlegm Symptoms), He Xi-Ting,
1978; Jiangsu Science and Technology Press.

《痰和痰症》，何熹廷

Tang Ye Ben Cao
(Materia Medica for Decoctions), Wang Hao-Gu,
c. 1246-1248.

《汤液本草》，王好古

The Foundations of Chinese Medicine:
A Comprehensive Text for Acupuncturists and
Herbalists, Giovanni Maciocia, Churchill
Livingstone, 1989.

The Theoretical Foundations of Chinese
Medicine, Manfred Porkert, MIT Press, 1974.

Tongue Diagnosis in Chinese Medicine, Giovanni
Maciocia, Eastland Press, Seattle, 1987.

Tong Su Shang Han Lun
(Popular Guide to the Discussion of Cold-induced
Disorders), Yu Gen-Chu, 1776.

《通俗伤寒论》，俞根初

Tong Xuan Zhi Yao Fu
(Ode on the Essentials for Penetrating the Dark
Mystery), Dou Mo, c. 1170.

《通玄指要赋》，窦默

Wai Ke Zheng Quan Sheng Ji
(The Complete Collection of Patterns and
Treatments in External Medicine), Wang Wei-De,
1740.

《外科证治全生集》，王维德

Wai Ke Zheng Zong
(True Lineage of External Medicine),
Chen Shi-Gong, 1617; People's Health
Publishing, 1979.

《外科正宗》，陈实功

Wai Tai Mi Yao
(Arcane Essentials from the Imperial Library),
Wang Tao, 752AD.

《外台秘要》，王焘

Wan Bing Hui Chun
(Restoration of Health from the Myriad Diseases),
Gong Ting-Xian, 1587.

《万病回春》，龚廷贤

Wen Bing Shu Ping
(Review of Warm Diseases), edited by Guo Qian-
Heng, 1987, Shaanxi Science and Technology
Press.

《温病述评》，郭谦亨

Wen Bing Tiao Bian
(Systematic Differentiation of Warm Diseases),
Wu Ju-Tong, 1798.

《温病条辨》，吴鞠通

Wen Bing Tiao Bian Bai Hua Jie
(Vernacular Explanation of the Systematic
Differentiation of Warm Diseases), edited by
Zhejiang TCM College; People's Health
Publishing, 1979.

《温病条辨白话解》
　　浙江中医学院

Wen Yi Lun
(Discussion of Epidemic Warm Diseases),
Wu You-Ke, 1642; edited by Zhejiang TCM
Research Institute, People's Health Publishing,
1985.

《温疫论》，吴又可

Wen Re Jing Wei
(Warp and Woof of Warm-febrile Diseases),
Wang Meng-Ying, 1852.

《温热经纬》，王梦英

Wen Re Lun
(Discussion of Warmth and Heat), Ye Tian-Shi,
c. 1766.

《温热论》，叶天士

Wu Shi Er Bing Fang
(Fifty-Two Formulas for Disease) c. 475BC.

《五十二病方》

Xiao Er Yao Zheng Zhi Jue
(Craft of Medical Treatments for Childhood
Disease Patterns), Qian Yi, 1119.

《小儿药证直诀》，钱乙

Xing Se Wai Zhen Jian Mo

《形色外诊简摩》，周学海

(Simple Study of Diagnosis from Body Forms and Facial Color), Zhou Xue-Hai, 1894; Jiangsu Science and Technology Press, 1984.

Xu Ming Yi Lei An
(Continuation of Famous Physicians' Cases Organized by Categories), Wei Zhi-Xu, 1770.

《续名医类案》，魏之琇

Xuan Ming Fang Lun
(Clear and Open Discussion of Formulas), Liu Wan-Su, 1172.

《宣明方论》，刘完素

Xue Zheng Lun
(Discussion of Bleeding Disorders), Tang Rong-Chuan, 1884; Shanghai Science and Technology Press, 1977.

《血证论》，唐容川

Yan Ke Da Quan
(A Complete Work on Opthalmology), Fu Yun-Ke, 1644. Also known as the Shen Shi Yao Han. (Scrutiny of the Precious Jade Case).

《眼科大全》，傅允科

《审视瑶函》

Yan Shi Ji Sheng Fang
(Formulas to Aid the Living from Master Yan), Yan Yong-He, 1253.
Also known as Ji Sheng Fang (Formulas to Aid the Living).

《严氏济生方》，严用和

《济生方》

Yao Pin Hua Yi
(Transformed Significance of Medicinal Substances), Jia Suo-Xue, 1644.

《药品化义》，贾所学

Yao Xing Ben Cao
(Materia Medica of Medicinal Properties), Zhen Li-Yan, c. 610AD. Also known as Ben Cao Yao Xing.

《药性本草》，甄立言

《本草药性》

Ye Shi Yi An Cun Zheng Shu Zhu
(Annotated True Cases of Ye Tian-Shi), by Peng Xian-Zhang, 1937; Sichuan Science and Technology Press, 1984.

《叶氏医案存真疏注》
彭宪彰

Yi Bian
(Fundamentals of Medicine), He Meng-Yao, 1751; Shanghai Science and Technology Press, 1982.

《医碥》，何梦瑶

Yi Fang Ji Jie
(Analytic Collection of Formulas), Wang Ang, 1682.

《医方集解》，汪昂

Yi Fang Ji Jie Bei Yao
(Essentials from the Analytic Collection of Formulas), ed. by Hu Yang-Ji, 1981; Chao Ren Publishing, Taichung.

《医方集解备要》，胡洋吉编

Yi Fang Kao
(Investigations of Medical Formulas), Wu Kun,
1584.

《医方考》，吴崑

Yi Guan
(Key Link of Medicine), Zhao Xian-Ke, 1647;
People's Health Publishing, 1982.

《医贯》，赵献可

Yi Jia Mi Ao
(Secrets of the Physicians), Chen Shu-Yu,
c. 1694.

《医家秘澳》，陈树玉

Yi Lin Gai Cuo
(Corrections of Errors Among Physicians), Wang
Qing-Ren, 1830; People's Health Publishing,
1985.

《医林改错》，王清任

Yi Men Fa Lu
(Precepts for Physicians), Yu Chang, 1658;
Shanghai Science and Technology Press, 1983.

《医门法律》，喻昌

Yi Shu
(The Medical Heritage), Cheng Wen-You, 1817.

《医述》，程文囿

Yi Xiao Mi Chuan
(Secret Transmission of Medical Efficacy),
Ye Tian-Shi, Qing Dynasty; Hong Kong, 1970.

《医效秘传》，叶天士

Yi Xue Fa Ming
(Medical Innovations), Li Dong-Yuan, Jin-Tartar
Period.

《医学发明》，李东垣

Yi Xue Gang Mu
(Outline of Medicine), Lou Ying, 1565.

《医学纲目》，楼英

Yi Xue Jian Neng
(Medical Ability on Sight), Tang Rong-Chuan,
1873.

《医学见能》，唐容川

Yi Xue Ru Men
(Introduction to Medicine), Li Chan, 1575;
Jiangxi Science and Technology Press, 1988.

《医学入门》，李梴

Yi Xue San Zi Jing
(The Three-Character Classic of Medicine),
Chen Xiu-Yuan, 1804; Shanghai Science and
Technology Press, 1982.

《医学三字经》，陈修园

Yi Xue Shi Zai Yi
(The Study of Medicine is Actually Easy),
Chen Xiu-Yuan, pub. 1844; Fujian Science and
Technology Press, 1982.

《医学实在易》，陈修园

Yi Xue Xin Wu
(Medical Revelations), Cheng Guo-Peng, 1732;
People's Health Publishing, Beijing, 1982.

《医学心悟》，程国彭

Yi Xue Zheng Chuan
(True Lineage of Medicine), Yu Tian-Min, 1515.

《医学正传》，虞天民

Yi Xue Chuan Xin Lu
(Record of the Transmission of the Heart of
Medicine), Li Zhen-Tong, Qing Dynasty.

《医学传心录》，李珍同

Yi Yi Bing Shu
(Book of Treatments for Doctors' Illnesses),
Wu Ju-Tong, 1831; Jiangsu Science and
Technology Press, 1985.

《医医病书》，吴鞠通

Yi Yuan
(Origin of Medicine), Shi Shou-Tang, 1861;
Jiangsu Science and Technology Press, 1985.

《医原》，石寿棠

You Ke Liang Fang
(Prescriptions for Pediatrics), He Meng-Yao, Qing
Dynasty.

《幼科良方》，何梦瑶

Yi Zong Bi Du
(Required Readings from the Masters of
Medicine), Li Zhong-Zi, 1637; reprint China
Bookstore, Beijing, 1991.

《医宗必读》，李中梓

Yi Zong Jin Jian
(Golden Mirror of the Medical Tradition), Wu
Qian et al., 1742; People's Health Publishing,
1992. (2 vol.).

《医宗金鉴》，吴谦

Yu Ji Wei Yi
(Subtle Meanings of the Jade Mechanism), begun
by Xu Yong-Cheng (d. 1358) and completed by
Liu Chun in 1396.

《玉机微义》，徐用诚

刘纯

Za Bing Yuan Liu Xi Zhu
(Wondrous Lantern for Peering into the Origin
and Development of Miscellaneous Diseases),
Shen Jin-Ao, 1773.

《杂病源流犀烛》，沈金鳌

Zhang Shi Yi Tong
(Comprehensive Medicine According to Master
Zhang), Zhang Lu, 1695.

《张氏医通》，张璐

Zhen Ben Tu Shu Ji Cheng
(Pearl Volume Medical Collection), Zhang Shou-
Kong, c. 1725.

《珍本医书集成》，张受孔

Zhen Jiu Da Cheng
(Great Compendium of Acupuncture and
Moxibustion), Yang Ji-Zhou, 1601; People's
Health Press, Beijing, 1984.

《针灸大成》，杨继洲

Zhen Jiu Ju Ying
(Collection of the Essentials of Acupuncture and

《针灸聚英》，高武

Moxibustion), Gao Wu, 1529; Shanghai Science and Technology Press, 1961.

Zhen Jiu Ge Fu Jiao Shi
(Comparative Explanation of the Songs of Acupuncture), Shi Shi-Sheng, 1987; Shanxi Science and Technology Press.

《针灸歌赋校释》，施士生

Zheng Yin Mai Zhi
(Symptoms, Cause, Pulse and Treatment), Qin Zhi-Zhen, 1706.

《症因脉治》，秦之桢

Zheng Zhi Hui Bu
(Supplement to Diagnosis and Treatment), Li Yong-Cui, 1687.

《证治汇补》，李用粹

Zheng Zhi Zhun Sheng
(Standards of Patterns and Treatments), Wang Ken-Tang, 1602.

《证治准绳》，王肯堂

Zhi Yi Lu
(Record of Questions and Doubts), Zhang Jing-Yue, 1687; Jiangsu Science and Technology Press, 1981.

《质疑录》，张景岳

Zhong Guo Yi Xue Shi
(History of Chinese Medical Studies), Pei-Chi Liu, 1974; Hwa Kang Press, Yang Ming Shan, Taiwan.

《中国医学史》，刘伯骥

Zhong Xi Yi Jie He Zhi Liao Chang Jian Wai Ke Ji Fu Zheng
(Combined Chinese-Western Treatment of Common Surgical Acute Abdominal Conditions), Zheng Xian-Li et al., 1982; Tianjin Science and Technology Press.

《中西医结合治疗
   常见外科急腹症》
   郑显理等

Zhong Yao Ying Yong Jian Bie
(Differentiations of Usage in Chinese Herbs), Weng Wei-Jian et al., 1984; Tianjin Science and Technology Press.

《中药应用鉴别》，翁维健等

Zhong Yi Da Ci Dian
(The Comprehensive Dictionary of Traditional Chinese Medicine), Ch'i Yeh Publishing, Taiwan, 1980.

《中医大辞典》

Zhong Yi Ji Chu Li Lun Xiang Jie
(Detailed Explanation of Traditional Chinese Medicine Basic Theory), Zhao Fen-Zhu, 1981; Fujian Science and Technology Press.

《中医基础理论详解》，赵棻主

Zhong Yi Li Dai Yi Lun Xuan
(Selected Medical Essays by Traditional Chinese Doctors of Past Generations), edited by Wang

《中医历代医论选》，王新华

Xin-Hua, 1983; Jiangsu Science and Technology Press.

Zhong Yi Ming Yan Lu
(Records of Famous Sayings in TCM), Deng Tie-Tao, 1986; Guangdong Science and Technology Press.

《中医名言录》，邓铁涛

Zhong Yi Fang Ji Yu Zhi Fa
(TCM Formulas and Treatment Methods), Chengdu TCM College; Sichuan Science and Technology Press, 1984.

《中医方剂与制法》

Zhong Yi Tan Bing Xue
(Study of TCM Phlegm Diseases), Zhu Ceng-Bo, 1984; Hubei Science and Technology Press.

《中医痰病学》，朱曾柏

Zhong Yi Zhen Duan Xue
(TCM Diagnostic Studies), Deng Tie-Tao, 1991, People's Health Publishing.

《中医诊断学》，邓铁涛

Zhong Yi Zheng Zhuang Jian Bie Zhen Duan Xue
(Diagnostic Studies of Symptom Differentiation in Chinese Medicine), Zhao Jin-Duo et al., 1985; People's Health Publishing, Beijing.

《中医症状鉴别诊断学》，赵金铎

Zhong Zang Jing
(Treasury Classic), attrib. Hua Tuo, c. Six Dynasties Period, 317-618AD; Jiangsu Science and Technology Press, 1985.

《中藏经》，华佗

Zhong Zang Jing Wu Yi
(Vernacular Translation of the Treasury Classic), Li Cong-Fu, 1990; People's Health Publishing.

《中藏经语译》，李聪甫

Zhou Hou Bei Ji Fang
(Emergency Formulas to Keep Up One's Sleeve), Ge Hong, 314AD.

《肘后备急方》，葛洪

Zhu Bing Yuan Hou Lun
(Generalized Treatise on the Etiology and Symptomatology of Disease), Chao Yuan-Fang, 610AD.

《诸病源候论》，巢元方

Zhu Bing Yuan Hou Lun Jiao Shi
(Annotated Explanation of the Zhu Bing Yuan Hou Lun), Nanjing TCM College, 1983; People's Health Publishing.

《诸病源候论校释》
　南京中医学院

Index of Formulas

To signal where a formula appears in full, the page reference is printed in bold.